Exercise Science and Sports Medicine

Exercise Science and Sports Medicine

Editor: Pablo De Souza

www.callistoreference.com

Callisto Reference,
118-35 Queens Blvd., Suite 400,
Forest Hills, NY 11375, USA

Visit us on the World Wide Web at:
www.callistoreference.com

ISBN: 978-1-63239-844-4 (Hardback)

The publisher's policy is to use permanent paper from mills that operate a sustainable forestry policy. Furthermore, the publisher ensures that the text paper and cover boards used have met acceptable environmental accreditation standards.

Printed in China.

Cataloging-in-publication Data

Exercise science and sports medicine / edited by Pablo De Souza.
p. cm.
Includes bibliographical references and index.
ISBN 978-1-63239-844-4
1. Physical education and training. 2. Sports medicine. 3. Exercise. 4. Sports--Physiological aspects.
5. Sports sciences. I. De Souza, Pablo.

RC1210 .E94 2017
613.711--dc23

Table of Contents

Preface

Exercise science and sports medicine deal with services and treatments availed by athletes who perform under high-levels of stress and intensity. This book deals with topics that are concerned with overall training, rigor and exercise practices that aim for optimum levels of health for athletes. Regular training and exercise cause tissue and nerve damage as well as nutritional drain that must be replenished through diet, medicine and physiotherapy. This book presents the complex subject of exercise science and sports medicine in the most comprehensible and easy to understand language. From theories to research and practical applications, case studies related to all contemporary topics of relevance of the field have been included in this book. Those with an interest in sports medicine field would find this book helpful. It will serve as a valuable source of reference for graduate and post graduate students.

This book is a comprehensive compilation of works of different researchers from varied parts of the world. It includes valuable experiences of the researchers with the sole objective of providing the readers (learners) with a proper knowledge of the concerned field. This book will be beneficial in evoking inspiration and enhancing the knowledge of the interested readers.

In the end, I would like to extend my heartiest thanks to the authors who worked with great determination on their chapters. I also appreciate the publisher's support in the course of the book. I would also like to deeply acknowledge my family who stood by me as a source of inspiration during the project.

Editor

1

Hypoxia and Exercise Increase the Transpulmonary Passage of ^{99m}Tc-Labeled Albumin Particles in Humans

Melissa L. Bates[1]*, Emily T. Farrell[1], Alyssa Drezdon[1], Joseph E. Jacobson[1,4], Scott B. Perlman[2], Marlowe W. Eldridge[1,3]

1 Department of Pediatrics, Critical Care Division and the John Rankin Laboratory of Pulmonary Medicine, University of Wisconsin School of Medicine and Public Health, Madison, Wisconsin, United States of America, **2** Department of Radiology, University of Wisconsin School of Medicine and Public Health, Madison, Wisconsin, United States of America, **3** Departments of Biomedical Engineering and Kinesiology, University of Wisconsin School of Medicine and Public Health, Madison, Wisconsin, United States of America, **4** Michigan State University College of Human Medicine, East Lansing, Michigan, United States of America

Abstract

Intrapulmonary arteriovenous anastomoses (IPAVs) are large diameter connections that allow blood to bypass the lung capillaries and may provide a route for right-to-left embolus transmission. These anastomoses are recruited by exercise and catecholamines and hypoxia. Yet, whether IPAVs are recruited via direct, oxygen sensitive regulatory mechanisms or indirect effects secondary to redistribution pulmonary blood flow is unknown. Here, we hypothesized that the addition of exercise to hypoxic gas breathing, which increases cardiac output, would augment IPAVs recruitment in healthy humans. To test this hypothesis, we measured the transpulmonary passage of ^{99m}Tc-macroaggregated albumin particles (^{99m}Tc-MAA) in seven healthy volunteers, at rest and with exercise at 85% of volitional max, with normoxic ($FIO_2 = 0.21$) and hypoxic ($FIO_2 = 0.10$) gas breathing. We found increased ^{99m}Tc-MAA passage in both exercise conditions and resting hypoxia. However, contrary to our hypothesis, we found the greatest ^{99m}Tc-MAA passage with resting hypoxia. As an additional, secondary endpoint, we also noted that the transpulmonary passage of ^{99m}Tc-MAA was well-correlated with the alveolar-arterial oxygen difference ($A\text{-}aDO_2$) during exercise. While increased cardiac output has been proposed as an important modulator of IPAVs recruitment, we provide evidence that the modulation of blood flow through these pathways is more complex and that increasing cardiac output does not necessarily increase IPAVs recruitment. As we discuss, our data suggest that the resistance downstream of IPAVs is an important determinant of their perfusion.

Editor: Tim Lahm, Indiana University, United States of America

Funding: This work was supported by funding from the National Institutes of Health (5R01HL086897 and 5T32HL007654) and the American Heart Association (Postdoctoral Fellowship, Bates). The funders had no role in study design, data collection and analysis, decision to publish, or preparation of the manuscript.

Competing Interests: The authors have declared that no competing interests exist.

* Email: mlbates@pediatrics.wisc.edu

Introduction

Inducible intrapulmonary arteriovenous anastamoses (IPAVs) are large diameter conduits that bypass the pulmonary capillary network. The existence of these pathways has been previously demonstrated with saline contrast echocardiography [1–3] and ^{99m}Tc-labeled albumin macroaggregates (^{99m}Tc-MAA) [4] in humans and solid latex microspheres in animals [5,6] and ex-vivo lung preparations [5–10]. While not typically perfused at rest, IPAVs open in ~90% of humans performing moderate to heavy intensity exercise [1,4]. These pathways are also recruited by hypoxia ($FIO_2 = 0.10$–0.08) [6,11] and their recruitment during exercise can be prevented or reversed by hyperoxia ($FIO_2 = 1.0$) [12,13]. Whether these observations are due to direct oxygen sensitive regulatory mechanisms or indirect effects secondary to redistribution pulmonary blood flow is unknown.

The mechanism by which IPAVs are recruited by exercise and hypoxia is not known. Several investigators have suggested that the transpulmonary passage of particles or bubbles through IPAVs is the result of elevated cardiac output and may occur in order to moderate pulmonary vascular pressure and decrease right ventricular stress [14–16]. Laurie, et al. observed right-to-left transpulmonary saline bubble passage through IPAVs in a group of healthy adults infused with epinephrine. The intensity of right-to-left bubble passage was correlated with cardiac output and these authors concluded that IPAVs recruitment was the result of a catecholamine-induced increase in cardiac output [13]. Additionally, Bryan, et al. demonstrated increases in cardiac output, intrapulmonary shunt (Q_S/Q_T), and transpulmonary bubble passage in healthy humans with dobutamine infusion [17]. Similarly, they found increased right-to-left bubble passage and also concluded that IPAVs recruitment was related to cardiac output.

It is possible, however, that the recruitment of IPAVs occurs only coincidentally with the elevation in cardiac output. The strongest evidence against a causative role for cardiac output is the fact that hyperoxia nearly universally reverses catecholamine-induced or exercise-induced IPAVs recruitment [12,13]. Furthermore IPAVs recruitment can occur at rest with alveolar hypoxia with a minimal increase in cardiac output and pulmonary vascular pressure [11]. Indeed, these data provide compelling evidence that IPAVs regulation is in part mediated by an oxygen sensitive mechanism and not primarily by mechanical factors such as increases pulmonary blood flow and driving pressure.

Given that IPAVs recruitment has never been quantified in the context of hypoxia or hypoxic exercise, it is also unknown if IPAVs recruitment is similar to that observed under other conditions. If IPAVs recruitment and cardiac output are indeed linked, then we would predict that their recruitment by hypoxia would be further enhanced by the addition of exercise. To test this hypothesis, we measured the transpulmonary passage of ^{99m}Tc-MAA particles at rest and at 85% of maximal exercise with normoxic and hypoxic gas breathing, according to previously described methods [4]. As a secondary endpoint, arterial blood gases were measured in each condition. By assessing IPAVs recruitment under these conditions, we are able to further contribute to our understanding of how these pathways are regulated. Surprisingly, and contrary to our hypothesis, we found the transpulmonary passage of ^{99m}Tc-MAA to be greatest with resting hypoxic gas breathing.

Methods

Ethics statement

Participants gave written, informed consent. The consent procedure and materials and the experimental protocol were approved by the Institutional Review Board at the University of Wisconsin School of Medicine and Public Health.

Subject population and screening

We recruited twelve individuals (18–35 years) from the general population of the University of Wisconsin-Madison. Data are available from the authors upon request.

Because a right-to-left intracardiac shunt could allow ^{99m}Tc-MAA to bypass the lung independent of IPAVs, we screened participants for septal shunts, including a patent foramen ovale (PFO). To observe these shunts, a saline contrast echocardiogram with a Valsalva maneuver was performed prior to participation. The Valsalva maneuver was standardized such that each participant donned nose clips and exhaled against a fixed resistance to generate +40 cmH$_2$O mouth pressure for 10–15 seconds, coinciding with the injection of saline contrast [18]. This pressure was then released and the transeptal passage of bubbles was assessed. This was repeated without Valsalva in order to exclude individuals with pathological pulmonary arteriovenous malformations. A PFO was observed in five individuals (42%) and they were excluded from participation.

Because ^{99m}Tc-MAA is contraindicated in pulmonary hypertension [19], the peak velocity of the tricuspid regurgitation jet [20,21] was evaluated in the remaining participants and found to be normal. Forced spirometry and single breath carbon monoxide diffusion capacity were measured using commercially-available equipment (Optima, Medgraphics, St. Paul, MN) using standardized techniques [22,23]. Percent predicted values were calculated using previously published regression equations [24–26]. Pulmonary function equipment was calibrated prior to each use with a 3L syringe and manufacturer-supplied carbon monoxide and neon control gases.

Overall study design

Participants visited the laboratory on five occasions with at least one week between visits. This interval was selected to ensure complete clearance of any previously-injected ^{99m}Tc-MAA (^{99m}Tc half-life = 6.0 hours). During visits 1&2, ^{99m}Tc-MAA was injected intravenously after ten minutes of FIO$_2$ = 0.21 or 0.10 breathing. During visits 3&4, ^{99m}Tc-MAA was injected while the participant breathed either FIO$_2$ = 0.21 or 0.10 while exercising at 85% of their maximal exercise capacity. On the 5th visit, ^{99m}Tc-MAA was again injected after ten minutes of FIO$_2$ = 0.21 breathing. Because the resting FIO$_2$ = 0.21 injection is used as a baseline by which changes in ^{99m}Tc-MAA passage in the other conditions are compared [4], the 5th visit served as a control in order to evaluate the reproducibility of transpulmonary ^{99m}Tc-MAA passage.

Preparation of the ^{99m}Tc-MAA injection

Briefly, ^{99m}Tc-MAA (Pulmolite, Pharmalucence, Bedford, MA) was prepared by a nuclear pharmacist such that each injection contained ~300,000 particles with 3–4 miC of activity. The fraction of unbound ^{99m}Tc was determined for each injection using thin-layer chromatography and was 4.8±2.8%. The same lot of MAA was used throughout the study. Microscopic analysis (ImageJ, National Institutes of Health, Bethesda, MD) of 1×10^6 particles, sampled from three different vials revealed a mean particle diameter of 29 μm. with 97% of particles greater than 10 μm on the shortest axis, but none was greater than 120 μm.

We investigated the feasibility of removing particles <20 μm by vacuum filtration prior to injection (Steriflip, Millipore, Billerica, MA). Vacuum filtration was highly effective in removing particles <20 μm, but resulted in the formation of several particles > 500 μm. Because the injection of particles >150 μm is not recommended in humans, we did not filter ^{99m}Tc-MAA prior to injection.

Study design – Visits 1, 2, & 5

A 22-gauge catheter was placed in an antecubital vein for the injection of ^{99m}Tc-MAA. Participants then laid supine, donned nose clips, and breathed FIO$_2$ = 0.21 or 0.10 (balance N$_2$) through a mouthpiece fitted to a 2-way non-rebreathing valve. After three minutes, arterial blood was drawn via radial arterial puncture. Participants were then seated upright and continued breathing for an additional seven minutes. At the end of the breathing trial, ^{99m}Tc-MAA was injected into the intravenous catheter. Whole body images were then acquired to quantify the fraction of ^{99m}Tc-MAA bypassing the pulmonary circulation.

During visits 1&2, participants also performed a graded exercise test, on a magnetically-braked cycle ergometer (Velotron, RacerMate, Seattle, WA) while breathing either FIO$_2$ = 0.21 or 0.10. Participants wore noseclips and a 2-way non-rebreathing mouthpiece for the measurement of ventilation and metabolic function. Beginning at 60 W, the workload was increased 25–50 W every five minutes. The exercise test was ended when the participant could no longer maintain a pedaling cadence ≥55 rpm for three minutes. Each test lasted 25–30 minutes. Stages longer than those of a typical max test were used to mirror the exercise performed in visits 3&4, where additional time was required to accommodate the ^{99m}Tc-MAA injection and to allow sufficient time for complete circulation of the ^{99m}Tc-MAA particles. A single ^{99m}Tc-MAA injection requires about two minutes, including agitation of the material, injection, and thorough flushing of the infusion line and syringe. Thus, a workload thought to be maintainable for the full duration of the 5-minute stage (85% of max wattage) was chosen. An exercise test was not performed at visit 5. The purpose of visit 5 was to evaluate the reproducibility of the ^{99m}Tc-MAA injection.

Study design – Visits 3&4

Prior to exercise, participants swallowed a pill-shaped core temperature probe (CorTemp, HQ Inc., Palmetto, FL). A 22-gauge catheter was placed in an antecubital vein for ^{99m}Tc-MAA injection and a 3F angiocath was placed in a brachial artery for blood sampling.

Participants were seated on the ergometer and fitted with noseclips. Ventilation and metabolic function were measured as in visits 1&2. After being seated at rest for 10 minutes, participants began exercising at 30% of the maximal wattage achieved during visit 1&2. They completed five minute stages at 30%, 45%, 60%, 75%, and 85% of maximal capacity. During the third minute of each stage, arterial blood gases were drawn. One participant during normoxic exercise and two participants during hypoxic exercise became exhausted prior to reaching 85% of max and measurements were made in the 75% stage. During the third minute of the final stage, ^{99m}Tc-MAA was injected into the intravenous catheter such that the ^{99m}Tc-MAA injection coincided with the drawing of arterial blood.

Imaging Methods

We have previously discussed, in detail, the use of ^{99m}Tc-MAA to detect IPAVs recruitment, including the limitations of this technique [4], and would direct the reader to this publication for further information. Participants were imaged supine with anterior and posterior whole body images acquired simultaneously by gamma camera (VPS-45, General Electric Medical Systems, Waukesha, WI) using a 20-minute "step and shoot" protocol. The anterior and posterior images were reconstructed into a single whole body image where each voxel represents the geometric mean of the anterior and posterior image (GE eNTEGRA software, GE Healthcare). The fraction of ^{99m}Tc-MAA traversing the pulmonary circulation was calculated by quantifying one minus the lung-to-whole body ratio from this unified image and correcting it for the amount of unbound ^{99m}Tc99. As described previously [4], the lung region of interest (ROI) was defined using the normoxic exercise scan and included all voxels with at least 3–5% of the peak voxel intensity. The ROI was then applied to the other images and visually inspected to ensure that the ROI contained the entirety of the lung. Because saline contrast and solid microsphere studies have repeatedly demonstrated that IPAVs are not recruited at rest in normoxia, the lung-to-whole body ratio in the normoxic resting condition was set as a baseline. Changes with hypoxia and exercise are described subsequently as relative to this baseline. Again, to verify the reproducibility of the resting normoxic injection, this procedure was repeated on a second occasion.

Blood gas and metabolic measurements

For each sampling, arterial blood was drawn into three airtight, heparinized syringes. Each syringe was analyzed once (pHOx Basic, Nova Biomedical, Waltham, MA) immediately after collection and corrected for body temperature. No more than five minutes passed between the collection and analysis. A three-point calibration was done prior to the study using manufacturer-supplied control solutions.

Equipment used to measure metabolic and ventilatory parameters (Optima, Medgraphics, St. Paul, MN) was calibrated prior to use with a 3L syringe and manufacturer-supplied carbon dioxide and oxygen control gases.

Alveolar PO_2 was calculated according to the following equation: $PAO_2 = PIO_2 - (PaCO_2/R) + [FIO_2 \times PaCO_2 \times (1-R)/R]$, where PIO_2 is the dry inspired partial pressure of oxygen and R is the respiratory exchange ratio [27]. The A-aDO_2 was then calculated as the difference between the alveolar and arterial PO_2.

Statistical Analysis

All data are displayed as ± standard deviation unless otherwise noted. Blood gas and metabolic parameters were compared using repeated measures ANOVA with post hoc analysis (Student's t-test) to compare differences between exercise and rest, as well as between normoxia and hypoxia. Paired t-tests were used to evaluate differences in ^{99m}Tc-MAA passage with hypoxia and exercise. Significance was determined when $p<0.05$ with a Bonferroni correction applied for multiple comparisons. Predictors of the A-aDO_2 during exercise were evaluated by repeated measures general linear model (Minitab, State College, PA) in which the participant was treated as a random variable, the FIO_2 as a fixed variable, and the ^{99m}Tc-MAA fraction as a covariate. Reproducibility of the baseline ^{99m}Tc-MAA injection was assessed by calculating the intra-class correlation coefficient between the repeated visits and the repeatability coefficient [28]. If ^{99m}Tc-MAA passage was beyond the repeatability coefficient, then it was concluded that the difference was outside of the measurement's error range.

Results

Anthropometric characteristics, pulmonary function, and exercise capacity data are given in Table 1.

Baseline transpulmonary ^{99m}Tc-MAA passage

Transpulmonary passage of ^{99m}Tc-MAA was 11.7±9.1% and 11.4±9.4% during repeated normoxic rest (visits 1 and 5, respectively) and were not statistically different ($p = 0.41$). This is consistent with the percentage of particles known to be ≤15 μm. The repeatability coefficient was 0.92%. As we have done previously [4], each individual's resting value was used as a correction factor for all subsequent scans. At rest, hypoxia increased the passage of ^{99m}Tc-MAA particles in 6/7 participants (Δ5.3±2.9%) (Figure 1). Normoxic exercise increased ^{99m}Tc-MAA passage in 5/7 participants (71%) (Δ3.5±2.3%) and hypoxic exercise increased ^{99m}Tc-MAA passage in 4/7 participants (57%) (Δ3.5±2.5). The overall population means in normoxic and hypoxic exercise were not different (Δ2.5±2.6% vs Δ1.7±3.0%, $p = 0.60$), nor were the percent changes in transpulmonary ^{99m}Tc-MAA passage correlated between the two conditions ($R^2<0.01$, $p = 0.996$), meaning that the same individuals did not necessarily recruit IPAVs similarly in both conditions (Figure 2A). While the percent changes in transpulmonary passage of ^{99m}Tc-MAA for each individual were well-correlated between hypoxic rest and hypoxic exercise ($R^2 = 0.82$, $p = 0.005$), the overall percentage of ^{99m}Tc-MAA passage was higher with hypoxic rest than hypoxic exercise (Δ4.6±3.1% vs Δ2.5±2.6%, $p = 0.001$) (Figure 2B).

Blood gas parameters for normoxic and hypoxic rest and exercise are given in Table 2. Exercise widened the A-aDO_2, although there was no difference between normoxic and hypoxic exercise ($p = 0.43$). The A-aDO_2 during the last exercise stage was significantly related to the fraction of transpulmonary ^{99m}Tc-MAA passage ($p = 0.01$) and 63% of the variance in the A-aDO_2 was accounted for by the percent passage of ^{99m}Tc-MAA (Figure 3).

Discussion

Our interest in intrapulmonary arteriovenous anastomoses (IPAVs) stems from the finding that these large diameter pathways can be recruited in ~90% of healthy individuals and may provide a conduit for right-to-left embolus transmission. Unlike our previous work investigating IPAVs recruitment with normoxic exercise [4], we have not directly quantified IPAVs recruitment with hypoxia or hypoxic exercise. To that end, our primary goal was to quantify the transpulmonary passage of ^{99m}Tc-MAA particles in the face of hypoxia. We aimed to further understand factors that influence their recruitment by specifically asking if exercise universally increases IPAVs recruitment. Here, we provide evidence suggesting that exercise, which increases cardiac

Table 1. Anthropometric characteristics of the seven participants completing the study.

	Age		Height	Weight	FEV_1		DL_{CO}	VO_2max $FIO_2=0.21$	VO_2max $FIO_2=0.10$
Subject	(yrs)	Sex	(cm)	(kg)	(L)	FEV_1/FVC	(mL/min/Torr)	(mL/kg/min)	(mL/kg/min)
01	23	F	165	56	3.54	0.83	30.74	30.9	20.6
					(113%)		(97%)	(92.3)	
02	22	M	183	80	5.10	0.85	45.06	56.5	32.4
					(101%)		(119%)	(117.1)	
03	21	F	171	61	3.98	0.88	32.12	43.3	30.2
					(116%)		(95%)	(98.4)	
04	31	M	172	88	4.02	0.88	37.14	33.6	18.6
					(106%)		(109%)	(76.4)	
05	33	F	171	62	3.90	0.83	32.57	57.1	32.3
					(121%)		(96%)	(132.4)	
06	21	M	178	76	4.42	0.86	34.59	45.2	23.8
					(95%)		(96%)	(93.3)	
07	20	M	184	72	4.36	0.75	42.92	58.0	30.5
					(103%)		(101%)	(118.6)	
Mean ±	24±5		175±7	71±12	4.19±0.50	0.84±0.04	36.45±5.57	46.4±11.3	26.9±5.8*
SD					(108±9)		(102±9)	(104±19)	

FVC, forced vital capacity; FEV_1, forced expired volume in 1 second; DL_{CO}, diffusion capacity for carbon monoxide; VO_2max; relative maximal oxygen uptake.
*indicates $p<0.05$. Values in parentheses are percent predicted (23–25).

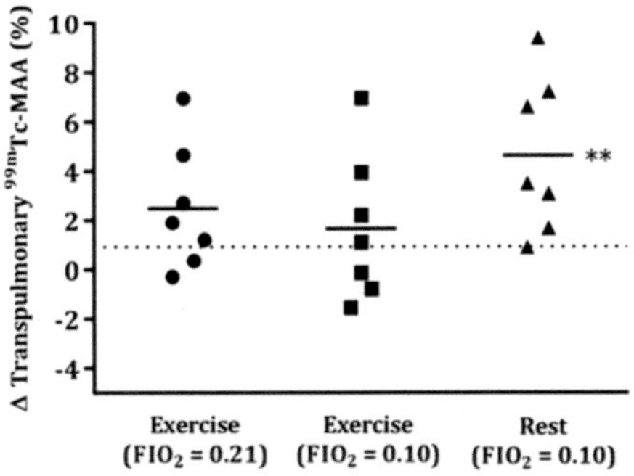

Figure 1. Change in the transpulmonary passage (%) of ^{99m}Tc-MAA compared to resting, normoxic gas breathing. Dashed line indicates the repeatability coefficient (0.92%) Transpulmonary ^{99m}Tc-MAA passage was noted in 6/7 participants performing exercise in normoxia and 4/7 participants performing exercise in hypoxia. Breathing hypoxic gas at rest increased ^{99m}Tc-MAA passage in all participants relative to hypoxic exercise. ** indicates a difference compared to hypoxic rest (p = 0.001).

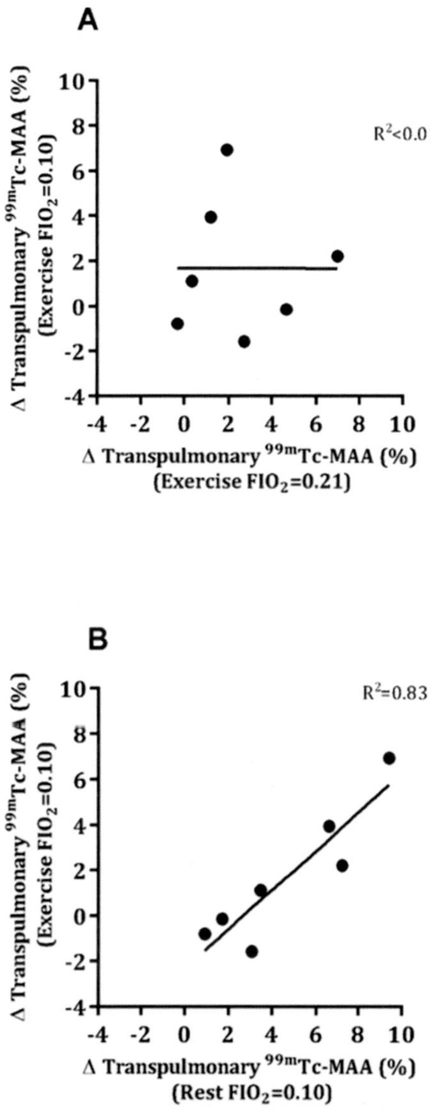

Figure 2. Relationship between transpulmonary ^{99m}Tc-MAA passage with exercise in normoxia vs. hypoxia (A) and between rest and exercise in hypoxia (B). The transpulmonary passage of ^{99m}Tc-MAA with exercise in hypoxia was well-correlated with that measured at rest with hypoxic gas breathing. Dashed line indicates the line of identity.

output, does not necessarily increase IPAVs recruitment. Indeed, if cardiac output were a major modulator of IPAVS recruitment in hypoxia, we would expect ^{99m}Tc-MAA passage to be higher during exercise than at rest. Instead, we found it to be greatest with resting hypoxia and similar between both exercise conditions.

Methodological considerations

We have previously validated the existence of IPAVs in intact rats and dogs and isolated rat, baboon, dog, and human lungs using solid latex particles of known diameter [5,7,29]. Although the lung is not permeable to solid latex particles 15–70 μm under resting conditions, these large particles traverse the lung with the addition of hypoxia or exercise [5,29]. A limitation of the study of IPAVs in humans is that, in contrast to our animal studies, we are unable to directly measure the size of the ^{99m}Tc-MAA particles that traverse the lung. However, we previously have demonstrated that the fraction of ^{99m}Tc-MAA particles that traverse the lung in exercising humans is similar to the fraction of radiolabeled latex particles that traverse the lungs of dogs performing similar exercise (1.3 and 1.4%, respectively) [4].

It has been suggested that small particles traverse the lung by "squeezing" through distended pulmonary capillaries when pulmonary vascular pressure is elevated [15,16]. Assuming that the pulmonary vascular distends 2% per mmHg increase in pulmonary vascular pressure [30], at physiological perfusion pressures we would expect a 6 μm pulmonary capillary to distend to no more than 8 μm. Manohar and Goetz demonstrated that the lung of the thoroughbred race horse, which apparently lacks IPAVs but is perfused at extraordinarily high pressure during exercise, is not permeable to 15μm microspheres, suggesting that the maximal capillary diameter is <15 μm [31]. Furthermore, the binding of ^{99m}Tc to albumin is proportional to the particle mass and our previous calculations demonstrate that the contribution of the additional ^{99m}Tc-MAA particles ≤15 μm that might pass through pulmonary capillaries during exercise is <0.4% of the total signal. [4]. Thus, we are confident that the additional ^{99m}Tc signal with exercise and hypoxia is the result of large diameter particles traversing IPAVs. Furthermore, if ^{99m}Tc-MAA is traversing the pulmonary capillaries, we would expect that the passage of ^{99m}Tc-MAA would be greatest during hypoxic exercise when pulmonary vascular pressures are highest and to increase in all participants. Instead, we found passage to be the greatest during resting hypoxia, suggesting that distended capillaries are not the primary source of transpulmonary capillary passage.

The excellent repeatability of the measurement in resting, normoxic individuals gives us confidence that the differences observed with hypoxia and exercise represent true increases in transpulmonary particle passage and are not caused by free pertechnate or inter-injection variability. Indeed, we took care to perform all scans within 10 minutes of the conclusion of exercise and found very little free label (<0.1% of the total extrapulmonary signal), in the bladder, gut, and thyroid, where free pertechnate accumulates. If our findings were caused by free pertechnate, we would expect to find substantial labeling of these organs [32]. It is also attractive to consider filtering very small particles from the injectate. However, in our hands this resulted in the significant aggregation of particles, resulting in the formation of large particles that are unsafe for injection in humans.

Table 2. Arterial blood gases, respiratory quotient (R), and the alveolar-arterial PO_2 difference (A-aDO_2), measured at rest and at 85% of the maximal attainable wattage during the resting and exercise visits.

	Condition	FIO_2	R	pH	PCO_2 [mmHg]	PO_2 [mmHg]	A-aDO_2 [mmHg]
Exercise Visit	Rest	0.21	0.86±0.11	7.46±0.02	38.8±4.9	102.1±8.3	−1.2±5.0
	Rest	0.10	1.34±0.15	7.48±0.02	34.3±3.9	43.8±3.6	−1.1±4.7
	85% Max Wattage	0.21	1.15±0.11*	7.38±0.07*	33.5±4.0*	101.3±5.7	14.1±5.2*
	85% Max Wattage	0.10	1.27±0.16*	7.39±0.07*	27.1±3.0*†	37.8±0.5*†	11.1±5.9*
Resting Visit	Rest	0.21	0.87±0.09	7.48±0.05	38.7±4.9	103.8±9.8	2.6±7.1
	Rest	0.10	1.19±0.11	7.48±0.01	37.9±3.3	42.1±5.0	−1.8±4.7

*indicates $p<0.05$ compared to values measured at rest on the same day.
†indicates $p<0.05$ compared to normoxic exercise.

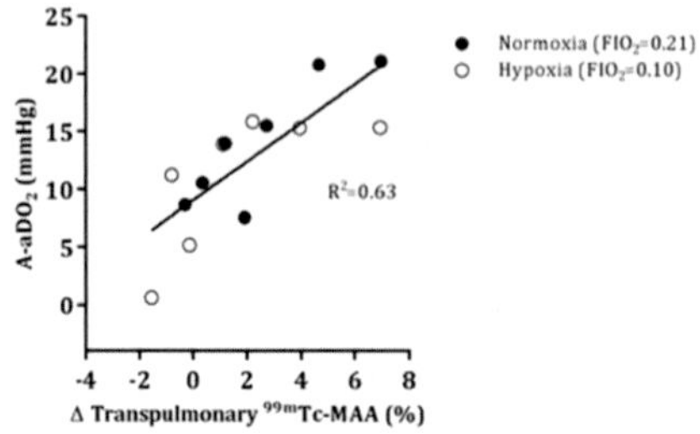

Figure 3. Relationship between transpulmonary ^{99m}Tc-MAA passage and the alveolar-arterial oxygen difference (A-aDO_2) in normoxic and hypoxic exercise. Line represents the result of a general linear model analysis in which the transpulmonary ^{99m}Tc-MAA passage was linearly correlated with the A-aDO_2 ($R^2=0.63$), but this relationship was not dependent on the FIO_2 ($p>0.05$).

What influences the recruitment of large diameter IPAVs?

In humans and experimental animal models with lesions that result in unventilated lung regions, increasing cardiac output typically increases physiological intrapulmonary shunt (Q_S/Q_T) [23,33–38]. It might, therefore, seem surprising and counterintuitive that we found a decrease in IPAVs perfusion with hypoxic exercise, where the cardiac output is higher, compared to rest. Our finding are, in fact, congruent with previous work in this area and understanding the interaction between FIO_2, cardiac output, and Q_S/Q_T provides insight into what factors may regulate IPAVs perfusion.

Many previous studies have relied on models of lung injury where the FIO_2 is normoxic or hyperoxic and injured regions of the lung are focally hypoxic because of the poor ventilation (ie, respiratory distress syndrome, pulmonary edema and atelectasis, arteriovenous malformation and methacholine challenge) [33–38]. However, Wagner, et al. measured the increase in Q_S/Q_T in a methacholine-challenged dog model with normoxic, hyperoxic, and hypoxic ventilation [39], thereby fundamentally improving our understanding of this phenomenon. In all conditions, methacholine challenge resulted in an initial 28% shunt. With normoxic and hyperoxic ventilation, this shunt increased 7% and 11% per L/min increase in cardiac output, but only 2% with hypoxic ventilation. The authors explain these different changes in Q_S/Q_T by asking the reader to consider a lung with two vascular compartments with parallel resistances – one that is normal and well-ventilated and one that is injured and poorly ventilated. Under normoxic and hyperoxic conditions, the poorly ventilated compartment is hypoxic, resulting in a high degree of vasoconstriction and high vascular resistance. The resistance in the well-ventilated compartment is lower than the injured compartment. As cardiac output increases, there is a greater fall in resistance in the poorly ventilated compartment relative to the well-ventilated compartment, thereby redistributing the cardiac output to the injured compartment. When both compartments are hypoxic, the resistances are similar and the cardiac output is distributed similarly between the compartments.

To understand our finding that IPAVs perfusion decreases with exercise, we would similarly ask the reader to consider a lung with two vascular compartments. Unlike Wagner et al.'s model, these resistances are morphometrically distinct. One compartment contains large diameter of IPAVs, which lie upstream of a second compartment of pulmonary arteries, capillaries, and veins. We have previously shown in rats that IPAVs are ≥70 μm [6], placing them early in the vascular tree and upstream of the primary resistance arterioles [40] that constrict in response to hypoxia. This location is further supported by anatomic studies that identify arteriovenous connections early in the vascular tree [41]. With resting hypoxia, large diameter IPAVs are open and there is also considerable vasoconstriction of the resistance arterioles, directing blood flow through IPAVs. With exercise, the post-IPAVs resistance falls tremendously [42]. Thus, following similar logic to that used by Wagner, et al. [39], we would expect the perfusion to IPAVs to fall as a function of the fall in resistance of the non-IPAVs compartment.

The strong correlation between the transpulmonary passage of ^{99m}Tc-MAA during hypoxic rest and hypoxic exercise supports this interpretation and suggests that when IPAVS are open, the fraction of the cardiac output that perfuses them is determined by two factors – 1) their relative abundance, which contributes to intersubject variability and 2) the downstream resistance, which redistributes blood flow through IPAVs and contributes to intercondition variability. Moreover, Tobin used a mechanism very similar to that we propose to identify IPAVs in isolated lungs [41]. By strategically elevating the downstream vascular resistance, he was able to preferentially fill these pathways with casting material. If IPAVs are located upstream of the vessels that are the largest contributors to the vascular resistance [43–45], then the tone of the resistance vessels could determine flow through IPAVs.

Eldridge, et al. [1] previously speculated that IPAVs exist as a "pressure relief valve" to normalize pulmonary pressure in the face of high cardiac output. Although this explanation seems physiologically plausible, it is not supported by these data and challenges our own previous ideas about IPAVs recruitment. It is possible that the recruitment of IPAVs is not caused by increased cardiac output and pressure, but by biochemical signals that directly impact their tone. Hyperoxia consistently prevents or reverses the recruitment of IPAVs, even in the face of high intensity exercise [12] and epinephrine and dobutamine infusion [13], suggesting that IPAVs regulation by hyperoxia occurs as a result of a distinct and secondary O_2-mediated mechanism. Further supporting a role for oxygen sensitivity, we found previously that $PvO_2<22$ mmHg is required for the recruitment of IPAVs in rats and we speculated that IPAVs are recruited via an oxygen-sensitive mechanism, in response to pulmonary arterial hypoxemia [6]. Epinephrine, dobutamine, and dopamine are vasoactive and may affect the tone of IPAVs independently of their effect on total pulmonary vascular flow. Isolated lung models may be valuable in future investigations, allowing the evaluation of biochemically-mediated effects while controlling pulmonary vascular pressure and flow.

The A-aDO$_2$ is related to the magnitude of transpulmonary ^{99m}Tc-MAA passage

Whether IPAVs contribute to exercise-induced arterial hypoxemia [46] has been a controversial question [47,48]. We have been motivated to use particles to quantify the recruitment of large diameter pathways that could contribute to anatomic shunt by the recognition of substantial pre-capillary gas exchange [49,50] that might confound measurements made with SF_6 or 100% O_2, thereby underestimating shunt under normoxic or hypoxic conditions. Although ^{99m}Tc-MAA passage has been related to SpO_2, it has not been related to the A-aDO$_2$. Thus, as a secondary endpoint of this study, we measured arterial blood gases in our participants and found the magnitude of IPAVs recruitment to be well-correlated with the A-aDO$_2$. Indeed, we were intrigued by the fact that the transpulmonary passage of ^{99m}Tc-MAA was quite similar to actual values of physiological shunt (Q_S/Q_T) reported elsewhere. Vogiatzis, et al. reported Q_s/Q_T in humans performing normoxic exercise at power outputs similar to ours and found Q_s/Q_T to be 3.5% [51]. This is similar to the 2.5% passage of ^{99m}Tc-MAA reported here. This is also similar to the amount of shunt that Gledhill et al. calculated [52] would be required to explain the remaining A-aDO$_2$ after accounting for ventilation-perfusion inequality. This suggests that the shunting of venous admixture through intrapulmonary pathways may, in fact, be an important contributor to Q_s/Q_T in normoxic exercise. However, we acknowledge that an important limitation of our work, and indeed the field at this point, is the inability to prevent IPAVs recruitment during exercise in an O_2-independent manner, thereby allowing the contribution of IPAVs to the A-aDO$_2$ to be evaluated during exercise without changes in FIO$_2$ that might alter IPAVs patency. We also recognize that it is possible that the increase in ^{99m}Tc-MAA occurs only coincidentally with the increased in A-aDO$_2$.

We note a similar increase in IPAVs recruitment proportional to the increase in A-aDO$_2$ in both normoxia and hypoxia, but the relative contributions of ventilation-perfusion inequality, diffusion limitation and shunt to the increased A-aDO$_2$ during exercise is certainly dependent on the FIO$_2$. Vogiatzis, et al. found a sevenfold increase in Q_s/Q_T with hypoxic exercise, yet we found no additional increase in IPAVs recruitment with our particle method. If we speculate that IPAVs do contribute to Q_s/Q_T, then additional contributors, including diffusion limitation, would need to account for the remaining A-aDO$_2$. While we note a positive relationship between A-aDO2 and the fractional IPAVs recruitment, future studies will be needed to separate the simultaneous contributions of IPAVs, ventilation-perfusion inequality, and diffusion limitation in normoxia and hypoxia, posing an interesting challenge to investigators motivated to understand the mechanism of the widened A-aDO$_2$ in exercising humans.

It may seem counterintuitive that the A-aDO$_2$ would be unchanged with resting hypoxia, despite the fact that the IPAVS recruitment was greatest in this condition. This is likely the result of the narrow arteriovenous oxygen difference in this condition. Relying on historical data obtained from resting humans breathing FIO$_2$ = 0.10 [53], we can estimate that the mixed venous saturation of hemoglobin (SO$_2$) is 50% in our participants. Using our participants own mean value of alveolar PO$_2$ and the Kelman equation to convert between PO$_2$ and SO$_2$ [54], we can estimate venous and alveolar oxygen content [27]. Using the standard shunt equation [27], we can then calculate the contribution of a 5% anatomic shunt on the A-aDO$_2$. Indeed, this calculation reveals that the impact of a 5% anatomic shunt on the A-aDO$_2$ is trivial under these conditions (1.2 mmHg), thereby demonstrating that IPAVs recruitment need not always result in a widened A-aDO$_2$.

We appreciate that, because of the number of visits required for the completion of this study, blood gases were obtained via arterial puncture preceding the resting injections rather than by placing an in-dwelling catheter. Our participants found this to be more comfortable in the supine position, which may impact the A-aDO$_2$ and limit our ability to interpret these data. There was, however, no significant difference between the A-aDO$_2$ measured during the resting visit in the supine position and the A-aDO$_2$ measured at rest in the upright position during the exercising visits.

Conclusion

Here, we demonstrate the perfusion of IPAVs is greatest in hypoxic individuals and that elevating the cardiac output with exercise does not increase IPAVs recruitment.

Author Contributions

Conceived and designed the experiments: MB SP ME EF JJ. Performed the experiments: MB ME EF JJ AD. Analyzed the data: MB SP ME EF JJ AD. Contributed reagents/materials/analysis tools: SP. Wrote the paper: MB SP ME EF JJ AD.

References

1. Eldridge MW, Dempsey JA, Haverkamp HC, Lovering AT, Hokanson JS (2004) Exercise-induced intrapulmonary arteriovenous shunting in healthy humans. J Appl Physiol 97: 797–805.
2. Elliott JE, Choi Y, Laurie SS, Yang X, Gladstone IM, et al. (2011) Effect of initial gas bubble composition on detection of inducible intrapulmonary arteriovenous shunt during exercise in normoxia, hypoxia, or hyperoxia. J Appl Physiol 110: 35–45.
3. Lovering AT, Romer LM, Haverkamp HC, Pegelow DF, Hokanson JS, et al. (2008) Intrapulmonary shunting and pulmonary gas exchange during normoxic and hypoxic exercise in healthy humans. J Appl Physiol 104: 1418–1425.
4. Lovering AT, Haverkamp HC, Romer LM, Hokanson JS, Eldridge MW (2009) Transpulmonary passage of ^{99m}Tc macroaggregated albumin in healthy humans at rest and during maximal exercise. J Appl Physiol 106: 1986–1992.
5. Stickland MK, Lovering AT, Eldridge MW (2007) Exercise-induced arteriovenous intrapulmonary shunting in dogs. Am J Respir Crit Care Med 176: 300–305.
6. Bates M, Fulmer B, Farrell E, Drezdon A, Pegelow D, et al. (2012) Hypoxia recruits intrapulmonary arteriovenous pathways in intact rats but not isolated rat lungs. J Appl Physiol.
7. Lovering AT, Stickland MK, Kelso AJ, Eldridge MW (2007) Direct demonstration of 25- and 50-microm arteriovenous pathways in healthy human and baboon lungs. Am J Physiol Heart Circ Physiol 292: H1777–1781.
8. Niden AH, Aviado DM Jr (1956) Effects of pulmonary embolism on the pulmonary circulation with special reference to arteriovenous shunts in the lung. Circ Res 4: 67–73.
9. Tobin CE (1966) Arteriovenous Shunts in Peripheral Pulmonary Circulation in Human Lung. Thorax 21: 197-&.
10. Prinzmetal M, Ornitz EM Jr, Simkin B, Bergman HC (1948) Arterio-venous anastomoses in liver, spleen, and lungs. Am J Physiol 152: 48–52.
11. Laurie SS, Yang X, Elliott JE, Beasley KM, Lovering AT (2011) Hypoxia-induced intrapulmonary arteriovenous shunting at rest in healthy humans (vol 109, pg 1072, 2010). J Appl Physiol 110: 1502–1502.
12. Lovering AT, Stickland MK, Amann M, Murphy JC, O'Brien MJ, et al. (2008) Hyperoxia prevents exercise-induced intrapulmonary arteriovenous shunt in healthy humans. J Physiol 586: 4559–4565.
13. Laurie SS, Elliott JE, Goodman RD, Lovering AT (2012) Catecholamine-induced opening of intrapulmonary arteriovenous anastomoses in healthy humans at rest. J Appl Physiol.
14. Lovering AT, Elliott JE, Beasley KM, Laurie SS (2010) Pulmonary pathways and mechanisms regulating transpulmonary shunting into the general circulation: an update. Injury 41 Suppl 2: S16–23.
15. La Gerche A, MacIsaac AI, Burns AT, Mooney DJ, Inder WJ, et al. (2010) Pulmonary transit of agitated contrast is associated with enhanced pulmonary vascular reserve and right ventricular function during exercise. J Appl Physiol 109: 1307–1317.
16. Lalande S, Yerly P, Faoro V, Naeije R (2012) Pulmonary vascular distensibility predicts aerobic capacity in healthy individuals. J Physiol 590: 4279–4288.
17. Bryan TL, van Diepen S, Bhutani M, Shanks M, Welsh RC, et al. (2012) The effects of dobutamine and dopamine on intrapulmonary shunt and gas exchange in healthy humans. J Appl Physiol 113: 541–548.
18. Marriott K, Manins V, Forshaw A, Wright J, Pascoe R (2013) Detection of Right-to-Left Atrial Communication Using Agitated Saline Contrast Imaging: Experience with 1162 Patients and Recommendations for Echocardiography. Journal of the American Society of Echocardiography 26: 96–102.
19. Pharmalucence (2010) Pulmolite, kit for the preparation of technetium Tc99m albumin aggregated for injection U.S. National Library of Medicine.
20. McLaughlin VV, Archer SL, Badesch DB, Barst RJ, Farber HW, et al. (2009) ACCF/AHA 2009 expert consensus document on pulmonary hypertension: a report of the American College of Cardiology Foundation Task Force on Expert Consensus Documents and the American Heart Association: developed in collaboration with the American College of Chest Physicians, American Thoracic Society, Inc., and the Pulmonary Hypertension Association. Circulation 119: 2250–2294.
21. Galie N, Hoeper MM, Humbert M, Torbicki A, Vachiery JL, et al. (2009) Guidelines for the diagnosis and treatment of pulmonary hypertension: the Task Force for the Diagnosis and Treatment of Pulmonary Hypertension of the European Society of Cardiology (ESC) and the European Respiratory Society (ERS), endorsed by the International Society of Heart and Lung Transplantation (ISHLT). Eur Heart J 30: 2493–2537.
22. Miller MR, Hankinson J, Brusasco V, Burgos F, Casaburi R, et al. (2005) Standardisation of spirometry. European Respiratory Journal 26: 319–338.
23. American Thoracic Society (1995) Single-breath carbon monoxide diffusing capacity (transfer factor). Recommendations for a standard technique–1995 update. Am J Respir Crit Care Med 152: 2185–2198.
24. Knudson RJ, Lebowitz MD, Burrows B (1980) The maximal expiratory flow-volume curve-Normal standards, variability and effects of age. American Review of Respiratory Disease 122: 990–991.
25. Cotes JE, Chinn DJ, Quanjer PH, Roca J, Yernault JC (1993) Standardization of the measurement of transfer-factor (diffusing capacity)-report working party standardization of lung-function tests European-community for steel and coal-official statement of the european respiratory society. European Respiratory Journal 6: 41–52.
26. Jones NL, Makrides L, Hitchcock C, Chypchar T, McCartney N (1985) Normal standards for an incremental progressive cycle ergometer test. Am Rev Respir Dis 131: 700–708.
27. West JB (2008) Respiratory Physiology: The Essentials 8th Edition. Philadelphia: Wolters Kluwer. 208 p.
28. Cleophas TJ, Zwinderman AH, Cleophas TF (2006) Statistics Applied to Clinical Trials: Springer.
29. Bates ML, Fulmer BR, Farrell ET, Drezdon A, Pegelow DF, et al. (2012) Hypoxia recruits intrapulmonary arteriovenous pathways in intact rats but not isolated rat lungs. J Appl Physiol 112: 1915–1920.
30. Reeves JT, Linehan JH, Stenmark KR (2005) Distensibility of the normal human lung circulation during exercise. Am J Physiol Lung Cell Mol Physiol 288: L419–425.
31. Manohar M, Goetz TE (2005) Intrapulmonary arteriovenous shunts of >15 mu m in diameter probably do not contribute to arterial hypoxemia in maximally exercising Thoroughbred horses. J Appl Physiol 99: 224–229.
32. Dogan AS, Rezai K, Kirchner PT, Stuhlmuller JE (1993) A scintographic sign for the detection of right-to-left shunts. Journal of Nuclear Medicine 34: 1607–1611.
33. Bishop MJ, Cheney FW (1983) Effects of pulmonary blood-flow and mixed venous O2 tension on gas-exchange in dogs. Anesthesiology 58: 130–135.
34. Breen PH, Schumacker PT, Hedenstierna G, Ali J, Wagner PD, et al. (1982) How does increased cardiac-output increase shunt in pulmonary edema. J Appl Physiol 53: 1273–1280.
35. Breen PH, Schumacker PT, Sandoval J, Mayers I, Oppenheimer L, et al. (1985) Increased cardiac-output increases shunt-role of pulmonary-edema and perfusion J Appl Physiol 59: 1313–1321.
36. Colley PS, Cheney FW (1977) Sodium nitroprusside increases QS-QT in dogs with regional atelectasis. Anesthesiology 47: 338–341.
37. Colley PS, Cheney FW, Hlastala MP (1979) Ventilation-perfusion and gas-exchange effects of sodium nitroprusside in dogs with normal and edematous lungs. Anesthesiology 50: 489–495.
38. Dantzker DR, Lynch JP, Weg JG (1980) Depression of cardiac-output is a mechanism of shunt reduction in acute respiratory failure Chest 77: 636–642.
39. Wagner PD, Schaffartzik W, Prediletto R, Knight DR (1991) Relationship among cardiac-output, shunt, and inspired O2 concentration J Appl Physiol 71: 2191–2197.
40. Jiang ZL, Kassab GS, Fung YC (1994) Diameter-defined Strahler system and connectivity matrix of the pulmonary arterial tree. J Appl Physiol 76: 882–892.
41. Tobin CE (1966) Arteriovenous shunts in the perопheral pulmonary circulation in the human lung. Thorax 21: 197–204.
42. Eldridge MW, Podolsky A, Richardson RS, Johnson DH, Knight DR, et al. (1996) Pulmonary hemodynamic response to exercise in subjects with prior high-altitude pulmonary edema. J Appl Physiol 81: 911–921.
43. Dingemans KP, Wagenvoort CA (1978) Pulmonary arteries and veins in experimental hypoxia. An ultrastructural study. Am J Pathol 93: 353–368.
44. Kato M, Staub NC (1966) Response of small pulmonary arteries to unilobar hypoxia and hypercapnia. Circ Res 19: 426–440.
45. Staub NC (1985) Site of hypoxic pulmonary vasoconstriction. Chest 88: 240S–245S.
46. Dempsey JA, Wagner PD (1999) Exercise-induced arterial hypoxemia. J Appl Physiol 87: 1997–2006.
47. Lovering AT, Eldridge MW, Stickland MK (2009) Counterpoint: Exercise-induced intrapulmonary shunting is real. J Appl Physiol 107: 994–997.
48. Hopkins SR, Olfert IM, Wagner PD (2009) Point: Exercise-induced intrapulmonary shunting is imaginary. J Appl Physiol 107: 993–994.
49. Tabuchi A, Styp-Rekowska B, Slutsky AS, Wagner PD, Pries AR, et al. (2013) Precapillary Oxygenation Contributes Relevantly to Gas Exchange in the Intact Lung. Am J Respir Crit Care Med 188: 474–481.
50. Conhaim RL, Staub NC (1980) Reflection spectrophotometric measurement of O_2 uptake in pulmonary arterioles of cats. J Appl Physiol 48: 848–856.
51. Vogiatzis I, Zakynthinos S, Boushel R, Athanasopoulos D, Guenette JA, et al. (2008) The contribution of intrapulmonary shunts to the alveolar-to-arterial oxygen difference during exercise is very small. J Physiol 586: 2381–2391.
52. Gledhill N, Froese A, Dempsey J (1977) Ventilation to perfusion distribution during exercise in health. In: Dempsey J, Reed C, editors. Muscular Exercise and the Lung. Madison, WI: University of Wisconsin Press. 325–344.
53. Motley HL, Cournand A, Werko L, Himmelstein A, Dresdale D (1947) The influence of short periods of induced acute anoxia upon pulmonary artery pressures in man. Am J Physiol 150: 315–320.
54. Kelman GR (1966) Digital computer subroutine for the conversion of oxygen tension into saturation. J Appl Physiol 21: 1375–1376.

2

Vitamin D and Exercise Performance in Professional Soccer Players

Nikolaos E. Koundourakis[1]*, Nikolaos E. Androulakis[2], Niki Malliaraki[3], Andrew N. Margioris[3]

1 Department of Clinical Chemistry, School of Medicine, University of Crete, Heraklion, Greece, **2** Department of Laboratory Haematology, University Hospital, Heraklion, Crete, Greece, **3** Departments of Clinical Chemistry, University of Crete, School of Medicine, and University Hospital, Heraklion, Greece

Abstract

Aim: The current study had two aims. The primary purpose was to examine the association between serum vitamin D levels and the ergometric evaluation of muscle strength, aerobic capacity, and speed in professional soccer players. The secondary aim was to evaluate the effects of the soccer off-season period on serum vitamin D levels.

Methods: Sixty-seven Caucasian male soccer players (age 25.6±6.2 and height 1.81±0.08 m), members of two Greek Superleague Soccer teams and one Football-league championship team participated in this study. Exercise performance testing for the determination of squat jump (SJ), countermovement jump (CMJ), 10 (10 m) and 20 meters (20 m) sprint performance, maximal oxygen consumption (VO_2max), anthropometry, and blood sampling were performed before (pre) and after (post) the six-week off-season period.

Results: Analysis of our results showed the following: (a) a significant correlations between serum vitamin D levels and performance parameters in both pre (SJ; $P<0.001$, CMJ; $P<0.001$, VO_2max; $P<0.001$, 10 m; $P<0.001$, and 20 m; $P<0.001$) and post (SJ; $P<0.001$, CMJ; $P<0.001$, VO_2max; $P=0.006$, 10 m; $P<0.001$, and 20 m; $P<0.001$) experimental sessions. (b) Vitamin D concentration increased significantly ($P<0.001$) following the six-week off-season period compared to baseline, while at the same time all measured performance parameters decreased (SJ; $P<0.001$, CMJ; $P<0.001$, 10 m; $P<0.001$, 20 m; $P<0.001$, VO_2max; $P<0.001$).

Discussion: Our findings suggest that vitamin D levels are associated with the ergometric evaluation of muscle strength, as expressed by SJ and CMJ, sprinting capacity, and VO_2max in professional soccer players, irrespective the levels of performance. Furthermore, our data reaffirm the importance of UVB on serum vitamin D levels. Moreover, reductions in exercise training stress may also have beneficial effects on vitamin D levels, suggesting a possible association of its levels and the training-induced stress. Our results indicate a possibly bidirectional interaction between soccer performance indices and vitamin D levels.

Editor: Markus M. Heimesaat, Charité, Campus Benjamin Franklin, Germany

Funding: These authors have no support or funding to report.

Competing Interests: The authors have declared that no competing interests exist.

* Email: nkoyndoy@hotmail.com

Introduction

Vitamin D is primarily synthesized endogenously following cutaneous exposure to ultraviolet B radiation (UVB) [1], [2]. Apart from its effect on calcium homeostasis and bone metabolism vitamin D exerts a host of other physiological effects on neural and muscular tissues, the immune system, and energy homeostasis, thus affecting among other parameters physical performance [3], [4], [5]. More specifically, it has been shown that vitamin D levels correlate with grip and quadriceps strength, physical fitness, and a decline of falls and bone fractures [5], [6]. Vitamin D deficiency predominantly affects the weight-bearing antigravity muscles of the lower limbs which are necessary for walking and postural balance [5], [7]. Furthermore, vitamin D supplementation boosts muscular strength and restores balance [7].

It should be noted that the majority of the above mentioned studies have been performed in the elderly [5], [7]. Nevertheless, similar findings have been reported in younger individuals. A recent study on adolescent girls reported a positive association between serum vitamin D levels and jump height, jump velocity, and power [2]. Similarly, early studies on collegiate athletes and students have documented that cardiovascular fitness, muscle endurance, and speed are enhanced following exposure to ultraviolet radiation [8], although other authors failed to document such associations [9]. Furthermore, a consisted literature indicates that physical and athletic performance is seasonal, it peaks when vitamin D levels peaks and declines as its levels decline [10], [11].

Paradoxically, a growing number of studies report a high prevalence of vitamin D insufficiency or downright deficiency even in regions with extensive sunlight in both athletic and non-athletic populations [12], [13]. The reason for this phenomenon is not entirely clear. It is mainly attributed to the limited exposure to sun, the types of clothing, and the declining ability of the skin to produce vitamin D precursors with advancing age [4]. Interestingly, a recent study reported that vitamin D levels also decline during strenuous military training [14]. This decrease was evident although training was performed outdoors in the summer and early autumn months during daylight hours and thus with adequate exposure under UVB. The latter data may indicate a possible relationship between exercise training stress and vitamin D levels.

Soccer is a sport where aerobic capacity, muscular strength and speed are of vital importance for most of the actions during playing. Indeed, players must perform repeated sprints, stops, jumps, and changes of direction with maximal force development, and in the shortest possible response time. Furthermore, top level players run approximately 10–12 km during a soccer game, and the total distance covered is linearly related to VO_2max [15]. Vitamin D seems to be involved on this type of activities. It is well documented that its levels are related with muscle strength [5], the proportion and the diameter of type II muscle fibers [16], and neuromuscular coordination [12], which are of paramount importance for explosive type human movements, such as sprints and jumps [17], [18], [19]. Moreover, the presence of vitamin D receptors (VDR) in the muscle cell appears to influence muscle strength. The discovery of VDR within the muscle indicates that vitamin D has the potential to impact upon muscle structure and function directly and has been identified as a regulator of skeletal muscle development and action [20]. In regard to aerobic capacity the findings from recent studies provide evidence that it could be affected by vitamin D levels through an effect of this vitamin on optimal lung function and/or erythropoietin resistance [21], [22].

Our study had two aims. The main objective was to examine the potential relationship between vitamin D levels and muscle strength, as expressed by squat jump (SJ) and countermovement jump (CMJ) [23], maximal oxygen consumption (VO_2max), 10 and, 20 meters sprint performance in two different occasions, prior to the beginning and at the end of the off-season soccer period. Our second aim was to examine the vitamin D response to the reduced exercise training during the six-week off-season transition period. We hypothesized that in both experimental sessions vitamin D levels would correlate with soccer players' jumping, sprinting, and aerobic capacity, and that the off-season transition period, of reduced training stress, would favorably affect vitamin D concentration. To the best of our knowledge, no published study has examined the relationship between vitamin D levels and muscle strength, VO_2max and speed in professional soccer players, and/or the effects off-season detraining soccer period on its levels in any kind of athletic population.

Materials and Methods

Participants

Initially, seventy seven professional players, members of three soccer teams, were evaluated for possible participation in the study. The exclusion criteria were as follow: a) any medical disorder that would affect vitamin D levels, b) players that their contract was ending before the conclusion of the study, and c) the consumption of supplements containing vitamin D. Ten (10) players failed to fulfill criteria b (8) and c (2) and were subsequently excluded from the study. Sixty seven Caucasian professional male soccer players, members of two Greek Super league teams (n = 45) and one Football league team (n = 22) were consecutively included in the study. The mean values of age (years) ± SD and height (m) ± SD were: age 25,6±6,2 and height 1,81±0,08 respectively.

Ethics Statement

Before testing verbal explanation of the aim of the study and the testing procedures were given to all participants, and written informed consent was obtained. The study was performed in strict accordance with the ethical guidelines of the Helsinki Declaration and was approved by the Ethical Scientific Committee of the University Hospital of Heraklion, Crete, Greece.

Experimental protocol

The duration of the off-season transition period was set to six-weeks, starting at the end of the competition period. During this recuperation period, participants were instructed to avoid any kind of exercise training for the first two weeks. After this two-week period, they were instructed to perform low intensity aerobic running (50%–60% of VO_2max) of 20 to 30 minute total duration (30, 20, 2×15, 3×10, 2×10) three times per week, divided by one day of rest. This type of activity was selected by the team coaches. All players were tested at two different occasions. Each experimental testing consisted of two days of consecutive measurements. The first experimental testing took place immediately after the end of the competition period in May (pre). The second experimental testing was performed at the beginning of July (post), just prior to the beginning of the preparation period for the forthcoming season. In each experimental periods testing consisted of anthropometric measurements (i.e. height, body weight, body fat percentage), blood testing for the assessment of vitamin D levels, and ergometry tests for the measurement of SJ (cm), CMJ (cm), VO_2max (ml/kg/min), 10 m, and 20 m sprint performance. The first day of each experimental period anthropometric characteristics were measured at 08:30 am. From 09:00 to 10:30 am, venous blood samples were obtained in order to determine the vitamin D concentration. In the afternoon of the same day (17:00 pm) the players were tested for SJ, CMJ, 10 m, and 20 m sprint performance. The second day of each experimental period, starting at 09:30 am, our participants were tested for the determination of VO_2max. During the study players were instructed to avoid consuming any vitamin D supplements. Before each experimental session, players were informed not to consume any supplement that could promote performance at least 2 days prior to the testing and to avoid any caffeine or alcohol beverages. Moreover, they were instructed to abstain from any exercise training sessions two days prior to each testing in order to avoid any fatigue effects. Detailed nutritional guidelines were given to all players in order to ensure a high (>60%) carbohydrate dietary intake during the study, including a list of a variety of foods, and based on individual resting metabolic rates and the calculated daily energy expenditure as per reported activities (24). Furthermore, players were also asked to maintain their hydration status. All players were familiarized with the testing protocol, as they had been previously tested with the same procedures on several occasions during the last soccer season. The study was performed in Crete, Greece, at latitude of 35,9°N.

Anthropometric Measurements and Body Composition

Height was measured using a stadiometer (Charder HM210D, Charder Electronics CO, LTD, Taiwan) and weight was obtained using an electronic weight scale (Seca Alpha 770, Seca Vogel, Hamburg, Germany). Body fat percentage was assessed by skinfold thickness measurement (Lange Skinfold Caliper, Cambridge Scientific Instruments, Cambridge, UK) using the 4 site formula by Durnin and Womersley [25].

Vitamin D measurement

Venus blood samples were obtained following a ten-minute period of rest in a lying position, after an overnight fast. Vitamin D levels were assessed using DiaSorin 25 hydroxy vitamin D (DiaSorin Inc. S.p.A, Italy), repeatability CV = 3–6% and reproducibility CV = 6–11%, according to the laboratory standard operating procedures. Calibrator 1 and 2 (human serum) concentrations are referenced to standard preparations containing highly purified 25(OH) vitamin D. According to the manufacturer the correlation of the immunoenzymatic assay with LC-MS/MS is described by the equation: concentration = 5,6+0,83*LC-MS/MS (R = 0,93). The intra assay coefficient of variation ranges between 3–6%. In our study vitamin D levels below 10 ng/ml were considered as severe deficiency, levels between 10–20 ng/ml as deficiency and levels between 20–30 ng/ml as insufficiency.

Ergometry tests

The jumping (SJ, CMJ) and sprinting ability (10 m, 20 m) of the soccer players were assessed with a jumping mat (Powertimer, Newtest Ltd., Oulu, Finland) and infrared photoelectric cells (Powertimer, Newtest Ltd., Oulu, Finland) respectively, according to standard procedures [24]. Maximal Oxygen Consumption (VO_2max) assessment was performed on a motorized treadmill using an automated gas-analysis system (VMAX29, Sensormedics, Yorba Linda, CA), with the use of set procedures of a standard protocol [24].

Statistical analysis

Statistical analysis was performed using the software program SPSS 17.0. Results are presented as means ± SD. The distribution of variables was tested by the Shapiro-Wilk statistical method. Then, Pearson's (for normally distributed variables) and Spearman's (for non-normally distributed variables) correlation coefficients were used to assess the linear relationship between quantative variables. The changes between the experimental periods in the measured parameters within the groups were analyzed by the paired samples t-test for normally-distributed data, and by Mann-Whitney test for non-normally-distributed data. Statistical power analysis was performed (Stata 13 software, StataCorp LP, USA) in order to attain 80% power. Analysis was carried out at a confidence level = 95% and confidence interval = 13,6 [26]. Our calculations showed that a sample size equal to 45, much lower than ours i.e. n = 67, was needed to attain 80% power in order to detect any differences in changes of the measured variables between the two experimental sessions. The level of significance was set at $p<0.05$.

Results

Correlation between vitamin D levels and exercise performance parameters

The correlations between vitamin D levels and exercise performance parameters, during the beginning and the end of the 6-week transition period, are presented in table 1. Analysis of our results revealed a significant positive correlation between vitamin D levels and SJ, CM, and VO_2max values at the beginning and at the end of the experimental period (table 1). A significant negative correlation was observed between vitamin D levels and 10 m, and 20 m sprint times at the beginning and at the end of the study (table 1).

Changes in vitamin D levels, exercise performance parameters, and body composition

The values of vitamin D and exercise performance parameters at baseline and after the six-week transition period are presented in table 2. Vitamin D levels increased significantly during the off season period compared to baseline (table 2). In contrast, analysis of our data revealed significant reductions in SJ, CMJ, VO_2max, 10m, and 20m values at the end of the study compared to baseline (table 2). Lastly, there was evident a significant increase in body weight (77,68±7,06 vs 79,08±7,24; $p=0.013$) and body fat (8,81±2,96 vs 10,05±3,56; $p<0.001$) at the end of the study compared to baseline.

Discussion

Our findings support our hypothesis. Analysis of our results showed that vitamin D levels are associated with neuromuscular performance and aerobic capacity in professional soccer players. Notably, to the best of our knowledge, for the first time our study provides evidence of a linear relationship between vitamin D serum levels, not only with jumping performance, but also with VO_2max and speed in non-supplemented soccer players. In addition, we have found that even the short off-season period of reduced training stress had a boosting effect on vitamin D levels. Interestingly, this increase in vitamin D levels was evident in parallel to a reduction in aerobic and neuromuscular performance parameters. The latter finding strengthens the well-documented concept that training plays the principal role for exercise adaptations and improvements in exercise performance, whereas all other parameters including vitamin D play a supportive role.

Vitamin D levels exhibited a positive linear relationship with the ergometric evaluation of muscular strength (SJ and CMJ) and speed at both experimental periods. Our observations are comparable to several studies showing that vitamin D is linearly associated with jumping ability and strength in pre-adolescent girls [2] and elderly individuals [7], [12], [27], and in agreement with the observation that 100 m performance was enhanced after a single biodose of ultraviolet radiation in collegiate women [28]. Moreover, a recent vitamin D supplementation-study on professional soccer players revealed that inadequate vitamin D concentration was detrimental to jumping and sprinting ability, whereas supplementation counteracted this effect [29]. Notably, regarding muscular strength, Hamilton et al. [9] reported that vitamin D levels were not associated with lower limb isokinetic muscle function in soccer players. However, this finding was attributed to the different mode of exercise used since, as the authors suggested, vitamin D could preferentially affect muscle groups that were not evaluated in their study. It should be mentioned that both SJ and CMJ are considered to be the most accurate field tests for the determination of the strength levels of the lower limps [23]. In order to perform SJ and CMJ the proximal muscles required are quadriceps, soleus, and gastrocnemius [7]. Those muscles have been found to be predominantly affected by vitamin D deficiency [7]. Furthermore, it is well established that sprint performance is linearly related with both SJ and CMJ [30], [31], suggesting a direct effect of strength levels on sprinting ability. Therefore, based on the aforementioned evidence, our findings indicate a possible effect of vitamin D on jumping ability and strength, which is in turn translated to an affected sprint performance in a similar manner.

The pathways via which vitamin D affects muscular strength (as measured by SJ and CMJ) and sprint performance are still hypothetical. However, there are several potential mechanisms conveying these effects. The ergogenic effects of vitamin D may be

Table 1. Correlations (correlation coefficients and p-values) between Vitamin D levels and exercise performance parameters.

Exercise Performance	Pre Vitamin D (ng/ml)	Post Vitamin D (ng/ml)
SJ (cm)	0.731 ($p<0.001$)	0.597 ($p<0.001$)
CMJ (cm)	0.740 ($p<0.001$)	0.476 ($p<0.001$)
VO_2max (ml/kg/min)	0.436 ($p<0.001$)	0.394 ($p=0.006$)
10 m (sec)	−0.649 ($p<0.001$)	−0.410 ($p<0.001$)
20 m (sec)	−0.673 ($p<0.001$)	−0.426 ($p<0.001$)

Pre: measurement prior to the beginning of the off-season transition period;
Post: measurement at the end of the off-season transition period.

related to the regulation of muscle protein synthesis which could affect muscle mass, thanks to the presence of vitamin D receptors on skeletal myocytes [5], [31], [32]. Furthermore, alterations in vitamin D levels also affect its receptors at the expression and activation levels [5], [20], and thus affecting muscle mass [5], [33], neuromuscular coordination [18], and the relative number and the cross-sectional area of type II muscle fibers [16]. Since it well documented that the major determinants of jumping and sprinting ability are muscle strength [31], [34], type II muscle fibers [35], [36] and neuromuscular coordination, [19], [37], any potential effect of vitamin D on these parameters would in turn affect jumping and sprinting capacity in a similar manner.

Analysis of our data revealed a linear association between vitamin D and VO_2max in both experimental sessions. This finding is supported by an early study which reported increased aerobic capacity as a result of exposure to ultraviolet radiation in collegiate students [8]. Furthermore, a recent study on adolescents observed a positive relationship between vitamin D and aerobic performance on adolescents [38]. Since VO_2max is related to soccer performance, as indicated by the well-documented relationship between this parameter and the distance covered during a soccer game [15], our findings suggest that in order to perform efficiently during a soccer game optimal vitamin D levels are needed. The observed association between vitamin D levels and VO_2max could be related to its protective effect on lung function. According to recently published evidence, low vitamin D levels are associated with lower indices of lung function [22] and increased airway reactivity [39]. Since exercise performance and especially aerobic capacity (VO_2max) is depended on optimal lung function [40], any protective and/or boosting effect of vitamin D on the function of this organ could beneficially influence aerobic performance during exercise [40]. Vitamin D could also influence VO_2max by affecting iron metabolism and erythropoietin [21], [41]. According to Li and associates [41] vitamin D deficiency results in dysregulation of innate immunity and inflammation which is affecting iron metabolism and contributes to erythropoietin resistance. It is well documented that erythropoietin is linearly associated with changes in red blood cells levels [42]. Thus, vitamin D could influence VO_2max via its effects on erythropoesis modifying the capacity of the oxygen supply to the exercising muscles and consequently affecting aerobic exercise performance [42].

Interestingly, analysis of our data showed that although vitamin D increased at the end of the off-season period all measured exercise performance parameters decreased. However, the observed linear correlation at baseline between vitamin D levels and performance was retained at the end of the study, suggesting that vitamin D is related to the ability to perform efficiently during exercise, irrespective the level of performance. These data clearly suggest that although vitamin D does seem to affect neuromuscular and aerobic performance, it does not play the primary role. Indeed, during periods of reduced training stimulus or training cessation (i.e. soccer transition period) there is deterioration in exercise performance [24]. Since this decline is widely accepted to be a result of the insufficient training stimulus [24], this finding demonstrates that the major determinant of exercise performance is the amount and the quality of training [15], [24]. The latter evidence documents that vitamin D plays a supportive role in exercise performance. However, this does not lessen the importance of vitamin D serum concentration since in elite soccer level even subtle changes in performance may determine the outcome of a competition.

In our study the six-week transition period had a boosting effect on vitamin D levels. Indeed, at the first experimental period,

Table 2. Vitamin D and Performance values in the two experimental periods.

Measurements	Pre	Post
Vitamin D (ng/ml)	34,41±7,08	47,24±13,50**
SJ (cm)	39,50±3,87	37,10±3,59**
CMJ (cm)	40,91±4,57	38,62±4,00**
VO_2max (ml/kg/min)	59,44±3,07	58,89±3,45**
10 m (sec)	1,74±0,07	1,79±0,08**
20 m (sec)	3,02±0,06	3,07±0,07**

Pre: measurement prior to the beginning of the off-season transition period;
Post: measurement at the end of the off-season transition period.*significant difference at the level of significance $p<0.05$**, significant difference at the level of significance $p<0.01$.

although none of our participants was vitamin D deficient (< 20 ng/ml) or severe deficient (<10 ng/ml), 55,22% of our players had insufficient vitamin D levels (<30 ng/ml), whereas at the second one only 4,47% were found to be below 30 ng/ml. In regard to the first experimental session our findings are in agreement with studies on soccer players (~50% <30 ng/ml) [43], and members of the American national football league [44] (~51% <30 ng/ml). Furthermore, our values were at the lower level of the range observed (30–84% vitamin D insufficiency) in several athletic and non-athletic population [9], [43], [45]. The most plausible explanation for the elevation of vitamin D levels at the second experimental session could be the consequence of an increased exposure to UVB during the off-season period [9]. Indeed, this transition period in Greek Superleague takes place during June and at the beginning of July at a favorable latitude (35,9°N). During this period UVB reaches its peak [46], resulting in increased vitamin D production. It is well demonstrated the extremely importance that UVB plays on vitamin D synthesis [1], [3] and the observation that its effectiveness is among other parameters, season dependent [32]. Furthermore, this off-season phase is actually a holiday period for professional soccer players. This could indicate increased time spend under sunlight, and also an increased exposure of a larger proportion of the players' body to UVB. Since all these parameters are related with vitamin D production, the observed increased in its levels at the end of our study could be partly accounted to these factors [3], [47]. The above mentioned suggestions are further supported by the observation that 84% of 342 Qatar soccer players were vitamin D insufficient (<30 ng/ml) [9], despite of the favorable latitude (25.4°N) and the period that the study was performed (i.e. July). This finding was attributed to inadequate exposure to the sun, since all outdoors training were performed after sunset, demonstrating the importance of UVB on vitamin D production.

Although our data reaffirm the importance of adequate exposure to UVB, recent evidence indicate that the exercise training -induced stress may play a regulatory role on vitamin D levels [14]. Andersen et al. [14] reported that intense military training resulted to reduced vitamin D levels in female soldiers, although these activities were performed outdoors in the summer and early autumn. This finding was unanticipated by the authors since they expected vitamin D levels to increase or at least to remain constant due to the adequate daily exposure to UVB during the whole study. Further support is coming from two recent studies on soccer players [43], [48]. The authors observed much lower vitamin D levels (30,82±9,04 [42], 32,83±6,64 [48]) and insufficiency values (83% <30 ng/ml [42], 65% <30 ng/ml [48]) during periods of training, compared to the ones we obtained after the six-week detraining period (45,67±13,70; 4,47<30 ng/ml). These low values were evident despite the fact that outdoor training sessions were performed at August [48] and during summer [43] under a sufficient daily exposure of a large proportion of their body to UVB. According to Holick [49], the participants of these two studies should have had sufficient vitamin D levels since the amount of sun exposure needed to maintain adequate vitamin D levels is approximately 5–30 minutes at least twice a week to the face, arms, and legs [49]. Based on the aforementioned evidence we could suggest that the exercise training-induced stress could play a regulatory role on vitamin D levels. Supporting to our hypothesis is the fact that our second testing was performed following a massive reduction of training stress, while the participants in these soccer studies were tested in pre-season and early in-season which are periods of high training stress (i.e. training sessions and games) [15]. This suggested impact of exercise-induced stress on vitamin D could be associated to the immune effects of the intense stress [50], since both vitamin D and exercise training are related with the immune system [50], [51]. Indeed, prolonged intense training sessions or intensified training periods, similar to the ones used repeatedly during a soccer season, suppresses athletes' immune system [50]. In our study, the first experimental session was performed at the end of competition season which according to the literature suppresses innate immunity [50]. On the contrary, the six-week period prior to the second testing our players were under minimal training stress, which could hypothetically have resulted in an enhanced innate immunity. Recently published data suggest a strong inverse correlation between inflammation and vitamin D concentration [8], [51], while elevated vitamin D levels boost immunity [52]. Therefore, we could hypothesize that any positive alteration in soccer players' immunity due to reduced training stress could be evident in conjunction with increased vitamin D status.

Our study provides evidence of an association between not supplemented vitamin D levels and parameters of aerobic and neuromuscular exercise performance in soccer. In particular, our findings indicated a linear relationship between vitamin D levels and muscle strength as evaluated by SJ and CMJ, sprinting ability (10 m, and 20 m), and VO_2max in professional soccer players. Moreover, our results indicate that, apart from increased exposure to UVB, reductions in exercise training stress may also have beneficial effects on vitamin D levels in elite soccer players. However in order to confirm this hypothesis additional research is needed, also examining indices of inflammation. Furthermore, our findings indicate that vitamin D plays, among other parameters, a secondary supportive role in athletic performance. However, this does not lessen its importance, especially in highly competitive athletes, since in elite athletic level slight changes in performance may determine the outcome of a competition. Our current data may provide an additional tool to sport scientists, coaches, and players to enhance soccer performance.

Author Contributions

Conceived and designed the experiments: NEK ANM. Performed the experiments: NEK NEA NM. Analyzed the data: NEK NM. Contributed reagents/materials/analysis tools: NEK NEA NM ANM. Contributed to the writing of the manuscript: NEK ANM.

References

1. Holick MF (2003) Vitamin D: a millennium perspective. J Cell Biochem 88: 296–307.
2. Muir SW, Montero-Odasso M (2011) Effect of vitamin D supplementation on muscle strength, gait and balance in older adults: a systematic review and meta-analysis. J Am Geriatr Soc 59: 2291–300.
3. Holick M (2002) Sunlight and Vitamin D. J Gen Intern Med 17: 733–5.
4. Moran SM, McClung JP, Kohen T, Lieberman HR (2013) Vitamin D and physical performance. Sports Med 2013 43: 601–11.
5. Bischoff-Ferrari HA, Dietrich T, Orav EJ, Hu FB, Zhang Y, et al. (2004) Higher 25-hydroxyvitamin D concentrations are associated with better lower-extremity function in both active and inactive persons aged > or =60 y. Am J Clin Nutr 80: 752–8.

6. Glerup H, Mikkelsen K, Poulsen L, Hass E, Overbeck S, et al. (2000) Hypovitaminosis D myopathy without biochemical signs of osteomalacic bone involvement. Calcif Tissue Int 66: 419–24.
7. Ward K, Das G, Berry J, Roberts S, Rawer R, et al. (2009) Vitamin D status and muscle function in postmenarchal adolescent girls. J Clin Endocrinol Metab 94: 559–63.
8. Cannell JJ, Hollis BW, Sorenson MB, Taft TN, Anderson JJ (2009) Athletic performance and vitamin D. Med Sci Sports Exerc 41: 1102–10.
9. Hamilton B, Whiteley R, Farooq A, Chalabi H (2014) Vitamin D concentration in 342 professional football players and association with lower limb isokinetic function. J Sci Med Sport17: 139–43.
10. Larson-Meyer DE, Willis KS (2010) Vitamin D and athletes. Curr Sports Med Rep 9: 220–6.
11. Cannell J, Hollis BW, Sorenson MB, Taft TN, Anderson JJ (2009) Athletic performance and vitamin D. Med Sci Sports Exerc 41: 1102–10.
12. Hamilton B (2010) Vitamin D and Skeletal muscle. Scand J Med Sci Sports 20: 182–90.
13. Maïmoun L, Manetta J, Couret I, Dupuy AM, Mariano-Goulart D, et al. (2006) The intensity level of physical exercise and the bone metabolism response. Int J Sports Med 27: 105–11.
14. Andersen NE, Karl JP, Cable SJ, Williams KW, Rood JC, et al. (2010) Vitamin D status in female military personnel during combat training. J Int Soc Sports Nutr 14: 7–38.
15. Stølen T, Chamari K, Castagna C, Wisløff U (2005) Physiology of soccer: an update. Sports Med 35: 501–36.
16. Young A, Edwards RHT, Jones DA, Brenton DP (1981) Quadriceps muscle strength and fibre size during the treatment of osteomalacia. In: Stokes IAF editor. Mechanical factors and the skeleton. London, Libbey: 137–45.
17. Missitzi J, Geladas N, Klissouras V (2004) Heritability in neuromuscular coordination: Implications for motor control strategies. Med Sci Sports Exerc 36: 233–40.
18. Dhesi JK, Jackson SH, Bearne LM, Moniz C, Hurley MV, et al. (2004) Vitamin D supplementation improves neuromuscular function in older people who fall. Age Ageing, 33: 589–95.
19. Ecker T (1996) Basic biomechanics of running. In: Eckert T editor. Basic Track & Field Biomechanics: Tafnews Press. 57–63.
20. Bischoff-Ferrari HA (2012) Relevance of vitamin D in muscle health. Rev Endocr Metab Disord 13: 71–7.
21. Christakos S, Hewison M, Gardner DG, Wagner CL, Sergeev IN, et al. (2013) Vitamin D: beyond bone. Ann N Y Acad Sci 1287: 45–58.
22. Zosky G, Berry L, Elliot J, James A, Gorman S, et al. (2011) Vitamin D deficiency causes deficits in lung function and alters lung structure. American Journal of Respiratory and Critical Care Medicine, 183: 1336–43.
23. Marcovic G, Dizdar D, Jukic I, Cardinale M (2004) Reliability and factorial validity of Squat and Countermovement jump tests. J Strength Cond Res 18: 551–5.
24. Koundourakis NE, Androulakis NE, Malliaraki N, Tsatsanis C, Venihaki M, et al. (2014) Discrepancy between Exercise Performance, Body Composition, and Sex Steroid Response after a Six-Week Detraining Period in Professional Soccer Players. PLoS ONE 9(2): e87803. doi:10.1371/journal.pone.0087803.
25. Durnin JV, Womersley J (1974) Body fat assessed from the total body density and its estimation from skinfold thickness: measurements on 481 men and women aged from 16 to 72 years. Br J Nutr 32: 77–97.
26. Izquierdo M, Ibañez J, González-Badillo JJ, Ratamess NA, Kraemer WJ, et al. (2007) Detraining and tapering effects on hormonal responses and strength performance. J Strength Cond Res 21: 768–75.
27. Geoff V (2005) Recent developments in vitamin D deficiency and muscle weakness among elderly people. BMJ330: 524–6.
28. Cheatum BA (1968) Effects of a single biodose of ultraviolet radiation upon the speed of college women Res Q. 39: 482–5.
29. Close GL, Russell J, Cobley JN, Owens DJ, Wilson G, et al. (2013) Assessment of vitamin D concentration in non-supplemented professional athletes and healthy adults during the winter months in the UK: implications for skeletal muscle function. J Sports Sci 31: 344–53.
30. Ingebrigtsen J, Jeffreys I (2012) The relationship between speed, strength and jumping abilities in elite junior handball players. Serb J Sports Sci 6: 83–8.
31. Perez-Gomez J, Rodriguez GV, Ara I, Olmedillas H, Chavarren J, et al. (2008) Role of muscle mass on sprint performance: gender differences? Eur J Appl Physiol 102: 685–94.
32. Pfeifer M, Begerow B, Minne HW (2002)Vitamin D and Muscle Function. Osteoporos Int 13: 187–94.
33. Lee GS, Choi KC, Park SM, An BS, Cho MC, et al. (2003) Expression of human Calbindin-D9k correlated with age, vitamin D receptor and blood calcium level in the gastrointestinal tissues. Clinical biochemistry, 36, 255–261.
34. Ziambaras K, Dagogo-Jack S (1997) Reversible muscle weakness in patients with vitamin D deficiency. West J Med 167: 435–9.
35. Stone MH, O'Bryant HS, McCoy L, Coglianese R, Lehmkuhl M, et al. (2003) Power and maximum strength relationships during performance of dynamic and static weighted jumps. J Strength Cond Res 17: 140–7.
36. Inbar O, Kaiser P, Tesch P, (1981) Relationships between leg muscle fiber type distribution and leg exercise performance. Int J Sports Med 2: 154–9.
37. Pereira R, Machado M, Miragaya dos Santos M, Pereira L, Sampaio-Jorge F (2008) Muscle activation sequence compromises vertical jump performance. Serb J Sports Sci 2: 85–90.
38. Lämmle L, Bergmann K, Bös K, Koletzko B (2013) Predictors of differences in vitamin D levels in children and adolescents and their relation to endurance performance. Ann Nutr Metab 62(1): 55–62.
39. Litonju A, Weiss S (2007) Is vitamin D deficiency to blame for the asthma epidemic? J Allergy Clin Immunol 120: 1031–5.
40. Fatemi R, Shakerian S, Ghanbarzade M, Habibi A, Moghaddam HF (2012) The comparison of dynamic volumes of pulmonary function between different levels of maximal oxygen uptake Intl Res J. Appl Basic Sci Vol 3: 667–74., 2012.
41. Li YC, Kong J, Wei M, Chen ZF, Liu SQ, et al. (2002) 1,25-dihydroxyvitamin D(3) is a Negative Endocrine Regulator of the Renin-Angiotensin System. J Clin Invest 110: 229–38.
42. Jones M, Tunstall-Pedoe DS (1989) Blood doping-a literature review. Br J Sports Med 23: 84–8.
43. Kopeć A, Solarz K, Majda F, Słowińska-Lisowska M, Mędraś M (2013) An evaluation of the levels of vitamin D and bone turnover markers after the summer and winter periods in polish professional soccer players. J Hum Kinet 38: 135–40.
44. Angeline ME, Gee AO, Shindle M, Warren RF, Rodeo SA (2013) The effects of vitamin D deficiency in athletes. Am J Sports Med 41: 461–4.
45. Shuler FD, Wingate MK, Moore GH, Giangarra C (2012) Sports Health Benefits of Vitamin D. Sports Health. 4: 496–501.
46. Galán I, Rodríguez-Laso A, Díez-Gañán L, Cámara E (2011) Prevalence and correlates of skin cancer risk behaviors in Madrid (Spain). Gaceta sanitaria 25: 44–9.
47. Hollis WB (2005) Circulating 25-Hydroxyvitamin D levels indicative of Vitamin D insufficiency: Implications of establishing a new effective dietary intake. Recommendations for Vitamin D. J Nutr 135: 317–22.
48. Morton JP, Iqbal Z, Drust B, Burgess D, Close GL, et al. (2012) Seasonal variation in vitamin D status in professional soccer players of the English Premier League. Appl Physiol Nutr Metab. 37: 798–802.
49. Holick MF (2007) Vitamin D deficiency. N Engl J Med 357: 266–81.
50. Gleeson M (2007) Immune function in sport and exercise. J Appl Physiol 103: 693–9.
51. Shroff R, Egerton M, Bridel M, Shah V, Donald AE, et al. (2008) A bimodal association of vitamin D levels and vascular disease in children on dialysis. J Am Soc Nephrol 19: 1239–46.
52. Christakos S, DeLuca HF (2011) Mini review: Vitamin D: is there a role in extraskeletal health? Endocrinology. 152: 2930–6.

Health in Elite Sports from a Salutogenetic Perspective: Athletes' Sense of Coherence

Jochen Mayer*, Ansgar Thiel

Institute of Sports Science, University of Tübingen, Tübingen, Germany

Abstract

Objective: Considering the high number of stressors encountered in the context of elite sports, a high sense of coherence (SOC) is crucial to allow athletes to maintain their health from both short- and long-term perspectives. The aim of this cross-sectional study was to investigate SOC in a population of elite athletes, focusing on identification of subsets of athletes with particularly high and low SOC scores, and any related predictors. The elite athletes' SOC scores were also evaluated for differences with those of the general population of Germany; whether a correlation between SOC and subjective health existed was additionally examined.

Method: In total, 698 male and female elite athletes, drawn from Germany's highest-level national track and field squads, and first and second division handball teams, completed a survey that included the SOC-L9 Scale and measures of subjective health, sociodemographic information, and the number of injury lay-offs experienced during the athletes' careers to date.

Results: Classification tree analysis reveals six contrast groups with varying SOC scores. Several interacting factors determine the group to which an athlete belongs. Together with overuse injuries, additional factors are age, gender, and completed/not completed apprenticeship/degree. Female athletes aged between 19 and 25, who had already been subject to lay offs due to overuse injuries, comprise the group with the lowest SOC scores. Overall, the SOC of elite athletes is slightly lower than in the general population. In accordance with other studies, a stronger SOC is also correlated significantly with better global subjective health.

Conclusion: The identification of contrast groups with varying SOC scores contributes to the development of more targeted salutogenetic health promotion programs. Such programs would ideally include learning modules pertaining to coping with overuse injuries, as well as social support systems aiming to effectively combine education and elite sport.

Editor: Mun Yin Ho, City University of Hong Kong, Hong Kong

Funding: The study was funded by the Federal Institute of Sports Science (BISp) as part of the German Ministry of the Interior. The funders had no role in study design, data collection and analysis, decision to publish, or preparation of the manuscript.

Competing Interests: The authors have declared that no competing interests exist.

* Email: jochen.mayer@uni-tuebingen.de

Introduction

Excellent health is essential for long-term, high performance levels in sports. At the same time, an athlete's health is always at risk. In addition to the common stressors of life, elite athletes are confronted with numerous sports-specific stressors. For example, they have to deal with high training loads and the physical demands of elite-level competition; management of injuries or illnesses; and coping with role conflicts generated by the differing expectations of sports organizations, families, and educational establishments. Therefore, staying healthy represents a huge challenge. From a salutogenetic perspective, elite athletes have to successfully cope with the state of tension created by these stressors in order to generate health. According to the medical sociologist Aaron Antonovsky, health is considered as a position on a health ease/disease continuum and a movement in the direction towards health [1]. In this regard, an important factor in successfully responding to stressors and staying healthy is one's sense of coherence (SOC).

SOC reflects a person's view of life and enables people to consider their external and internal resources, to identify and mobilize them, to promote effective coping by finding solutions, and to resolve tension in a health-promoting manner [2]. SOC is defined as "a global orientation that expresses the extent to which one has a pervasive, enduring though dynamic feeling of confidence that (1) the stimuli deriving from one's internal and external environments in the course of living are structured, predictable, and explicable; (2) the resources are available to one to meet the demands posed by these stimuli; and (3) these demands are challenges worthy of investment and engagement" [1].

When confronted with a stressor, a person with a strong SOC will be motivated to cope (meaningfulness) and believe that the situation may be understood (comprehensibility) and that resources to cope are available (manageability) [3]. To date, research on health in elite sport has mainly focused on biomedical perspectives, although many recent studies with non-athlete populations have demonstrated that a strong SOC promotes resilience and the development of a positive subjective state of health, especially mental health [2]. The relationship between SOC and perceived health is manifested in study populations regardless of age, gender, ethnicity, nationality, or study design. There are also strong positive correlations between SOC and different measures of well-being, as well as negative correlations with distress, maladaptation, depression, and subjective complaints [2]. Longitudinal studies employing the SOC scale reveal a relatively high degree of predictability of future health in both the short and long term. For example, a strong SOC was the most important predictor of differences between employees with serious "burnout," and those without burnout, in a 10-year follow-up study [4]. A strong SOC was also associated with reduced risk of psychiatric disorders in a 19-year follow-up study [5].

For elite athletes in particular, who we define as athletes competing at least at the top level nationally, a high SOC should be considered a central factor for maintaining both health and performance levels in sports. Considering both the role of the SOC as a key health resource, and the extreme strain engendered by intense exercise and competition, it appears intuitive to assume that athletes with a low SOC will have serious difficulties staying healthy and being able to perform. Although there exist many studies pertaining to several aspects of SOC in different populations (and in different countries), there has been, to our knowledge, no research on elite athletes' health in this field. The only study conducted with an elite athlete population focused on the relationship between mental skills in Swedish elite athletes and the concepts of locus of control (LOC) and SOC, but not on aspects of health [6]. In light of the existing deficit in research, several theoretical considerations will first be made regarding the possible characteristics and development of SOC in elite athletes.

According to Antonovsky's theoretical assumptions, SOC develops during childhood and adolescence and stabilizes around the age of 30 [1]. In order for a strong SOC to develop, people must continually have coherent life experiences. The strength of a person's SOC, according to Antonovsky's theory [3], is shaped by different kinds of life experiences characterized by consistency, underload-overload balance, and participation in socially valued decision-making. The extent of such experiences is underpinned by many factors, ranging from one's position in society to one's culture, vocation, and family structure. Additional factors can also play a major role in a person's life experience, such as gender, ethnicity, chance occurrences, and even genetics.

It has thus far been assumed that the strength of an individual's SOC is related to their age and gender. A recent study, with 43,598 respondents, underlines the fact that males have a stronger SOC than do females. In terms of age, a stronger SOC is also observable in older age groups [7]. Both gender and age are therefore taken into consideration when calculating standard values for certain population groups [8]. Considering the dynamic nature of the development of SOC, it should be stated that SOC is not as stable as Antonovsky assumed. Evidence shows that SOC tends to increase with age and that the level of SOC achieved in adulthood is most relevant in terms of its stability. Particularly among individuals with an initially high SOC, SOC is more stable than it is in individuals with a lower initial SOC [9].

Theoretical Considerations on the Development of Elite Athletes' SOC

Considering that SOC "is partly determined by an individual's position in the social structure and partly by current work conditions, social network, and support, rather than predominantly by experiences made in his early life" [10,11], it may be expected that the social context of elite sport influences the strength of SOC. In the course of socialization occurring via elite sports participation, athletes are increasingly bound to the sport system. The life of an elite athlete is highly structured, through training and competition commitments, and adherence to the formal structures of elite sport. Sport networks comprised of coaches, physicians, therapists, and managers teach athletes appropriate health management in addition to the basic moral and normative concepts of elite sport [12]. Furthermore, athletes are exposed to specific health risks, principally various kinds of sports injuries.

It appears that an initially high SOC is required in order to manage the demands of elite sports and that repeated, successful management of health problems contributes to a stabilization of, or even an increase in, SOC. This is true particularly in terms of subsequent athletic success in competitions and the social recognition that stems from such efforts. This argument is supported by studies of athletes in college student populations. Athletes in a large Japanese college sample possessed a higher SOC score than did non-athletes. Furthermore, the results suggest that engaging in sporting activities for several successive years enhances SOC [13]. Another study, based on a small, non-elite sample of US college varsity athletes and college non-athletes, also reveals higher SOC scores in the athlete subpopulation [14].

Despite the above discussion, it should also be noted that SOC can be weakened. Traumatic life events as well as the appearance of severe health problems [15] can decrease SOC in both genders [16]. In the context of elite athletes, injuries have to be categorized as critical life events that place high demand on psychological ability to cope [17,18]. In a study on the quality of life of US elite collegiate athletes, for example, injuries which required a hiatus from athletics had a negative effect on all indices of quality of life [19]. Elite athletes do not experience injury lay-offs only owing to traumatic injuries; as a result of discrepancies between stress and individual resilience, over-training syndrome and overuse injuries can also occur, sometimes leading to chronic symptoms and enforced training and competition absences. Accordingly, it may be assumed that a strong SOC can be weakened when athletes repeatedly experience instability in their athletic career and a lack of control over their health due to risk of injury. One can therefore also assume that there are certainly elite athletes with a low SOC, who do not possess the optimal conditions for coping with further elite athletic demands.

With respect to the foregoing discussion, we hypothesize that elite athletes will have a higher mean SOC than age-matched controls, but that there will still exist groups of athletes with particularly low SOC scores. In addition, we expect a strong correlation between SOC and subjective health in athlete populations.

Objective

In summary, the primary objective of the present study is to investigate SOC in a sample of elite athletes focusing on three aspects: determination of SOC in a sample of German handball players and track and field athletes versus the general population; assessing the relationship between SOC and subjective health; and identifying subsets of athletes with either particularly high or low SOC via the method of classification tree analyses (main study objective). Therefore, the question is raised as to whether there exist subsets of elite athletes with notably different SOC values and, if so, which variables predict such differences. In addition to the influence of general sociodemographic and sport-specific characteristics, the role of injuries as a specific type of critical life event in an athlete's career progression is of major interest.

Materials and Methods

Study Design

Analyses are based upon data drawn from a larger multi methodical study pertaining to health management in Germany's elite handball and track and field teams. In the quantitative section of the study, a cross-sectional survey was conducted with a questionnaire covering health-related topics including SOC, subjective health, sports injuries, attitudes towards health, risk and pain, and sociodemographic and sports-specific characteristics.

Ethics Statement

Our research was approved by the Institutional Review Board of the Faculty for Economics and Social Sciences. We adhered to the principles expressed in the Declaration of Helsinki. All participants were informed in writing about the study's aims and procedures, the confidential treatment of the data, voluntary nature of participation, and use of anonymous data in analyses. Informed consent was implied through the act of completing and returning the questionnaire. All data obtained was anonymized before it was received and therefore not connected to the athletes' personal information when entered in SPSS.

Participants and Procedure

German male and female elite athletes meeting the following criteria were included in the study: (a) engaged in handball or track and field, (b) member of one of the highest-level national squads (i.e., A, B, C to D/C squad) and/or (c) competing in the first or second division of Germany's professional handball league. The study was supported by the National Handball Federation, the National Handball League and the National Track and Field Federation. The survey was administered in 2006. Due to sports-specific organizational differences, it was necessary to distribute the questionnaire in the following manner. (1) Track and field athletes were contacted by mail via an existing mailing list comprising all of the squad members. In total, 328 of 559 athletes completed and returned the questionnaire (58.50%). (2) For the handball players, a complete mailing list did not exist; thus, contact was made via their home teams: packages containing sealable questionnaires were sent to all 30 premier league teams and to the best 26 teams in the second division (either to the headquarters of the home teams or directly to team physicians). In total, 395 players, from 43 different teams, responded. We approximated a response rate of 50.38% based on an estimated 14 German players within each of the 56 contacted teams. 25 of the total of 723 male and female athletes who responded did not complete the SOC section and were therefore excluded from the analysis. The final study population consisted of 698 elite athletes (380 handball players and 318 track-and field athletes) with an average age of 22.85 years (see Table 1). There are slightly more male athletes (58.8%) in our sample. 36.7% of respondents consider themselves professional athletes, who make their living from their sport. 55.3% of respondents attained the highest level of school education available in Germany'; 19.8% still attend school. 34.4% have completed vocational training or a tertiary degree, and 18% currently attend university. The majority of respondents are single (85.8%). Athletes' average weekly training load amounts to 13.95 hours (season and off-season) with an average of 28.2 competitions entered per season. Athletes had experienced an average of 4.81 injury lay-offs due to traumatic injuries and 3.17 injury lay-offs due to overuse injuries, during their entire career.

Measures

SOC. The SOC scale is considered a reliable, valid, cross-culturally applicable instrument measuring how people manage stress and remain healthy [20]. It is also considered a useful screening tool to identify individuals with inadequate coping capabilities who are particularly vulnerable to distress [21].

Alongside the SOC-29 and the SOC-13, the shorter SOC-L9 is increasingly being used [22]. An additional factor in favor of these various scales is the fact that values for population-representative random samples exist for comparison. To measure SOC, the Leipzig Short Scale SOC-L9 was utilized presently [23]. Here, SOC is measured one-dimensionally, and with a comparable rating, as per the 29-item scale, but is determined with less diagnostic effort. The Leipzig Short Scale contains the 9 items of the 29-item scale that correlate most closely with the original total scale. The one-dimensionality of the scale has been borne out via factor-analysis. The postulated subcomponents of SOC (comprehensibility, manageability and meaningfulness) are not therefore separately assessed, owing to their being unsatisfactorily replicated in many empirical studies [23]. This scale also exhibits good reliability in our elite athlete population (Cronbach's alpha = 0.82).

Subjective health. As variables of subjective health, athletes' general perception of their health, and subjective health complaints, were also included. Global self-reported health was measured according to the HBSC studies [24]. Athletes were required to respond to the question "Would you say your health is…?" on a 4-point scale, as to whether their subjective health was poor, fair, good, or excellent. Global self-reported health is regarded as a valid predictor of mortality and future morbidity [25].

Subjective health complaints were measured by the HBSC Symptom Check List (HBSC-SCL) [26]. This includes the following 8 items: headache, abdominal pain, backache, feeling low, irritability or bad mood, feeling nervous, sleeping difficulties, and dizziness. Athletes reported, via a 5-point scale, if each symptom was experienced most days, more than once a week, about once every month, seldom, or never. Non-occurrence of a symptom corresponded to 0; occurrence most days corresponded to 4. Total scores were calculated for each athlete between a minimum of 0 and a maximum of 32 [27]. The reliability and validity of the instrument has been confirmed, and the overall scale is considered to measure one-dimensional, latent psychosomatic complaints [26]. Within our elite athlete population this scale also has acceptable reliability (Cronbach's alpha = 0.74).

Variables used in the classification tree analysis. Eleven variables from three categories were incorporated into the classification tree analysis. This method will be described in more detail in the data analysis section. Table 2 displays the characteristics of the dependent and independent variables. In addition to common sociodemographic statistics such as age, gender and marital status, and educational and vocational status, sports-specific sociodemographic variables, such as type of sport engaged in, squad level, professional status, career duration, training load, and number of competitions entered were incorporated. To identify injuries as a specific type of critical life event in an athlete's career, the number of severe injury lay-offs due to overuse and traumatic injuries was assessed. According to Bird, Black, and Newton [28], traumatic injuries are those which occur due to an accident with or without an external influence such as tears (torn ligaments, ruptured muscle fiber, etc.), breaks, strains, bruises, or open wounds. Overuse injuries were categorized as physical symptoms caused by improper or excessive biomechanical stress; for example joint pain owing to enthesitis, tendinitis, or

Table 1. Sociodemographic Data and Descriptive Statistics for Health Related Variables (N = 698).

Category	Subcategory	Absolute (N)	%	M (SD), [Range]
Sex	Female	283	40.5	-
	Male	410	58.8	-
	Missing	5	0.7	-
Age	Valid	674	-	22.85 (5.41), [14–41]
	Missing	24	-	
Education	Student (No Degree yet)	138	19.8	-
	University Entrance Degree (*Abitur*)	386	55.3	-
	Secondary School Certificate (*Mittlere Reife*)	126	18.1	-
	Secondary Modern School (*Hauptschule*)	21	3.0	-
	No degree	5	0.7	-
	Missing	22	3.2	-
Family status	Single	599	85.8	-
	Married	80	11.5	-
	Missing	19	2.7	-
Vocational Status	School Student	140	20.1	-
	University Student	131	18.8	-
	Apprenticeship	13	1.9	-
	Completed Apprenticeship/University Degree	242	34.4	-
	No Apprenticeship/University Degree	12	1.7	-
	Missing	160	22.9	-
Type of Sport	Handball	380	54.4	
	Track and Field	318	45.6	
Professional Athlete	Yes	256	36.7	-
	No	421	60.3	-
	Missing	21	3.0	-
Performance Level	A-, B-Squad/Premier league/National team (Level 1)	367	52.6	-
	C-, D/C-Squad/Second division league (Level 2)	321	46.0	-
	Missing	10	1.4	-
Career Length in Elite Sports (Years)	Valid	676	-	6.94 (4.66), [1–26]
	Missing	22	-	
Training in Hours/Week in Past Season	Valid	684	-	13.95 (4.86), [2–36]
	Missing	14	-	
Competitions in Past Season	Valid	664	-	28.2 (16.67), [1–90]
	Missing	34	-	
Traumatic Injuries: Lay-offs >1 Week	Valid	667	-	4.81 (5.09), [0–37]
	Missing	31	-	
Overuse Injuries: Lay-offs >1 Week	Valid	668	-	3.17 (5.26), [0–46]
	Missing	30	-	
Global Subjective Health	Valid	692	-	3.26 (0.73), [1–4]
	Missing	6	-	
Subjective Complaints (Score from 0 to 32)	Valid	680	-	4.00 (4.05), [0–21]
	Missing	18	-	
Current Competition Lay-off due to Injury or Illness	Yes	102	14.6%	-
	No	593	85.0%	-
	Missing	3	0.4%	-
Current Limitation on	Yes	358	44.1%	-
Athletic Performance	No	308	51.3%	-
	Missing	32	4.6%	-

bursitis. To calculate the overall prevalence of each type of injury, an extensive list of self-developed filter questions pertaining to previous career injuries (differentiated according to location) was employed. If a filter question was answered with a "yes," athletes were then asked how often they had been "laid off" for at least 1 week due to the injury. Athletes' answers were separated according to type of injury (traumatic/overuse): results were summed to obtain a total score.

Analysis

Descriptive statistics and group differences. Descriptive statistics are herein based on mean, standard deviation, and range values. To determine group differences in SOC, between the elite athlete population and an age-appropriate, representative comparison group, drawn from German-speaking countries [22], one-sample t-tests were calculated for both males and females. The confidence interval was set at 95%, and alpha at 0.05. Moreover, effect sizes were calculated using Cohen's *d*.

Correlation calculations. Correlations between SOC, subjective health, incidence of subjective symptoms, and the necessity of an injury-induced lay-off from sport were assessed, where only correlation coefficients with a significance of $p<.001$ were considered relevant, in light of the large sample.

Classification tree analysis. Classification tree analysis is considered a promising research tool for identification of at-risk populations in public health research and outreach [29]. However, this method is not yet commonly used in public health or sports science. Classification tree analysis allows for exploratory identification of contrast groups, based on potential factors influencing the development of SOC. Compared to other multivariate methods, classification tree analyses have the following three main advantages [30–32]: the ability to separate a population into subgroups whose members share common characteristics; simultaneous treatment of interactions among independent variables; and high flexibility, conferred by handling a variety of variable types simultaneously (continuous, ordinal, or nominal) and not requiring the stringent theoretical and distributional assumptions of more traditional methods (such as cluster analysis, discriminant analysis, and regression models).

One commonly used classification tree technique is the so-called Chi-Squared Automatic Interaction Detector (CHAID), which was originally utilized as a data mining technique in the field of marketing, in order to segment large samples into homogenous subgroups. Owing to the successful implementation of data mining techniques in business-related contexts, these techniques have increasingly been used to analyze patterns in health care and rehabilitation contexts [32], clinical and surgical settings [33], and epidemiology [30]. Given the complex nature of the development of SOC, with potential interactions between several different independent variables, classification tree analysis employing the exhaustive CHAID algorithm is an appropriate way to identify and characterize contrast groups in larger samples. It is important to note that, in addition to exhaustive CHAID, there are several varieties of decision tree method. These methods, including CHAID, Quick, Unbiased, Efficient Statistical Trees (QUEST) and Classification and Regression Trees (C&RT), refer to various algorithms which differentially affect the way in which the tree is "grown" [29]. A recent study modeling landslide hazard via decision trees demonstrated that the exhaustive CHAID algorithm had the highest degree of classification accuracy [34].

Table 2. Classification Tree Analysis: Description of Dependent and Independent Variables.

Target Variable	Type	Description
Sense of Coherence	Interval	SOC-L9; Scale from 9 to 63. Higher values represent a stronger sense of coherence.
Independent Variables	**Type**	**Description**
Sociodemographic Characteristics		
Sex	Nominal	Male, Female
Age	Ratio	Age at time of the survey
Education	Nominal	University Entrance Degree (*Abitur*), Secondary School Degree (*Mittlere Reife*), Secondary Modern School Degree (*Hauptschulabschluss*), No School Degree (Student), Other School Degree
Family Status	Nominal	Single, Married
Vocational Training	Nominal	School Student, University Student, Apprenticeship, Completed Apprenticeship/University Degree, No Completed Apprenticeship/University Degree
Elite Sport-Specific Sociodemographic Characteristics		
Type of Sport	Nominal	Handball (Team Sport), Track and Field (Individual Sport)
Professional Athlete	Nominal	Full-time employment in elite sport (yes/no)
Performance Level	Ordinal	Level 1: A-/B-Squad (T&F) and National/Junior National/Premier League Team (HB), Level 2: C- & D/C-Squad (T&F) & Second Division League (HB)
Career Length in Elite Sports	Ratio	Performance-oriented participation in sport in years
Training Length	Ratio	Average length of training per week in hours
Competition Frequency	Ratio	Total number of completed competitions in the previous season
Traumatic & Overuse Injuries in the Athletes' Career as Sports-Specific Critical Life Events		
Training and Competition Lay-offs >1 Week due to traumatic injuries	Ratio	Total number of necessary training and competition lay-offs lasting longer than 1 week in the athletes' career to date due to traumatic injuries (e.g. tears, breaks, sprains, open wounds).
Training and Competition Lay-offs >1 Week due to overuse injuries	Ratio	Total number of necessary training and competition lay-offs lasting longer than 1 week due to overuse injuries (physical complaints because of too much or improper biomechanical stress, e.g. enthesitis, tendonitis, or bursitis).

The present classification tree analysis was performed via SPSS for Windows (SPSS, Ver. 19.0, Chicago, IL., USA) using the method of exhaustive CHAID. Exhaustive CHAID uses a systematic algorithm to detect the strongest association between the target variable and independent variables. At each step, the independent variable with the strongest interaction with the dependent variable is chosen. The categories of each independent variable are merged if they are not significantly different with respect to the dependent variable. Exhaustive CHAID is a modification of the CHAID algorithm that examines all possible splits for each dependent variable, thereby effecting greater precision [35,36]. The starting point of the analysis is the so-called "root node" at the top of a tree model, which contains the whole data set of the target variable. If a node splits to form part of a new level, it is referred to as a "parent node." Nodes splitting even further from the parent node are termed "child nodes." Each node at the end of a branch is labeled a "terminal node." Terminal nodes represent the identified contrast groups. Nodes are represented by boxes including the mean value, standard deviation, absolute numbers, and percentage of the sample contained therein. Above each node, the name of the most significant predictor variable, the p-value, chi-squared value, and degrees of freedom are illustrated.

The SOC-L9 score was employed as the target variable, with possible outcomes ranging between 9 and 63. The 11 predictor variables included in the analyses are displayed in Table 2. For continuous dependent variables, data are automatically divided into approximate deciles and used as ordinal variables in the analysis [36]. The following parameters were chosen in order to "grow" the tree: a maximum tree depth of 3, a minimum parent node size of 100, a minimum child node size of 40, and a significance threshold of 0.05 for splitting. Because the dependent variable (SOC) is neither nominal nor ordinal, the overall misclassification risk in the tree cannot be calculated using the correctly classified individuals. The misclassification risk was therefore given by calculating the proportion of variance explained through the model using the risk estimators and the total variance of the root node [36].

Results

SOC of Elite Athletes in Relation to the General Population and Subjective Health

As can be seen in Table 3, elite athletes' mean SOC scores are slightly lower than are those of the general population group (aged 17 to 40). With alpha set at 0.05, the one-sample t-test reveals that mean differences (female: 1.86; male: 0.97) are statistically significant (female: $t = -3.95$ (282), $p < 0.001$ and male: $t = -2.83$ (409), $p = 0.005$). The 95% confidence interval indicated that the populations' mean difference is likely to fall within −2.79 and −0.93 for females and −1.65 and −0.3 for males. However, the differences have little practical relevance considering the effect sizes (female: Cohen's $d = 0.24$ and male: Cohen's $d = 0.13$).

To test the correlation between SOC and subjective health, which has been previously documented in many populations, correlations between SOC scores and global assessment of current health, incidence of subjective complaints, and necessity of an acute injury lay-off were calculated. The correlation coefficients displayed in Table 4, for the elite athlete population, confirm the expected correlations between SOC and general health perception, as well as subjective health complaints. However, the correlation coefficients have low values.

Contrast Groups with Varying SOC-Scores: Predictors Using Classification Tree Analysis

On the basis of the most significant factors, which split the data set, the tree model depicted in Figure 1 was constructed. The tree model demonstrates that the SOC value is predicted by four interacting factors from three different levels. The variable with the strongest influence on SOC is the number of lay-offs due to a severe overuse injury (level 1). Age has the second strongest influence (level 2). In the 19 to 25 years age group, gender is the next best predictor (level 3), and in the age group of athletes older than 25, SOC score is significantly influenced by vocational status (level 3). All the other variables, for example the type of sport participated in or level of school education, have no significant influence on SOC. The proportion of variance explained by the classification tree model is 9.12%, which dictates that there are additional influencing variables that were not included in our study.

The tree model indicates that the age of athletes is only a significant factor when athletes have experienced two or more overuse injury lay-offs. Gender and vocational status are significant influencing factors on SOC only in specific age groups. For example, a gender difference in the 19 to 25 year-olds was only observable among those athletes who had already experienced multiple injury hiatuses owing to overuse injuries. Regarding the terminal nodes, six different contrast groups with specific SOC scores and characteristics were identified (Table 5).

(1) The group with the highest SOC score, of 51.65, consists of athletes who experienced at least two severe overuse injury lay-offs during their career, who are older than 25, and who have already completed their apprenticeship/degree. In total, 11.7% of the study subjects belong to this group (node 8).

(2) The largest identified group has the second highest mean SOC score, of 49.97. This group is characterized by athletes who have never, or only on one occasion, experienced a severe overuse injury lay-off. 48.7% of the study subjects belong to this group (node 1).

(3) The third-highest SOC score (48.07) occurred for those athletes who have experienced at least two 1-week lay-offs due to overuse injuries, and who are under 19 years of age. 12.9% of the study subjects belong to this group (node 3).

(4) Another group consisted of male athletes aged between 19 and 25 years who had an overuse injury-related lay-off at least twice. The mean SOC for this group was the third lowest at 47.59, and where this group size comprised 11.60% of the total respondents (node 6).

(5) The group with the second-lowest SOC scores comprised athletes who have had at least two overuse injury lay-offs during their career, are older than 26 years, and have not completed an apprenticeship or tertiary degree. 6.3% of the respondents belong to this group, with a mean SOC score of 46.96 (node 9).

(6) The lowest mean SOC score, by some distance (of 43.08), was seen in the group characterized by female athletes aged between 19 and 25 years, who have experienced two or more severe overuse injury hiatuses during their career. 8.7% of the total respondents belong to this group (node 7).

Comparison of the contrast group mean SOC scores with the total mean SOC scores for the athlete population (cf. Table 3) indicates that only nodes 8 and 1 have above-average SOC scores. The mean for nodes 6, 9, and 7 are all less than the total sample mean, and are less than the mean for the female athletes alone.

Table 3. Sense of Coherence in Comparison to Population Representative Norm Values.

Athletes SOC-L9	**N**	**M**	**SD**		**Median**
Total Sample[1]	698	48.85	7.41		50
Female	283	47.82	7.93		49
Male	410	49.52	6.96		51
German Norm Sample SOC-L9 (Hannöver et al., 2004)	**N**	**M**	**SD**		**Median**
Age Group 17–40: Female	1022	49.68	7.88	(p = 0.000)*	51
Age Group 17–40: Male	1012	50.49	7.77	(p = 0.005)*	51

[1]This study's sample of athletes has an average age of 22.85. 88.1% of the athletes surveyed are aged between 17 and 40. In the German general population sample SOC-L9 (cf. Hannöver et al. 2004), only gender-specific values exist for the age group 17–40.
*Significant at $p<0.05$. One-sample t-test calculated for both genders and for both general population samples. Confidence interval 95%.

Discussion

From a salutogenetic perspective, successfully coping with stressors is highly relevant for both elite athletes' health and their performance in sports. It is evident that SOC plays a fundamental role in this regard. The main purpose of the study was identification of contrast groups with high and low SOC scores, using the promising method of classification tree analysis, based on a large population of Germany's elite handball and track and field athletes. Analyzing elite athletes contributes to our understanding of how extreme physical and psychological demands in a highly competitive social context affect an individual's SOC. Accordingly, athletes' SOC scores were additionally compared with SOC scores in the general population. In order to examine the health-related relevance of an individual's SOC to coping with physical and psychological stressors in elite sports, the correlation between SOC and subjective health was also analyzed.

SOC of Elite Athletes in Relation to the General Population and Subjective Health

Our analysis demonstrates that the SOC of elite athletes is slightly lower than that of the general population. Although these differences are significant, they should not be over-interpreted due to the small effect sizes and large study population. Nevertheless, this finding is surprising considering that good physical and mental health is a key factor for achieving high performance levels in sports, and also that a high SOC is normally associated with above-average health. It can therefore be argued that elite athletes do not have better preconditions for good health than do the general population. Furthermore, the athlete population exhibits a similar SOC to clinical populations, in which patients with psychological challenges score lower than do random samples [2]. The generally lower SOC scores observed in elite athletes may be explained by the instability of their athletic careers, engendered by constant pressure to perform in combination with a permanent risk of injury. Sports injuries, which are accompanied by a decrease in athletic performance, can lead to a perceived lack of control over life and challenge athletes' overall identity. Additionally, the need to permanently exist on the boundary between overload and optimal performance can lead to a discrepancy between stress and individual resilience.

Our findings differ from those of other studies of college athletes, who had higher SOC values than did college non-athletes [13,14]. This could be explained by the greater career length and number of stressors that manifest at an elite level, compared to average college athletes. Health problems, particularly due to overuse, often pose huge career risks to the future career development of elite-level athletes. Furthermore, athletes have to cope with demanding environments (e.g. sponsors, journalists, and officials) and many different stressors (e.g. competing for positions in national teams, contract negotiations, and attaining a professional education for life after their sporting career finishes).

Our findings confirm that SOC and subjective health also correlate in elite athletes. As in other cross sectional studies with different populations across several countries, a strong SOC positively correlates with better global subjective health and negatively correlates with subjective health complaints [2,7,37]. A stronger SOC also negatively correlates with subjective performance limitations due to injury and illness. This could be interpreted as further evidence that SOC is a general health-related source of resistance [2].

Contrast Groups with Varying SOC Scores

To our knowledge, classification tree analysis has not been applied to SOC research thus far. As our results show, this method is useful for identifying subpopulations at risk for developing future biopsychosocial health problems. Although our study population should to be regarded as very specialized, we identified contrast

Table 4. Correlation Between Sense of Coherence and Indicators of Subjective Health.

Scale	**Sense of Coherence SOC-L9**
Global subjective health	0.281*
Subjective complaints (Score)	−0.384*
Current competition lay-off due to injury or illness	−0.072
Current limitation to athletic performance ability due to injury/illness	−0.135*

*The correlation is significant at the level of 0.01 (2-sided).

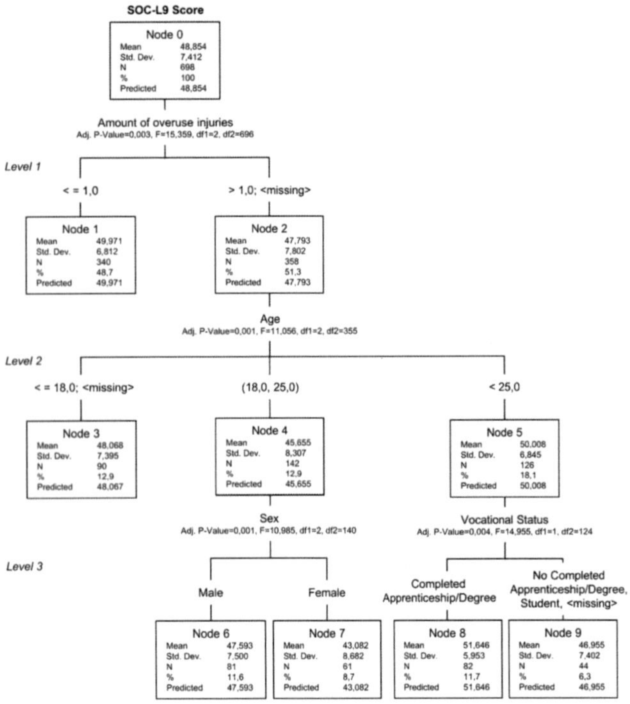

Figure 1. Classification Tree of Predictors Associated with SOC.

groups with higher and lower than average SOC scores. According to our results, classification tree analysis can help us better understand the simultaneous interaction of different factors which influence SOC. Several interacting factors determined the group to which an athlete belonged; in addition to overuse injuries, age, gender, and whether athletes had completed their vocational training or educational degree were also factors. This is in line with previous research demonstrating that SOC relates to age and gender [7], the appearance of severe health problems [15,16] and professional career events [11]. Nevertheless, as the identification of contrast groups demonstrates, these factors only play a role in certain instances. When compared to previous studies, this provides new insight into the interplay which exists between several factors when predicting SOC.

A direct link exists between SOC and previous overuse injury experiences in the group with the second highest overall score. This could be because these athletes have had very few overuse injuries. Here, we see neither large deviations from the German general population, for men or women, nor differences in the influence of age, gender, or apprenticeship status. That overuse injury lay-off experiences have an influence on SOC is consistent with salutogenetic theory: an initial, already well-established SOC is further stabilized if no incidents occur that endanger the functionality of general resistance resources [3]. The successful management of tension engendered by the demands of the elite sports system, without experiencing stress and developing overuse injuries, indirectly stabilizes SOC through the consolidation of generalized resistance resources. In this regard, the social support system plays an important role. Both training control systems designed to minimize overloads, and experienced team doctors who detect and successfully treat early symptoms of overuse, can contribute to the development and maintenance of a strong SOC.

Our results further demonstrate that experiencing multiple overuse injury lay-offs is associated with a decrease in SOC. However, this only pertains to certain constellations of age, gender, and educational degree status. Among athletes who have experienced multiple overuse injury lay-offs during their career, those aged 18 and below had a greater SOC than 19–25-year-old athletes. This may be owing to the cumulative impact of overuse injuries over the course of an athlete's entire career: if an injury

Table 5. Classification Tree Analyses: Gains Chart.

Knot	Description	N	Size	SOC-L9 Mean (SD)
8	Two or more severe overuse injury lay-offs, 26 years or above, completed apprenticeship/university degree	82	11.7%	51.65 (5.95)
1	Less than one severe overuse injury lay-off	340	48.7%	49.97 (6.81)
3	Two or more severe overuse injury lay-offs, 18 years or below	90	12.9%	48.07 (7.39)
6	Two or more severe overuse injury lay-offs, 19–25 years, male	81	11.6%	47.59 (7.50)
9	Two or more severe overuse injury lay-offs, 26 years or above, no completed apprenticeship/university degree	44	6.3%	46.96 (7.40)
7	Two or more severe overuse injury lay-offs, 19–25 years, female	61	8.7%	43.08 (8.68)

occurs during an elite athlete's prime (typically their mid-20s), the impact is more significant than if it occurs during the earlier stages of their career. Moreover, adolescents are more focused on the "here and now," which dictates that the possible consequences of overuse injuries have probably not yet been fully realized. Furthermore, given the fact that many athletes under 18 still attend school, the biographical fixation on elite sports is probably not yet as strong as it is for adult athletes.

Female athletes aged between 19 and 25 who have experienced overuse injuries are a high-risk group for low SOC scores and indeed had the lowest SOC scores in this study. In this age group, crises and career insecurities, along with overuse injuries, are felt most acutely by female athletes. In contrast to the large study of Nilsson et al. [7] who employed more common statistical methods, and where males had a stronger SOC than females, we identified gender differences only in one age group. The significantly lower SOC in females, in contrast to men in the same age group, may be because, in this age group, women's SOC scores are particularly vulnerable to overuse injuries. This corresponds with the fact that a downturn in the health of women has a stronger effect on SOC than it does for men [7]. Moreover, and in relation to the influence of life events, gender-specific differences are reported, which vary according to the type of life event [16].

Our findings also support the theoretical assumption that successfully coping with stressors leads to an increase in SOC under certain conditions. In our study, athletes aged 26 years and above, and who have completed an apprenticeship, exhibit the highest SOC scores, despite having experienced two or more overuse injuries. These athletes were obviously able to both successfully cope with overuse injuries and to successfully manage non-athletic career challenges.

In the case of professional insecurity owing to an incomplete education, older athletes who have already experienced overuse injuries have distinctly lower SOC scores, even compared to the general population. For older athletes who have not completed their education, life appears less meaningful, less comprehensible, and less manageable. Accordingly, this group is expected to have more difficulties in maintaining health than athletes with a completed education.

Antonovsky's assumption that SOC automatically increases with age does not hold true for our elite athlete population [1]. Nevertheless, the findings confirm Antonovsky's assumption that SOC develops until approximately the age of 30 and further that it can be influenced by critical life events. However, against the background of our findings it has to be assumed that in elite sports age only influences SOC development indirectly. This is in line with research demonstrating that a high SOC, rather than greater age, seems to effect stable development of the SOC [9]. Given the important influence of overuse injuries, and the role of vocational status, it can also be stated that SOC is less stable than was assumed by Antonovsky. Our data concords with a longitudinal study that reports a general lack of stability in SOC [38].

Of particular interest are the factors in the classification tree analysis that have no significant influence on SOC strength. The type of sport engaged in plays no role in our analysis, perhaps because the general principles and basic structures of the elite sports system are applicable to all athletes. For example, a set of regulations, defined competition calendar, and structured training units apply to all types of sports. In addition, career length; performance level; extent of training; frequency of competition; and professional, educational, and family status have no influence on SOC. A comparison with athletes from lower-level leagues or without squad status might lead to different results, however. Interestingly, crisis events such as frequent traumatic injuries, play no, or only a minor role, in contrast to overuse injuries. This may be due to a selection effect, however, as it can be assumed that only athletes who were able to achieve their previous level of performance after a traumatic injury participated in the study. Athletes whose traumatic injuries led to an inability to continue to engage in their sport, or resulted in a severe limitation of their ability to participate in elite sports, are unlikely to be in the sample because they ended their career prematurely. From an athletes' point of view, this could also be the result of improved knowledge and management of traumatic injuries, in terms of diagnostics, treatment strategies, and rehabilitation procedures, in comparison to overuse injuries [39]. The overall results therefore suggest that, in particular, the occurrence of overuse injuries should be considered as a critical life event for athletes because they have a profound effect on SOC strength.

Limitations and Directions for Future Research

The study underlines the fact that identifying mutually exclusive groups, by summarizing and segmenting large datasets using exhaustive CHAID, is useful in SOC research. Nevertheless, some limitations must also be considered. As the intention of the exhaustive CHAID procedure is to identify distinct population subgroups, it does not allow for the estimation of the net effects of a single independent variable on the dependent variable, while accounting for other factors, as is the case with common regression techniques [29]. Therefore, it is not possible to predict increases or decreases in SOC, for example, in relation to the number of overuse injuries experienced. Nevertheless, and in contrast to more conventional methods of regression analysis, it is possible to model multilevel interactions and to simultaneously include more independent variables, for a more complex model that is still relatively easy to interpret [30,32]. Due to its exploratory character, it is necessary that the present study be replicated with other samples of elite athletes in order to corroborate the predictive capacity of the model.

Another limitation of our study concerns the sample, which only consists of elite athletes drawn from two sporting disciplines. This may limit the representativeness of our results for all elite athletes. However, and at least for the sports in question, the study achieved representativeness by contacting all of the elite athletes who were active in these sports.

Regarding the interpretation of the SOC scores observed, another general problem emerged: it is not yet clear at which point SOC loses its protective effect on health and the development of severe health problems begins [2]. This complicates the interpretation of the identified groups with regard to their risk of developing future health problems. A further limitation of our study concerns its cross-sectional design, which does not allow for conclusions about causal relations to be drawn. The long-term stability of SOC in elite sports can therefore not be evaluated with the present study, nor can the question of the extent to which overuse injuries may be connected to a low initial SOC. This study also has the typical limitations characteristic of survey studies, which rely on self-report variables. Particularly in terms of assessment of the extensive medical history of injury events via questionnaire, it can be assumed that not all events will be remembered and that incomplete answers may be provided. This may be especially pertinent for questions pertaining to critical life events, where a bias can be expected leading to underestimation of the importance of these events [40].

For future research, it is recommended that longitudinal studies, examining the influence of different factors on SOC throughout an entire athletic career, be conducted. By doing so, interrelations between SOC, other general resistance resources, and health outcomes may be analyzed in detail, along with the dynamics of possible changes in athletes' SOC. Here, the impact of sports-specific critical life events, such as injuries or a career coming to an end, should be analyzed more thoroughly. In particular, time elapsed subsequent to retirement appears potentially impactful on changes in SOC. The role of SOC in successfully overcoming sports and chronic overuse injuries is also of particular interest. Overuse injuries should be measured using more recently developed and elaborate methods [41], as should the relationship between SOC, health status, and ability to perform. It is conceivable that ability to perform in training and competition is the decisive factor determining whether athletes view their lives as meaningful, comprehensible, and manageable. Follow-up studies might focus on extreme cases of highly resilient athletes, such as elite athletes with greatly above average SOC scores, who are successfully pursuing dual careers. Analysis of highly resilient athletes appears particularly promising for ascertaining what exactly confers such fortitude. Analyzing highly gifted elite athletes could therefore contribute to the general understanding of how people manage extreme stress and pressure in order to perform and remain healthy. In this context, qualitative methods employing athletes' biographies should be applied along with quantitative methods.

Conclusion and Recommendation

Salutogenetic research on health generally adds important knowledge to the prevalent pathogenetic point of view, with its focus on the risk factors for, and causes of, specific injuries or diseases. To our knowledge, this study is the first to analyze SOC as the principal concept of salutogenetic research in an elite athlete population, and the first to use classification tree analyses to this end. Classification tree analysis should be emphasized in SOC research, because it allows for identification of sub-populations at risk for a low SOC and the attendant risk of developing future health problems. Moreover, identification of contrast groups with high and low SOC scores supports the development of health promotion programs that are more directly targeted at specific groups. Based on our study, a particular risk group for a low SOC comprises female athletes aged between 19 and 25 years who have already experienced several enforced absences due to overuse injuries. For this group specific, tailored interventions, such as general stress management courses or educational programs concerned with coping and prevention strategies are required. Furthermore, highly individualized and controlled training frameworks aimed at avoidance of systematic overload experiences should be provided. Tailored interventions are also needed for athletes older than 26 years who have had two or more overuse injury lay-offs, and who have not completed an apprenticeship or university degree. This group could be supported through individual career counseling, optional apprenticeships for post-career purposes, and more effective synchronization of educational and sportive schedules.

The present study's results have further implications for relevant stakeholders. Sports organizations, such as federations and clubs, should generally facilitate athletes to complete a dual-career, through combining education with high performance sport. They should also provide team doctors, physiotherapists and sports psychologists who have expertise in attending to overuse injuries. Injury rehabilitation processes should be highly person-centered and systematically employed to educate athletes with regard to preventive health, such that occurrence of an injury might lead to even greater resilience and SOC. Coaches could further contribute to the development of constitutional and psychosocial resistance resources by strengthening athletes' general athletic abilities and buffering the extreme social pressure situations which occur in sports. Concerning reduction of risk of chronic or recurring injuries, coaches should in particular try to temper the social expectations that lead to training and competing despite the presence of acute health problems. Albeit that initial studies demonstrate the positive effects of salutogenetic concepts on inpatient psychosomatic treatments and health outcomes [42], the effects of different salutogenetic health promotion interventions in elite sports have not yet been evaluated. It is hoped that future research will address this knowledge gap.

Author Contributions

Conceived and designed the experiments: JM AT. Performed the experiments: JM AT. Analyzed the data: JM AT. Contributed reagents/materials/analysis tools: JM AT. Wrote the paper: JM AT.

References

1. Antonovsky A (1987) Unraveling the Mysteries of Health: How People Manage Stress and Stay Well. San Francisco: Jossey Bass. 238 p.
2. Eriksson M, Lindstrom B (2006) Antonovsky's sense of coherence scale and the relation with health: a systematic review. Journal of Epidemiology & Community Health 60: 376–381.
3. Antonovsky A (1996) The salutogenic model as a theory to guide health promotion. Health Promotion International 11: 11–18.
4. Kalimo R, Pahkin K, Mutanen P, Toppinen-Tanner S (2003) Staying well or burning out at work: work characteristics and personal resources as long-term predictors. Work & Stress 17: 109–122.
5. Kouvonen AM, Väänänen A, Vahtera J, Heponiemi T, Koskinen A, et al. (2010) Sense of coherence and psychiatric morbidity: a 19-year register-based prospective study. Journal of Epidemiology & Community Health 64: 255–261.
6. Fallby J, Hassmén P, Kenttä G, Durand-Bush N (2006) Relationship between locus of control, sense of coherence, and mental skills in swedish elite athletes. International Journal of Sport and Exercise Psychology 4: 111–120.
7. Nilsson KW, Leppert J, Simonsson B, Starrin B (2010) Sense of coherence and psychological well-being: improvement with age. Journal of Epidemiology & Community Health 64: 347–352.
8. Singer S, Brähler E (2007) Die Sense of Coherence Scale. Testhandbuch zur deutschen Version (The Sense of Coherence Scale. Test manual for the German version). Göttingen: Vandenhoeck & Ruprecht. 103 p.
9. Feldt T, Leskinen E, Koskenvuo M, Suominen S, Vahtera J, et al. (2011) Development of sense of coherence in adulthood: a person-centered approach. The population-based HeSSup cohort study. Quality of Life Research 20: 69–79.
10. Krantz G, Ostergren PO (2004) Does it make sense in a coherent way? Determinants of sense of coherence in swedish women 40 to 50 years of age. International Journal of Behavioral Medicine 11: 18–26.
11. Liukkonen V, Virtanen P, Vahtera J, Suominen S, Sillanmaki L, et al. (2010) Employment trajectories and changes in sense of coherence. Eur J Public Health 20: 293–298.
12. Nixon HL (1992) A Social Network Analysis of Influences on Athletes to Play with Pain and Injury. Journal of Sport & Social Issues 16: 127–135.
13. Endo S, Kanou H, Oishi K (2012) Sports Activities and Sense of Coherence (SOC) among College Students. International Journal of Sport and Health Science 10: 1–11.
14. Skirka N (2000) The relationship of hardiness, sense of coherence, sports participation, and gender to perceived stress and psychological symptoms among college students. Journal of Sports Medicine and Physical Fitness 40: 63–70.
15. Caap-Ahlgreen M, Dehlin O (2004) Sense of coherence is a sensitive measure for changes in subjects with Parkinson's disease during 1 year. Scandinavian Journal of Caring Sciences 18: 154–159.
16. Volanen SM, Suominen S, Lahelma E, Koskenvuo M, Silventoinen K (2007) Negative life events and stability of sense of coherence: A five-year follow-up study of Finish women and men. Scandinavian Journal of Psychology 48: 433–441.
17. Petrie G (1993) Injury from the athlete's point of view. In: Heil J, editor. Psychology of Sport Injury. Champaign: Human Kinetics. pp. 17–24.
18. Leddy MH, Lambert MJ, Ogles BM (1994) Psychological consequences of athletic injury among high-level competitors. Research Quarterly for Exercise and Sport 65: 347–354.

19. McAllister DR, Motamedi AR, Hame SL, Shapiro MS, Dorey FJ (2001) Quality of Life Assessment in Elite Collegiate Athletes. The American Journal of Sports Medicine 29: 806–810.
20. Eriksson M, Lindstrom B (2005) Validity of Antonovsky's sense of coherence scale: a systematic review. Journal of Epidemiology & Community Health 59: 460–466.
21. Kenne Sarenmalm E, Browall M, Persson LO, Fall-Dickson J, Gaston-Johansson F (2013) Relationship of sense of coherence to stressful events, coping strategies, health status, and quality of life in women with breast cancer. Psycho-Oncology 22: 20–27.
22. Hannöver W, Michael A, Meyer C, Rumpf HJ, Hapke U, et al. (2004) Die Sense of Coherence Scale von Antonovsky und das Vorliegen einer psychiatrischen Diagnose: Ergänzungen zu den deutschen Normwerten aus einer bevölkerungsrepräsentativen Stichprobe (Antonovsky's Sence of Coherence Scale and presentation of a psychiatric diagnosis. Complements to German norms from a representative population survey). Psychotherapie Psychosomatik medizinische Psychologie 54: 179–186.
23. Schumacher J, Wilz G, Gunzelmann T, Brähler E (2000) Die Sense of Coherence Scale von Antonovsky – Testatische Überprüfung in einer repräsentativen Bevölkerungsstichprobe und Konstruktion einer Kurzskala. (The Antonovsky Sense of Coherence Scale. Test statistical evaluation of a representative population sample and construction of a brief scale). Psychotherapie Psychosomatik medizinische Psychologie 50: 472–482.
24. Ravens-Sieber U, Torsheim T, Hetland J, Vollebergh W, Cavallo F, et al. (2009) Subjective health, symptom load and quality of life of children and adolescents in Europe. International Journal of Public Health 54: 151–159.
25. Idler EL, Benyamini Y (1997) Self-related health and mortality: a review of twenty-seven community studies. Journal of Health and Social Behavior 38: 21–37.
26. Ravens-Sieber U, Erhart M, Torsheim T, Hetland J, Freeman J, et al. (2008) An international scoring system for self-reported health complaints in adolescents. European Journal of Public Health 18: 294–299.
27. Haugland S, Wold B, Stevenson J, Aaroe LE, Woynarowska B (2001) Subjective health complaints in adolescence. European Journal of Public Health 11: 4–10.
28. Bird S, Black N, Newton P (1998) Sport injuries. Causes, diagnosis, treatment and prevention. Musselburgh: Scotprint Ltd. 320 p.
29. Lemon SC, Roy J, Clark MA, Friedmann PD, Rakowski W (2003) Classification and regression tree analysis in publich health: methodological review and comparison with logistic regression. The society of behavioral medicine 26: 172–181.
30. Camp N, Slattery M (2002) Classification tree analysis: a statistical tool to investigate risk factor interactions with an example for colon cancer (United States). Cancer Causes Control 13: 813–823.
31. Chen JA, Shih CC, Lin PF, Chen JJ, Lin KC (2012) Collaborative evaluation and management of students' health-related physical fitness: applications of cluster analysis and the classification tree. International Journal of Public Health 24: 153–159.
32. Chan F, Cheing G, Chan JYC, Rosenthal DA, Chronister J (2006) Predicting employment outcomes of rehabilitation clients with orthopedic disabilities: A CHAID analysis. Disability and Rehabilitation 28: 257–270.
33. Zangger P, Detsky A (2000) Computer-assisted decision analysis in orthopedics: resurfacing the patella in total knee arthroplasty as an example. Journal of Arthroplasty 15: 283–288.
34. Alkhasawneh MS, Ngah UK, Tay LT, Isa NAM, Al-Batah MS (2014) Modeling and Testing Landslide Hazard Using Decision Tree. Journal of Applied Mathematics.
35. Bühl A (2012) SPSS 20: Einführung in die moderne Datenanalyse (SPSS 20: Introduction to modern data analysis). München: Pearson. 1056 p.
36. SPSS Inc. (n.d.) PASW Desicion Trees 18. Chicago: SPSS Inc. pp. 106.
37. Simonsson B, Nilsson KW, Leppert J, Diwan VK (2008) Psychosomatic complaints and sense of coherence among adolescents in a county in Sweden: a cross sectional school survey. BioPsychoSocial Medicine 2.
38. Smith PM, Breslin CF, Beaton DE (2003) Questioning the stability of sense of coherence. The impact of socio-economic status and working conditions in the Canadian population. Social Psychiatry and Psychiatric Epidemiology 38: 475–484.
39. Mayer J (2010) Verletzungsmanagement im Spitzensport (Injury management in elite sports). Hamburg: Czwalina.
40. Wolff AC, Ratner PA (1999) Stress, Social Support, and Sense of Coherence. Western Journal of Nursing Research 21: 182–197.
41. Clarsen B, Myklebust G, Bahr R (2013) Developement and validation of a new method for the registration of overuse injuries in sports injury epidemiology: the Oslo Sports Trauma Research Center (OSTRC) Overuse Injury Questionnaire. British Journal of Sports Medicine 47: 495–502.
42. Hinterberger T, Auer J, Schmidt S, Loew T (2013) Evaluation of a salutogenetic concept for inpatient psychosomatic treatment. Evid Based Complement Alternat Med 2013: 735731.

4

The Effects of Chronic Exercise on Attentional Networks

Laura Pérez[1,2], Concepción Padilla[1,2], Fabrice B. R. Parmentier[1,2], Pilar Andrés[1,2]*

1 Neuropsychology and Cognition Group, Research Institute on Health Sciences and Department of Psychology of the University of the Balearic Islands, Palma, Spain,
2 Neuropsychology and Cognition Group, Instituto de Investigación Sanitaria de Palma, Palma, Spain

Abstract

The aim of this study was to test the hypothesis that chronic physical exercise improves attentional control in young healthy participants. To do this, we compared the performance of physically active and passive participants in the Attentional Network Task, which allows for the assessment of the executive, orienting and alerting networks. The results showed a selective positive effect of exercise on the executive network. These results extend the evidence gathered in children, older adults and certain clinical populations suggesting that exercise can also improve attentional control in healthy young adults.

Editor: Giuseppe di Pellegrino, University of Bologna, Italy

Funding: This work was supported by a grant from the Spanish Ministry of Science and Innovation (PSI2010-21609-C02-02). Concepción Padilla was granted with a FPI predoctoral studentship from the Spanish Ministry of Economy and Competitivity (BES-2011-043565). Fabrice Parmentier is an External Research Associate and an Adjunct Senior Lecturer at the School of Psychology, University of Western Australia, and was supported by a Ramón y Cajal Fellowship (RYC-2007-00701) from the Ministry of Economy and Competitiveness and Plan E from the Spanish Ministry of Science and Innovation, and the Campus of International Excellence Program from the Ministry of Education, Culture and Sports. The funders had no role in study design, data collection and analysis, decision to publish, or preparation of the manuscript.

Competing Interests: The authors have declared that no competing interests exist.

* Email: pilar.andres@uib.es

Introduction

Attention, widely defined as the faculty of focusing the mind on a task or object, is at the heart of the cognitive system and regulates other cognitive functions such as memory and language. Its breakdown has major consequences in everyday life functioning and has been linked to a number of outcomes such as academic failure, human error in numerous work environments (e.g., air traffic control settings), or cognitive deficits in a range of pathological conditions (e.g., attention deficit disorder, dementia).

Attention has been categorised in different ways through history [1,2]. In one of the most prominent theories of attention, Posner and Petersen [3,4] suggested that the human attentional system can be subdivided into three functionally and anatomically independent networks. In this model, the alerting network allows maintenance of a vigilant and alert state, the orienting network is responsible for the movement of attention through space to attend to sensory events, and the executive network allows for the monitoring and conflict resolution in situations of interference. A neuroimaging analysis revealed very little overlap between the neuroanatomical systems associated with alerting, orienting, and conflict resolution [5]. Alerting showed strong thalamic involvement and the activation of anterior and posterior cortical sites, whereas orienting activated parietal sites and frontal eye fields, and response conflict resolution implicated the anterior cingulated cortex and the dorsolateral prefrontal cortex.

The Attention Network Test (ANT [6]) is a quick and simple computerised task developed to measure independently the efficiency of the three attention networks (see Figure 1). This task has contributed to the better characterisation of developmental trends [7] and certain attention disorders such as attention deficit disorder [8] or Borderline personality disorder [9].

Given the importance of attentional functions in efficient everyday cognitive functioning, it is of both theoretical and practical interest not to limit research to conditions in which attentional functions are impaired but also to investigate whether these can improve in certain circumstances. Interestingly, physical exercise has recently been suggested as a factor enhancing attention (see [10], for a review). However, its positive effect on attention has thus far only been reported in old age or certain clinical populations [10,11]. In contrast, there has been very little research investigating such benefits in young healthy adults [11,12]. One of the few studies that have investigated the role of exercise on the attentional networks in young adults was carried out by Huertas, Zahonero, Sanabria and Lupiáñez [13]. These authors considered the impact of acute (as opposed to chronic o regular) exercise on attentional functions. A group of highly experienced cyclists performed the Attention Network Test [14] at rest and during aerobic exercise (a bout of intense cycling). Results indicated that acute exercise reduced the alerting effect. However, it did not modulate the functioning of either the orienting and executive attentional networks. The authors concluded that acute aerobic exercise modulates the functioning of phasic alertness by increasing the general state of tonic vigilance.

In contrast to acute exercise, chronic exercise refers to exercise routines carried out for a number of years. Because chronic exercise is more likely to induce more permanent changes in the brain and to create cognitive reserve [15–17], one may hypothesize that it should benefit executive functions. To our knowledge, only a few behavioural studies have focused on the topic of chronic exercise and executive functions in young healthy adults and these have been inconclusive, as described below.

Several studies failed to find any effect of chronic exercise on executive functions. For example, using a flanker task, Hillman,

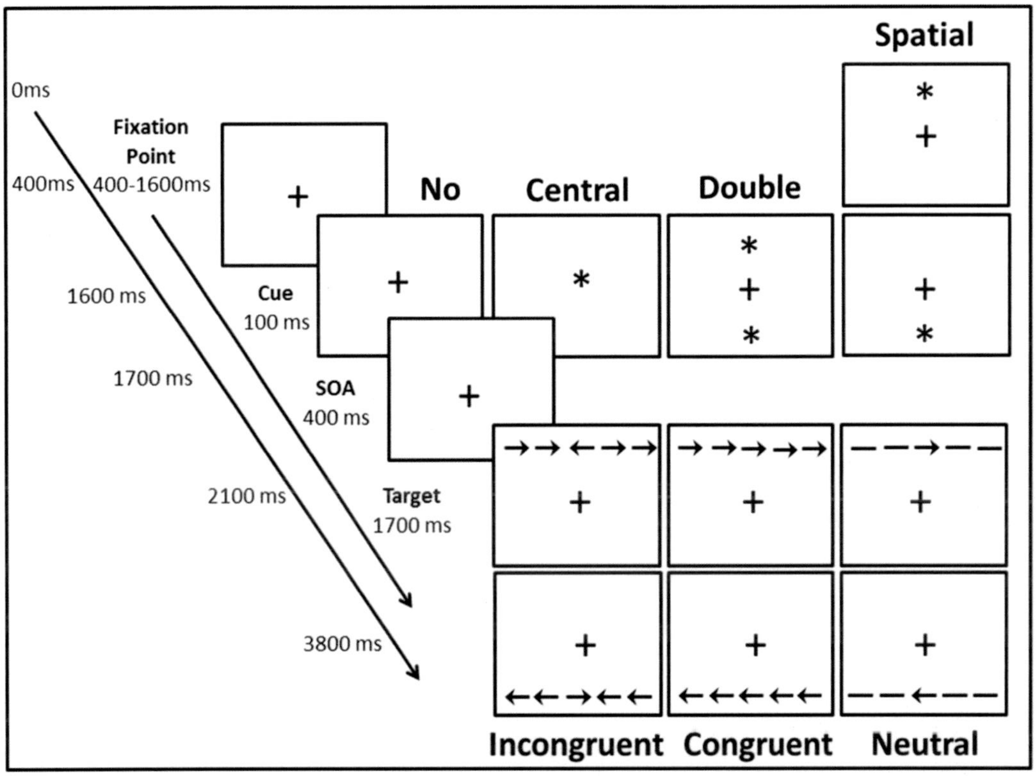

Figure 1. Attention Network Test (ANT). ANT design and procedure with the four warning cue conditions (no cue, central cue, double cue and spatial cue) and the three flanker conditions (Incongruent, Neutral and Congruent). The timing of events is presented on the left.

Kramer, Belopolsky and Smith [18] found that increased levels of chronic exercise reduced the negative impact of incongruent stimuli in older but not in the younger participants. The absence of effect of exercise on executive functioning in young adults was replicated by Hillman et al. [18] using the same task, and similar conclusions were reported by Boucard et al. [19] in several executive tasks (e.g. Stroop, task switching, random generation, Simon).

Potential reasons why some studies failed to measure an impact of exercise in young adults may stem from the complexity and multi-determined nature of executive functions, as well as the difficulty to operationalize their measurement [20]. It has also been argued that it is difficult to observe such effects in young people because their cognitive functioning is at its peak [21]. Furthermore, and perhaps most critically, tasks designed to measure executive functions typically exhibit low reliability [22] and sufficient statistical power is required to detect group effects, particularly when working with healthy participants instead of clinical samples. Finally, the selection criteria must be established in a way that passive and active participants present with clearly different cardiovascular fitness levels.

In contrast to the studies described above, more recent studies found a link between chronic exercise and executive control. Padilla et al. [12] compared physically active participants (practiced exercise regularly for the last 10 years) to sedentary participants in a stop signal task [23]. This task measures motor inhibitory control, which is strongly related to the functioning of the frontal lobe [24]. The results revealed better inhibitory abilities in active participants, but only when the task was more executively demanding (*strategic* version). These results were recently replicated by Padilla, Pérez and Andrés [25], who also reported that the better inhibitory capacity observed in active participants was, at least in part, related to their larger working memory capacity.

The aim of the present study was to look for the first time at the effects of chronic exercise on attentional networks in healthy young adults using the Attention Network Task (ANT, [6]). More precisely, we investigated whether the improvement previously observed in executive inhibition [26] in active participants [12] could be extended to the type of inhibition required by the conflict resolution involved in a flanker task. Indeed, it has been shown that perceptual and motor inhibition (the first type being involved in the flanker task and the second in the stop signal task) can be dissociated [27]. It is therefore possible that the effects of exercise on inhibition may also be dissociated. Furthermore, we wondered whether the possible effect of exercise would be selective to executive functioning or would also affect the orienting and alerting networks.

Methods

Participants

Participants were recruited through advertisements placed across the campus and the sports center at the University of the Balearic Islands, as well as in other sports facilities throughout Mallorca. They were categorised as physically active or inactive by completing a questionnaire that estimated their level of physical activity (Physical Activity Questionnaire, Appendix S1). Those who had performed cardiovascular activity for a period greater than 10 years for an average of 6 or more hours per week distributed across at least three days a week, and continued doing sport activity at the time of testing were considered active. The inclusion criterion for the passive participants was that they should not have practiced exercise more than 2 hours per week for the last 4 years. The type of exercise that had been practiced could not be cardiovascular (e.g. yoga, stretching, etc. were allowed). History of neurological disease, psychiatric illness, head injury, stroke, substance abuse (excluding nicotine), learning disabilities, or any difficulty that could interfere with behavioral and cognitive testing were criteria for exclusion. None of the participants were aware of the purpose of the experiment before testing and all reported normal or corrected-to-normal vision. A sample of 64 healthy young adults took part in the study (*M* age = 24.12, *SD* = 3.26, range 20–30 years, 38 females). Thirty one of them were considered physically active (*M* age = 24.29, *SD* = 3.48, 11 females) and thirty three were physically inactive (*M* age = 23.97, *SD* = 3.07, 27 females). The assessment was carried out in a single 60 minutes session. Written informed consent was obtained from each participant prior to the study and they received a payment or course credit for taking part in the experiment. The experiment was performed in accordance with the ethical standards of the 1964 Declaration of Helsinki and received ethical approval by the Ethics committee from the University of the Balearic Islands.

Cardiorespiratory capacity

In addition to the questionnaire used to assess the history of physical activity, the Rockport 1-mile Fitness Walking test [28] was used to assess cardiorespiratory fitness. This sub maximum cardiovascular stress test provides an accurate estimate of the maximum level of oxygen consumption (VO_2max), with a correlation coefficient of.88 between VO_2max estimated based on performances during the test and a direct measure of VO_2max during an increment test on a treadmill [28–30]. Higher values of VO_2max are considered to reflect higher aerobic capacity, since it means greater oxygen consumption. The Rockport Test was performed in the University Campus surroundings.

The Vocabulary Subtest of Wechsler Adult Intelligence Scale-III (WAIS-III, [31]) was administered to assess the degree of verbal ability.

The Attention Network Test (ANT) was downloaded from https://www.sacklerinstitute.org/cornell/assays_and_tools/. It was programmed using E-Prime software [32] and running on a PC computer. Stimuli were presented on a19 inches color screen with a resolution of 1024×768 pixels. Participants were seated approximately 50 cm away from the screen. Their responses were collected via two keyboard keys. Stimuli consisted of a row of five visually presented black lines, with arrowheads pointing leftward or rightward, against a white background where the target was a leftward or rightward arrowhead at the center. The stimuli (one central arrow plus four flankers) fell into three different conditions: the target was flanked on either side by two arrows in the same direction (congruent condition), or of the opposite direction (incongruent condition), or by two dashed lines (neutral condition). The participant's task was to identify the direction of the central arrow as fast and as accurately as possible, by pressing the left button of the mouse with the index finger of the right hand if that arrow pointed left, or the right button of the mouse with the middle finger of the right hand if that arrow pointed right. The target stimulus remained on the screen until the participant responded or until 1700 ms had elapsed. Each trial began with a fixation point (a plus sign) presented for 400–1600 ms in the center of the screen (see Figure 1). Next, one of the four possible cues was presented. Cues consisted of the appearance of an asterisk for 100 ms that was presented 400 ms before the presentation of the target. The four cue-related conditions were as follows: (1) no cue: the fixation point was not replaced by an asterisk (cue) so that participants were not warned that the target was about to appear; (2) central: the fixation point was substituted by an asterisk; (3) double cue: two asterisks were presented above and below the fixation central point; and (4) a spatial cue: an asterisk above or below the fixation point informed the subject that the target was coming and also, where it would be presented (up or down). In total, each trial lasted 3800 ms.

Results

Demographic variables and Rockport Test scores are presented in Table 1. The two groups did not differ significantly in terms of age [t (62) = 0.391, p = .697], years of formal education [t (62) = 0.275, p = .784] or vocabulary levels [t (62) = 0.516, p = .608]. However, the Rockport Test revealed better scores in the active compared to the passive participants [t (62) = 4.989, $p<$ .001], revealing, as predicted, a higher cardiovascular fitness (estimated VO_2max; see Appendix S2) in active participants.

Mean RTs in the ANT task (see Table 2) were analysed with a 2 (Group: Actives - Passives)×3 (Flanker Type: Congruent - Incongruent - Neutral)×4 (Cue Type: No Cue - Cue Central - Double Cue - Spatial Cue) ANOVA for repeated measures. The results revealed significant main effects of flanker [F (1, 360) = 485.980, MSE = 1091853.6, $p<.001$, $\eta p^2 = .887$] and cue [F (2, 648) = 322.969, MSE = 235349.007, $p<.001$, $\eta p^2 = .839$]. There was also a significant interaction between flanker and cue [F (4, 971) = 15.223, MSE = 7077.968, $p<.001$, $\eta p^2 = .197$] and between group and flanker [F (1, 360) = 4.325, MSE = 9716.247, p = .029, $\eta p^2 = .065$]. There was however no significant effect of group [F (1, 62) = 2.498, MSE = 113317.592, p = .119, $\eta p^2 = .039$] or group×flanker×cue interaction [F (4, 971) = .656, MSE = 304.947, p = .656, $\eta p^2 = .010$]. The group×cue interaction approached significance [F (2, 648) = 2.653, MSE = 1933.338, p = .058, $\eta p^2 = .041$].

Error rates (see Table 3) were analyzed with a 2 (Group: Actives - Passives)×3 (Flanker Type: Congruent- Incongruent– Neutral)×4 (Cue Type: No Cue - Cue Central - Double Cue - Spatial Cue) ANOVA for repeated measures. The results revealed significant effects of flanker [F (1, 132) = 46.821, MSE = .111, $p<$ .001, $\eta p^2 = .430$], cue [F (2, 546) = 4.730, MSE = .004, $p<.01$, $\eta p^2 = .071$] and a significant flanker×cue interaction [F (3, 648) = 6.298, MSE = .007, $p<.001$, $\eta p^2 = .092$]. There was no significant effect of group [F (1, 62) = 1.594, MSE = .006, p = .212, $\eta p^2 = .025$], group×flanker [F (1, 132) = 2.042, MSE = .005, p = .156, $\eta p^2 = .032$], group×cue interaction [F (2, 546) = 1.656, MSE = .001, p = .186, $\eta p^2 = .026$] or group×flanker×cue interaction [F (3, 648) = 2.126, MSE = .002, p = .085, $\eta p^2 = .033$].

Repeated ANOVA measures were also carried out for each component of the attentional system (alerting, orientating and executive networks, see Figure 2). To establish whether our results might be mediated by gender, this factor was introduced as an independent variable. This factor was introduced following a request from a reviewer. The alerting effect was calculated as the difference between the no cue and double cue conditions. The orienting effect was calculated as the difference between the central and spatial cue conditions. The conflict effect was calculated as the difference between the congruent and incongruent conditions.

Alerting

The 2 (group)×2 (condition)×2 (gender) ANOVA on RTs revealed a significant effect of condition [F (1, 60) = 169.079, MSE = 41918.808, $p<.001$, $\eta p^2 = .738$], indicating that, as expected, the double cue acted as a warning and speeded RTs relative to the no cue condition. There was also a significant effect of gender

Table 1. Demographic Variables (Means and SDs) and Rockport Test, * $p<.01$.

	Active	Passive
n	31	33
Age	24.3 (3.48)	24 (3.07)
Education	13.3 (2.34)	13.4 (2.42)
Vocabulary	44.7 (6.99)	43.8 (6.36)
Rockport (VO_2max)	57 (7.33)*	47 (8.34)

[F (1, 60) = 4.099, MSE = 30642.041, p = .047, ηp^2 = .064] revealing that male participants were generally (no cue and double cue conditions) faster than female participants. However, neither the main effect of group [F (1, 60) = .235, MSE = 1759.751, p = .629, ηp^2 = .004], nor the condition×group [F (1, 60) = .034, MSE = 8.358, p = .855, ηp^2 = .001], condition×gender [F (1, 60) = 1.636, MSE = 405.616, p = .206, ηp^2 = .027], gender×group [F (1, 60) = .034, MSE = 253.407, p = .855, ηp^2 = .001] or condition×gender×group [F (1, 60) = .756, MSE = 187.344, p = .388, ηp^2 = .012] interactions were significant.

Error scores for the alerting network revealed no main effect of condition [F (1, 60) = .009, MSE = 2680000, p = .923, ηp^2<.001] or group [F (1, 60) = .705, MSE<0.001, p = .404, ηp^2 = .012]. The condition×group interaction was not significant [F (1, 60) = 1.995, MSE = .001, p = .163, ηp^2 = .032]. The main effect of gender was not significant, and it did not interact significantly with condition, group or condition×group (all ps>.23).

Orienting

The 2 (group)×2 (condition)×2 (gender) ANOVA showed significantly shorter RTs in the spatial cue condition [F (1, 60) = 282.923, MSE = 53232.221, p<.001, ηp^2 = .825). The effect of group was not significant [F (1, 60) = .069, MSE = 520.083, p = .793, ηp^2 = .001], but the condition×group interaction was [F (1, 60) = 4.583, MSE = 862.324, p = .036, ηp^2 = .071]. The analysis of this interaction with Newman Keuls post hocs revealed that, while both groups showed significant orienting effects (both ps< .001), the orienting effect was greater for the passive (M = 51.60; SD = 16.73) than for the active (M = 40.25; SD = 22.22) participants (p<.001). However, as visible in Figure 3, this interaction may have reflected the fact that smaller room for improvement was available to active participants as they produced faster responses than the passive participants in the central cue condition (p = .04). In order to examine orienting outside the potential limitation of a ceiling effect, we carried out two complementary analyses. First, we compared the orienting effect in the slowest active participants from the active group (n = 16; M = 49.3, SD = 20.15) and the fastest participants of the passive participants (n = 16; M = 47.8, SD = 17.73). This comparison was not statistically significant (t (30) = 0.22; p = 0.82), demonstrating that the two groups showed equivalent levels of orienting when eliminating the risk of a ceiling effect. Second, in order to reduce to a minimum the inter-subject variability, we also computed orienting using median RTs (instead of mean RTs) for all participants. Again, the orienting effect was equivalent in both groups (t (62) = 1.074, p = .287) (Note: for safety we also conducted all other analyses reported in this manuscript using median RTs and that the results were identical to those found using mean RTs). Overall, therefore, the data revealed no difference between active and passive participants in terms of orienting. The main effect of gender was not significant, and it did not interact significantly with condition, group or condition×group (all p>.58).

The orienting effect for errors was significant [F (1, 60) = 9.756, MSE = .002, p<.005, ηp^2 = .140], revealing that participants committed fewer errors in the spatial than in the central condition. However, neither the group [F (1, 60) = 1.851, MSE = .002, p = .179, ηp^2 = .030] nor the condition×group interaction were significant [F (1, 60) = .000, MSE<.001, p = .987, ηp^2 = .000]. The main effect of gender was not significant, and it did not interact with condition, group or condition×group (all p>.15).

Executive network

The 2 (group)×2 (condition)×2 (gender) ANOVA on RTs revealed a significant effect of condition [F (1, 60) = 501.287, MSE = 198746.078, p<.001, ηp^2 = .893], with faster RTs for congruent than for incongruent trials. There was no significant main effect of group [F (1, 60) = 186, MSE = 1591.82, p = .668, ηp^2 = .003]. The condition×group interaction was significant, however [F (1, 60) = 5.290, MSE = 2097.284, p = .025, ηp^2 = .081], revealing a smaller difference between incongruent and congruent trials for active participants (see Figure 4), while both groups did show significant conflict effects (both ps<.001). Also, the difference between active and passive participants was significant for the incongruent (p = .04) but not for the congruent condition (p = .35).

Table 2. Mean RTs (ms) and standard deviations in the different Flanker and Cue conditions.

	Congruent		Incongruent		Neutral	
	Active	**Passive**	**Active**	**Passive**	**Active**	**Passive**
No	512 (59)	536 (76)	582 (75)	623 (81)	509 (60)	532 (63)
Central	473 (66)	492 (66)	568 (76)	614 (82)	465 (58)	485 (58)
Double	464 (58)	481 (64)	556 (75)	589 (74)	459 (49)	479 (59)
Spatial	439 (53)	451 (63)	509 (72)	534 (75)	435 (47)	448 (62)

Table 3. Mean proportions of errors and standard deviations in the different Flanker and Cue conditions.

	Congruent		Incongruent		Neutral	
	Active	**Passive**	**Active**	**Passive**	**Active**	**Passive**
No	.0013 (.01)	.0085 (.02)	.0308 (.04)	.0257 (.04)	.0143 (.02)	.0085 (.02)
Central	.0026 (.01)	.0024 (.01)	.0409 (.05)	.0631 (.07)	.0052 (.01)	.0107 (.03)
Double	.0066 (.02)	.0012 (.01)	.0196 (.03)	.0442 (.05)	.0066 (.02)	.0134 (.03)
Spatial	.0026 (.01)	.0036 (.01)	.0159 (.03)	.0259 (.05)	.0066 (.02)	.0112 (.03)

The main effect of gender was not significant, and it did not interact significantly with condition, group or condition×group (all *p*s>.14).

The conflict effect for errors was significant [$F\,(1, 60) = 41.869$, $MSE = .024$, $p < .001$, $\eta p^2 = .411$], revealing that participants committed more errors in incongruent than in congruent trials. However, neither the effect of group [$F\ (1,\ 60) = 2.337$, $MSE = .002$, $p = .132$, $\eta p^2 = .037$] nor the condition×group interaction were significant [$F\ (1,\ 60) = 3.518$, $MSE = .005$, $p = .07$, $\eta p^2 = .055$]. The main effect of gender was not significant, and it did not interact significantly with condition, group or condition×group (all $p > .42$).

Discussion

The aim of this study was to examine the extent to which exercise can modulate attentional functions in healthy young active adults using the ANT task [6]. We were interested in extending the results from Padilla et al. [12,25] showing that active participants presented with better inhibition in the strategic version of the stop signal task to tasks measuring alerting, orienting and executive control.

Our study is original in a number of respects. First, we concentrated on the effect of chronic exercise as opposed to acute exercise as examined in past studies [13,33,34]. This is important because chronic exercise is more likely to induce brain cognitive reserve [17] and is accompanied by more permanent physiological changes in the cortical areas supporting executive functions. We used a strict selection criterion for the recruitment of participants, with active participants having practiced aerobic exercise for at least 10 years with a frequency of at least 6 hours a week distributed in at least 3 days a week over and above the minimum dose recommended by the American Centre for Disease Control & Prevention [35] and stricter than the criteria adopted in previous studies. Furthermore, we corroborated the significant difference in fitness levels between our two groups of participants by using an objective estimation of cardiovascular capacity (Rockport test, [28]). Such measure is useful to compare our results with those of Boucard et al. [19], who also looked at the effect of aerobic exercise on executive control in young and older healthy adults. These authors found no beneficial effect of exercise in young adults, but a close examination of the VO_2max levels measured in their active and passive participants revealed that their groups were not as distinct as ours. Indeed, Boucard et al. [19] reported values of 48.4 and 44.2 (mL/min/kg) for the active and passive groups, while our values were 57 and 47 respectively. Not only the difference in VO_2max in our study was over twice that reported by Boucard et al. [19], but the value they reported for their active

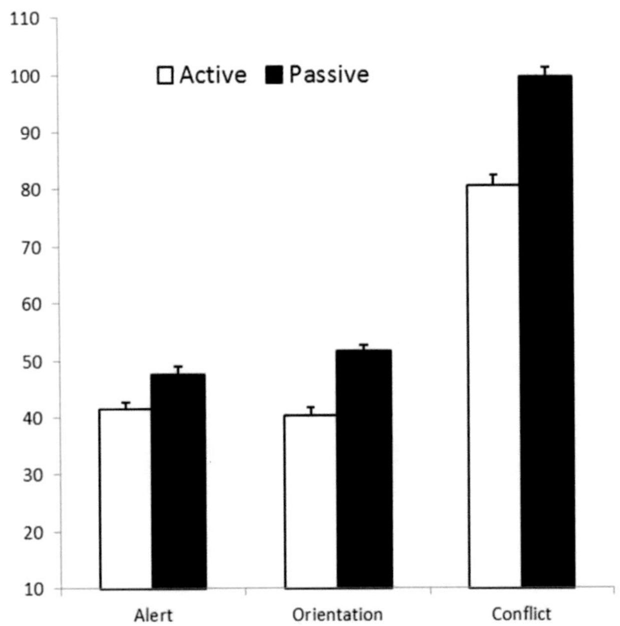

Figure 2. Attentional Network Effects. Difference scores in active and passive participants for RTs. The error bars represent one standard error of the mean.

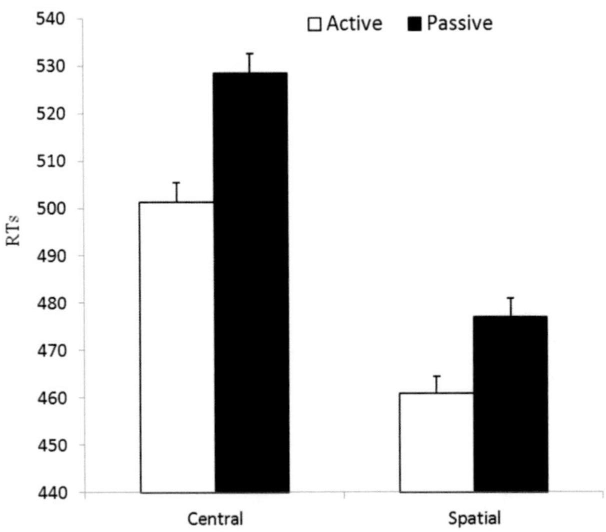

Figure 3. Orienting. Mean RTs in the central and spatial conditions associated to the orienting network, for active and passive participants. The error bars represent one standard error of the mean.

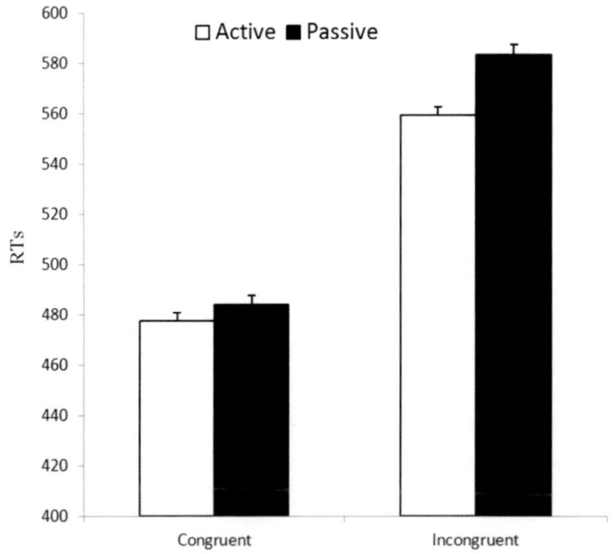

Figure 4. Conflict. Mean RT in the congruent and incongruent conditions associated to the executive network, for active and passive participants. The error bars represent one standard error of the mean.

group is virtually that we observed in our passive participants, suggesting that Boucard et al.'s [19] active participants may not have sufficiently active for differences in executive control to be detected.

The finding of a smaller conflict effect in our active participants fits with Padilla et al.'s [12,25] results showing a selective positive effect of aerobic exercise on inhibitory performance in the stop signal task and, more generally, points to a consistent and reliable effect of chronic exercise in executive functioning in young participants. The fact that previous studies have not found such an effect in young participants may be due to factors such as the type of exercise (acute instead of chronic in Huertas et al.'s study [13]) or the insufficient amount of exercise practice by active participants [19].

In contrast with the results of the executive function measure, active and passive participants revealed equivalent levels of alerting and orienting. While response times for the measurement of orienting might have been affected by a ceiling effect, our complementary analyses (restricting the analysis to the fastest passive and the slowest active participants, and using medians instead of means) suggest that it did not affect our findings. Nevertheless, and as suggested by one reviewer, a replication of our study involving a more sensitive version of the ANT task giving rise to longer RTs (for example by emphasizing the need for accuracy) would help to ascertain further this issue.

The observation of a selective effect of chronic exercise on executive control network fits well with previous reports showing such selective effects in aging and neuroimaging studies [36–38]. This conclusion is bolstered by the fact that differences in executive functioning in the ANT are statistically more difficult to measure than differences in alerting or orienting. Indeed, in a study investigating the psychometrical properties of the ANT task, Macleod, Lawrence, McConnell, Eskes, Klein and Shore [39] showed that in the context of a between-subjects design, the executive control network affords the least statistical power compared to alerting and orienting, despite providing the highest reliability. According to Macleod et al. [39] the failure to find such differences in the alerting and orienting networks in the present study supports genuine selective between groups differences in the executive network only.

Our sample included more active men than active women and more passive women than passive men. We think this did not affect our results for two key reasons, however. First, it is important to note that research has shown that females are more efficient in their use of executive and inhibitory control to reduce the magnitude of response conflict [40]. Therefore, if anything, this would go against the direction of the effect we found for the executive network (since we had more women in the passive group). Second, and most importantly, our analyses showed no interaction of gender with group or condition for any of the three networks, suggesting that gender did not modulate the effect of physical activity in our study.

One factor that has been strongly linked with conflict resolution is inhibition. It is suggested that inhibitory mechanisms are put in place to restrain irrelevant information and unwanted stimulus-driven response tendencies. Age-related differences in conflict resolution and inhibitory mechanisms have been, in turn, linked to neurophysiological maturation of the frontal cortex [41,42]. Interestingly, cumulating evidence is revealing that the effects of chronic exercise are more easily found in inhibitory functions, particularly if the inhibitory task requires executive control. For example, Boucard et al. [19] revealed that higher levels of physical activity were specifically associated with better inhibition functioning in older adults. Taken together, these elements suggest that the inhibition function may be particularly sensitive to factors like age and/or physical activity level because of its elemental and ubiquitous properties in the executive function construct [19,43].

Previous results have revealed that older adults with higher cardiovascular fitness exhibit significant volumetric and functional improvements particularly in prefrontal areas and anterior cingulate cortex [44–46]. Interestingly, these brain structures underpin inhibition and executive processes (see [47,48]). For example, Weinstein et al. [24] recently revealed that gray matter volume of the right inferior frontal gyrus mediates the relationship between higher cardiovascular fitness and inhibition (Stroop interference) in older adults. Hence, the functional network specialized in the function of inhibition could be preferentially boosted by the cardiovascular effects of physical activity, which is consistent with the pattern of results observed in our studies and revealing a relatively specific effect of chronic exercise on tasks requiring inhibitory control.

Several mediating factors have been proposed to explain the nature of the relationship between aerobic exercise and cognition. First, physiological factors, such as increased levels of neurotrophins (e.g., brain-derived neurotrophic factors -BDNF-, insulin-like growth factor type 1 -IGF-1- and vascular endothelial growth factor -VEGF-) have been observed in humans after exercising. Second, evidence also indicates that angiogenesis and neurogenesis are upregulated with exercise (see [49,50] for reviews). In addition, it has been shown that chronic exercise is associated with an increase in prefrontal volume [44,45], the main area involved in executive control. In this vein, Weinstein et al. [24] revealed that higher fitness levels were associated with better performance on executive tasks and greater gray matter volumes in the dorsolateral prefrontal cortex (DLPFC). They also showed that prefrontal volume mediates the relationship between cardiovascular fitness and executive functions. Finally, greater neural connectivity has been observed in physically active compared to physically passive participants [51,52].

There may also be other non-physiological factors mediating the benefits of exercise on cognition. For example, it has been found that people's beliefs regarding their capacity to accomplish a goal plays an important role in their performance. Self-efficacy, a primary variable in social cognitive theory, concerns the individual's beliefs in his or her capabilities to successfully execute necessary courses of action to satisfy situational demands, and is the most salient variable affecting well-being and psychological health [53]. Links between self-efficacy and cognitive performance and between physical activity and self-efficacy have also been reported [54]. It is therefore possible that the physically active people included in the present study present with better self-efficacy levels than passive participants, and that this might have had an effect on tasks requiring relatively high levels of controlled attentional resources.

The study of the interaction between these factors remains in its infancy, however, and the degree and direction of these interactions needs further investigation. One important direction for future work would be to examine the effects of exercise within a multi-factorial framework in which these various factors can be measured or manipulated.

From an applied perspective, our results should encourage public authorities to consider exercise as a protective or cognitive reserve factor [17]. Our data reveal that young adults practising regular exercise exhibit better executive control, a cognitive function playing a central role in many aspects of everyday life cognitive functioning. By demonstrating that physical exercise does not only enhance executive control in old age but also in young adults, our study suggests that exercise may have positive effects on learning and academic achievement and be of interest to health policy makers.

Acknowledgments

We are grateful to the volunteers who participated in our study and to Pablo Rodríguez, Pedro Reus and Antonio Martin for their help with data collection. This study was part of Laura Pérez's doctoral thesis.

Author Contributions

Conceived and designed the experiments: PA LP CP. Performed the experiments: LP CP. Analyzed the data: LP CP FP PA. Contributed reagents/materials/analysis tools: LP CP FP PA. Wrote the paper: LP PA.

References

1. LaBerge D (1995) Attentional Processing: The Brain's Art of Mindfulness. Cambridge, MA: Harvard University Press.
2. Parasuraman R, Davis DR (1984) *Varieties of Attention.* Orlando: Academic Press.
3. Posner MI, Petersen SE (1990) The attention system of the human brain. Annu Rev Neurosci 13: 25–42.
4. Petersen SE, Posner MI (2012) The attention system of the human brain: 20 years after. Annu Rev Neurosci 35: 73–89.
5. Fan J, McCandliss BD, Fossella J, Flombaum JI, Posner MI (2005) The activation of attentional networks. Neuroimage 26: 471–479.
6. Fan J, McCandliss BD, Sommer T, Raz A, Posner MI (2002) Testing the efficiency and independence of attentional networks. J CognNeurosci 14: 340–347.
7. Rueda MR, Fan J, McCandliss BD, Halparin JD, Gruber DB, et al. (2004) Development of attentional networks in childhood. Neuropsychologia 42: 1029–1040.
8. Johnson KA, Robertson IA, Barry E, Mulligan A, Dáibhis A, et al. (2008) J Child PsycholPsychiat 49: 1339–1347.
9. Posner MI, Rothbart MK, Vizueta N, Levy KN, Evans DE, et al. (2002) Attentional mechanisms of the borderline personality disorder. Proc Natl Acad Sci U S A 99: 16366–16370.
10. Hillman CH, Erickson KI, Kramer AF (2008) Be smart, exercise your heart: exercise effects on brain and cognition. Nat Rev Neurosci 9: 58–65.
11. Guiney H, Machado L (2013) Benefits of regular aerobic exercise for executive functioning in healthy populations. Psychon Bull Rev 20: 73–86.
12. Padilla C, Pérez L, Andrés P, Parmentier FBR (2013) Exercise improves cognitive control: Evidence from the Stop-Signal Task. Appl Cogn Psychol 27: 505–511.
13. Huertas F, Zahonero J, Sanabria D, Lupiáñez J (2011) Functioning of the attentional networks at rest vs. during acute bouts of aerobic exercise. J Sport ExercPsychol 33: 649–65.
14. Callejas A, Lupiañez J, Tudela P (2004) The three attentional networks: on their independence and interactions. Brain Cogn 54: 225–227.
15. Dishman RK, Berthoud HR, Boot FW, Cotman CW, Edgerton VR, et al. (2006) The neurobiology of exercise. Obes Res 14: 345–356.
16. Kempermann G (2008) The neurogenic reserve hypothesis: what is adult hippocampal neurogenesis good for? Trends Neurosci 31: 163–169.
17. Stern Y (2009) Cognitive reserve. Neuropsychologia 47: 2015–2028.
18. Hillman CH, Kramer AF, Belopolsky AV, Smith P (2006) A cross-sectional examination of age and physical activity on performance and event-related brain potentials in a task switching paradigm. Int J Psychophysiol 59: 30–39.
19. Boucard G, Albinet C, Bugaiska A, Bouquet C, Clarys D, et al. (2012) Impact of Physical Activity on Executive Functions in Aging: A Selective Effect on Inhibition Among Old Adults. J Sport Exerc Psychol 34: 808–827.
20. Burgess PW (1997) Theory and methodology in executive function research. In: Rabbitt P, editors. Methodology of Frontal and Executive Function. 79–108.
21. Bialystok E, Craik FIM, Luk G (2012) Bilingualism: Consequences for mind and brain. Trends Cogn Sci 16: 240–250.
22. Rabbitt P (1997) Methodologies and models in the study of executive function. In: Rabbitt P, editors. Methodology of Frontal and Executive Function. 1–38.
23. Verbruggen F, Logan GD, Stevens MA (2008) Windows executable software for the stop-signal paradigm. Behav Res Methods 40: 479–483.
24. Weinstein AM, Voss MW, Prakash RS, Chaddock L, Szabo A, et al. (2012) The association between aerobic fitness and executive function is mediated by prefrontal cortex volume. Brain Behav Immun 7: 811–819.
25. Padilla C, Pérez L, Andrés P (2014) Chronic exercise keeps working memory and inhibitory capacities fit. Front Behav Neurosci, 8: 49. doi:10.3389/fnbeh.2014.00049.
26. Andrés P, Guerrini C, Phillips L, Perfect T (2008) Differential effects of aging on executive and non executive inhibition. Dev Neuropsychol 33: 101–123.
27. Nassauer KW, Halperin JM (2003) Dissociation of perceptual and motor inhibition processes through the use of novel computerized conflict tasks. J Int Neuropsychol Soc 9: 25–30.
28. Kline GM, Porcari JP, Hintermeister R, Freedson PS, Ward A, et al. (1987) Estimation of VO_2max from a one-mile track walk, gender, age and body weight. Med Sci Sports Exerc 19: 253–259.
29. McAuley E, Szabo AN, Mailey EL, Erickson KI, Voss M, et al. (2011) Non-exercise estimated cardiorespiratory fitness: associations with brain structure, cognition, and memory complaints in older adults. Ment Health Phys Act 4: 5–11.
30. Weiglein L, Herrick J, Kirk S, Kirk E (2011) The 1-mile walk test is a valid predictor of VO_2 max and is a reliable alternative fitness test to the 1.5-mile run in U.S. Air Force males. Military Medicine 176: 669–673.
31. Wechsler D (1999) Wechsler adult intelligence scale-third edition - UK. London: The Psychological Corporation.
32. Schneider W, Eschman A, Zuccolotto A (2002) *E-Prime user's guide.* Pittsburgh, PA: Psychology Software Tools Inc.
33. Sibley BA, Etnier JL, Le Masurier GC (2006) Effects of an acute bout of exercise on cognitive aspects of Stroop performance. J Sport Exerc Psychol 28: 285–299.
34. Sibley BA, Beilock SL (2007) Exercise and working memory: an individual differences investigation. J Sport Exerc Psychol 29: 783–791.
35. Kuczmarski RJ, Ogden CL, Grummer-Strawn LM, Flegal KM, Guo SS, et al. (2000) CDC growth charts: United States. National Center for Health Statistics (NCHS) Advance Data 314: 1–27.
36. Colcombe SJ, Kramer A (2003) Fitness effects on the cognitive function of older adults. A meta-analytic study. Psychol Sci 14: 125–130.
37. Hall CD, Smith AL, Keele SW (2001) The impact of aerobic activity on cognitive function in older adults: A new synthesis based on the concept of executive control. Eur J Cogn Psychol 13: 279–300. doi:10.1080/09541440126012.
38. Prakash RS, Voss MW, Erickson KI, Lewis JM, Chaddock L, et al. (2011). Cardiorespiratory fitness and attentional control in the aging brain. Front Hum Neurosci 4: 229. doi:10.3389/fnhum.2010.00229.
39. MacLeod JW, Lawrence MA, McConnell MM, Eskes GA, Klein RM, et al. (2010) Appraising the ANT: Psychometric and theoretical considerations of the Attention Network Test. Neuropsychology 24: 637–651.
40. Yucell M, Fornito A, Youssef G, Dwyer D, Whittle S, et al. (2012). Inhibitory control in young adolescents: the role of sex, intelligence, and temperament. Neuropsychology 26: 347–356.

41. Bunge SA, Dudukovic NM, Thomanson ME, Vaidya C, Gabrieli JD (2002) Immature frontal lobe contributions to cognitive control in children: Evidence from fMRI. Neuron 33: 301–311.
42. Chao LL, Knight RT (1997) Prefrontal deficits in attention and inhibitory control with aging. Cereb Cortex 7: 63–69.
43. Miyake A, Friedman NP, Emerson MJ, Witzki AH, Howerter A, et al. (2000) The unity and diversity of executive functions and their contributions to complex "frontal lobe" tasks: A latent variable analysis. Cogn Psychol 41: 49–100.
44. Colcombe S, Kramer AF, Erickson KI, Scalf P, McAuley E, et al. (2004) Cardiovascular fitness, cortical plasticity, and aging. Proc Natl Acad Sci U S A 101: 3316–3321.
45. Colcombe Erickson KI, Raz N, Webb AG, Cohen NJ, et al. (2003) Aerobic fitness reduces brain tissue loss in aging humans. J Gerontol A Biol Med Sci 58: M176–M180. doi:10.1093/Gerona/58.2M176.
46. Voelcker-Rehage C, Godde B, Staudinger UM (2011) Cardiovascular and coordination training differentially improve cognitive performance and neural processing in older adults. Front Hum Neurosci, 5. doi:10.3389/fnhum.2011.00026.
47. Aron AR, Robbins TW, Poldrack RA (2004) Inhibition and the right inferior frontal cortex. Trends Cogn Sci 8: 170–177.
48. Braver TS, Barch DM, Gray JR, Molfese DL, Snyder A (2001) Anterior cingulated cortex and response conflict: effects of frequency, inhibition and errors. Cereb Cortex 11: 825–836.
49. Kramer AF, Erickson KI (2007) Capitalizing on cortical plasticity: influence of physical activity on cognition and brain function. Trends Cogn Sci 11: 342–348.
50. Zoeller R (2010) Exercise and cognitive function: can working out train the brain too? Am J Lifestyle Med 4: 397–409.
51. Voss MW, Erickson KI, Prakash RS, Chaddock LC, Kim JS, et al. (2013) Neurobiological markers of exercise-related brain plasticity in older adults. Brain Behav Immun 28: 90–99. doi:10.1016/j.bbi.2012.10.021.
52. Voss MW, Heo S, Prakash RS, Erickson KI, Alves H, et al. (2013) The influence of aerobic fitness on cerebral white matter integrity and cognitive function in older adults: results of a one-year exercise intervention. Hum Brain Mapp 34: 2972–85.
53. Bandura A (1991) Self-efficacy mechanism in physiological activation and health-promoting behaviour. In: J Madden, editors. Neurobiology of learning, emotion, and affect. New York: Raven Press. 229–269.
54. Netz Y, Wu MJ, Becker BJ, Tenenbaum G (2005) Physical Activity and Psychological Well-Being in Advanced Age: A Meta-Analysis of Intervention Studies. Psychol Aging 20: 272–284. doi:10.1037/0882-7974.20.2.272.

5

Chronic Aerobic Exercise Associated to Dietary Modification Improve Endothelial Function and eNOS Expression in High Fat Fed Hamsters

Beatriz C. S. Boa[1]*, Maria das Graças C. Souza[1], Richard D. Leite[1], Simone V. da Silva[2], Thereza Christina Barja-Fidalgo[2], Luiz Guilherme Kraemer-Aguiar[1,3], Eliete Bouskela[1]

1 Laboratory for Clinical and Experimental Research on Vascular Biology (BioVasc), Biomedical Center, State University of Rio de Janeiro - Rio de Janeiro, RJ – Brazil, **2** Department of Cell Biology, Institute of Biology Roberto Alcântara Gomes, Biomedical Center, State University of Rio de Janeiro - Rio de Janeiro, RJ – Brazil, **3** Department of Internal Medicine, Faculty of Medical Sciences, Biomedical Center, State University of Rio de Janeiro – Rio de Janeiro, RJ – Brazil

Abstract

Obesity is epidemic in the western world and central adipose tissue deposition points to increased cardiovascular morbidity and mortality, independently of any association between obesity and other cardiovascular risk factors. Physical exercise has been used as non-pharmacological treatment to significantly reverse/attenuate obesity comorbidities. In this study we have investigated effects of exercise and/or dietary modification on microcirculatory function, body composition, serum glucose, iNOS and eNOS expression on 120 male hamsters treated for 12 weeks with high fat chow (HF, n = 30) starting on the 21st day of birth. From week 12 to 20, animals were randomly separated in HF (no treatment change), return to standard chow (HFSC, n = 30), high fat chow associated to an aerobic exercise training program (AET) (HFEX, n = 30) and return to standard chow+AET (HFSCEX, n = 30). Microvascular reactivity in response to acetylcholine and sodium nitroprusside and macromolecular permeability increase induced by 30 minutes ischemia followed by reperfusion were assessed on the cheek pouch preparation. Total body fat and aorta eNOS and iNOS expression by immunoblotting assay were evaluated on the experimental day. Compared to HFSC and HFSCEX groups, HF and HFEX ones presented increased visceral fat [(mean±SEM) (HF)4.9±1.5 g and (HFEX)4.7±0.9 g vs. (HFSC)*3.0±0.7 g and (HFSCEX)*1.9±0.4 g/100 g BW]; impaired endothelial-dependent vasodilatation [Ach 10^{-8} M (HF)87.9±2.7%; (HFSC)*116.7±5.9%; (HFEX)*109.1±4.6%; (HFSCEX)*105±2.8%; Ach10^{-6} M (HF)95.3±3.1%; (HFSC)*126±6.2%; (HFEX)*122.5±2.8%; (HFSCEX)*118.1±4.3% and Ach10^{-4} M (HF)109.5±4.8%; (HFSC)*149.6±6.6%; (HFEX)*143.5±5.4% and (HFSCEX)*139.4±5.2%], macromolecular permeability increase after ischemia/reperfusion [(HF)40.5±4.2; (HFSC)*19.0±1.6; (HFEX)*18.6±2.1 and (HFSCEX)* 21.5±3.7 leaks/cm^2), decreased eNOS expression, increased leptin and glycaemic levels. Endothelial-independent microvascular reactivity was similar between groups, suggesting that only endothelial damage had occurred. Our results indicate that an aerobic routine and/or dietary modification may cause significant improvements to high fat fed animals, diminishing visceral depots, increasing eNOS expression and reducing microcirculatory dysfunction.

Editor: Erik Svensjo, Universidade Federal do Rio de Janeiro (UFRJ), Brazil

Funding: This study was supported by grants from the National Research Council (CNPq - 474116/2008-5) and the Research Supporting Agency of Rio de Janeiro State (FAPERJ - E-26/111.732/2011). Further information concerning those agencies are founded on the following URLs: CNPq: http://www.cnpq.br/web/guest/geral;jsessionid = 7C28AB306E0BE450036DAE00943FFEB0, FAPERJ: http://www.faperj.br/. The funders had no role in study design, data collection and analysis, decision to publish, or preparation of the manuscript.

Competing Interests: The authors have declared that no competing interests exist.

* Email: beatrizcsb@gmail.com

Introduction

Life style changes seem to mark contemporary men, from active to sedentary and from healthy alimentation to high fat/salt one. With that, now is clear that the adipose tissue represents much more than simply an energy storage site, being also a powerful endocrine organ with numberless functions. The Western profile of high fat feeding is directly related to adipocyte hypertrophy, hypoxia and, as consequence, its dysfunction comprising anatomic and functional disturbances due to prolonged positive caloric balance in genetic susceptible individuals [1]. Consequences of adipose tissue dysfunction involve systemic effects such as micro/macrovascular dysfunction, type 2 diabetes mellitus (T2DM), hypertension and cardiovascular diseases (CVD). In obesity, there is an increased production of free fatty acids, angiotensinogen, leptin, resistin and inflammatory mediators that might be involved in mechanisms of obesity-associated microvascular dysfunction [2]. In fact, visceral and truncal subcutaneous adipose tissues are associated to microvascular dysfunction even in lean subjects [3] and weight loss improves endothelial function and decreases inflammation in an obese population [4].

Endothelial dysfunction (ED), reduction of bioavailability of vasodilators, mainly NO, may also be characterized by a state of endothelial activation where pro-inflammatory, proliferative and pro-coagulant milieu predominates [5]. Therewith, ED is a clinical syndrome able to predict and also be associated to cardiovascular events [6]. Indeed, the immense endothelium surface area in the microcirculation compared to conductance vessels makes this region more vulnerable to effects of its dysfunction. Therefore, microvascular dysfunction emerges as an independent predictor of cardiovascular risk and systemic inflammation [7] and it has been associated to hypertension [8], presence of chest pain in absence of coronary artery disease [9] and classical cardiovascular risk markers [6]. The cheek pouch, an invagination of the oral mucosa that extends under the subcutaneous tissue down to the shoulder region, is an appropriate preparation to study microcirculatory function/dysfunction due to its clarity and stability.

Physical activity has gained visibility since it is seen as non-pharmacological treatment of excessive weight and adiposity as well as its co-morbidities, and far more accessible to several patient populations. The skeletal muscle constitutes approximately 40% of total body weight, responsible for 30% of energy expenditure and considered the most important determinant of peripheral vascular sensibility to insulin [10]. It is also an important place for uptake, storage and liberation of glucose [11]. Regular exercise practice reduces primary [12] and secondary [13] vascular events. Therewith, it is the best non-pharmacological treatment for the vasculature inasmuch it exerts several of its physiological improvements through modification of laminar shear stress, as a result increased eNOS expression (endothelium nitric oxide synthase), arterial stiffness and decreased oxygen reactive species (ROS) production [14–15]. These effects reflect a direct interaction between exercise's actions and the microcirculation.

Both exercise and dietary modifications culminate in changes of the energetic balance, which modify adiposity and improve metabolic parameters [15–17], but data in experimental literature concerning microcirculatory analysis when these two treatments are combined are scarce. In this study we have investigated effects of an aerobic exercise training (AET) associated or not to dietary modification on microcirculatory function, body composition, serum glucose, iNOS and eNOS expression on male hamsters to evaluate if these non-pharmacological treatments, namely exercise and diet, could attenuate/reverse the consequences of high fat feeding.

Experimental Methods

Experiments were performed on male Syrian golden hamsters (n = 120; *Mesocricetus auratus*, ANILAB, Paulínea, SP, Brazil), acclimatized at 20±1°C, with 12 hours cycles of day/night controlled by timer and light from 6:00AM to 18:00PM. On the 21th day after birth, hamsters started to be feeding with high fat (HF) chow [18] for twelve weeks. From the twelfth to the twentieth week, animals were randomly divided into four different groups: HF (20 weeks, fed with high fat chow), HF + Standard Chow (HFSC – from 12 to 20th week animals returned to standard chow), HF + Exercise (HFEX – similar to HF associated to an exercise routine in the last eight weeks) and HF+SC/Exercise (HFSCEX – similar to HFSC, associated to an exercise routine in the last eight weeks). Nutritional characteristics of used high fat chow may be seen on table 1, in detail. The experimental design and the aerobic exercise training protocol [19] can be seen on figure 1. Animals had unrestricted access to food and water.

On the day of experiment, the right femoral vein and the left femoral artery were cannulated (0.28 mm internal/0.61 mm outer diameters) for drug injection and mean arterial pressure (MAP) and heart rate (HR) measurements (Biopac, Santa Barbara, CA, USA, Spectramed pressure transducer). A tracheal tube was inserted to facilitate spontaneous breathing (room air). The cheek pouch was gently everted and mounted on an experimental chamber as previously described [20]. All preparations were superfused at a rate of 4.0 ml/min by a HEPES-supported HCO_3^--saline solution [composition in mM: NaCl 110.0, KCl 4.7, $CaCl_2$ 2.0, $MgSO_4$ 1.2, $NaHCO_3$ 18.0, N-2-hydroxyethylpiperazine-N′-2- ethanesulfonic acid (HEPES) 15.39 and HEPES Na^+-salt 14.61] bubbled with 5% CO_2–95% N_2, to maintain the superfusion solution with pH at 7.4 and the temperature at 36.5°C. Preparations were placed under an intravital microscope (Leica DMLFS, Wetzlar, Germany, magnification x600, NA 0.65) coupled to a closed-circuit TV system and allowed to rest for 30 min before measurements were taken. Images were recorded in sVHS and analyzed after the experiment.

Ethics Statement

The protocol was approved by the Ethical Committee of the State University of Rio de Janeiro (CEUA/061/2010). The investigation was strictly conducted according to the *Guide for Care and Use of Laboratory Animals* published by the US National Institute of Health (NIH Publication No. 85–23, revised in 1996). Animals were euthanized through cardiac puncture, under anesthesia, for blood analysis. All efforts were made to minimize their suffering.

All surgical procedures were performed under anesthesia induced by an intraperitoneal injection of 0.1–0.2 ml of sodium pentobarbital (Pentobarbital sodique, 60 mg/ml, Sanofi Santé Animale, Paris, France) and maintained with α-chloralose [100 mg/kg body weight (Sigma Chemicals, St. Louis MO, USA)] given. Throughout surgery and experiment, hamsters were placed on a heating pad, controlled by a rectal thermistor, in order to maintain their body temperature at 36.5°C (LTB 750 Thermostat System, Uppsala, Sweden).

Microvascular research model

The hamster cheek pouch is an appropriate preparation to study effects of dietary change associated to aerobic exercise. This preparation consists on an invagination of the oral mucosa under the subcutaneous tissue down to the shoulder region. Its blood supply comes mainly from the carotid arteries, although some blood is diverged to the retractor muscle, also part of the cheek pouch structure. The preparation remains stable for 5–6 h for arteriolar reactivity to acetylcholine (ACh) [21], for macromolecular permeability increase induced by bradykinin [22] and for spontaneous arteriolar vasomotion [20]. There are several advantages related to the use of this preparation: 1) ease and relatively non-traumatic access make it useful in studies requiring repeated observations of the same site; 2) highly vascularized with all classes of microcirculatory vessels visible within the microscopic field, allowing observation and comparison of various segments; 3) clarity and optical properties are good when compared to other densely vascularized tissues; 4) presence of skeletal muscle and cutaneous microcirculatory beds [21].

Microvascular reactivity and macromolecular permeability

Three 2nd to 3rd order arterioles were selected and studied in each preparation, taking into account its position, in order to return exactly to the same sites for consecutive evaluations after topical application of vasoactive drugs (e.g. presence of fat cells and bifurcations). As a precaution, a conversion ruler (mm to μm) was used to guarantee that recorded vessels encompassed 2nd to 3rd order and mean luminal diameter of 100 μm was considered as upper limit. Such choices were important to keep homogeneity of microvessels' response after topical application of vasoactive agents

Table 1. Nutritional composition and comparison between experimental chows.

	Standard Chow (%)	High Fat Chow (%)
Standard Chow[a]	100	60
Hydrogenated Vegetable Fat[b]	-	25
Condensed Milk[c]	-	15
Macronutrients		
Protein	23	12
Fat	6	50
Carbohydrates	71	38
Total Energy		
KJ/Kg	17.9	23

[a]Standard chow for rodents; Nuvital, Nuvilab - Colombro Paraná - Brazil;
[b]Shortening Primor: Gaspar, Santa Catarina - Brazil; c Condensed Milk Moça Nestlé, São Paulo – Brazil.
[c]Condensed Milk Moça Nestlé, São Paulo – Brazil.

(e.g. acetylcholine). Mean internal microvessel diameter was determined using an Image Shearing device (Vista Electronics, model 908, San Diego, CA, USA), at baseline and after topical application, 10 min each, of three concentrations of either acetylcholine [Ach 10^{-8}, Ach 10^{-6} and Ach 10^{-4} M (Sigma Chemicals, St. Louis, MO, USA)] or sodium nitroprusside [SNP 10^{-8}, SNP 10^{-6} and SNP 10^{-4} M (Sigma Chemicals, St. Louis, MO, USA)] in a cumulative dose-response curve.

Induction of ischemia/reperfusion-induced changes was made with an air inflatable tourniquet placed distally of the preparation

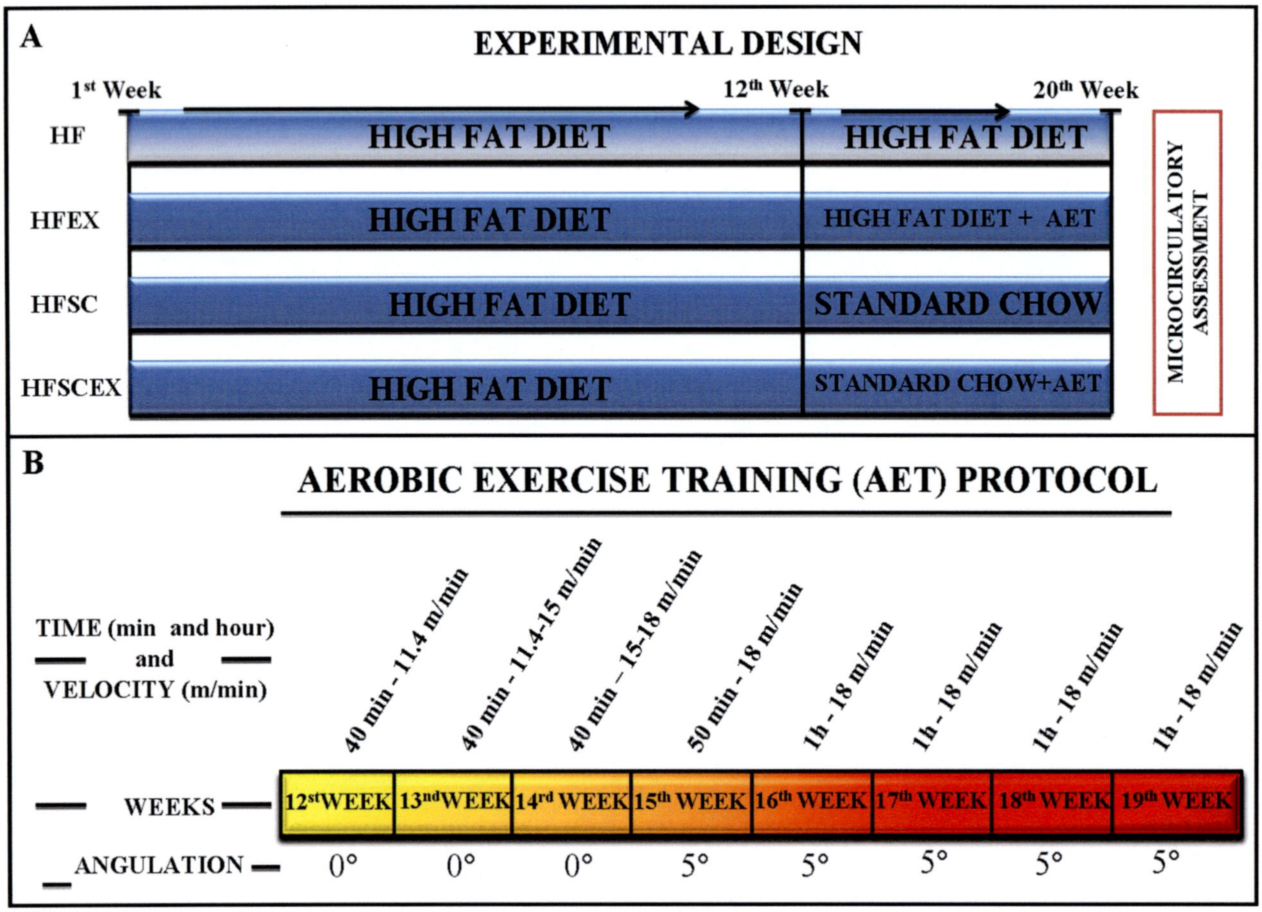

Figure 1. Experimental design and Aerobic Exercise Training. (A) Experimental design with dietary modification and aerobic exercise training, after week 12. (B) Aerobic Exercise Training (AET) performed by hamsters, organized by weeks, time, speed and angulations. High fat fed hamsters were subjected to AET in the last two months associated or not to diet modification.

around the neck of the pouch (HCP) and inflated for 30 min to suppress local blood flow as previously described, Persson et al [23]. FITC-dextran (150 kDa, TdB Consultancy, Uppsala, Sweden) was injected i.v. 25 mg/100 g body weight for measurements of macromolecular permeability changes. FITC-dextran (150 kDa, 25 mg/100 g body weight, 5% solution, TdB Consultancy, Uppsala - Sweden). Permeability for large molecules was quantified by counting the number of leaky sites (leaks) in the prepared area (1 cm^2) using an UV-light microscope (40× magnification). Leaks are defined as visible extravascular spots (diameter>100 μm) of FITC-dextran in post-capillary venules seen under fluorescent light. The number of leaks was counted at baseline, during reperfusion and after 30 min ischemia in times 0, 5 and 10 min (T0, immediately after; T_5; 5 min after and T_{10}; 10 min after tourniquet release). Preparations presenting more than 10 spontaneous leaks or petechiae at baseline were excluded due to previous damage to the tissue.

Adipose tissue collection

Urogenital, mesenteric and retroperitoneal fat depots were collected according to Cinti [24], weighed and store at −80°C.

Blood samples analysis

Blood samples were collected before the experimental protocol from the saphenous vein, using a capillary tube containing heparin (Heparina Perfecta, 75 mm length – São Paulo, SP - Brazil) for glucose analysis (One touch ultra - Johnson e Johnson, Medical Brazil) [25]. Immediately after the sacrifice of the animal, blood was collected by cardiac puncture, centrifuged [3000 r min−1 (1157×g) for 10 min at 4°C] and stored at −80°C for total triglycerides (TG), total cholesterol (TC), and high-density lipoprotein (HDL) determinations using the Biosystem kit with sensitivity of 0.7 mMol l−1, 0.14 mMol l−1, and 0.5 mMol l−1, respectively. Low-density lipoprotein (LDL) = TC−HDL−(TGL×0.2) and very low density lipoprotein (VLDL) = TGL/5) were calculated by Friedwald's equation [26].

Preparation of the aortic extract

After the experimental protocol and microvascular study, the thoracic aorta was dissected from six animals per group, excised and its strips lysed in 50 mM HEPES (pH 6.4), 1 mM $MgCl_2$, 10 mM EDTA, 1% Triton X-100, 1 mg/ml DNase, 0.5 mg/ml RNase containing the following protease inhibitors: 1 mM PMSF, 1 mM benzamidine, 1 mM leupeptin, and 1 mM soybean trypsin inhibitor (Sigma Chemicals, St. Louis, MO, USA).

Immunoblotting essay

Total protein content of aortic extracts was determined by Bradford's method [27]. Samples (30 μg in total) were resolved by 10% SDS-PAGE and proteins were transferred to PVDF membranes (Hybond- P, Amersham Pharmacia Biotech, San Francisco, CA, USA). Rainbow markers (Amersham Pharmacia Biotech, San Francisco, CA, USA) run in parallel to estimate molecular weights. Membranes were blocked with Tween-PBS (0.1% Tween-20 in PBS) containing 5% bovine serum albumin and incubated with specific primary antibody: anti-iNOS (1:500; Santa Cruz Biotechnology, Santa Cruz, CA, USA) and anti-eNOS (1:500; Santa Cruz Biotechnology, Santa Cruz, CA, USA). After extensive washings in Tween-PBS, PVDF sheets were incubated with appropriate secondary biotin-conjugated antibody conjugated to biotin (Santa Cruz Biotechnology, Santa Cruz, CA, USA) for 1 h and then incubated with horseradish peroxidase conjugated to streptavidin (1:10000; Caltag Laboratories, Burlingame, CA, USA). Immunoreactive proteins were visualized using ECL system (Pierce ECL Chemiluminescent Substrate; Thermo Scientific, Rockford USA). Membranes were stripped with buffer containing 62.5 mM Tris–HCl, 2% SDS and 100 mM β-mercaptoethanol and re-probed similarly with anti-ERK2 antibody (1:1000; Santa Cruz Biotechnology, Santa Cruz, CA, USA). Films were scanned and analyzed semi quantitatively and iNOS and eNOS were normalized to actin levels. Bands were quantified by densitometry, using Image J 1.34 s Software (NIH, USA).

Exercise protocol

After 12 weeks of HF feeding, hamsters (5 to 6 months of age) were randomly assigned to an exercise practice (n = 60). One week before the beginning of the exercise protocol, they were placed in the treadmill machine at lower speed for a short time for adaptation. The exercise training consisted of 8 weeks of running on a motor treadmill (INSIGHT – EP 131 – Ribeirão Preto, SP, Brazil), 5 times/week, raising weekly time and speed until the limit of 60 min at 18 m/min (Figure 1) [19]. Exercise was conducted at 50–70% of VO_2 maximum, featuring the overall AET protocol as of moderate intensity. Measures of RQ (respiratory quotient) were set at 1 to designate respiratory exhaustion and conducted in 0.89, characterizing the exercise as aerobic. Animals did not pass through exercise training 24–36 h before the experimental day.

Leptin evaluation

Leptin levels were evaluated in blood serum obtained by heart puncture (centrifugation −2.500 rpm for 12 minutes – Eppendorf, Centrifuge 5804R,Hamburg – Germany) using an ELISA kit (Peprotech ELISA Development Kit, 900-K76 Lot# 0608076 – London, UK). The assay sensitivity was 20 pg/ml. Inter and intra-assay coefficient of variation were, respectively, 6.4% and 5.1%, Samples were assayed in triplicate.

Data analysis

Statistical analysis was performed initially using Kolmogorov-Smirnov normality test and homoscedasticity tests (Bartlett criterion). Body mass, fat percentage, fat depots, lipid profile and blood measures presented normal distribution and are reported as means±standard error of the mean (S.E.M.). Microvascular reactivity and macromolecular permeability did not show normal distribution and are reported as median [10–90 percentiles]. Microvessel diameters are presented as relative changes, normalized to baseline. Microcirculatory data between groups were analyzed using Kruskal-Wallis test, followed by post hoc Dunn test. Group differences in arteriolar diameter responses to Ach were determined by Friedman's test. Variables with normal distribution were analyzed using One Way ANOVA to compare differences between groups, followed by post hoc Tukey test. Statistical analysis was performed using Prism 5.01 (Graphpad Inc., San Diego, CA, USA). Results were considered statistically different when $p<0.05$.

Results

One hundred and twenty male hamsters used were randomly distributed into four experimental groups: high fat (HF, n = 30), high fat + Exercise (HFEX, n = 30), high fat +Standard chow (HFSC, n = 30), high fat + Standard chow + exercise (HFSCEX, n = 30). Most data are shown as mean±SEM, except for microcirculatory assessments presented as median (10–90 percentiles).

Fat overload elicits significant increase on body weight that could be altered after interventions (experimental design shown on figure 1). Treated groups (HFSC and HFSCEX) showed significant reduction not only on body weight [HFSC vs. HF and HFEX reduction of 10.24% and 9.56% respectively, HFSCEX vs. HF and HFEX reduction of 9.66% and 8.8% respectively; $p<0.0001$], but also on naso-anal length [HFSC vs. HF and HFEX reduction of 9.0% and 6.9% respectively, HFSCEX vs. HF and HFEX reduction of 6.1% and 2.9% respectively; $p = 0.0011$] and fat depots [fat% HFSC vs. HF and HFEX with differences of 29.7% and 32.3% respectively, HFSCEX vs. HF and HFEX with differences of 26.6% and 29.2% respectively, $p<0.001$; visceral HFSC vs. HF and HFEX with differences of 30% and 31.4% respectively, HFSCEX vs. HF and HFEX with differences of 28% and 29.4% respectively, $p< 0.0001$]. Concerning hemodynamic responses, mean arterial pressure (MAP) and heart rate (HR) showed linear improvements on all treated groups (HFSC, HFEX and HFSCEX) {[MAP – HFEX vs. HF and HFSC with differences of 20.2% and 9.2% respectively; HFSCEX vs. HF and HFSC with differences of 31.1% and 21.7% respectively, $p<0.001$]; [HR - HFEX vs. HF and HFSC with differences of 8.9% and 11.6% respectively; HFSCEX vs. HF and HFSC with differences of 15% and 16.4% respectively $p<0.01$]}. These results are shown on table 2. In terms of blood analysis, no difference could be found between groups concerning total cholesterol, LDL, HDL and triglycerides, but fasting blood glucose began to show a tendency towards reduction on treated groups (HFEX and HFSCEX) as seen on table 3. HF animals had significantly higher levels of leptin (figure 2), that gradually decreased from HF to HFSCEX [(HF) 222±15.5 ng/dl, (HFSC) 181±13.1 ng/dl, (HFEX) 146.2±8.3 ng/dl and [(HFSCEX)*99.4±23.4 ng/dl; *significantly different from HF group; $p = 0.0039$].

The vasomotor activity was studied in more detail on two hundred and forty 2nd to 3rd order arterioles with baseline mean internal diameter ranging from 40 to 90 µm. No significant differences on baseline diameter were observed in any group and all of them presented robust blood flow and single flowing red blood cells were not discernible at any time. Changes in the microvasculature consisted on reverting most endothelial-dependent microvascular dysfunction demonstrated by Ach responses on arteriolar diameter on HFSC, HFEX and HFSCEX animals, while on HF ones it has been observed even a contractile phenotype. Data are shown as median (1st and 4th quartiles). This scenario was observed in all doses utilized, in values compared to baseline, considered as 100% [10^{-8} M - HF 90.70(78.00–97.80)%, HFSC *113.5(104.0–156.5)%, HFEX *108.3(101.6–138.3)%, HFSCEX *103.8(96.59–115.2)%; *significantly different from the HF group - $p<0.0001$]; [10^{-6} M - HF 99.04 (86.80–107.2)%, HFSC *118.7 (106.5–144.6)%, HFEX *121.7 (108.7–138.5)%, HFSCEX *122.8(106.4–141.5)%; *significantly different from the HF group - $p<0.0001$]; [10^{-4} M - HF 106.8(89.14–125.5)%, HFSC *145.9 (115.3–181.2)%, *HFEX 138.8(118.3–161.6)%, *HFSCEX 147.0(115.2–164.1)%; *significantly different from the HF group - $p<0.0001$] (Figure 3). No significant differences between groups could be observed with topical application of sodium nitroprusside, as seen on figure 4.

Macromolecular permeability after ischemia/reperfusion procedure, measured at 10 minutes after the onset of reperfusion, was significantly higher on HF animals and, after all intervention protocols (HFSC, HFEX and HFSCEX groups), animals showed significantly lower number of leaks at 10 minutes [HF 40.5(32–49)leaks/cm^2, HFSC *19.0 (17–22)leaks/cm^2, HFEX *18.6(16–23)leaks/cm^{2}and HFSCEX *16.0(13.5–25)leaks/cm^2, *Significantly different from the HF group; $p<0.0057$ - as visualized on figure 5].

eNOS expression assay showed a linear increase in all treated groups, but significant differences compared to HF were only found on HFSCEX ($p = 0.032$- figure 6). No significant differences were found on iNOS evaluations.

Discussion

Our initial hypothesis was confirmed since microcirculatory dysfunction induced by fat overload was significantly attenuated by chronic moderate aerobic exercise training program (AET) associated or not to dietary modification. This study represents a continuation of our previous work [28] in which 16 weeks HF feeding was responsible for inciting visceral obesity, insulin resistance and microvascular damage.

In order to evaluate AET's and dietary modification effects, the chosen microcirculatory assessment technique was the cheek pouch preparation. This preparation represents a trustworthy technique since it displays robust, stable blood flow and responsiveness to topic vasoactive drugs. Although the microcirculatory bed observed in the cheek pouch in this investigation was mostly the cutaneous part of it, it is conceivable to consider that it

Table 2. Assessments performed on experiment day.

	HF	HFSC	HFEX	HFSCEX
Body mass (g)	171.8±2.8	*+154.2±2.6	170.5±2.8	*+155.5±1.9
Naso-anal length (cm)	18±0.29	*16.2±0.32	17.4±0.18	*16.9±0.23
Body Fat (%)	15.8±0.6	*+11.1±0.33	16.4±0.53	*+11.6±0.28
Uro Depot	2.6±0.37	2.5±0.29	3.0±0.24	2.6±0.28
Vis Depot	5.0±0.79	*+3.5±0.39	5.1±0.54	*+3.6±0.52
Ret depot	1.5±0.23	1.1±0.11	1.4±0.11	1.2±0.11
MAP	159.5±3.4	*140.3±5.8	*127.3±5.7	#*109.8±5.9
HR	378.9±6.8	386±13.7	#*344±9	#*322.7±9.2

All values are presented as mean±standard error of the mean. HF = High Fat diet. HFSC = High Fat Diet + Standard Chow. HFEX = High Fat Diet+Exercise. HFSCEX = High Fat Diet +Standard Chow/Exercise (n = 10/per group). Fat (%) = Fat percentage; Uro depot = Urogenital fat depot (g/100 g of body mass); Vis depot = Visceral fat depot (g/100 g of body mass); Ret depot = Retroperitoneal fat depot (g/100 g of body mass). MAP = Mean arterial pressure. HR = Heart rate.
*Significantly different from HF group ($p<0.001$).
+Significantly different from the HFEX group ($p<0.01$).
#Significantly different from the HFSC group ($p<0.01$).

Table 3. Lipid profile and Glucose evaluation of high fat chow (HF), High fat+Standard chow (HFSC), High fat +Aerobic Exercise (HFEX) and High fat +Standard Chow/Exercise (HFSC/EX) groups.

	HF	HFSC	HFEX	HFSCEX
TC (mmol/l)	2.380	1.890	1.990	2.070
HDL(mmol/l)	1.580	1.345	1.500	1.505
LDL(mmol/l)	0.4950	0.3300	0.1850	0.1800
VLDL(mmol/l)	0.2800	0.3400	0.3050	0.3300
TGL(mmol/l)	1.415	1.718	1.515	1.650
Glycemia (mg/dL)	94.5±8.4	91±6.8	86.2±5.1	81.2±5.8

All values are presented as mean±S.E.M. No significant difference was found between groups. HF = High Fat Diet. HFSC = High Fat Diet +Standard Chow. HFEX = High Fat Diet +Exercise. HFSCEX = High Fat Diet +Standard Chow/Exercise (n = 10/per group). TC = total cholesterol; HDL = high density lipoprotein; LDL = low density lipoprotein; VLDL = very low density lipoprotein; TGL = triglycerides.

represents systemic alterations. Experiments in humans using laser Doppler and intravital videomicroscopy to examine the skin of the dorsum of the middle finger have shown a good correlation between cutaneous microcirculation and systemic alterations [29]. Microvascular alterations observed on cutaneous tissue attributed to microvascular dysfunction are not only local, but also a systemic process, and studies concerning the cutaneous vascular bed may reproduce alterations on tissues such as muscle [30–31].

Enhanced fat depots, features of obese states, incite a unique shift in adipocytes with the installation of an inflammatory and vasoconstrictor profiles. Mature adipocytes secrete an ever-increasing number of growth factors that participate in diverse metabolic processes, particularly insulin resistance. Numberless compounds such as lipoprotein lipase, angiotensinogen, aldosterone, adiponectin, TNF-α and nitric oxide participate in different metabolic and vascular processes, including adipogenesis [32]. The combination of abdominal obesity, impaired glucose and insulin metabolism, dyslipidemia and hypertension is known as metabolic syndrome, an important risk factor for cardiovascular and coronary heart disease mortality. Insulin resistance is a metabolic defect present in this syndrome, associated to type 2 diabetes, obesity, hypertension and dyslipidaemia [33]. In this context, the microcirculation represents an important site to evaluate the profile of adipocytes since systemic inflammation, observed in dysfunctional adipose tissues, can harm the microcirculatory function before perceptible changes on body composition and comorbidities may be observed.

Our findings demonstrated that HF feeding elicited microvascular dysfunction and AET was able to reverse/attenuate most of fat overload damage. Animals from HFEX group presented an important restoration of endothelial function as well as body composition modifications after AET program since these animals did not show any significant changes in either body weight or fat deposition (see in table 2). It is interesting to notice that diet is a necessary component in our study, since microvascular improvements are leashed to reductions on body composition and fat depots stimulated by dietary modifications. Animals that return to standard diet with or without AET presented significantly increased responses to endothelium-dependent vasodilator, indicating an improvement of their endothelial function. Our work showed that there was a significant improvement on HFEX, but more explicit on HFSC and HFSCEX groups concerning vascular reactivity, reflected on vasodilator responses elicited by acetylcholine in all concentrations tested (10^{-8} M, 10^{-6} M and 10^{-4} M - see in figure 3).

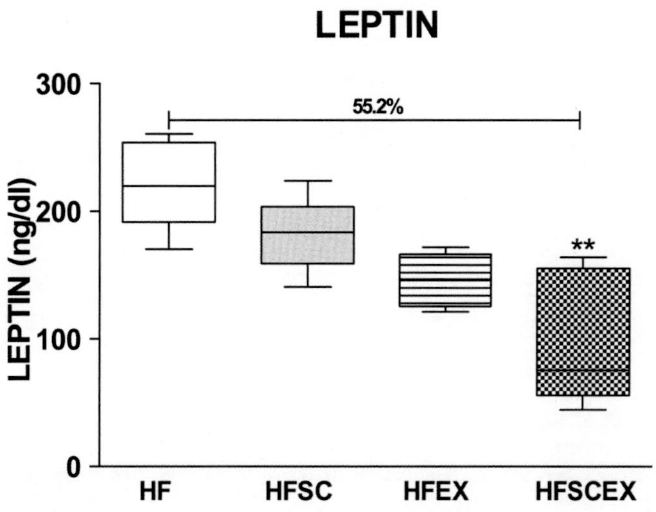

Figure 2. Leptin evaluation. Data are presented as mean±standard error of the mean HF = High Fat Diet. HFSC = High Fat Diet + Standard Chow. HFEX = High Fat Diet + Exercise. HFSCEX = High Fat Diet +Standard Chow/Exercise. *Significantly different from the HF group (p<0.01).

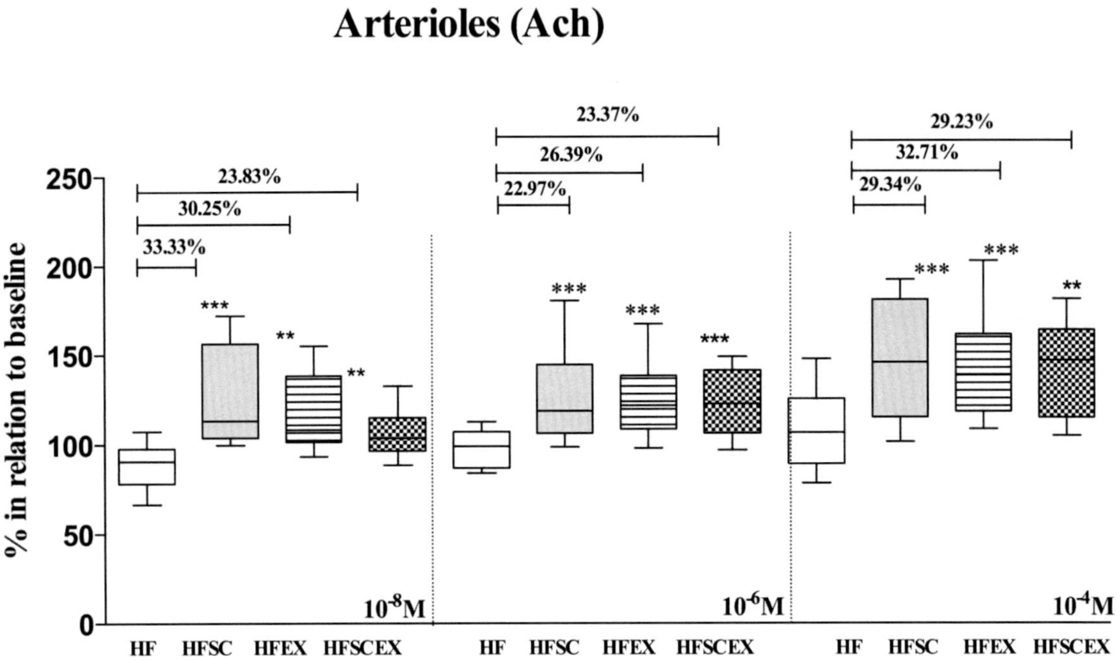

Figure 3. Mean arteriolar diameters after topical application of three concentrations of acetylcholine (10^{-8}, 10^{-6} and 10^{-4} M) to the cheek pouch of hamsters fed with high fat diet (HF and HFEX, n = 10 each) and that had dietary modification associated or not to AET (HFSC and HFSCEX, n = 10 each) during 20 weeks. Data are shown as changes relative to baseline considered as 100%. Data are expressed as median±10–90 percentile, represented by vertical bars. *Significantly different from sedentary obese control group ($p<0.001$ and $p<0.01$, respectively) in all concentrations of Ach.

Endothelial dysfunction (ED) is characterized by blunted vasodilator responses to a number of stimuli responsible for increasing production or release of endothelial NO such as activation of muscarinic receptors or increase on shear stress by raising blood flow. ED reflects alterations in the endothelial barrier and is consider an early marker of cardiovascular risk that precedes any visible structural atheromatous plaques and traditional cardiovascular risk factors, such as hypertension [34], diabetes mellitus, hypercholesterolemia and obesity [35]. Therefore, studies concerning ED could be applied as therapeutic strategies to prevent these diseases. Fat distribution, in this sense, has been found to be an important determinant of endothelial dysfunction and a strong modulator of microvascular reactivity [36], which reinforces the benefits obtained in the present

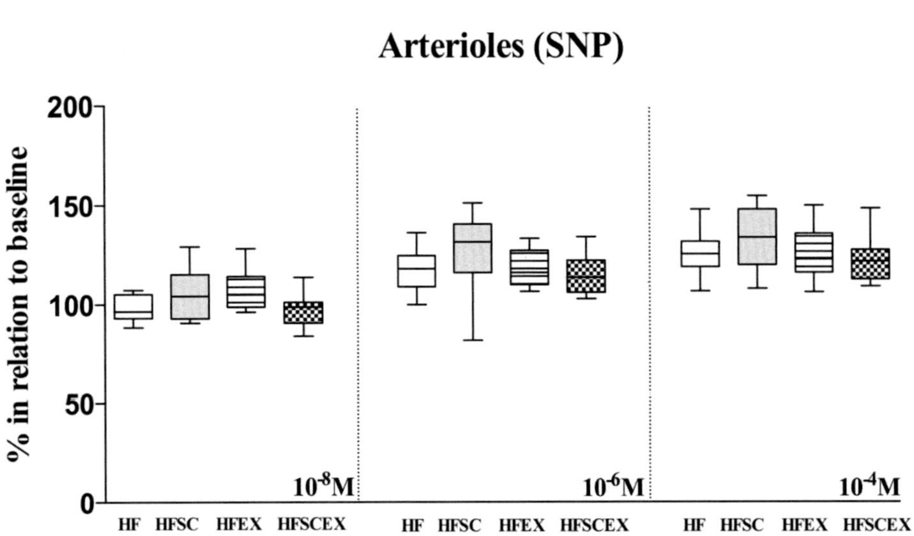

Figure 4. Mean arteriolar diameters after topical application of three concentrations of sodium nitroprusside (10^{-8}, 10^{-6} and 10^{-4} M) to the cheek pouch of hamsters fed with high fat diet (HF and HFEX, n = 10 each) and that had dietary modification associated or not to AET (HFSC and HFSCEX, n = 10 each) during 20 weeks. Data are shown as changes relative to baseline considered as 100%. Data are expressed as median±10–90 percentile. No difference was found between groups for sodium nitroprusside. HF = High Fat Diet. HFSC = High Fat Diet + Standard Chow. HFEX = High Fat Diet + Exercise. HFSCEX = High Fat Diet +Standard Chow/Exercise.

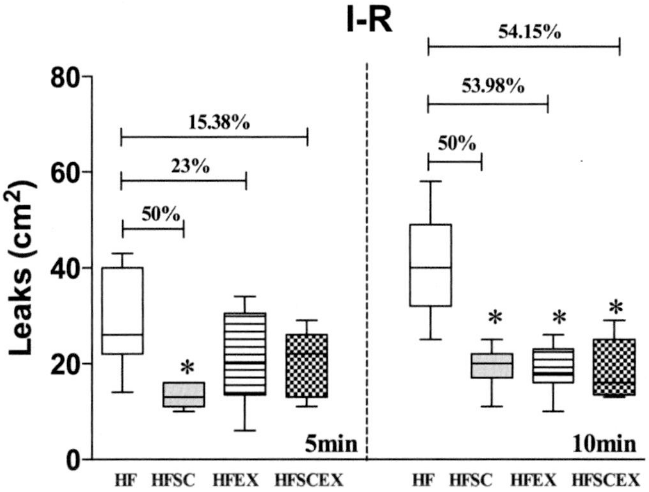

Figure 5. Macromolecular permeability at post capillary venules after 30 minutes ischemia of the cheek pouch of hamsters fed with high fat chow (HF and HFEX, n = 10 each) and with dietary modification associated or not to AET (HFSC and HFSCEX, n = 10 each) during 20 weeks. T5, 5 minutes after and T10, 10 minutes after tourniquet release. Data are expressed as median ± 10–90 percentile, represented by vertical bars. * Significantly different from the HF group ($p<0.05$). HF = High Fat Diet. HFSC = High Fat Diet + Standard Chow. HFEX = High Fat Diet + Exercise. HFSCEX = High Fat Diet +Standard Chow/Exercise.

investigation. High fat diets can be successfully used as inciter of ED, although this model is not only related to ED but also to prostanoid- mediated vasoconstriction in conductance vessels of mice [37] and atherosclerosis in hamsters exposed to high cholesterol diet [38]. Nitric oxide plays an important role on insulin's vasodilator effect as well as in states of insulin resistance, such as obesity and diabetes, characterized by reduced insulin-mediated vasodilatation subsequent to endothelial dysfunction. The mechanisms underlying impaired vascular responses later in life probably involves nitric oxide (NO) and other factors that could interfere with insulin vasodilator effects such as pro-inflammatory adipocytokines like IL-6 and TNF-α [39–40].

Ischemia/reperfusion-induced macromolecular permeability increase obtained after 30 min ischemia showed significant reduction on the number of leaks in peak time (10 min) on groups that passed through intervention protocols (HFSC, HFEX and HFSCEX), reflecting improvements on endothelial dysfunction state. Although not significant, there was a higher decrease on leaks in animals exposed to both interventions. Diet and exercise (HFSCEX), showed the highest difference when compared to HF, suggesting that not only the protective effects of exercise, but also the reduction of deleterious effects caused by fat consumption achieved by dietary modification is necessary (HFSC and HFSCEX – see in figure 5). The investigation combining diet changes and moderate aerobic exercise indicates that mediators well known to increase endothelial permeability, such as thrombin, reactive oxygen species, vascular endothelial growth factor (VEGF) and TNF-α, augmented in obesity, could be reduced after exposure to these protocols [41–42]. Endothelial properties are affected by mechanical stress and macromolecular permeability increase induced by ischemia/reperfusion demonstrated opposite effects when acute and chronic enhance of shear stress occurred. An acute increase in shear stress promotes an increase of macromolecular permeability count in endothelial cells monolayer, while a chronic increase is responsible for protecting the endothelial monolayer [43], as demonstrated by our findings.

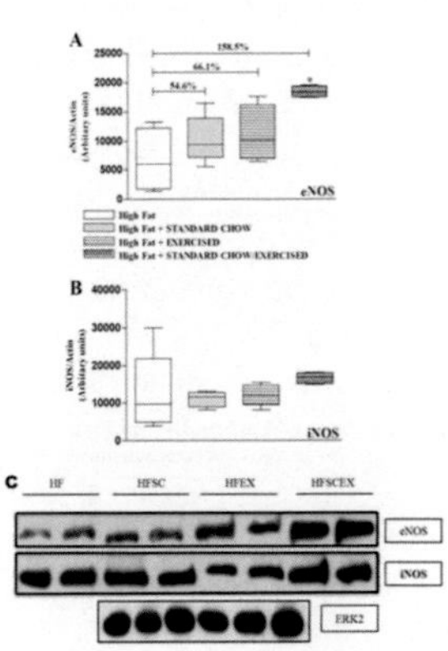

Figure 6. Western blot essays of eNOS (A and B) and iNOS (A and C) in the thoracic aorta of hamsters fed with high fat (HFD) or standard diet (Control) during 16 weeks. Data are expressed as means±S.E.M represented by vertical bars. *Significantly different from the control group ($p<0.05$). HF = High Fat Diet. HFSC = High Fat Diet + Standard Chow. HFEX = Obese + Exercise. HFSCEX = High Fat Diet + Standard Chow/Exercise.

The premise that fat overnutrition after weaning increased body weight and body fat mass could be confirmed in the present investigation. Urogenital, visceral and retroperitoneal fat depots and naso-anal length were greater in HF group at 20th week when compared to HFSC, HFEX and HFSCEX ones. Exercise and dietary implementation proved to be important non-pharmacological ways of treatment, since they were able to decrease body mass after 12 weeks of HF. Data on the literature corroborate our findings since diet-induced obesity in rats chronically subjected to exercise showed that they developed lower levels of adiposity and body mass [44]. Although AET was able to reverse most damages caused by HF feeding, it was not the only effective treatment and dietary modification has proved once again that reduction in caloric intake was essential for changes/improvements not only on body composition but also on microcirculatory dysfunction as seen on modifications observed in groups HFSC and HFSCEX. According to guidelines of the American College of Sports Medicine from 2001 [45] and 2009 [46], changes in caloric intake are necessary to lose and, most importantly, maintain weight. In simplistic terms, when energy intake is reduced below the current needs of the body, weight loss will occur. Obese subjects normally regain their lost weight, showing even worsen body composition scenario after the first weight loss. Therefore, it is necessary not only to enhance the amount of exercise which those subjects are exposed to, but also tailor constantly the diet to each patient needs [Weight management. J. Am Diet Assoc. 2009;109(2):330–46], in order to acquire better responses from exercise. Guidelines point to 150 min.wk^{-1} to 250 min.wk^{-1} to guarantee that lost weight will not be regained [46]. For that purpose, our experimental design matched most guidelines directions, since increased intensity and time of endurance were made, concomitantly with a dietary approach (see AET program and experimental design in figure 1). In order to make a parallel to human intervention it adds an important bias, not usually present in animal experiments, the failure of exercise and dietary interventions in either maintenance and reduction of body weight or fat and to achieve patients' purpose drugs are usually prescribed. These drugs usually act (1) in the central nervous system, decreasing the appetite, (2) reducing the absorption of nutrients or (3) raising body energy expenditure [47]. Their efficiency is related to the capacity of reducing fat depots, maintaining weight loss, diminishing risks related to obesity and ultimately improving life quality. Nowadays the most indicated ones are tesofensin, successor of sibutramine, and orlistat, the first two enhance satiation and thermogenesis [48], and the last one reduces fat absorption through inhibition of gastrointestinal and pancreatic lipases. High cost and serious side effects (psycho-stimulatory, depression, addiction, cardio-excitatory effects, pulmonary hypertension, and valve disease) demand surveillance. Antiobesity agents that possess cardio-excitatory and psycho-stimulatory effects (e.g., phentermine, ephedrine, and caffeine mixture) are still available for the short-term use in some countries and have been abolished in others. To summarize, the rationale of obesity treatment in humans is far more complicated than in animal models.

Several mechanisms are associated to exercise improvements, and some of them are worthwhile mention. Exercise has a close relation to increasing blood flow velocity, modifying laminar shear stress that has an intimate connection to endothelial cell monolayer genetic expression. In fact, blood flow is responsible for the constitutive genetic pattern of endothelial cells [49]. Mechanical agonist stimulus provoked by exercise augments target endothelial genes (e.g. eNOS, MnSOD and NADPH oxidase) and blood flow followed by upregulation of eNOS and Ca^{2+}-dependent K^{+} channel 4 (KCNN4) genes [49]. Generally, prolonged unidirectional chronic shear stress elevation is atheroprotective because it increases endothelial anti-inflammatory and antioxidative profiles. The cross-talk between exercise and endothelial cells is important to explain how shear stress acts on the cell surface. Furthermore mechanical alterations of endothelium result in decreased β-adrenergic vascular responsiveness, and consequently attenuated sympathetic outflow [50]. Concomitantly, the skeletal muscle acts as an endocrine organ secreting IL-6, a classical myokine, which increases in an exponential fashion with exercise according to its intensity, duration, recruited mass and endurance capacity. Exercise-derived IL-6 is related to reduction of TNF-α, enhanced s-TNF-r (TNF-α soluble receptor) and IL-10, indicating important anti-inflammatory effects [51] from exercise that could influence the microcirculation. These downstream effects of exercise found in our study could explain the improvements seen in hemodynamic parameters where animals exposed to AET showed a decrease in mean arterial pressure and heart rate.

Adiposopathy reflects a chronic inflammatory state and increased iNOS expression in the aorta of HF group points towards such inflammatory profile. Chronic blockade of NO synthesis in HFD-induced obese mice reduced inflammation and improved insulin signaling to skeletal muscle [52]. Therefore, increased iNOS expression might be a factor associated to endothelial dysfunction in obese groups. It should be mentioned that iNOS expression was not significantly different between groups, probably due to the short intervention time.

Other important marker that may contribute to reduce endothelium-dependent vasodilatation on HF is the lipid profile, strongly associated to an increased risk of cardiovascular disease and atherogenic profile. Nevertheless, studies concerning aerobic training and its effects on lipid profile markers diverge between improvements and neuter consequences, depending on modality and intensity [53]. In our study, no significant differences were found on lipid profile on treated groups, again probably due to the short intervention time. Another factor to be considered was the dietary modification, since those animals that did not passed through calorie reduction (return to normal rodent chow) the damages elicited by high fat exposure could not be completely restored.

Besides the lipid profile, leptin has shown a linear reduction according to the interventions, achieving a significant difference in HFSCEX group, compared to HF. Leptin is produced by fat tissues and it has a clear role in weight control. Obese subjects develop leptin resistance and in our work a significant relationship between plasma leptin and body weight was found. After the exercise protocol there was a linear reduction of these levels, suggesting an increase on leptin sensibility. Our results could be confirmed by data on obese rats subjected to treadmill routine for four weeks [54].

Limitations of our study deal with animal and methodology choices (1) low compatibility to measurement kits, which prevented the evaluation of important adipokines such as TNF-α, MCP-1 and others and (2) the lack of tail, important for blood collection and analysis during exercise exposure. Although attempts to measure blood lactate, pO_2, pCO_2 and bicarbonate were made, these failed due to lack of blood drops during the exercise protocol. The last limitation concerned the chosen microcirculatory method, as mention above the cheek pouch present a robust blood flow, clarity and stability, notwithstanding the overriding analyzed tissue, e.g. the window of observation, was the cutaneous one and only few parts of skeletal muscle composed the overall observation, reflecting systemic alterations and improvements.

In summary, we have presented evidence suggesting that the damage elicited on the endothelium by an inflammatory scenario, observed in high fat fed animals, may be attenuated with interventions such as returning to standard chow associated or not to aerobic exercise training, leading to reduction of adipose tissue accumulation and improvement on microvascular reactivity.

Acknowledgments

Authors would like to thank Mr. Claudio N. Ribeiro and Mr. Paulo José F. Lopes for their help with animal care.

Author Contributions

Conceived and designed the experiments: BCSB EB. Performed the experiments: BCSB MGCS SVS TCBF. Analyzed the data: BCSB EB. Contributed reagents/materials/analysis tools: RDL LGKA. Contributed to the writing of the manuscript: BCSB EB.

References

1. Bays HE (2011) Adiposopathy. Is "Sick Fat" a Cardiovascular Disease? Journal of the Am College of Cardiology 57, N°25.
2. Jonk AM, Houben AJ, de Jongh RT, Serné EH, Schaper NC, et al. (2007) Microvascular dysfunction in obesity: a potential mechanism in the pathogenesis of obesity-associated insulin resistance and hypertension. Physiology (Bethesda) 22, 252–260.
3. de Jongh RT, Ijzerman RG, Sernè EH, Voordouw JJ, Yudkin JS, et al. (2006) Visceral and truncal subcutaneous adipose tissue are associated with impaired capillary recruitment in healthy individuals. J Clin Endocrinol Metab 91, 5100–5106.
4. Ziccardi P, Nappo F, Giugliano G, Esposito K, Marfella R, et al. (2002) Reduction of inflammatory cytokine concentrations and improvement of endothelial functions in obese women after weight loss over one year. Circulation 105, 804–809.
5. Anderson TJ (1999) Assessment and treatment of endothelial dysfunction in humans. J Am Coll Cardiol 34, 631–638.
6. Bonetti PO, Lerman LO, Lerman A (2003) Endothelial dysfunction: a marker of atherosclerotic risk. Arterioscler Thromb Vasc Biol 23, 168–175.
7. Huang AL, Silver AE, Shvenke E, Schopfer DW, Jahangir E, et al. (2007) Predictive value of reactive hyperemia for cardiovascular events in patients with peripheral arterial disease undergoing vascular surgery. Arterioscler Thromb Vasc Biol 27, 2113–2119.
8. Kullo IJ, Malik AR, Santos S, Ehrsam JE, Turner ST (2007) Association of cardiovascular risk factors with microvascular and conduit artery function in hypertensive subjects. Am J Hypertens 20, 735–742.
9. Reis SE, Holubkov R, Conrad Smith AJ, Kelsey SF, Sharaf BL, et al. (2001) Coronary microvascular dysfunction is highly prevalent in women with chest pain in the absence of coronary artery disease: results from the NHLBI WISE study. Am Heart J 141, 735–741.
10. Smith AG, Muscat GE (2005) Skeletal muscle and nuclear hormone receptors: implications for cardiovascular and metabolic disease. The International Journal of Biochemistry & Cell Biology v.37, n.10, p.2047–2063.
11. Nuutila P, Koivisto VA, Knuuti J, Ruotsalainen U, Teräs M, et al. (1992) Glucose-Free Fatty Acid Cycle Operates in Human Heart and Skeletal Muscle In Vivo. J Clin Invest 89, 1767–1744.
12. Myers J, Prakash M, Froelicher V, Do D, Parlington S, et al. (2002) Exercise capacity and mortality among men referred for exercise testing. N Engl J Med 346: 793–801.
13. Piepoli MF, Corrà U, Benzer W, Bjarnason-Wehrens B, Dendale P, et al. (2010) Secondary prevention through cardiac rehabilitation: from knowledge to implementation. A position paper from the Cardiac Rehabilitation Section of the European Association of Cardiovascular Prevention and Rehabilitation 17(1):1–17.
14. Gu Q, Wang B, Zhang X-F, Ma YP, Liu JD, et al. (2014) Chronic aerobic exercise training attenuates aortic stiffening and endothelial dysfunction through preserving aortic mitochondrial function in aged rats. Exp Gerontology, S0531-5565(14)00071-0.
15. Collier SR, Sandberg K, Moody AM, Frechette V, Curry CD, et al. (2014) Reduction of plasma aldosterone and arterial stiffness in obese pre- and stage 1 hypertensive subjects after aerobic exercise. J Hum Hypertens doi:10.1038/jhh.2014.33.
16. Dias IB, Panazzolo DG, Marques MF, Paredes BD, Souza MG, et al. (2013) Relationships between emerging cardiovascular risk factors, z-BMI, waist circumference and body adiposity index (BAI) on adolescents. Clin Endocrinol (Oxf) 79(5):667–74.
17. Cho JK, Lee SH, Lee JY, Kang HS (2011) Randomized Controlled Trial of Training Intensity in Adiposity. Int J Sports Med ISSN 0172–4622.
18. Pinheiro AR, Cunha AR, Aguila MB, Mandarim-de-Lacerda CA (2007) Beneficial effects of physical exercise on hypertension and cardiovascular adverse remodeling of diet-induced obese rats. Nutrition, Metabolism & Cardiovascular Diseases 17, 365–375.
19. Heunks LMA, Bast AALT, Van Herwaarden CLA, Haenen GR, Dekhuijzen PN (2000) Effects of emphysema and training on glutathione oxidation in the hamster diaphragm. J Appl Physiol 88: 2054–2061.
20. Bouskela E, Grampp W (1992) Spontaneous vasomotion in hamster cheek pouch arterioles in varying experimental conditions. Am J Physiol 262, H478–H485.
21. Duling BR (1973) The preparation and use of the hamster cheek pouch for studies of the microcirculation. Microvasc Res 5, 423–429.
22. Svensjõ E, Arfors KE, Arturson G, Rutili G (1978) The hamster cheek pouch preparation as a model for studies of macromolecular permeability of the microvasculature. Ups J Med Sci 83(1):71–9.
23. Persson NH, Erlansson M, Svensjö E, Takolander R, Berqqvist D (1985). The hamster cheek pouch-an experimental model to study postischemic macromolecular permeability. Int J Microcirc Clin Exp 4(3):257–63.
24. Cinti S (2005). The adipose organ. Prostaglandins, Leukotrienes and Essential Fatty Acids 73: 9–15.
25. Beeton C, Garcia A, Chandy KG (2007) Drawing blood from rats through the saphenous vein and by cardiac puncture. J Vis Exp (7) 266.
26. Friedewald WT, Levy RI, Fredrickson DS (1972) Estimation of the concentration of low-density lipoprotein cholesterol in plasma, without use of the preparative ultracentrifuge. Clin Chem 18, 499–502.
27. Bradford MM (1976) A rapid and sensitive method for the quantitation of microgram quantities of protein utilizing the principle of protein-dye binding. Analytical Biochemistry 72 248–254.
28. Costa RRS, Villela NR, Souza MGC, Boa BC, Cyrino FZ, et al. (2011) High fat diet induces central obesity, insulin resistance and microvascular dysfunction in hamsters. Microvasc Res doi:10.1016/j.mvr.2011.08.007.
29. Antonios TFT, Kaski JC, Hasan KM, Brown SJ, Singer DR (2001) Rarefaction of skin capillaries in patients with anginal chest pain and normal coronary arteriograms. Eur Heart J 22: 1144–1148.
30. Ijzerman RG, Serne EH, van Weissenbruch MM, de Jongh RT, Stehouwer CD (2003) Cigarette smoking is associated with an acute impairment of microvascular function in humans. Clinical Sci 104; 247–252.
31. Sax FL Cannon RO, Hanson C, Epstein SE (1987) Impaired Forearm Vasodilator Reserve in Patients with Microvascular Angina. Evidence of a Generalized Disorder of Vascular Function? N Engl J Med 317: 1366–1370.
32. Van Gaal LF, Mertens IL, De Block CE (2006) Mechanisms linking obesity with cardiovascular disease. Nature Vol 444. doi:10.1038/nature05487.
33. Wilson PW, D'Agostino RB, Parise H, Sulivan L, Meigs JB (2005) Metabolic syndrome as a precursor of cardiovascular disease and type 2 diabetes mellitus. Circulation 112, 3066–3072.
34. Kullo IJ, Malik AR, Santos S, Ehrsam JE, Turner ST (2007) Association of cardiovascular risk factors with microvascular and conduit artery function in hypertensive subjects. Am. J. Hypertens. 20, 735–742.
35. de Jongh RT, Sernè EH, Ijzerman RG, de Vries G, Stehouwer CD (2004) Impaired microvascular function in obesity: implications for obesity-associated microangiopathy, hypertension, and insulin resistance. Circulation 109, 2529–2535.
36. Singer G, Granger DN (2007) Inflammatory responses underlying the microvascular dysfunction associated with obesity and insulin resistance. Microcirculation 14, 375–387.
37. Traupe T, Lang M, Goettsch W, Münter K, Morawietz H, et al. (2002) Obesity increases prostanoid-mediated vasoconstriction and vascular thromboxane receptor gene expression. J. Hypertens 20, 2239–2245.
38. Mawatari K, Kakui S, Harada N, Ohnishi T, Niwa Y, et al. (2004) Endothelin-1(1–31) levels are increased in atherosclerotic lesions of the thoracic aorta of hypercholesterolemic hamsters. Atherosclerosis 175, 203–212.
39. Bourgoin F, Bachelard H, Badeau M, Mélançon S, Pitre M, et al. (2008) Endothelial and vascular dysfunctions and insulin resistance in rats fed a high-fat, high-sucrose diet. Am. J. Physiol. Heart Circ Physiol 295, H1044–H1055.
40. Steinberg HO, Brechtel G, Johnson A, Fineberg N, Baron AD (1994). Insulin-mediated skeletal muscle vasodilation is nitric oxide dependent. A novel action of insulin to increase nitric oxide release. J Clin Invest 94, 1172–1179.
41. Ay L, Kopp HP, Brix JM, Ay C, Quehenberger P, et al. (2010) Thrombin generation in morbid obesity: significant reduction after weight loss. J Thromb Haemost 8, 759–765.
42. Miyazawa-Hoshimoto S, Takahashi K, Bujo H, Hashimoto N, Yaqui K, et al. (2005) Roles of degree of fat deposition and its localization on VEGF expression in adipocytes. Am. J. Physiol. Endocrinol. Metab. 288, E1128–E1136.
43. Warboys CM, Eric Berson R, Mann GE, Pearson JD, Weinberg PD (2010) Acute and chronic exposure to shear stress have opposite effects on endothelial permeability to macromolecules. Am J Physiol Heart Circ Physiol 298: H1850–H1856.
44. Levin BE, Dunn-Meynell AA (2004) Chronic exercise lowers the defended body weight gain and adiposity in diet-induced obese rats. Am J Physiol Regul Integr Comp Physiol 286: R771–R778.
45. Jakicic JM, Clark K, Coleman E, Donnelly JE, Foreyt J, et al. (2001) Appropriate intervention strategies for weight loss and prevention of weight regain for adults. Med Sci Sports Exerc 33(12):2145–56.
46. Donnelly JE, Blair SN, Jakicic JM, Manore MM, Rankin JW, et al. (2009) Appropriate physical activity intervention strategies for weight loss and prevention of weight regain for adults. Med Sci Sports Exerc 41(2):459–71.
47. Hainer V (2011) Comparative Efficiency and Safety of Pharmacological Approaches to the Management of Obesity Diabetes Care Vol 34: Sup2.
48. Bravata DM, Sanders L, Huang J, Krumholz HM, Olkin I, et al. (2003) Efficacy and safety of low-carbohydrate diets—a systematic review. JAMA 289: 1837–50.
49. Zhang J, Friedman MH (2012) Adaptive response of vascular endothelial cells to an acute increase in shear stress magnitude. Am J Physiol Heart Circ Physiol 302: H983–H991.
50. Laughlin MH, Korthuis RJ, Duncker DJ, Bache RJ (1996) Chapter 16: control of blood flow to cardiac and skeletal muscle during exercise. In: Powelland LB, Shepherd JT, editors. Handbook of physiology, section 120. Exercise: regulation and integration of multiple systems. New York: American Physiological Society and Oxford University Press.
51. Petersen AMW, Pedersen BK (2005) The anti-inflammatory effect of exercise. J Appl Physiol 98: 1154–1162.
52. Tsuchiya K, Sakai H, Suzuki N, Iwashima F, Yoshimoto T, et al. (2007) Chronic blockade of nitric oxide synthesis reduces adiposity and improves insulin resistance in high fat-induced obese mice. Endocrinology 148, 4548–4556.
53. Mann S, Beedie C, Jimenez A (2014) Differential Effects of Aerobic Exercise, Resistance Training and Combined Exercise Modalities on Cholesterol and the Lipid Profile: Review, Synthesis and Recommendations. Sports Med 44: 211–221.
54. Kowalska I, Straczkowski M, Górski J, Kinalska I (1999) The effect of fasting and physical exercise on plasma leptin concentrations in high-fat fed rats. J Physiol Pharmacol Jun 50(2):309–20.

Reduced Oxygen Uptake Efficiency Slope in Patients with Cardiac Sarcoidosis

Wilhelm Ammenwerth[1], Henrik Wurps[1], Mark A. Klemens[2], Catharina Crolow[1], Jeanette Schulz-Menger[3], Nicolas Schönfeld[1], Roland C. Bittner[2], Torsten T. Bauer[1]*

1 Department of Pneumology, Lungenklinik Heckeshorn, HELIOS Klinikum Emil von Behring, Berlin, Germany, **2** Institute of Radiology and Nuclear Medicine, HELIOS Klinikum Emil von Behring, Berlin, Germany, **3** WG Cardiac MRI ECRC a joint institution of the MDC and Charité Medical University Berlin and HELIOS Klinikum Berlin-Buch Department of Cardiology and Nephrology, Berlin, Germany

Abstract

Background: The non-invasive diagnosis of cardiac sarcoidosis (CS) is difficult. Cardiovascular magnetic resonance (CMR) has become a very valuable diagnostic tool in patients with suspected CS, but usually a combination of different tests is used. Oxygen uptake efficiency slope (OUES) is a parameter of cardiopulmonary exercise testing (CPET), which is used as an indicator for cardiovascular impairment. We investigated the predictive value of OUES for the diagnosis of myocardial involvement in sarcoid patients.

Methods: Retrospectively 37 consecutive patients (44.9±13.8 years) with histologically confirmed sarcoidosis and clinical suspicion of heart involvement underwent noninvasive diagnostic testing including CMR. CS was diagnosed according to the guidelines from the Japanese Society of Sarcoidosis and other Granulomatous Disorders with additional consideration of CMR findings. Furthermore, CPET with calculation of predicted OUES according to equations by Hollenberg et al. was carried out.

Results: Patients with CS (11/37; 30%) had a worse cardiovascular response to exercise. OUES was significantly lower in CS-group compared to non-CS-group (59.3±19.1 vs 88.0±15.4%pred., $p<0.0001$). ROC curve method identified 70%pred. as the OUES cut-off point, which maximized sensitivity and specificity for detection of CS (96% sensitivity, 82% specificity, 89% overall accuracy). OUES <70%pred. was the single best predictor of CS (Odds ratio: 100.43, 95% CI: 1.99 to 5064, $p<0.001$) even in multivariate analyses.

Conclusion: OUES assessed in CPET may be helpful in identifying patient with cardiac involvement of sarcoidosis. Patient selection for CMR may be assisted by CPET findings in patients with sarcoidosis.

Editor: Vincenzo Lionetti, Scuola Superiore Sant'Anna, Italy

Funding: The study was supported by the Oskar-Helene-Heim Foundation, Berlin, Germany and HELIOS Research Center, Berlin, Germany. The funders had no role in study design, data collection and analysis, decision to publish, or preparation of the manuscript.

Competing Interests: All authors are employees of the HELIOS Clinic. The HELIOS Research Center is a 100% daughter of HELIOS Clinic and supported this study with a grant. This does not alter adherence to PLOS ONE policies on sharing data and materials.

* Email: torsten.bauer@helios-kliniken.de

Introduction

Sarcoidosis is a multisystemic disease of unknown origin in usually young patients. Lung (90%), liver (30–40%), skin (20–35%), eyes (20–30%), musculoskeletal (2–38%) and nervous system (1–5%) are the organs most commonly affected. Cardiac involvement is associated with a poor prognosis and is extremely difficult to detect. Although cardiac involvement is present in 5–30% of patients with systemic sarcoidosis, only about 5% of these patients are symptomatic [1]. The absence of clinical symptoms does not rule out cardiac sarcoidosis, which is documented by the high rate of unexpected cardiac sarcoidosis in postmortem studies [2,3]. The clinical presentation of sarcoid heart disease includes congestive heart failure, arrhythmias, conduction disturbances, pericardial effusion and also sudden death [4]. The diagnosis can be made by several diagnostic approaches [5] but is confirmed by either noncaseating granulomas in myocardial biopsy or diagnosed by evidence of granulomas in any extracardiac tissue in association with cardiac abnormalities unexplained by other causes. Cardiac sarcoidosis is much more common in the Japanese population compared to other regions and is e.g. the leading cause of death from sarcoidosis in Japan. Therefore, the Japanese Ministry of Health and Welfare published in 1993 guidelines for diagnosing cardiac sarcoidosis [6], which were revised in 2006 by the Japanese Society of Sarcoidosis and other Granulomatous Disorders (Table 1) [7]. These guidelines combine the results of various diagnostic tests and provide an useful framework, particularly for patients with proven systemic sarcoidosis in whom cardiac involvement is suspected. However, cardiovascular magnetic resonance imaging (CMR) has become a diagnostic tool of growing impact for noninvasive assessment of myocardial inflammation in patients with suspected cardiac sarcoidosis[8–11]. Thus, CMR was included in the revised Japanese guidelines, but is currently an expensive method with usually limited access.

Table 1. Summary of the 2006 revised guidelines of diagnosing cardiac sarcoidosis of the Japanese Society of Sarcoidosis and Other Granulomatous [7].

I. Histologic diagnosis group:
Endomyocardial biopsy demonstrates noncaseating epithelioid granulomata.
II. Clinical diagnosis group:
Cardiac sarcoidosis is diagnosed in the absence of an endomyocardial biopsy specimen when extracardiac sarcoidosis has been proven and a combination of major or minor diagnostic criteria has been satisfied as follows:
- More than 2 of 4 major criteria are satisfied, OR
- 1 of the 4 major criteria and 2 or more of the minor criteria are satisfied
Major criteria
(1) Advanced AV block
(2) Basal thinning of the ventricular septum
(3) Positive cardiac gallium uptake
(4) Left ventricular ejection fraction less than 50%
Minor criteria
(1) Abnormal electrocardiogram findings including ventricular tachycardia (VT), multifocal frequent premature ventricular contractions (PVC), complete right bundle branch block (RBBB), pathologic Q waves or abnormal axis deviation
(2) Abnormal regional wall motion, ventricular aneurysm or unexplained increase in wall thickness
(3) Perfusion defects detected by myocardial scintigraphy
(4) Delayed gadolinium enhancement of the myocardium (LGE) on CMR
(5) Interstitial fibrosis or monocyte infiltration greater than moderate grade by endomyocardial biopsy

RBBB = complete right bundle branch block. VT = ventricular tachycardia. PVC = premature ventricular contraction.

Cardiopulmonary exercise testing (CPET) is a widely accessible method for measuring physical performance including cardiovascular function. The oxygen uptake efficiency slope (OUES) is a novel parameter derived from oxygen uptake (VO_2) and minute ventilation (VE)[12]. OUES measures cardiopulmonary functional reserve and may serve for screening of cardiovascular dysfunction[13]. To our knowledge, this tool has never been applied to patients with sarcoidosis in order to assess cardiac function. The aim of this investigation was to find out whether the OUES is a clinically useful predictor of cardiac involvement in patients with biopsy specimen-proven sarcoidosis.

Methods

The patient records was anonymized and de-identified prior to analysis. The study was approved by the ethics committee of the Charité-University Medicine Berlin, Germany. We studied retrospectively 37 consecutive patients (44.9±13.8 years) with biopsy proven sarcoidosis and clinical evidence for cardiac involvement. Studies on the issue of cardiac involvement included electrocardiography (ECG), transthoracic echocardiography and Holter-ECG. Further investigation in suspected cardiac sarcoidosis was cardiovascular magnetic resonance (CMR), in case of unclear findings a coronary angiography was performed. In brief, cardiac sarcoidosis was diagnosed according to revised guidelines from the Japanese Society of Sarcoidosis and other Granulomatous Disorders (Table1) [7] and additional consideration of clearly defined CMR-criteria in 11 patients [14]. The study was approved by the ethics committee of the Charité-University Medicine Berlin, Germany.

CMR Studies were performed using a 1.5-T MRI-Scanner (Achieva, Philips Medical Systems, Amsterdam', The Netherlands) with a cardiac-dedicated, five element phased array coil (SENSE), respectively with a body coil at sequences for semiquantitative analysis of myocardial inflammation following the recommendations as described by an International Consensus Group on CMR Diagnosis of Myocarditis [14]. We examined cardiac function (i.e., left ventricular ejection fraction = LVEF, wall motion) with a steady state free precession gradient echo cine sequence (three long axis images and at least three short axis images).

T2-weighted triple-inversion-recovery (STIR) images were acquired during the patient's breath hold by using the body coil in short axis. The following parameters were used: 15-mm section thickness, TE-time of 61-msec. Evidence for regional edema, or a signal intensity ratio of ≥2.0 (signal intensity normalized to skeletal muscle in the same slice), renders T2 findings positive.

EGE was performed before and after the intravenous injection of 0.2 ml of Gadoteridol (ProHance®, Bracco IMAGING Deutschland GmbH, Konstanz, Germany) per kilogram of body weight for acquisition of transverse sections. The following parameters were used: repetition time of one R-R interval, TE-time of 14-msec, 15-mm section thickness. An additional T1-weighted fast spin-echo saturation section was positioned across the atria to reduce the blood-signal. Quantitative evaluation of the signal enhancement (skeletal-muscle normalized myocardial enhancement ratio of ≥4.0 or an absolute enhancement of ≥45%) has been considered as a positive criterion.

LGE images were acquired, on average, 10 minutes after the intravenous administration of a second bolus of Gadoteridol (0.2 ml/kg) by using a look-locker-sequence to clarify the TI-time then recovery of two-dimensional inversion-recovery gradient-echo sequence and a PSIR-sequence on a complete set of short-axis sections (encompassing the entire LV) and three long-axis sections (four-, three- and two-chamber views). LE images were acquired by using 8-mm section thickness. Presence of at least 1 focal lesion with nonischemic regional distribution in inversion recovery-prepared gadolinium-enhanced T1-weighted images was considered a positive criterion.

Data were analyzed using software for evaluating CMR images (cmr[42], Circle Cardiovascular Imaging Inc., Calgary, Canada).

All patients received a complete pulmonary function test (PFT) according to international recommendations [15–17]. The measurements were obtained by using a MasterScreen® Body/Diffusion (CareFusion, Hoechberg, Germany). All collected PFT-parameters were expressed as a percentage of the predicted values, which were obtained from regression equations by Quanjer et al [18] and Cotes et al [19].

CPET was carried out on an electromagnetically braked cycle ergometer (Excalibur Sport, Lode B.V. Groningen, The Netherlands) with respiratory gas exchange analysis on a breath-by-breath basis (MasterScreen® CPX, CareFusion, Hoechberg, Germany) and additional blood gas analysis according to a standardized procedure [20]. The used reference values for peak VO_2/kg (ml/min/kg) are based on the recommendations of Cooper et al. (women: VO_2 max/kg = 42.83– (0.371 * years); men: VO_2 max/kg = 50.02– (0.394 * years)) [21].

OUES was computed by a linear least squares regression from the oxygen uptake (VO_2) on the logarithm of the minute ventilation (VE) according to the following equation: $VO_2 = a * \log_{10} VE + b$. Constant 'a' is called the OUES, as it represents the rate of absolute increase in oxygen uptake in response to a change in minute ventilation. To compare the OUES results from our study group with reference values, we estimated the predicted OUES for age, body surface area (BSA) and sex-matched normal participants according to the equations published by Hollenberg et al. (for women: OUES = 1175–15.8 * age +841 * BSA; for men: OUES = 1320–26.7 * age +1394 * BSA) [22].

Data were analyzed using IBM® SPSS® Statistics 19 for Windows® computer software. All values were reported as mean ± standard deviation except when specified otherwise. Unpaired Student's t-test and Wilcoxon signed-rang-test were used for appropriate comparisons. Relationships between variables were assessed by the Pearson's correlation coefficient (r). The receiver operating characteristic (ROC) curve method was used to plot the true positive rate (sensitivity) in function of the false positive rate (1-specificity) for different cut-off points of predicted OUES values.

To test the simultaneous influence of other independent predictor variables on the dependent target variable (cardiac sarcoidosis) and to reduce the risk of overfitting the data we used a binary logistic regression model with stepwise forward selection ($p_{in}<0.05$; $p_{out}>0.1$). The following candidate variables were used: radiographic stage (Typ 0 through Typ IV), FEV_1 (absolute value in L), DLCO/VA (%pred), LVEF (%),VO_2max (absolute value in ml/min/kg), OUES (absolute value in ml/min/log(ml/min)). This analysis was repeated with the cut-off value identified in the ROC-analyses in order to yield maximal clinical applicability. Results of the multivariable analysis are reported as β-coefficient, 95% confidence intervals and p-value. A *p*-value of less than 0.05 was reported as significant for all analyses.

Results

A total of 37 patients (mean age 44.9±13.8 years; 11 female) was assessed. Demographic, clinical and diagnostic findings for the groups with cardiac sarcoidosis (11/37, 30%) and without cardiac sarcoidosis are shown in Tables 2 and 3. Age, gender, height, weight, Body Surface Area and Body Mass Index did not differ significantly between the two groups. Only the radiographic distribution of pulmonary stages was unevenly distributed with more advanced stages among patients with cardiac involvement ($p = 0.031$).

Only 1/37 patients (3%) could not be examined by CMR during the study because he presented a symptomatic 2nd degree AV block (Mobitz II), and a pacemaker had to be implanted. However, in this case a transthoracic echocardiography was performed and showed regional wall motion abnormalities with normal LV-function and exclusion of pericardial effusion, so that the patient was not excluded from the study. Of the other 36 patients, 4/36 (11%) had pericardial effusion, 9/36 (25%) patients had increased global myocardial early gadolinium enhancement (EGE) ratio in T1-weighted images, 8/36 (22%) patients had regional or global myocardial SI increase in T2-weighted images and 6/36 (17%) had local myocyte injury and/or scar, confirmed by myocardial late gadolinium enhancement (LGE) with typical nonischemic regional distribution [23].

In 5 patients (14%) cardiac involvement was diagnosed according to revised guidelines of diagnosing cardiac sarcoidosis from the Japanese Society of Sarcoidosis and Other Granulomatous Disorders including CMR-findings (Tab. 1) [7]. The remaining 6 patients (17%) of the cardiac sarcoidosis group presented at least two of the three tissue-based CMR-findings for myocardial inflammation and fulfilled the proposed diagnostic CMR criteria (i.e., Lake Louise Consensus Criteria) for myocarditis [14]. It is likely that abnormalities on CMR in these patients represent cardiac sarcoidosis even in the absence of clinical cardiac abnormalities[24].

Cardiac function (LVEF) was mildly impaired on average, but significantly poorer in the patient group with cardiac sarcoidosis compared to the group without cardiac sarcoidosis due to the sarcoidosis associated heart failure after exclusion of other possible causes (57±7 vs 68±5%, $p<0.0001$). Nevertheless, both groups were in the range of preserved ejection fraction.

No significant differences in the preserved lung function parameters between the two groups (CS-group vs non-CS-group) were observed (Tab. 2). 10/37 (27%) patients presented a ventilatory dysfunction as defined by ATS/ETS guidelines [17] (4/11, 36% in CS-group vs 6/26, 23% in non-CS-group, $p = 0.544$). 22/37 (59%) patients showed a decreased transfer factor (i.e., DLCO corrected for Hb <80% of predicted; 8/11, 73% in CS-group vs 14/26, 54% in non-CS-group, $p = 0.384$).

All patients completed the cardiopulmonary exercise test (CPET) without any complication. Mean peak respiratory exchange ratio (RER) was 1.14±0.11. Only two patients stopped the exercise test before reaching the metabolic exertion (i.e., peak RER <1.0) due to pulmonary limitations (1/11, 9% in CS-group vs 1/26, 4% in non-CS-group, $p = 0.806$).

Mean peak VO_2 values were 22.1±5.8 and 68.5±19.3 when expressed respectively in ml/min/kg and as percent of predicted value. In comparison to the patient group without cardiac sarcoidosis the patients with cardiac involvement had lower peak VO_2-values (18.3±5.9 vs 23.7±5.1 ml/min/kg, $p = 0.014$) and significantly lower percentage of predicted peak VO_2-values (55.9±21.2 vs 73.9±16.0%pred., $p = 0.005$) (Figure 1 upper left and right panel).

Mean maximal $AaDO_2$ was 36.2±11.3 mmHg and showed no significant difference between both groups (38.9±12.5 vs 35.1±10.8 mmHg, $p = 0.358$).

In the entire study population, OUES could be calculated and ranged from 855.79 to 4756.39 [ml/min/log(ml/min)] (mean ± SD: 2177.56±824.15). Absolute OUES values and percentage of predicted OUES values according to the equations released by Hollenberg et al. were significantly poorer in the patient group with evidence of cardiac sarcoidosis (1669.70±635.82 vs 2392.43±809.25 [ml/min/log(ml/min)], $p = 0.013$ and 59.3±19.1

Table 2. Summary of Demographic, CMR-, Pulmonary function tests and CPET-Data (n = 37).

	Group with Cardiac Sarcoidosis	Group without Cardiac Sarcoidosis	p-value
	(n = 11)	(n = 26)	
Mean age [yrs]	44.3±14.6	45.1±13.7	NS
Pulmonary stage (0/I/II/III/IV)	(0/1/4/3/3)	(1/5/18/1/1)	0.031‡
height [cm]	177.5±12.6	175.7±10.8	NS
weight [kg]	82.4±15.4	84.7±15.2	NS
BMI [kg/m2]	26.0±3.2	27.5±4.8	NS
BSA [m2]	1.99±0.24	2.00±0.21	NS
CMR-findings	**(n = 10)**	**(n = 26)**	
Myocardial EGE (SI)	4.4 (3.0–22.2)	2.9 (1.2–6.6)	0.006‡
T2 signal intensity (SI)	2.0 (1.6–2.7)	1.7 (1.2–2.0)	0.013§
LGE (n)	6/10 (60%)	0/26 (0%)	<0.0001‡
Abnormal wall motion (n)	6/10 (60%)	2/26 (7.7%)	<0.0001‡
Mean LVEF [%]	56±9	67±6	<0.0001§
Pericardial effusion (n)	2/10 (20%)	2/26 (7.7%)	NS
Pulmonary function tests	**(n = 11)**	**(n = 26)**	
FEV1 (%pred)	78.7±16.4	86.9±19.8	NS
VC (%pred)	77.1±21.9	89.7±13.5	NS
TLC (%pred)	88.4±18.8	100.8±14.8	NS
DLCO (%pred)	61.1±23.6	78.0±18.0	NS
CPET	(n = 11)	(n = 26)	
Peak VO2 abs. [ml/min/kg]	18.3±5.9	23.7±5.1	0.014§
Peak VO2 (%pred)*	55.9±21.2	73.9±16.0	<0.005§
RER max.	1.19±0.14	1.12±0.08	NS
AaDO2 max. [mmHg]	38.9±12.5	35.1±10.8	NS
OUES abs. [l/min/log(l/min)]	1669.70±635.82	2392.43±809.25	0.013§
OUES (%pred)†	59.3±19.1	88.0±15.4	<0.0001§

BMI = body mass index; BSA = body surface area; CMR = cardiovascular magnetic resonance; LVEF = left ventricular ejection fraction; CPET = cardiopulmonary exercise testing; EGE = Early gadolinium enhancement; LGE = Late gadolinium enhancement.
*Reference values according to equations published by Cooper et al. [21]
†Reference values according to equations published by Hollenberg et al [22].
‡Wilcoxon signed-rang-test.
§Unpaired Student's t-test.

vs 88.0±15.4%pred., *p<0.0001*, respectively) (Figure 1, lower left and right panel).

When related to the resting cardiac function, LVEF showed a positive correlation with predicted peak VO_2 values ($r = 0.414$, $p = 0.012$). Moreover, LVEF was significantly and directly related to predicted OUES values ($r = 0.443$, $p = 0.007$).

In order to assess and compare operative characteristics of OUES for the distinctions between patients with and without cardiac sarcoidosis, ROC-curves were plotted. The area under curve (AUC) was 0.879 (95% CI: 0.73 to 1.03, $p<0.0001$) (Figure 2). 70% of predicted OUES as cut-off point had the largest diagnostic discriminatory power for diagnosing cardiac sarcoidosis (96% sensitivity, 82% specificity and 89% overall accuracy) (Table 4).

Multivariable Analyses

When all candidate variables were included in the regression model only OUES and LVEF were significantly associated with the presence of cardiac sarcoidosis (Table 5). When the cut off point (70% of predicted) for OUES was used in the model, it returned as the strongest predictor of cardiac sarcoidosis (Odds ratio: 100.43, 95% CI: 1.99 to 5064, $p<0.001$). LVEF remained as a clinical predictor (Odds ratio: 0.776, 95% CI: 0.578 to 1.042, $p = 0.092$) in both models, but contributed little improvement (correct classified with OUES (70%pred) 91.7%, adding LVEF 94.4%).

Radiographic findings (i.e., pulmonary stage of sarcoidosis according to chest x-ray) did not fulfill inclusion criteria of this method. In addition, neither PFT-parameters associated with ventilatory impairment nor PFT-parameters associated with gas exchange disorder qualified for the regression model with cardiac sarcoidosis as the dependent variable (p_{in} <0.05).

Discussion

The main findings of the present study were: (1) cardiac sarcoidosis is associated with a poor cardiovascular response to exercise and can be verified by CPET. (2) Patients with cardiac sarcoidosis had significantly lower levels of OUES due to the sarcoidosis associated heart failure. (3) A cut-off point of OUES (70% of predicted according to equations published by Hollenberg et al) was able to discriminate between patients with and without

Table 3. Eleven patients with evidence for Cardiac Sarcoidosis (CS).

Patient #	Age (yrs)/Sex	Chest x-ray	CMR-criteria (tissue marker)	T2-STIR/EGE/LGE	ECG	Decreased LVEF/abnormal wall motion	LVEF	Pericardial effusion	OUES	OUES
		(Pulmonary stage)					[%]		[ml/min/log]	[%pred.]
1	46/w	4	(2/3)	no/yes/yes	normal	no/yes	54	no	855.79	47
2*	51/m	4	(1/3)	no/no/yes	1st AV block, PVC	yes/yes	45	no	900.70	35
3	61/m	3	(3/3)	yes/yes/yes	left-axis deviation	no/no	61	no	2381.76	99
4*	71/m	4	(1/3)	no/yes/no	complete RBBB	yes/yes	43	no	1436.38	57
5	30/m	1	(2/3)	yes/yes/no	normal	no/yes	61	yes	1521.59	45
6	51/w	3	(2/3)	no/yes/yes	normal	no/no	65	no	964.73	56
7*	33/m	2	(1/3)	no/yes/no	pathological Q	yes/yes	60	no	1336.43	40
8	47/m	2	(2/3)	no/yes/yes	LBBB	no/no	67	no	2372.60	82
9	45/m	3	(1/3)	no/no/yes	normal	yes/yes	49	yes	2335.01	67
10	22/m	2	(2/3)	yes/yes/no	normal	yes/yes	54	no	1787.81	53
11†	30/m	2	no CMR	no CMR	2nd AV block, PVC, left-axis deviation	no/yes	no CMR	no	2473.88	71

CMR = Cardiovascular Magnetic Resonance; EGE = Early myocardial Gadolinium Enhancement; LGE = Late myocardial Gadolinium Enhancement; LVEF = Left Ventricular Ejection Fraction; ECG = Electrocardiogram; OUES = oxygen uptake efficiency slope; RBBB = right bundle branch block; LBBB = left bundle branch block; PVC = premature ventricular contraction.
*Coronary angiography excluded significant obstructive coronary artery disease.
†no CMR because of implanted pacemaker.

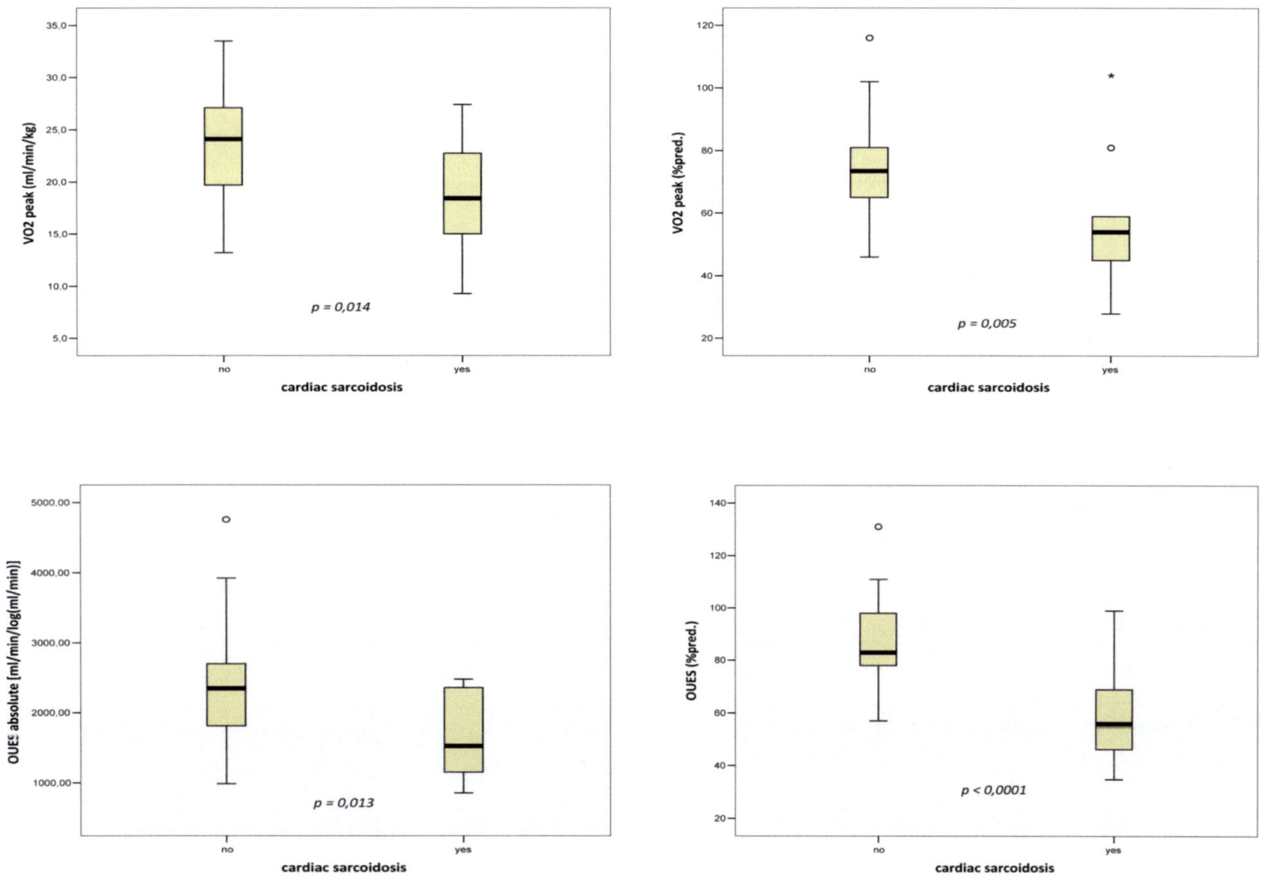

Figure 1. Comparison of CPET parameters in patients with and without cardiac sarcoidosis (CS). Peak VO_2 [ml/min/kg] upper left, peak VO_2 [% of predicted] upper right, OUES [ml/min/log(ml/min)] lower left, and OUES (% of predicted) lower right panel. All panels: Outliers (values that are between 1.5 and 3 times the interquartile range) are represented by circles beyond the whiskers. Extreme values (values that are more than 3 times the interquartile range) are represented by asterisk beyond the whiskers. P-values are given for the univariable comparison.

cardiac sarcoidosis (Odds ratio: 100.43, 95% CI: 1.99 to 5064, $p < 0.001$).

In order to identify and treat patients with cardiac involvement in histologically proven sarcoidosis at an early stage a screening-series of noninvasive diagnostic approaches is recommended. However, the incidence of cardiac involvement is much higher when specific cardiac tests are performed in unselected patients with sarcoidosis [25–27]. This finding underscores the fact, that patients with cardiac sarcoidosis are often asymptomatic and a potentially dangerous cardiac involvement may remain undetected. Several studies showed that cardiovascular magnetic resonance (CMR) imaging improves the sensitivity and specificity of diagnosis of cardiac sarcoidosis [14,28–30]. Late gadolinium enhancement has emerged as the dominant CMR sequence for evaluation of cardiac sarcoidosis [28–30]. Preliminary observations suggest that monitoring gadolinium enhancement may also be helpful in the assessment of the efficacy of steroid therapy [11]. Patel et al. compared late gadolinium enhancement CMR with Japanese Ministry of Health and Welfare (JMH) criteria in a series of 81 patients with biopsy proven extracardiac sarcoidosis [30]. In this study late gadolinium enhancement was more than twice as sensitive for CS as JMH criteria.

In order to assess best diagnostic accuracy of CS, revised Japanese guidelines including late gadolinium enhancement CMR and the CMR criteria according to the International Consensus Group on CMR Diagnosis of Myocarditis were applied in our study [7,14].

The present study investigated the usefulness of CPET with calculation of OUES for the evaluation of patients with sarcoidosis in a setting that could become part of a routine screening.

In line with previous studies, we found that cardiac function (i.e., LVEF) was closely related to OUES [31,32]. Interestingly, we also demonstrated that in patients with sarcoidosis cardiac involvement was associated with a poor cardiovascular exercise performance, both in terms of oxygen uptake (peak VO_2) and oxygen uptake efficiency slope (OUES). Peak VO_2 is strongly influenced by the motivation of the patient, the selected exercise protocol and the tester's subjective choice of the test end point [33]. In contrast, the OUES is an objective and reproducible measure of cardiopulmonary function reserve that can also be measured with submaximal exercise [34]. Therefore, OUES is a better parameter of CPET in order to evaluate patients with sarcoidosis and should be calculated and recorded with peak VO_2.

In the present study, we found that evidence for sarcoid heart failure was associated with decreased levels of oxygen uptake efficiency during exercise. The chance to diagnose cardiac sarcoidosis in patients with an OUES <70% of predicted was 67-times higher than in patients with an OUES >70% of predicted. In addition, only OUES remained in the multiple regression model with cardiac sarcoidosis as the dependent variable, when possible confounders were offered in the statistical

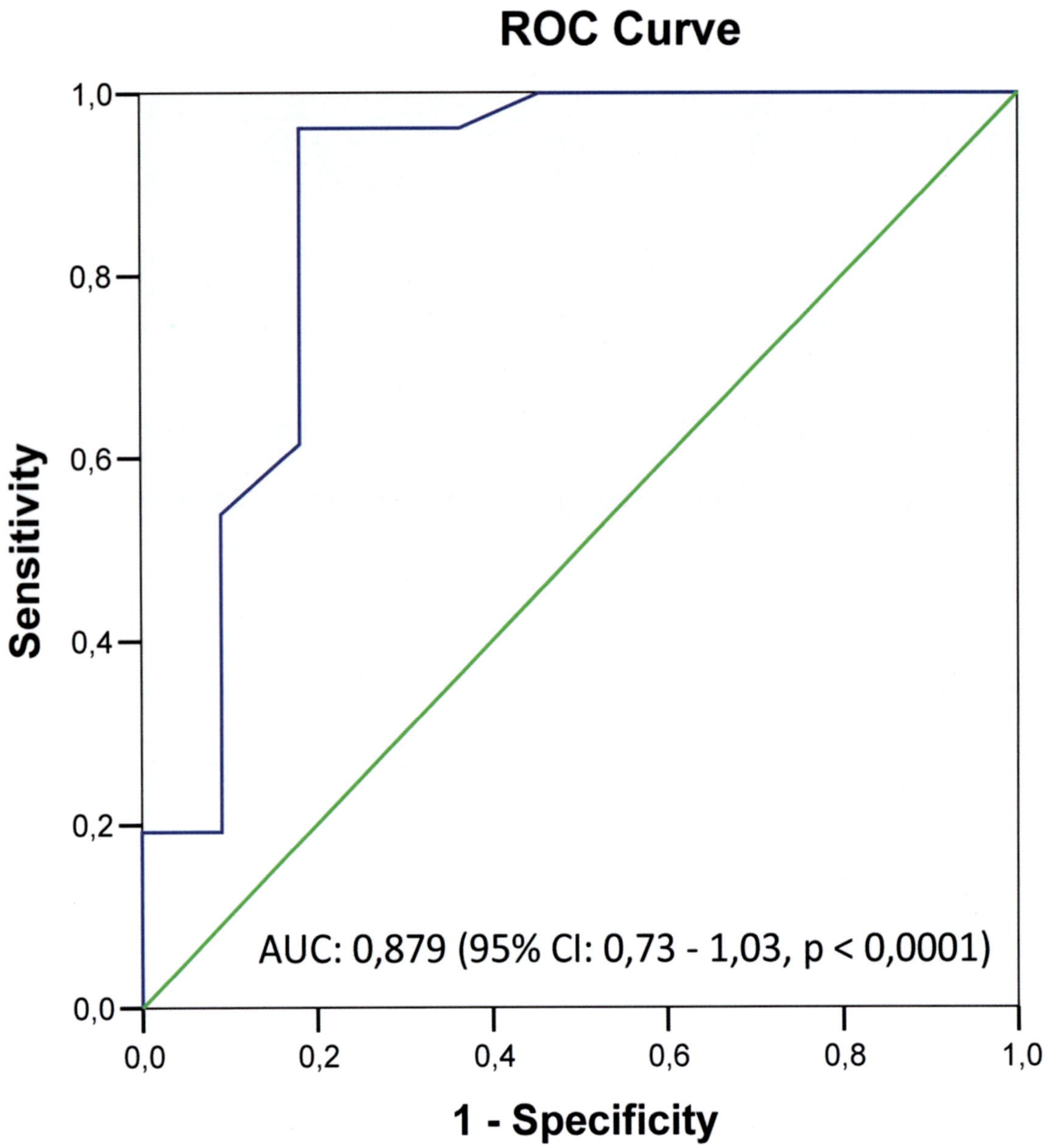

Figure 2. The Receiver Operating Characteristic (ROC) curve of different OUES cut-off points (%pred) and CS diagnosis. A OUES < 70% of predicted as cut-off point had the largest diagnostic discriminatory power for diagnosing cardiac sarcoidosis.

Table 4. Association between observed and predicted cardiac sarcoidosis according to the best OUES cut-off point at 70% of predicted.

	Predicted			
	No Cardiac sarcoidosis (n = OUES >70%pred)	*Cardiac sarcoidosis* (n = OUES <70%pred)	*Total* (n)	*Percentage* correct (%)
Observed				
No cardiac sarcoidosis (n)	25 (true negative)	1 (false positive)	26	96.2
Cardiac sarcoidosis (n)	3 (false negative)	8 (true positive)	11	72.7
Overall correct (%)				89.2

Table 5. Results of the multivariable analyses (stepwise forward $p_{in}<0.05$; $p_{out}>0.1$).

Variable	Values	β-coefficient	95% Confidence interval	p-value
Continuous Values				
OUES	% predicted	0.942	0.886–1.01	0.056
LVEF	continuous	0.751	0.591–0.944	0.014
radiographic stage	Stage 0–4	Excluded from the model	-	0.234
FEV1	continuous	Excluded from the model	-	0.326
VO2max	continuous	Excluded from the model	-	0.069
DLCO/VA	% predicted	Excluded from the model	-	0.206
Categorical Values				
OUES	categorical (cut-off 70% pred)	100.434	1.992–5064	0.021
LVEF	continuous	0.776	0.578–1.042	0.092
radiographic stage	Stage 0–4	Excluded from the model	-	0.215
FEV1	continuous	Excluded from the model	-	0.911
VO2max	continuous	Excluded from the model	-	0.871
DLCO/VA	% predicted	Excluded from the model	-	0.807

Two models were calculated with either OUES in continuous (upper table) or as categorical values (70% predicted, lower table).

model. Therefore these findings strongly suggest that a reduced cardiovascular performance measured by OUES is associated with cardiac sarcoidosis.

In the interpretation of our study results, some possible limitations have to be discussed. First, the number of included patients was limited and our results should be prospectively confirmed in a larger cohort, before CPET and OUES is introduced into the assessment routine of patients with sarcoidosis. However, the predictive power of OUES for results of CMR was strong (OR 67) and plausible which makes controversial future findings unlikely. Secondly, we cannot rule out that the degree of physical fitness and the extent of pulmonary impairment may also affect the relationship between oxygen uptake and ventilation during exercise in individual patients with sarcoidosis [35]. For example, the false positive tested patient in our study showed a moderate restrictive ventilatory impairment and a significant gas exchange disorder in rest and during exercise. Third, we did not analyze complete medication history and future longitudinal studies are needed to determine whether a therapy with corticosteroids or other immunosuppressants is also associated with an increase of OUES in patients with cardiac sarcoidosis. The effect of drug intervention could be a plausible reason for the false negative findings in our study. But we felt that the diagnosis of cardiac sarcoidosis was only firmly established when patients with less than three CMR-criteria also fulfilled the Japanese Society Criteria. The may have biased the results towards sicker patients. However, we wanted to focus on patients with possible clinical consequences, such as high dose corticosteroid treatment. On one hand, we could therefore include the patient who had already cared for with a cardiac pacemaker and thus clinically cardiac sarcoidosis. On the other hand, the absence of significant functional cardiac disorders could explain the elevated OUES values in the false negative tested patients. It is well known that the clinical manifestations of cardiac sarcoidosis depend upon the location and the extent of the myocardium involved [3]. Roberts et al. reported the result of 113 necropsy patients with cardiac sarcoidosis. They found that the left ventricular free wall is the most common location for granulomas and scars (96%), followed by the intra-ventricular septum (73%). Cardiac infiltration by sarcoid granulomas in these locations may cause diminished systolic contractile function or diastolic dysfunction more frequently.

The diagnosis of cardiac involvement through MRI was limited due to the retrospective nature of this study. This was possibly the absence of a complete stack of short axis images to calculate LV volumes and function and the relative high slice thickness (15 mm) of STIR and EGE images, with consequent low spatial resolution, compared to the current gold standard (6–10 mm, as used for LGE).

Furthermore, recent research pointed out the importance of biomarkers for the prognosis of patients with cardiac involvement of sarcoidosis. Therefore the inclusion of e.g. plasma NT-proBNP [36], high-sensitive cardiac troponin T [37], and NT-proatrial natriuretic peptide [38] in future prospective studies may improve the results.

Conclusion

In conclusion, cardiopulmonary exercise test (CPET) potentially improves detection of cardiac sarcoidosis and should be implemented in the routine evaluation of patients with histologically proven sarcoidosis. Low OUES (<70%pred.), was the single best predictor of cardiac sarcoidosis in our study. Therefore, OUES should be assessed at each examination, also in submaximal tests. Future studies need to confirm OUES as a clinically useful and powerful predictor of cardiac sarcoidosis. In addition, the role of OUES in monitoring of drug-treatment effects in patients with cardiac sarcoidosis will be subject to further investigations.

Acknowledgments

The authors would like to thank Leonore Leischner, Sabrina Moehring, Marina Haesler-Wegener, and Gabriele Schreiber for organizing and performing PFT and CPET in our patients.

Author Contributions

Conceived and designed the experiments: WA JSM TB. Performed the experiments: WA HW CC NS JSM MK RB HW. Analyzed the data: WA TB. Wrote the paper: WA TB CC. Substantial involvement in the revision of the manuscript prior to submission: WA TB NS JSM HW. Study coordinator: WA.

References

1. Iwai K, Sekiguti M, Hosoda Y, DeRemee RA, Tazelaar HD, et al. (1994) Racial difference in cardiac sarcoidosis incidence observed at autopsy. Sarcoidosis 11: 26–31.
2. Silverman KJ, Hutchins GM, Bulkley BH (1978) Cardiac sarcoid: a clinicopathologic study of 84 unselected patients with systemic sarcoidosis. 58: 1204–1211.
3. Roberts WC, McAllister HA, Ferrans VJ (1977) Sarcoidosis of the heart. A clinicopathologic study of 35 necropsy patients (group 1) and review of 78 previously described necropsy patients (group 11). The American journal of medicine 63: 86–108.
4. Kim JS, Judson MA, Donnino R, Gold M, Cooper LT, et al. (2009) Cardiac sarcoidosis. Am Heart J 157: 9–21.
5. Smedema JP, Snoep G, van Kroonenburgh MPG, van Geuns RJ, Dassen WRM, et al. (2005) Cardiac involvement in patients with pulmonary sarcoidosis assessed at two university medical centers in the Netherlands. Chest 128: 30–35.
6. Hiraga H, Yuwai K, Hiroe M (1993) Guideline for the Diagnosis of Cardiac Sarcoidosis: Study Report on Diffuse Pulmonary Diseases (in Japanese)Tokyo, Japan: The Japanese Ministry of Health and Welfare. 23–24.
7. Soejima K, Yada H (2009) The Work Up and Management of Patients with Apparent or Subclinical Cardiac Sarcoidosis: With Emphasis on the Associated Heart Rhythm Abnormalities. Journal of cardiovascular GÇª 578–583.
8. Tadamura E, Yamamuro M, Kubo S, Kanao S, Saga T, et al. (2005) Effectiveness of delayed enhanced MRI for identification of cardiac sarcoidosis: comparison with radionuclide imaging. Am J Roentgenol 185: 110–115.
9. Schulz-Menger J, Wassmuth R, bdel-Aty H, Siegel I, Franke A, et al. (2006) Patterns of myocardial inflammation and scarring in sarcoidosis as assessed by cardiovascular magnetic resonance. Heart 92: 399–400.
10. Iannuzzi MC, Rybicki BA, Teirstein AS (2007) Sarcoidosis. The New England Journal of Medicine 357: 2153–2165.
11. Vignaux O, Dhote R, Duboc D, Blanche P, Dusser D, et al. (2002) Clinical Significance of Myocardial Magnetic Resonance Abnormalities in Patients With SarcoidosisA 1-Year Follow-up Study. Chest 122: 1895–1901.
12. Baba R, Nagashima M, Goto M, Nagano Y, Yokota M, et al. (1996) uptake efficiency slope: a new index of cardiorespiratory functional reserve derived from the relation between oxygen uptake and minute ventilation during incremental. JACC 28: 1567–1572.
13. Van Laethem C, Bartunek J, Goethals M, Nellens P, Andries E, et al. (2005) Oxygen uptake efficiency slope, a new submaximal parameter in evaluating exercise capacity in chronic heart failure patients. Am Heart J 149: 175–180.
14. Friedrich MG, Sechtem U, Schulz-Menger J, Holmvang G, Alakija P, et al. (2009) Cardiovascular Magnetic Resonance in Myocarditis: A JACC White Paper. JACC 53: 1475–1487.
15. Miller MR, Hankinson J, Brusasco V, Burgos F, Casaburi R, et al. (2005) Standardisation of spirometry. The European respiratory journal 26: 319–338.
16. Wanger J, Clausen JL, Coates A, Pedersen OF, Brusasco V, et al. (2005) Standardisation of the measurement of lung volumes. The European respiratory journal 26: 511–522.
17. Laszlo G (2006) Standardisation of lung function testing: helpful guidance from the ATS/ERS Task Force. Thorax 61: 744–746.
18. Quanjer PH, Tammeling GJ, Cotes JE, Pedersen OF, Peslin R, et al. (1993) Lung volumes and forced ventilatory flows. Report Working Party Standardization of Lung Function Tests, European Community for Steel and Coal. Official Statement of the European Respiratory Society. The European respiratory journal Suppl 16: 5–40.
19. Cotes JE, Chinn DJ, Quanjer PH, Roca J, Yernault JC (1993) Standardization of the measurement of transfer factor (diffusing capacity). European Respiratory Journal Suppl 16: 41–52.
20. Weisman IM, Marciniuk D, Martinez FJ, Sciurba F, Sue D, et al. (2003) ATS/ACCP Statement on cardiopulmonary exercise testing. Am J Respir Crit Care Med 167: 211–277.
21. Cooper CB, Storer TW (2001) Exercise Testing and Interpretation: A Practical Guide. Cambridge: Cambridge University Press.
22. Hollenberg M, Tager IB (2000) Oxygen uptake efficiency slope: an index of exercise performance and cardiopulmonary reserve requiring only submaximal exercise. JACC 36: 194–201.
23. Codreanu A, Djaballah W, Angioi M, Ethevenot G+, Moulin F, et al. (2007) Detection of myocarditis by contrastGÇÉenhanced MRI in patients presenting with acute coronary syndrome but no coronary stenosis. Journal of Magnetic Resonance Imaging 25: 957–964.
24. Dubrey SW, Falk RH (2010) Diagnosis and management of cardiac sarcoidosis. Progress in cardiovascular diseases 52: 336–346.
25. Tellier P, Paycha F, Antony I, Nitenberg A, Valeyre D, et al. (1988) Reversibility by dipyridamole of thallium-201 myocardial scan defects in patients with sarcoidosis. American Journal of Medicine 85: 189–193.
26. Ishimaru S, Tsujino I, Takei T, Tsukamoto E, Sakaue S, et al. (2005) Focal uptake on 18F-fluoro-2-deoxyglucose positron emission tomography images indicates cardiac involvement of sarcoidosis. Eur Heart J 26: 1538–1543.
27. Fahy GJ, Marwick T, McCreery CJ, Quigley PJ, Maurer BJ (1996) Doppler echocardiographic detection of left ventricular diastolic dysfunction in patients with pulmonary sarcoidosis. Chest 109: 62–66.
28. Shimada T, Shimada K, Sakane T, Ochiai K, Tsukihashi H, et al. (2001) Diagnosis of cardiac sarcoidosis and evaluation of the effects of steroid therapy by gadolinium-DTPA-enhanced magnetic resonance imaging. American Journal of Medicine 110: 520–527.
29. Smedema JP, Snoep G, van Kroonenburgh MPG, van Geuns RJ, Cheriex EC, et al. (2005) The additional value of gadolinium-enhanced MRI to standard assessment for cardiac involvement in patients with pulmonary sarcoidosis. Chest 128: 1629–1637.
30. Patel MR, Cawley PJ, Heitner JF, Klem I, Parker M, et al. (2009) Detection of myocardial damage in patients with sarcoidosis. Circulation 120: 1969–1977.
31. Davies LC, Wensel R, Georgiadou P, Cicoira M, Coats AJS, et al. (2006) Enhanced prognostic value from cardiopulmonary exercise testing in chronic heart failure by non-linear analysis: oxygen uptake efficiency slope. Eur Heart J 27: 684–690.
32. Baba R, Tsuyuki K, Kimura Y, Ninomiya K, Aihara M, et al. (1999) Oxygen uptake efficiency slope as a useful measure of cardiorespiratory functional reserve in adult cardiac patients. Eur J Appl Physiol Occup Physiol 80: 397–401.
33. Andreacci JL, LeMura LM, Cohen SL, Urbansky EA, Chelland SA, et al. (2002) The effects of frequency of encouragement on performance during maximal exercise testing. Journal of Sports Sciences 20: 345–352.
34. Van Laethem C, Van De Veire N, De Sutter J, Bartunek J, De Backer G, et al. (2006) Prospective evaluation of the oxygen uptake efficiency slope as a submaximal predictor of peak oxygen uptake in aged patients with ischemic heart disease. Am Heart J 152: 297.
35. Gademan MG, Swenne CA, Verwey HF, van de Vooren H, Haest JC, et al. (2008) Exercise training increases oxygen uptake efficiency slope in chronic heart failure. Eur J Cardiovasc Prev Rehabil 15: 140–144.
36. Handa T, Nagai S, Ueda S, Chin K, Ito Y, et al. (2010) Significance of plasma NT-proBNP levels as a biomarker in the assessment of cardiac involvement and pulmonary hypertension in patients with sarcoidosis. Sarcoidosis Vasc Diffuse Lung Dis 27: 27–35.
37. Baba Y, Kubo T, Kitaoka H, Okawa M, Yamanaka S, et al. (2012) Usefulness of high-sensitive cardiac troponin T for evaluating the activity of cardiac sarcoidosis. Int Heart J 53: 287–292.
38. Magri D, Agostoni P, Ricotta A, Pisani L, Cauti FM, et al. (2013) NT-proatrial natriuretic peptide as a possible biomarker of cardiopulmonary involvement in sarcoidosis. Eur J Intern Med 24: 278–284.

Blood Born miRNAs Signatures that Can Serve as Disease Specific Biomarkers Are Not Significantly Affected by Overall Fitness and Exercise

Christina Backes[1*⁹], Petra Leidinger[1⁹], Andreas Keller[2], Martin Hart[1], Tim Meyer[3], Eckart Meese[1¶], Anne Hecksteden[3¶]

1 Department of Human Genetics, Medical School, Saarland University, Homburg/Saar, Germany, **2** Department of Clinical Bioinformatics, Saarland University, Saarbruecken, Germany, **3** Institute of Sports and Preventive Medicine, Saarland University, Saarbruecken, Germany

Abstract

Blood born micro(mi)RNA expression pattern have been reported for various human diseases with signatures specific for diseases. To evaluate these biomarkers, it is mandatory to know possible changes of miRNA signatures in healthy individuals under different physiological conditions. We analyzed the miRNA expression in peripheral blood of elite endurance athletes and moderatly active controls. Blood drawing was done before and after exhaustive exercise in each group. After Benjamini-Hochberg adjustment we did not find any miRNA with significant p-values when comparing miRNA expression between the different groups. We found, however, 24 different miRNAs with an expression fold change of minimum 1.5 in at least one of the comparisons (athletes before vs after exercise, athletes before exercise vs controls and athletes after exercise vs controls). The observed changes are not significant in contrast to the expression changes of the blood born miRNA expression reported for many human diseases. These data support the idea of disease associated miRNA patterns useful as biomarkers that are not readily altered by physiological conditions.

Editor: Szabolcs Semsey, Niels Bohr Institute, Denmark

Funding: This work was supported in part by DFG grants. The funders had no role in study design, data collection and analysis, decision to publish, or preparation of the manuscript.

Competing Interests: The authors have declared that no competing interests exist.

* Email: c.backes@mx.uni-saarland.de

⁹ These authors contributed equally to this work as first authors.

¶ These authors contributed equally to this work as senior authors.

Introduction

A yet increasing number of microRNAs (miRNAs) is identified in various species including *Caenorhabditis elegans* for which the first report on miRNAs has been published in 1993 [1]. As of now, a total of 24,521 entries representing hairpin precursor miRNAs, expressing 30,424 mature miRNA products in 206 species are deposited in miRBase [2,3] (release 20), including more than 2,500 different mature miRNAs for *Homo sapiens*. MiRNAs exert their effect by each regulating hundreds of genes post-transcriptionally and are, thus, involved in a manifold of biological processes including proliferation and differentiation. Beyond their physiological role they are also central to many pathological processes [4]. To better understand the physiological and pathological role of miRNAs, many studies do no longer focus on the effects of single miRNAs but analyze the effects of multiple miRNAs in cellular networks. To this end, expression patterns are determined and signatures are derived for various tissues and for specific diseases. While the overwhelming majority of miRNA expression profiles are reported for solid tissues, there are also numerous studies on miRNA profiles in body fluids [5,6]. In blood, miRNA signatures have been determined both in blood cells and in plasma where they are protected by associated proteins are by inclusion in lipid or lipoprotein complexes [7,8]. Due to their high stability miRNAs are increasingly explored as future biomarkers for a large variety of human diseases including cancer [9–12] but also non cancer diseases [13]. We and others have recently employed standardized operating procedures for measuring blood born miRNA profiles in patients with common adult tumors like lung cancer, childhood cancer like Wilms tumor, and multiple non cancer diseases like multiple sclerosis, chronic obstructive pulmonary disease (COPD), and acute myocardial infarction [14–16]. In a comparative study of 863 microRNAs in 454 blood samples from human individuals with 14 different diseases, we found on average for each disease 103 significantly deregulated miRNAs ($P<0.05$; *t*-test after Benjamini-Hochberg adjustment) [17]. In addition, we recently identified miRNA expression profiles in blood samples of healthy individuals including long-lived individuals with a mean age of 96.4 years. The miRNA expression data revealed a distinct separation between the long-lived individuals and younger controls (P-value $<10^{-5}$) [18]. To better understand the meaning of altered miRNA expression pattern both in diseased and in healthy individuals, it is important to also analyze the effect of physiological challenges to the healthy individuals. As of now there are only very few studies analyzing miRNA expression changes in healthy individuals under various conditions [19,20]. Recently, studies have analyzed the changes of miRNA expression in peripheral blood mononuclear cells [21] and neutrophils after acute exercise [22,23]. Here we set out to determine the impact of acute exercise and long-term exercise training on miRNA expression in peripheral blood of elite endurance athletes and matched controls before and after exhaustive exercise.

Material and Methods

Participants

12 elite endurance athletes (6 males, 6 females; 10 triathletes, 2 cyclists) and 12 age- and sex-matched, moderately active controls participated in the present study. Subject characteristics are summarized in Table 1. All athletes compete on an international level and were mostly recruited at the Olympic training center Saarbrücken. Two of the study subjects participated in the 2012 Olympic Games. Controls were matched for sex and age (±2 years) and are engaged in recreational physical activties only.

All subjects gave written informed consent prior to participation. The study was approved by the local ethics commitees (Ärztekammer des Saarlandes; ID 115/12).

Blood sampling

Participants reported to the laboratory between 8 and 10 a.m. after abstaining from physical exercise for at least 36 hours (A fasting period was not required to enable the recruitment of elite athletes). After a supine rest period of 10 minutes venous blood samples were collected from the antecubital vein by standard techniques. Samples for the determination of miRNA expression were collected in special tubes (PAXgene blood RNA tube, Becton Dickinson, Germany) and stored at −20°C until analysis. Post-exercise blood samples were collected in the same way 30 min after cessation of exercise.

Exercise testing protocol

An exhaustive, stepwise exercise test was conducted on a calibrated cycle ergometer (Excalibur Sport, Lode B.V., Groningen, Netherlands). Initial load was 50 W for women and 100 W for men. Step duration and increment were 3 min and 50 W, respectively. Verbal encouragement was given to all subjects during the final stages of the exercise test. Capillary blood samples for the determination of blood lactate concentration were taken from the hyperemizied earlobe at rest, during the last 15 seconds of each step as well as 1, 3, 5, 7 and 10 min after cessation of exercise. Samples were immediately hemolyzed and analysis carried out using an enzymatic-amperometric system (Super GL, Greiner, Flacht, Germany).

Objective criteria of exhaustion (maximal blood lactate concentration of >8 mmol/l and maximal heart rate of >200-age (years)) were met by all subjects.

RNA Isolation

Total RNA including miRNA was isolated using the PAXgene Blood miRNA Kit (Qiagen GmbH, Hilden, Germany) following the manufacturer's recommendations. Isolated RNA was stored at −80°C. RNA integrity was analysed using Bioanalyzer 2100 (Agilent Technologies, Böblingen, Germany) and concentration and purity was measured using NanoDrop 2000 (Thermo Fisher Scientific, Schwerte, Germany).

miRNA Microarray

Microarray analysis was peformed with samples from 8 endurance atheletes and 8 controls according to the manufacturer's instructions using SurePrint 8×60K Human v16 miRNA microarrays (Agilent, CatNo G4870A) that contain 40 replicates of each of the 1,205 miRNAs of miRBase v16 (http://www.mirbase.org/). In brief, a total of 100 ng total RNA was processed using the miRNA Complete Labeling and Hyb Kit to generate fluorescently labeled miRNA. This method involves the ligation of one Cyanine 3-pCp molecule to the 3′ end of a RNA molecule with greater than 90% efficiency. First, the RNA is dephosphorylated using Calf Intestinal Alkaline Phosphatase (CIP). After the dephosphorylation step, dimethylsulfoxide (DMSO), which is an effective RNA denaturant, is added to the samples and the RNA is heat denaturated to minimize the effect of structure and sequence differences among miRNAs. Using T4 RNA ligase and a 3′, 5′-cytidine bisphosphate which is labelled by a cyanine dye at its 3′ phosphate (pCp-Cy3) miRNA molecules with an additional 3′-cytidine and exactly one cyanine dye on its 3′end are produced. After the labelling reaction, the mixture is dryed in a vacuum centrifuge and resuspended in the hybridization mixture containing hybridization buffer and blocking reagent. Then the microarrays were loaded and incubated for 20 h at 55°C and 20 rpm. To check if the labelling and hybridization was successful, labeling and hybridization spike-in controls were added in the appropriate steps. After several washing steps microarrays were scanned with the Agilent Microarray Scanner at 3 microns in double path mode. Microarray scan data were further processed using Feature Extraction software.

Table 1. Anthropometric data and physical capacity.

	Athletes	Controls	p-value
Sex (♀/♂)	6/6	6/6	n.a.
Age (years)	24±5	25±3	0.73
Heigth (cm)	176±10	173±9	0.52
Body mass (kg)	65±10	69±12	0.41
BMI (kg/m^2)	21±1	23±3	**0.04**
Pmax (W/kg)	5,2±0,5	3,5±0,7	**<0.01**

BMI = body mass index; Pmax = maximal workload attained during the stepwise incremental exercise test.
means ± standard deviation; Statistical testing of differences between groups: 1-way ANOVA.

Statistical data evaluation of microarrays

Using the raw totalProbeSignals generated by the Agilent Feature Exraction Software, we applied quantile normalization and log2 transformed the expression values. After that we kept only miRNAs that were expressed (flagged as detected from the Feature Extraction Software) in all samples of at least one group in a comparison. We carried out parametric t-test (two-tailed, paired for samples from same individuals before and after exercise, unpaired otherwise) for each miRNA separately to detect miRNAs that show different behavior in different groups of blood donors. The resulting p-values were adjusted for multiple testing by Benjamini-Hochberg adjustment [24,25].

Quantitative Real Time Polymerase Chain Reaction (qRT-PCR)

The qRT-PCR was performed with samples from 12 endurance atheletes and 12 controls. Using the miScript PCR System (Qiagen), we analyzed the expression of three miRNAs that were expressed in all 32 samples from the microarray experiment, namely hsa-miR-181a-5p, hsa-let-7c, and hsa-miR-24-3p. RNU48 was used as endogenous control [26–30]. In brief, 100 ng RNA was reverse transcribed using miScript HiSpec Buffer following manufacturers recommendations, but in a final vomlume of 10 µl. The PCR was run in a final volume of 10 µl with 2 µl diluted (1:100) cDNA.

Results

Subject characteristics

Anthropometrical and physical performance data are summarized in Table 1. A significantly lower BMI in elite athletes is caused by slight numerically differences in body weight and height in opposite directions. Maximum performance values for the two groups substantiate the expected contrast in physical capacity.

MicroRNA expression analysis

We analysed the expression of 1,205 different miRNAs in blood of 8 elite endurance athletes and 8 age and sex matched controls. Out of 1,205 tested miRNAs 901 miRNAs were not expressed in any of the analyzed blood samples. A total of 154 miRNAs were expressed in all 32 analyzed blood samples. In detail, in the blood of controls obtained before and after exercise we detected 167 and 161 miRNAs, respectively, and in the blood of athletes obtained before and after exercise we detected 172 and 173 miRNAs, respectively. Overall, we found 173 miRNAs that were expressed in more than 90% of all analyzed samples. Table 2 lists the number of miRNAs that were not expressed in any sample and expressed in only one sample, two samples, etc. of each group.

We grouped all blood samples according to whether they were obtained from controls or endurance athletes and whether they were drawn before or after the exertion. Furthermore, we grouped the samples according to the time point of blood withdrawal (before or after exercise) regardless of the study participants. We did not find any miRNA yielding significant p-values after Benjamini-Hochberg adjustment for the comparisons athletes before vs after exercise, athletes before vs controls before exercise, and athletes after vs controls after exercise. The only significant miRNA hsa-miR-320b after adjustment was found for the comparisons controls before vs controls after exercise (fold change: 1.4) and all samples before vs all samples after exercise (fold change 1.6).

For further analyses, we extracted all miRNAs that showed an absolute expression fold change of at least 1.5 in any of the above mentioned comparisons. This revealed a total of 29 miRNAs

Table 2. Number of miRNAs expressed in 0–8 samples of each group.

	0	1	2	3	4	5	6	7	8	in minimum 1 sample
controls before	940	20	15	13	12	17	7	14	167	265
controls after	917	33	15	17	13	9	20	20	161	288
athletes before	935	20	12	16	8	9	14	19	172	270
athletes after	929	25	14	9	13	13	14	15	173	276

(including 24 different miRNAs). Table 3 lists these miRNAs with fold changes >1.5 for the different comparisons. Figure 1 shows a venn diagram indicating the overlapping miRNAs between the different comparisons.

We found five miRNAs that were differentially expressed based on the fold change criterion in blood samples of the endurance athletes due to heavy exercise. Of those, 2 miRNAs were upregulated and three miRNAs were downregulated. In the control group, heavy exercise resulted in >1.5 fold deregulation of six miRNAs, with three upregulated and three downregulated miRNAs. Interestingly, we found no overlap between the deregulated miRNAs of those two comparisons. Most deregulated miRNAs were found for the comparison of endurance athletes and controls before exercise and likewise for the comparison of endurance athletes and controls after exercise. This fold change based analysis shows that more miRNAs are differentially expressed between controls and endurance-trained athletes than between probands before and after the exhaustive exercise.

We obtained nine miRNAs differentially expressed between endurance athletes and controls comparing all samples obtained before exercise, and also nine miRNAs differentially expressed between endurance athletes and controls comparing all samples obtained after exercise. The comparison of all samples obtained before versus all samples obtained after exercise revealed only one deregulated miRNA.

To validate the microarray results we performed qRT-PCR using blood samples obtained before and after exercise from 12 endurance athletes and 12 controls. Of those, samples from 8 endurance athletes and 8 controls were already used for microarray analysis. In detail, we analyzed the expression of hsa-miR-181a that was >1.5 fold more expressed in controls compared to endurance athletes after exercise (p-value 0.0390), and of hsa-let-7c that was >1.5 fold more expressed in controls compared to endurance athletes before exercise (p-value 0.0275). Furthermore, we analyzed hsa-miR-24, that was only about 1.2 times more expressed in endurance athletes before vs endurance athletes after exercise (p-value 0.0257), controls before vs controls after exercise (p-value 0.0319), and all samples before vs all samples after exercise (p-value 0.0011). These three miRNAs were expressed in all 32 analyzed blood samples according to the microarray analysis. The results of the qRT-PCR were also not significant, but confirmed the results of the microarrays. Although the fold changes were smaller than those revealed by microarray, the direction of regulation was the same (see Figure 2).

Target gene analysis

We extracted the predicted targets from miRDB v4.0 [31] for the 25 miRNAs with fold changes >1.5 for the different comparisons and performed an over-representation analysis using GeneTrail [32]. We found 5 KEGG categories with p-values below 0.05 and FDR adjustment.

We compared the list of predicted targets for the 25 miRNAs with gene expression data of white blood cells published by Büttner et al [33]. In their study they identified 39 upregulated transcripts of 30 different genes and 7 downregulated transcripts of 4 different genes as exercise marker genes. We selected these transcripts and examined whether they are possible targets of the miRNAs that were found to be deregulated in different comparisons in our study. This analysis revealed 35 transcripts from 13 different genes, namely the upregulated *CGI-58, TGFA, F5, SLC2A3, REPS2, MME, MOSC1, ABAT, TRIB1*, and *IL1RAP* and the downregulated *PTGDR, FAM115A*, and *YES1*, that might be targeted by the deregulated miRNAs identified in our study (see Table 4).

Comparison of the miRNA expression profile of athletes with published data

We extracted the microarray data from Radom-Aizik et al. [21] deposited in the GEO database (GSE28745) and compared their results to ours. A total of 17 out of 34 miRNAs deregulated in the Radom-Aizik study were expressed in all of the 32 tested samples of our study, 10 miRNAs were expressed in 22 to 31 samples, one miRNA was only expressed in two samples, and six miRNAs were not expressed in any of the tested samples. Only miRNA hsa-miR-181a, significantly deregulated in the Radom-Aizik study was also more than 1.5-fold deregulated in our study. We have to point out that the study designs differed in that Radom-Aizik et al. analyzed the expression of 723 miRNAs in peripheral mononuclear cells (PBMC) from untrained individuals before and after exercise whereas we analyzed the expression of 1205 miRNAs in whole blood of athletes before and after exertion. We found an overlap of 700 miRNAs present on both microarray types. To determine only the influence of the different sample types (PBMC vs whole blood) and participants (untrained vs athletes) independent of the exercise protocols, we compared the microarray data of both studies. Of the 700 miRNAs present on the microarrays of both studies, 202 were expressed in all samples from Radom-Aizik before exercise and 125 were expressed in our study in all 8 endurance athletes and 119 were expressed in all 8 control samples before physical activity. Out of the 202 miRNAs expressed in all samples before exercise from Radom-Aizik, a total of 53 and 52 miRNAs were not expressed in our samples from endurance and controls before exercise, respectively. Figure 3 shows a heatmap for the 50 miRNAs with highest variance and all samples obtained before and after exercise analyzed in our study and by Radom-Aizik et al. and clearly illustrates the differences between both studies relying on the different study designs.

Discussion

In our study we set out to examine the effect of exhaustive exercise on the miRNome of whole blood of both elite endurance athletes and sex and age matched moderately active controls. We identified a total of 25 miRNAs that were >1.5-fold differentially expressed between blood samples obtained from elite endurance athletes and controls. However, their deregulation was in most cases not statistically significant after adjustment. In detail, we found five miRNAs deregulated after exhaustive exercise in elite endurance athletes, namely hsa-miR-144*, hsa-miR-150, hsa-miR-320b, hsa-miR-3656, and hsa-miR-494. Some of those miRNAs have already been reported to be involved in haematopoiesis. The miR-451/miR-144 cluster has been found to play a crucial role in erythropoiesis and the miRNA hsa-miR-150 is involved in myelopoiesis, megakaryopoiesis, B- and T-cell development, and NK cell development [34–36]. Six miRNAs were altered in expression due to exhaustive exercise in controls, namely hsa-miR-1260, hsa-miR-27a, hsa-miR-30e, hsa-miR-320c, hsa-miR-320d, and hsa-miR-320e. Besides others, the miR-30 family regulates the expression of *BCL6* and *PRDM1* that are involved in interleukine and interferone production [35]. Interestingly, there was no overlap in the miRNAs deregulated after exercise in endurance athletes and controls. However, samples from elite endurance athletes and controls in rest differed in nine miRNAs. After exhaustive exercise the differences in eight of nine miRNAs disappeared, but eight additional other miRNAs were differentially expressed. The one overlapping miRNA hsa-miR-98 is part of the let-7 cluster and is deregulated in activated human platelets [36].

Table 3. miRNAs with fold change >1.5 in the different comparisons.

		median group 1	median group 2	logqmedian	median fold change	ttest rawp	AUC	
athletes	hsa-miR-494	5,184173398	5,896861896	−0,712688498	−1,638855321	0,097997900	0,7578125	up
before vs	hsa-miR-150	10,72359337	11,4038118	−0,680218429	−1,602382343	0,268030702	0,6328125	up
althletes after	hsa-miR-3656	7,282186154	6,694879568	0,587306586	1,502439175	0,057284503	0,3828125	down
	hsa-miR-144*	6,180073597	5,502584859	0,677488738	1,599353377	0,560463180	0,3984375	down
	hsa-miR-320b	10,00967385	9,325617772	0,684056075	1,60665044	**0,030736681**	0,359375	down
athletes	*hsa-miR-563*	2,311943693	3,209581359	−0,897637666	−1,863012902	0,171494856	0,75	up
before vs	*hsa-miR-3180-3p*	3,69575586	4,352516391	−0,656760531	−1,576538641	0,30978821	0,609375	up
controls	hsa-miR-629	3,389998045	2,795845641	0,594152404	1,509585431	**0,043596785**	0,2109375	down
before	hsa-let-7b	11,80686722	11,15338943	0,653477739	1,572955427	0,166432114	0,296875	down
	hsa-miR-182	3,920389491	3,258942332	0,661447159	1,581668391	0,194567263	0,3203125	down
	hsa-let-7c	7,881850981	7,204856236	0,676994746	1,598805838	**0,027465882**	0,1640625	down
	hsa-miR-98	4,53605938	3,81236171	0,72369767	1,651409226	0,050531661	0,203125	down
	hsa-miR-144*	6,180073597	5,406467128	0,773606459	1,709537973	0,675212368	0,4921875	down
	hsa-miR-183	6,461844278	5,678446337	0,783397941	1,721179952	0,0590943	0,234375	down
athletes after	*hsa-miR-27a*	3,65966376	4,551620012	−0,891956253	−1,855690681	0,346005439	0,6484375	up
vs controls	*hsa-miR-1274a*	3,539826718	4,399130323	−0,859303605	−1,814162396	0,233977017	0,6484375	up
after	hsa-miR-4286	4,34102114	5,161308005	−0,820283864	−1,76575706	0,281432877	0,65625	up
	hsa-miR-148a	3,115085426	3,930077176	−0,814991751	−1,759288093	0,203644838	0,71875	up
	hsa-miR-30e	4,214221792	4,910975925	−0,696754133	−1,620853986	0,80986352	0,5	up
	hsa-miR-98	4,308581136	3,706456759	0,602124377	1,517950112	0,220850161	0,296875	down
	hsa-miR-181a	6,218547498	5,588206679	0,630340819	1,54793063	**0,039032053**	0,1953125	down
	hsa-miR-197	6,814805493	6,130665142	0,684140351	1,606744296	0,354239372	0,359375	down
	hsa-miR-320b	10,00967385	9,325617772	0,684056075	1,60665044	**0,00004845**	0,3515625	down
all samples before vs all samples after	hsa-miR-1260	3,866717805	4,579511597	−0,712753792	−1,638974936	0,185206743	0,75	up
controls	hsa-miR-30e	4,222505424	4,910975925	−0,688470501	−1,611574073	0,210651178	0,6015625	up
before vs	*hsa-miR-27a*	3,906470607	4,551620012	−0,645149405	−1,563901235	0,138004582	0,65625	up
controls after	hsa-miR-320d	9,473326877	8,858763331	0,614563545	1,531094729	**0,001930516**	0,28125	down
	hsa-miR-320e	8,814483484	8,194836789	0,619646596	1,536498859	**0,015668754**	0,25	down
	hsa-miR-320c	8,609153145	7,937844648	0,671308497	1,592516696	**0,002253772**	0,2109375	down

miRNAs in italics are not expressed in all 32 tested samples. Numbers in bold are statistically significant p-values.

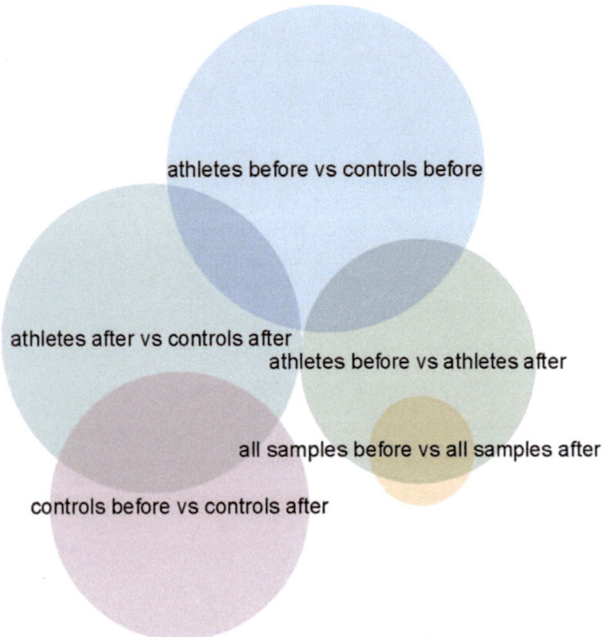

Figure 1. Venn diagram of the miRNAs with fold changes >1.5 in the different group comparisons.

The identification of miRNAs that are indicative for the individual fitness level or training load and the knowledge on the target genes that are regulated by those miRNAs might give insight into the physiological aspects connected with sports. A target gene analysis for the 25 miRNAs that were >1.5-fold deregulated in the different comparisons of our study revealed influences on five KEGG pathways. Most interestingly, we found a significant enrichment (p-value 0.0018) of genes involved in the neurotrophin signaling pathway. Neurotrophins are involved in the proliferation, differentiation, survival and death of neuronal and non-neuronal cells and are implicated in neurodegenerative disorders [37]. It is known that physical activity positively influences mental function. Several neurotrophic factors are increased due to physical activity [38].

Radom-Aizik et al. analyzed the expression of miRNAs in peripheral blood mononuclear cells (PBMC) obtained from untrained individuals before and after exercise and identified 34 significantly >1.2-fold deregulated miRNAs. We only found a small overlap of deregulated miRNAs identified in their study compared with our results. This might be explained by the differences in study design, as we analyzed the miRNA expression pattern of whole blood obtained from athletes. As PBMC account for only about 1% of cells in whole blood it is conceivable that slight changes in miRNA content of leucocytes might be masked. These discrepancies are also underlined by the heatmap of the 50 miRNAs with highest variance and all samples of our study and the Radom-Aizik study. The heatmap is separated into 4 clusters with one cluster comprising miRNAs that are known to be enriched in red blood cells, namely hsa-miR-451, hsa-miR-486-5p, and hsa-miR-92a [39] or involved in erythropoiesis, namely hsa-miR-185 [40]. On the other hand, our findings might also indicate that heavy exhaustive exercise has a lower effect on athletes than on untrained individuals, suggesting a general influence of the fitness level on the miRNA expression pattern in blood. This hypothesis is underlined by the findings that the samples obtained before exercise from endurance athletes and controls differ in 9 miRNAs and that we did not find any overlap between the comparisons of samples obtained before and after exercise from endurance athletes and controls, respectively. We hypothesize that the individual fitness level impacts the dimension of miRNA expression changes due to exercise.

The observed changes of the miRNA expression in the present study were, however, not statistically significant. In a multicenter study we previously compared the blood expression profiles of 863

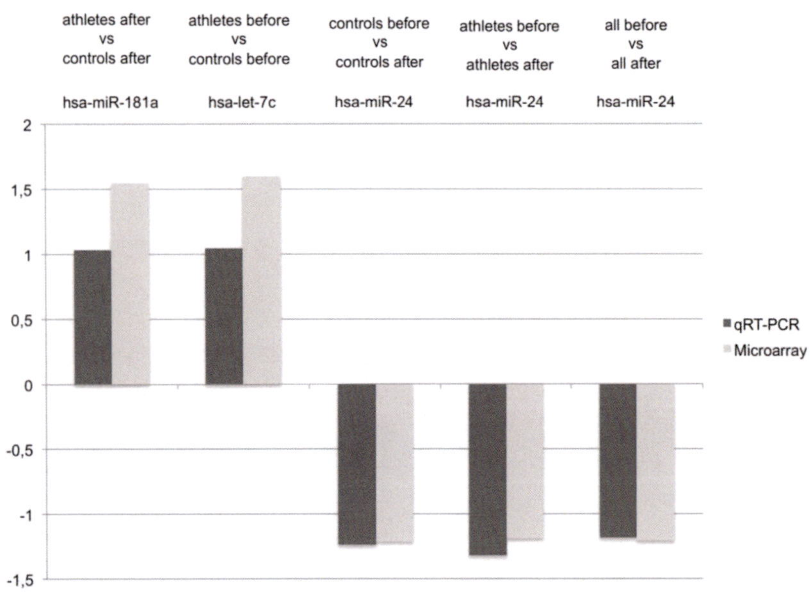

Figure 2. Comparisons of the fold change of the qRT-PCR and the microarray results. Comparison of the fold changes of three miRNAs found deregulated in different comparisons in the microarray experiment and the corresponding qRT-PCR results. A fold change means an upregulation of the respective miRNA In the first group of the comparison; a negative fold change means a downregulation of the respective miRNA in the first group of the comparison.

Table 4. Genes deregulated after exercise extracted from Büttner et al. [33] and the miRNAs deregulated in different comparisons in our study that are predicted to regulate these genes.

miRNA	Comparison	Transcript	GeneID	GeneName	gene Regulation	miRNA Regulation
hsa-miR-183-5p	athletes before vs controls before	NM_000663	18	ABAT	up	down
hsa-miR-183-5p	athletes before vs controls before	NM_020686	18	ABAT	up	down
hsa-miR-183-5p	athletes before vs controls before	NM_001127448	18	ABAT	up	down
hsa-miR-30e-5p	athletes after vs controls after/controls before vs controls after	NM_016006	51099	CGI-58	up	up/up
hsa-miR-181a-5p	athletes after vs controls after	NM_000130	2153	F5	up	down
hsa-miR-494	athletes before vs athletes after	NM_000130	2153	F5	up	up
hsa-miR-4286	athletes after vs controls after	NM_014719	9747	FAM115A	down	up
hsa-miR-629-5p	athletes before vs controls before	NM_014719	9747	FAM115A	down	down
hsa-miR-181a-5p	athletes after vs controls after	NM_001167930	3556	IL1RAP	up	down
hsa-miR-181a-5p	athletes after vs controls after	NM_134470	3556	IL1RAP	up	down
hsa-miR-197-3p	athletes after vs controls after	NM_001167930	3556	IL1RAP	up	down
hsa-miR-197-3p	athletes after vs controls after	NM_134470	3556	IL1RAP	up	down
hsa-miR-27a-3p	athletes after vs controls after/controls before vs controls after	NM_001167928	3556	IL1RAP	up	up/up
hsa-miR-27a-3p	athletes after vs controls after/controls before vs controls after	NM_001167929	3556	IL1RAP	up	up/up
hsa-miR-27a-3p	athletes after vs controls after/controls before vs controls after	NM_002182	3556	IL1RAP	up	up/up
hsa-miR-494	athletes before vs athletes after	NM_001167928	3556	IL1RAP	up	up
hsa-miR-494	athletes before vs athletes after	NM_001167929	3556	IL1RAP	up	up
hsa-miR-494	athletes before vs athletes after	NM_002182	3556	IL1RAP	up	up
hsa-miR-181a-5p	athletes after vs controls after	NM_007287	4311	MME	up	down
hsa-miR-181a-5p	athletes after vs controls after	NM_000902	4311	MME	up	down
hsa-miR-181a-5p	athletes after vs controls after	NM_007289	4311	MME	up	down
hsa-miR-181a-5p	athletes after vs controls after	NM_007288	4311	MME	up	down
hsa-miR-27a-3p	athletes after vs controls after/controls before vs controls after	NM_022746	64757	MOSC1	up	up/up
hsa-miR-27a-3p	athletes after vs controls after/controls before vs controls after	NM_000953	5729	PTGDR	down	up/up
hsa-miR-30e-5p	athletes after vs controls after/controls before vs controls after	NM_000953	5729	PTGDR	down	up/up
hsa-miR-1260a	controls before vs controls after	NM_000953	5729	PTGDR	down	up
hsa-miR-181a-5p	athletes after vs controls after	NM_004726	9185	REPS2	up	down
hsa-miR-181a-5p	athletes after vs controls after	NM_001080975	9185	REPS2	up	down
hsa-miR-4286	athletes after vs controls after	NM_004726	9185	REPS2	up	up
hsa-miR-4286	athletes after vs controls after	NM_001080975	9185	REPS2	up	up
hsa-miR-182-5p	athletes before vs controls before	NM_006931	6515	SLC2A3	up	down
hsa-miR-148a-3p	athletes after vs controls after	NM_003236	7039	TGFA	up	up
hsa-miR-148a-3p	athletes after vs controls after	NM_001099691	7039	TGFA	up	up
hsa-miR-150-5p	athletes before vs athletes after	NM_025195	10221	TRIB1	up	up
hsa-miR-182-5p	athletes before vs controls before	NM_005433	7525	YES1	down	down

For certain genes several transcripts are listed. The direction of regulation of the miRNAs and the target genes is given in the last two columns.

miRNAs in 454 analyzed blood samples from 14 different human diseases and found disease-specific alterations of the miRNA pattern [17]. In detail we found miRNA signatures for lung cancer, prostate cancer, pancreatic ductal adenocarcinoma, melanoma, ovarian cancer, gastric tumors, Wilms tumor, pancreatic tumors, multiple sclerosis, chronic obstructive pulmonary disease (COPD), sarcoidosis, periodontitis, pancreatitis, and acute myocardial infarction. For each disease we found an average of 103 deregulated miRNAs ($P<0.05$; *t*-test after Benjamini-Hochberg adjustment). The according blood-borne 'miRNome' data are deposited in the Gene Expression Omnibus and available at http://genetrail.bioinf.uni-sb.de/wholemirnomeproject/. In contrast to the diseases, the miRNome of healthy individuals does not seem to be significantly changed neither by acute exhaustive exercise nor by the long-term effects of training performed by elite endurance athletes.

Conclusions

Although the overall fitness and the exercise do seem to impact the miRNA expression level in human blood cells, the observed changes are not comparable to the expression changes found for human diseases. The deregulation of the miRNAs identified in the present study was in most cases not statistically significant after

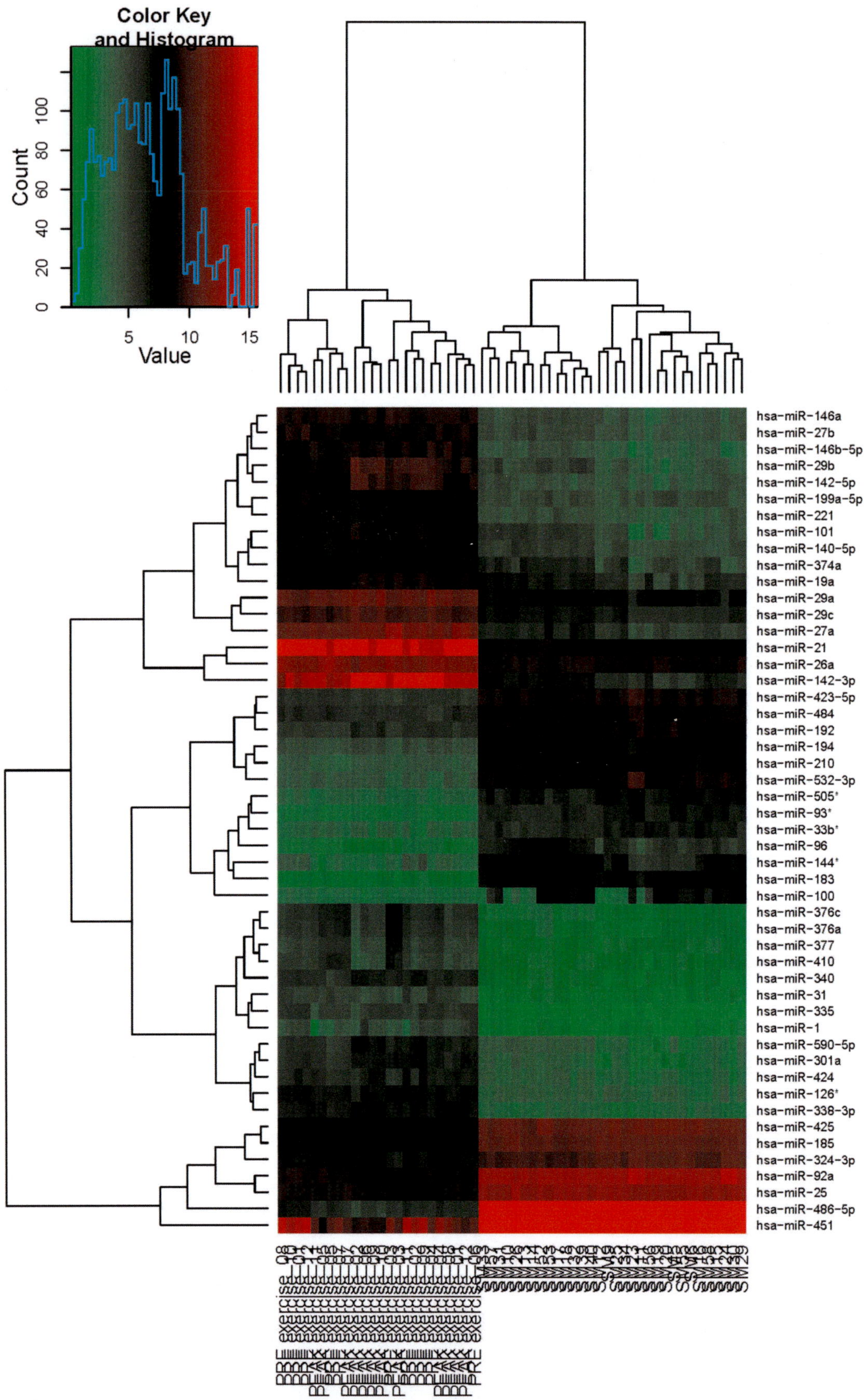

Figure 3. Heatmap for the 50 miRNAs with highest variance and all samples analyzed in the study by Radom-Aizik [21] and in our study.

adjustment. MiRNA patterns appear to be rather robust at least against the influence of training effects. This observation lends further support to the employment of miRNA signatures as disease associated biomarkers.

Author Contributions

Conceived and designed the experiments: TM EM AH. Performed the experiments: PL. Analyzed the data: CB AK. Contributed to the writing of the manuscript: CB PL MH EM AH. Collected blood samples: TM AH.

References

1. Lee RC, Feinbaum RL, Ambros V (1993) The C. elegans heterochronic gene lin-4 encodes small RNAs with antisense complementarity to lin-14. Cell 75: 843–854.
2. Kozomara A, Griffiths-Jones S (2011) miRBase: integrating microRNA annotation and deep-sequencing data. Nucleic Acids Res 39: D152–157.
3. Griffiths-Jones S, Grocock RJ, van Dongen S, Bateman A, Enright AJ (2006) miRBase: microRNA sequences, targets and gene nomenclature. Nucleic Acids Res 34: D140–144.
4. Taft RJ, Pang KC, Mercer TR, Dinger M, Mattick JS (2010) Non-coding RNAs: regulators of disease. J Pathol 220: 126–139.
5. Mitchell PS, Parkin RK, Kroh EM, Fritz BR, Wyman SK, et al. (2008) Circulating microRNAs as stable blood-based markers for cancer detection. Proc Natl Acad Sci U S A 105: 10513–10518.
6. Otaegui D, Baranzini SE, Armananzas R, Calvo B, Munoz-Culla M, et al. (2009) Differential micro RNA expression in PBMC from multiple sclerosis patients. PLoS ONE 4: e6309.
7. Kosaka N, Iguchi H, Ochiya T (2010) Circulating microRNA in body fluid: a new potential biomarker for cancer diagnosis and prognosis. Cancer Sci 101: 2087–2092.
8. Cortez MA, Calin GA (2009) MicroRNA identification in plasma and serum: a new tool to diagnose and monitor diseases. Expert Opin Biol Ther 9: 703–711.
9. Wang ZX, Bian HB, Wang JR, Cheng ZX, Wang KM, et al. (2011) Prognostic significance of serum miRNA-21 expression in human non-small cell lung cancer. J Surg Oncol 104: 847–851.
10. Keller A, Leidinger P, Gislefoss R, Haugen A, Langseth H, et al. (2011) Stable serum miRNA profiles as potential tool for non-invasive lung cancer diagnosis. RNA Biol 8: 506–516.
11. Gotte M (2010) MicroRNAs in breast cancer pathogenesis. Minerva Ginecol 62: 559–571.
12. Yin Y, Li M, Li H, Jiang Y, Cao LY, et al. (2010) [Expressions of 6 microRNAs in prostate cancer]. Zhonghua Nan Ke Xue 16: 599–605.
13. Fu Y, Yi Z, Wu X, Li J, Xu F (2011) Circulating microRNAs in patients with active pulmonary tuberculosis. J Clin Microbiol 49: 4246–4251.
14. Schmitt J, Backes C, Nourkami-Tutdibi N, Leidinger P, Deutscher S, et al. (2012) Treatment-independent miRNA signature in blood of Wilms tumor patients. BMC Genomics 13: 379.
15. Keller A, Leidinger P, Steinmeyer F, Stahler C, Franke A, et al. (2014) Comprehensive analysis of microRNA profiles in multiple sclerosis including next-generation sequencing. Mult Scler 20: 295–303.
16. Meder B, Keller A, Vogel B, Haas J, Sedaghat-Hamedani F, et al. (2011) MicroRNA signatures in total peripheral blood as novel biomarkers for acute myocardial infarction. Basic Res Cardiol 106: 13–23.
17. Keller A, Leidinger P, Bauer A, ElSharawy A, Haas J, et al. (2011) Toward the blood-borne miRNome of human diseases. Nat Meth advance online publication.
18. ElSharawy A, Keller A, Flachsbart F, Wendschlag A, Jacobs G, et al. (2012) Genome-wide miRNA signatures of human longevity. Aging Cell 11: 607–616.
19. Bye A, Rosjo H, Aspenes ST, Condorelli G, Omland T, et al. (2013) Circulating microRNAs and aerobic fitness–the HUNT-Study. PLoS One 8: e57496.
20. Baggish AL, Hale A, Weiner RB, Lewis GD, Systrom D, et al. (2011) Dynamic regulation of circulating microRNA during acute exhaustive exercise and sustained aerobic exercise training. J Physiol 589: 3983–3994.
21. Radom-Aizik S, Zaldivar F, Jr., Leu SY, Adams GR, Oliver S, et al. (2012) Effects of exercise on microRNA expression in young males peripheral blood mononuclear cells. Clin Transl Sci 5: 32–38.
22. Radom-Aizik S, Zaldivar F, Jr., Leu SY, Galassetti P, Cooper DM (2008) Effects of 30 min of aerobic exercise on gene expression in human neutrophils. J Appl Physiol 104: 236–243.
23. Radom-Aizik S, Zaldivar F, Jr., Oliver S, Galassetti P, Cooper DM (2010) Evidence for microRNA involvement in exercise-associated neutrophil gene expression changes. J Appl Physiol 109: 252–261.
24. Benjamini Y, Drai D, Elmer G, Kafkafi N, Golani I (2001) Controlling the false discovery rate in behavior genetics research. Behav Brain Res 125: 279–284.
25. Hochberg Y (1988) A sharper bonferroni procedure for multiple tests of significance. Biometrica 75: 185–193.
26. Bryant RJ, Pawlowski T, Catto JW, Marsden G, Vessella RL, et al. (2012) Changes in circulating microRNA levels associated with prostate cancer. Br J Cancer 106: 768–774.
27. Hirata H, Ueno K, Shahryari V, Deng G, Tanaka Y, et al. (2013) MicroRNA-182-5p promotes cell invasion and proliferation by down regulating FOXF2, RECK and MTSS1 genes in human prostate cancer. PLoS One 8: e55502.
28. Li SC, Essaghir A, Martijn C, Lloyd RV, Demoulin JB, et al. (2013) Global microRNA profiling of well-differentiated small intestinal neuroendocrine tumors. Mod Pathol 26: 685–696.
29. Ratert N, Meyer HA, Jung M, Mollenkopf HJ, Wagner I, et al. (2012) Reference miRNAs for miRNAome analysis of urothelial carcinomas. PLoS One 7: e39309.
30. Srivastava A, Goldberger H, Dimtchev A, Ramalinga M, Chijioke J, et al. (2013) MicroRNA profiling in prostate cancer–the diagnostic potential of urinary miR-205 and miR-214. PLoS One 8: e76994.
31. Wang X (2008) miRDB: a microRNA target prediction and functional annotation database with a wiki interface. RNA 14: 1012–1017.
32. Backes C, Keller A, Kuentzer J, Kneissl B, Comtesse N, et al. (2007) GeneTrail–advanced gene set enrichment analysis. Nucleic Acids Res 35: W186–192.
33. Buttner P, Mosig S, Lechtermann A, Funke H, Mooren FC (2007) Exercise affects the gene expression profiles of human white blood cells. J Appl Physiol 102: 26–36.
34. Edelstein LC, Bray PF (2011) MicroRNAs in platelet production and activation. Blood 117: 5289–5296.
35. Lawrie CH (2013) MicroRNAs in hematological malignancies. Blood Rev 27: 143–154.
36. Osman A, Falker K (2011) Characterization of human platelet microRNA by quantitative PCR coupled with an annotation network for predicted target genes. Platelets 22: 433–441.
37. Chao MV, Rajagopal R, Lee FS (2006) Neurotrophin signalling in health and disease. Clin Sci (Lond) 110: 167–173.
38. Cotman CW, Berchtold NC (2002) Exercise: a behavioral intervention to enhance brain health and plasticity. Trends Neurosci 25: 295–301.
39. Pritchard CC, Kroh E, Wood B, Arroyo JD, Dougherty KJ, et al. (2011) Blood cell origin of circulating microRNAs: a cautionary note for cancer biomarker studies. Cancer Prev Res (Phila).
40. Choong ML, Yang HH, McNiece I (2007) MicroRNA expression profiling during human cord blood-derived CD34 cell erythropoiesis. Exp Hematol 35: 551–564.

Health-Related Behaviors and Effectiveness of Trivalent Inactivated versus Live Attenuated Influenza Vaccine in Preventing Influenza-Like Illness among Young Adults

Tabitha Woolpert[1]**, Christopher J. Phillips**[2*]**, Carter Sevick**[2]**, Nancy F. Crum-Cianflone**[2]**, Patrick J. Blair**[1]**, Dennis Faix**[1]

1 Operational Infectious Diseases, Naval Health Research Center, San Diego, California, United States of America, **2** Deployment Health Research, Naval Health Research Center, San Diego, California, United States of America

Abstract

Background: Vaccination is the preferred preventive strategy against influenza. Though health behaviors are known to affect immunity and vaccine delivery modes utilize different immune processes, data regarding the preferred influenza vaccine type among adults endorsing specific health-related behaviors (alcohol use, tobacco use, and exercise level) are limited.

Methods: The relative effectiveness of two currently available influenza vaccines were compared for prevention of influenza-like illness during 2 well-matched influenza seasons (2006/2007, 2008/2009) among US military personnel aged 18–49 years. Relative vaccine effectiveness was compared between those self-reporting and not reporting recent smoking history and potential alcohol problem, and by exercise level using Cox proportional hazard modeling adjusted for sociodemographic and military factors, geographic area, and other health behaviors.

Results: 28,929 vaccination events and 3936 influenza-like illness events over both influenza seasons were studied. Of subjects, 27.5% were smokers, 7.7% had a potential alcohol-related problem, 10.5% reported minimal exercise, and 4.4% reported high exercise levels. Overall, the risk of influenza-like illness did not significantly differ between live attenuated and trivalent inactivated influenza vaccine recipients (hazard ratio, 0.98; 95% confidence interval, 0.90–1.06). In the final adjusted model, the relative effectiveness of the 2 vaccine types did not differ by smoking status ($p = 0.10$), alcohol status ($p = 0.21$), or activity level ($p = 0.11$).

Conclusions: Live attenuated and trivalent inactivated influenza vaccines were similarly effective in preventing influenza-like illness among young adults and did not differ by health-related behavior status. Influenza vaccine efforts should continue to focus simply on delivering vaccine.

Editor: Mohammed Alsharifi, The University of Adelaide, Australia

Funding: This work was supported by the US Military Vaccine Agency (MILVAX). The funder had no role in study design, data collection and analysis, decision to publish, or preparation of the manuscript.

Competing Interests: The authors have declared that no competing interests exist.

* Email: chris.phillips@med.navy.mil

These authors contributed equally to this work.

Introduction

Certain risky health behaviors, such as tobacco use and significant alcohol consumption, are known to affect disease risk by impairing the immune response. Studies have documented impaired mucosal immunity among smokers compared with nonsmokers [1] and negative cellular and innate immune system effects among excessive alcohol consumers [2–10], providing a basis for a differential vaccine effectiveness of the available influenza vaccines that use different delivery methods. Since smoking and alcohol use are associated with a higher risk of respiratory infections including influenza, defining optimal vaccine strategies among these groups is important for both patient care and public health strategies [11–13].

Vaccination against influenza virus has been a common practice since the vaccine's development in 1945 [14], and is the single most effective prevention strategy [15–17]. Since it is expected that the majority of individuals worldwide will remain susceptible to one or more circulating influenza strains at any given time, continued understanding of optimal vaccine practices is essential. Two of the influenza vaccine types currently licensed in the United States include the trivalent inactivated influenza vaccine (TIV), an older formulation, and live, attenuated influenza vaccine (LAIV), licensed since 2003. TIV is prepared by killing influenza viruses and isolating subvirion or purified surface antigens to create "split" or subunit vaccines [16], while LAIV comprises attenuated live viruses. Vaccine antigens contained in LAIV and TIV are presented to an individual's immune system through markedly different routes: TIV is injected, causing rapid distribution into the bloodstream and induction of a humoral response, while LAIV virions are delivered to the nasopharyngeal epithelial cells where they appear to induce both humoral (mucosal IgA antibody) and cell-mediated immune responses [18].

Because various immune mechanisms are involved to differing degrees between the two vaccine methods, the immune response induced by each could differ among individuals with altered immunity. In addition to smoking and alcohol use, intense exercise may alter immunity through various mechanisms including transient reduced salivary IgA levels [19–24], providing a basis for a potential differential vaccine response to LAIV versus TIV. Likewise, though its immune effects are not well established, a sedentary lifestyle may result in adverse health consequences, while exercise has been shown to boost immunity [25–27]. Hence, differential vaccine responses by exercise level are plausible.

Given the high prevalence of adverse health-related behaviors in the general population [28], a statistical difference in vaccine effectiveness between LAIV and TIV in these risk groups would likely correspond to a significant influenza disease burden that could be eliminated with tailored vaccine protocols. The risk of influenza-like illness (ILI) by vaccine type received among smokers, those with a potential alcohol problem, and those reporting varying levels of exercise was evaluated in this study.

Methods

Study Population and Data Sources

A retrospective cohort study was conducted during 2012–2013 among US military members who completed a health survey for a large prospective Department of Defense study (Millennium Cohort Study) [29] within 2 years of influenza vaccination. Subjects were active-duty members stationed in the United States at the beginning of the influenza season who received influenza vaccination during the 2006/2007 and/or 2008/2009 seasons. These seasons were chosen because vaccine strains were well matched to circulating influenza strains, according to surveillance data published by the Centers for Disease Control and Prevention (CDC) [30–32]. Although 66% of influenza A (H1N1) viruses were found to be similar to the vaccine strain, the 2007/2008 influenza season was excluded as 77% of influenza A (H3N2) and 98% of B viruses were poorly matched [33]. All participants were aged 18–49 years at the time of vaccination since LAIV use is limited to adults ≤49 years of age. Exclusion criteria included a diagnosis of asthma, chronic bronchitis, emphysema, history of shortness of breath, diabetes mellitus, HIV infection, or pregnancy, since LAIV use may have been contraindicated and these conditions may result in suboptimal vaccine responses. Data on preexisting medical diagnoses were obtained from the Millennium Cohort survey and medical records. Additionally, pharmacy records (Pharmacy Data Transaction Service) were used to exclude subjects receiving medications for diabetes mellitus or HIV. Non–active duty military personnel, personnel deployed at the time of study, and members stationed on ships or overseas were excluded because these groups may be exposed to influenza strains not covered in the vaccine and outcomes of interest may not be captured in existing databases. Additionally, military recruits were excluded given their unique risks for respiratory illnesses [34–37].

The type and date of influenza vaccinations were obtained from military records maintained by the Defense Manpower Data Center (DMDC). Annual influenza vaccination is mandatory for active-duty members, though the type of vaccine (TIV or LAIV) is often based on available supply. The study was approved by the Institutional Review Board at the Naval Health Research Center (protocol NHRC.2010.0027), in accordance with 32 CFR §219. 1 16(d) and classified as minimal risk. The IRB waived the requirement to obtain informed consent because it is impractical with numerous record holders that are geographically widely-dispersed, and the decision to waive informed consent will not adversely affect the rights and welfare of the record holders of this study population.

Study Outcome

The outcome of interest was ILI, chosen because laboratory testing for influenza virus is not commonly employed and because ILI has both medical and occupational significance. The diagnosis of ILI was determined by review of *International Classification of Diseases, 9th Revision* (ICD-9) codes in the Military Health System Data Repository, which contains all outpatient and inpatient encounters from military treatment facilities and care provided by TRICARE network providers. An ILI case was defined by the presence of specific ICD-9 codes (Table 1) shown in previous studies to be related to culture-confirmed influenza in military service members [38,39]. Independent of the presence of these ICD-9 codes, anti-influenza medication dispensing (i.e., oseltamivir, zanamivir, amantadine, or rimantadine) documented in pharmacy records was also considered to represent a case.

Outcomes were captured beginning September 1 of each season, and only the first ILI event per subject in each season was considered in the analyses. Subjects with an event during the current influenza season occurring prior to 14 days post vaccination were excluded from analyses to ensure that only vaccinated individuals with adequate time for development of an immune response and no recent influenza infection were studied. Subjects were followed from the time of influenza vaccination (administered September 1–November 30 of each season) until the end of the influenza season (May 19, 2007, and March 28, 2009; the latter season truncated given the emergence of the pandemic H1N1 strain) for occurrence of an ILI outcome, or censoring event [32,40]. Individuals were right-censored if they deployed by land or aboard ship or transferred outside the continental United States. Subjects could contribute to both influenza seasons if they received vaccine and met the inclusion/exclusion criteria during each season.

Exposures of Interest

Three specific exposures of interest were evaluated: recent smoking history, potential alcohol problem, and exercise level. Exposure data were obtained from self-reported survey information from the Millennium Cohort Study. Recent smoking history was defined as reporting both ≥100 cigarettes in a lifetime and cigarette use within the last year. Potential alcohol problems were defined as an affirmative answer to 1 or more of the 5 alcohol questions on the Patient Health Questionnaire [41], which represents a positive screen for alcohol abuse [42]. Exercise was categorized based on the current CDC physical activity recommendations [43]: the number of days exercised per week at a moderate level multiplied by time (in minutes) plus twice the number of days per week of vigorous exercise multiplied by time. If the result was <150 minutes then the exercise level was minimal, and if 6–7 days per week of vigorous activity was reported then the

Table 1. ICD-9 Codes Used To Identify Influenza-like Illness.

ICD-9 Code	Description
079.99	Viral infection, NOS
382.9	Otitis media, NOS
460.0	Nasopharyngitis, acute
461.9	Acute sinusitis, unspecified
465.8	Upper respiratory infection, other multiple sites
465.9	Upper respiratory infection, acute NOS
466.0	Bronchitis and bronchiolitis, acute
486.0	Pneumonia, organism unspecified
487.0	Influenza with pneumonia
487.1	Influenza with other respiratory manifestations
487.8	Influenza with other manifestations
490.0	Bronchitis, not specified as acute or chronic
780.6	Fever
786.2	Cough

level was high; otherwise, the classification was moderate. Those with missing exercise activity data were denoted as unknown.

Covariates

Information on sociodemographic and military-related characteristics were obtained from DMDC and included age, sex, self-reported race/ethnicity, marital status, service branch, military pay grade (enlisted, officer), duty station (coded into four geographic areas), occupation, and deployment history.

Statistical Analyses

Descriptive statistics are presented as numbers (percentages) for categorical variables and medians (interquartile range, IQR) for continuous variables. The univariable associations between the covariates and vaccine type were assessed using logistic regression (for categorical variables) and the Wilcoxon rank-sum test for age (continuous). Crude incidence rates of ILI per 1000 persons per season were compared between the LAIV- and TIV-immunized groups. Cox proportional hazard modeling was used to evaluate the unadjusted and adjusted risk (time to event) for ILI by vaccine type (LAIV vs TIV) as well as other covariates of interest (sociodemographic, military, geographic, and behavioral factors). To test the hypothesis that relative vaccine effectiveness is differential by specific health behavior (smoking, alcohol, and exercise level), an interaction term with vaccine type was added to the model for each behavior. In addition, interactions were evaluated between vaccine type and 3 covariates: sex, service branch, and influenza season. In order to adjust for the potential effects of individuals contributing to multiple seasons, a robust variance estimator was used. To account for individuals receiving the vaccination at different times in relation to the influenza season, a left-truncated model was developed starting survival time at September 1 of the influenza season and truncating on date of vaccination plus 14 days. Follow-up time was measured from September 1 of each influenza season until an outcome was observed or the censor date. A final multivariable model was derived using a backward, stepwise approach and was adjusted for covariates significantly associated with the outcome ($p<0.05$) or that confounded the relationship between vaccine type and ILI by ≥10%. Results of the Cox models are presented as hazard ratios (HRs) and 95% confidence intervals (CIs). All statistical analyses were performed using SAS software, version 9.3 (SAS Institute, Inc., Cary, NC).

Results

Overall, 28,929 vaccination events were studied during the 2 influenza seasons (2006/2007 and 2008/2009), including 22,734 (79%) LAIV and 6195 (21%) TIV administrations. The median age of the cohort was 27 years (IQR, 23–34), 73% were white, and 73% male. Regarding health-related behaviors, 27.5% subjects reported a recent smoking history and 7.7% a potential alcohol problem. Exercise levels were distributed as follows: 10.5% minimal, 70.3% moderate, 4.4% high, and 14.7% unknown (Table 2).

Women, officers, those with a potential alcohol problem, those serving in the Navy or Marine Corps (vs Army or Air Force), those residing in the US Southwest (vs each other region) and in a health care occupation (vs combat or other occupation) were less likely than comparison groups to have received LAIV ($p<0.0001$). Additionally, compared with 2006/2007, those vaccinated in 2008/2009 were more likely to have received LAIV ($p = 0.04$). Vaccine type did not significantly differ by age, smoking status, exercise level, marital status, or race/ethnicity.

During the 2 seasons, 3936 ILI events were diagnosed, for an overall crude ILI incidence rate of 136.1 cases per 1000 person-seasons. Weekly ILI case volume demonstrated a pattern similar to that of positive influenza isolates in the general population reported by CDC over the same time period [30,32]. ILI rates for LAIV and TIV were 138.5 and 127.0 cases per 1000 person-seasons, respectively. The ILI rate by vaccine type did not significantly vary by season.

In the univariable model, type of vaccine was not associated with the development of ILI (HR, 1.02; 95% CI, 0.95–1.11) (Table 3). Factors associated with an increased risk of ILI included recent smoking history, younger age, female sex, other race/ethnicity, and health care occupation. Those serving in the Army or Marine Corps (compared with the Air Force), officers, and combat specialists had a lower risk (Table 3).

In the final multivariate model, adjusted for all significant covariates and using average values for health behaviors in vaccine type interaction terms, the risk of ILI did not significantly differ between LAIV and TIV (HR, 0.98; 95% CI, 0.90–1.06) (Table 4). In the final adjusted model, the relative effectiveness of the 2 vaccine types did not differ by smoking status ($p = 0.10$), alcohol status ($p = 0.21$), or activity level ($p = 0.11$). In addition, ILI risk did not significantly differ by vaccine type among smokers (n = 7955) (HR, 1.09; 95% CI, 0.94–1.27), nonsmokers (n = 20,974) (HR, 0.94; 95% CI, 0.85–1.03), those with a potential alcohol problem (n = 2221) (HR, 1.19; 95% CI, 0.86–1.63), those without an alcohol problem (n = 26,708) (HR, 0.96; 95% CI, 0.89–1.05), those reporting a high exercise level (n = 1283) (HR, 1.12; 95% CI, 0.71–1.76), and those reporting a minimal exercise level (n = 3039) (HR, 1.08; 95% CI, 0.85–1.36) in the model adjusting for sociodemographic factors and the other adverse health behaviors of interest. Similar findings resulted from examining health behaviors by vaccine type for each season separately.

Discussion

This study demonstrated that the relative effectiveness of LAIV versus TIV in preventing ILI among young adults did not vary by health-related behaviors (tobacco, alcohol use, or exercise level) using data from the 2006/2007 and 2008/2009 influenza seasons. These findings are in accordance with current recommendations

Table 2. Population Characteristics[a] Among US Service Members, 18–49 Years of Age, During Two Influenza Seasons (2006/2007, 2008/2009).

	Total Study	2006/2007		2008/2009		Combined Seasons	
Characteristic	**Population**	**TIV**	**LAIV**	**TIV**	**LAIV**	**TIV**	**LAIV**
Number	28,929	2905	10,316	3290	12,418	6195	22,734
ILI event	3936 (13.6)	383 (13.2)	1477 (14.3)	404 (12.3)	1672 (13.5)	787 (12.7)	3149 (13.9)
Recent smoking history	7955 (27.5)	776 (26.7)	2814 (27.3)	941 (28.6)	3424 (27.6)	1717 (27.7)	6238 (27.4)
Potential alcohol problem	2221 (7.7)	292 (10.1)	760 (7.4)	274 (8.3)	895 (7.2)	566 (9.1)	1655 (7.3)
Exercise level							
Minimal	3039 (10.5)	345 (11.9)	1062 (10.3)	360 (10.9)	1272 (10.2)	705 (11.4)	2334 (10.3)
Moderate	20,345 (70.3)	2021 (69.6)	7243 (70.2)	2292 (69.7)	8789 (70.8)	4313 (69.6)	16,032 (70.5)
High	1283 (4.4)	139 (4.8)	461 (4.5)	137 (4.2)	546 (4.4)	276 (4.5)	1007 (4.4)
Unknown	4262 (14.7)	400 (13.8)	1550 (15.0)	501 (15.2)	1811 (14.6)	901 (14.5)	3361 (14.8)
Age, years	27 (23–34)	25 (22–32)	25 (22–33)	28 (24–35)	27 (24–35)	27 (23–34)	27 (23–34)
Sex							
Male	21,003 (72.6)	2046 (70.4)	7537 (73.1)	2241 (68.1)	9179 (73.9)	4287 (69.2)	16,716 (73.5)
Female	7926 (27.4)	859 (29.6)	2779 (26.9)	1049 (31.9)	3239 (26.1)	1908 (30.8)	6018 (26.5)
Race/ethnicity							
White/non-Hispanic	21,090 (72.9)	2195 (75.6)	7520 (72.9)	2345 (71.3)	9030 (72.7)	4540 (73.3)	16,550 (72.8)
Black/non-Hispanic	3620 (12.5)	286 (9.8)	1305 (12.7)	446 (13.6)	1583 (12.7)	732 (11.8)	2888 (12.7)
Hispanic	2077 (7.2)	206 (7.1)	714 (6.9)	261 (7.9)	896 (7.2)	467 (7.5)	1610 (7.1)
Other/unknown	2142 (7.4)	218 (7.5)	777 (7.5)	238 (7.2)	909 (7.3)	456 (7.4)	1686 (7.4)
Marital status							
Married	17,857 (61.7)	1605 (55.2)	5847 (56.7)	2233 (67.9)	8172 (65.8)	3838 (62.0)	14,019 (61.7)
Other	11,072 (38.3	1300 (44.8)	4469 (43.3)	1057 (32.1)	4246 (34.2)	2357 (38.1)	8715 (38.3)
Service branch							
Air Force	14,291 (49.4)	1168 (40.2)	5469 (53.0)	1215 (35.9)	6439 (51.9)	2383 (38.5)	11,908 (52.4)
Army	9405 (32.5)	651 (22.4)	3639 (35.3)	923 (28.1)	4192 (33.8)	1574 (25.4)	7831 (34.5)
Marine Corps	2974 (10.3)	774 (26.6)	679 (6.6)	651 (19.8)	870 (7.0)	1425 (23.0)	1549 (6.8)
Navy	2259 (7.8)	312 (10.7)	529 (5.1)	501 (15.2)	917 (7.4)	813 (13.1)	1446 (6.4)
Rank							
Enlisted	21,931 (75.8)	2117 (72.9)	7914 (76.7)	2421 (73.6)	9479 (76.3)	4538 (73.3)	17,393 (76.5)
Officer	6998 (24.2)	788 (27.1)	2402 (23.3)	869 (26.4)	2939 (23.7)	1657 (26.8)	5341 (23.5)
Occupation							
Combat	5231 (18.1)	478 (16.5)	1821 (17.7)	542 (16.5)	2390 (19.2)	1020 (16.5)	4211 (18.5)
Health care	4280 (14.8)	592 (20.4)	1449 (14.0)	724 (22.0)	1515 (12.2)	1316 (21.2)	2964 (13.0)
Other	19,418 (67.1)	1835 (63.2)	7046 (68.3)	2024 (61.5)	8513 (68.6)	3859 (62.3)	15,559 (68.4)
US geographic area							

Table 2. Cont.

Characteristic	Total Study	2006/2007		2008/2009		Combined Seasons	
	Population	TIV	LAIV	TIV	LAIV	TIV	LAIV
Southwest	8746 (30.2)	1101 (37.9)	2997 (29.1)	1348 (41.0)	3300 (26.6)	2449 (39.5)	6297 (27.7)
Southeast	8992 (31.1)	966 (33.3)	3322 (32.2)	954 (29.0)	3750 (30.2)	1920 (31.0)	7072 (31.1)
Northeast	6367 (22.0)	537 (18.5)	2013 (19.5)	667 (20.3)	3150 (25.4)	1204 (19.4)	5163 (22.7)
Northwest	4824 (16.7)	301 (10.4)	1984 (19.2)	321 (9.8)	2218 (17.9)	622 (10.0)	4202 (18.5)

Abbreviations: ILI, influenza-like illness; IQR, interquartile range; LAIV, live, attenuated influenza vaccine; TIV, trivalent inactivated influenza vaccine.
[a]Numbers (percentages) for all data except age, which is reported as median (IQR).

regarding influenza vaccine from the Advisory Committee on Immunization Practices [44] and indicate that tailoring vaccine type recommendations to these specific health behavior groups is not warranted.

The effectiveness of the influenza vaccine depends on the recipient's immunocompetence, the similarity of vaccine strains to circulating strains in a population (ie, the "match"), the outcome measured, and possibly the mode of vaccine delivery. The role of immunocompetence, since it may be modulated by particular health behaviors, and its interaction with the mode of vaccine delivery were explored by controlling for both the vaccine match (by selecting 2 well-matched seasons) and the outcome measured (ILI). Several health behaviors that may have differential effects on vaccine effectiveness against influenza-related events were examined.

Tobacco and alcohol misuse have been associated with a higher risk for influenza and related complications [11,12], hence data on the optimal vaccine type in this group are important for patient care and public health strategies. Tobacco use is known to result in respiratory tract (impaired ciliary action) and immune (altered humoral and cell-mediated immunity) dysfunction from exposure to carcinogens, toxins, and lipopolysaccharide [1]. Further, a tobacco dose-related decrease in salivary IgA levels among smokers, a decrease in serum IgG, and alterations in immune cell counts (including lymphocytes, monocytes, B cells, and helper and suppressor T cells) have been described [1]. Hence, impaired mucosal immunity among smokers offers a biologically plausible reason for smokers to respond differently to LAIV (administered to the nasal mucosa) compared with TIV. Prior to this study, a single study had found a significant interaction between cigarette smoking and influenza vaccination by circulating influenza antibodies [45], however, no difference in protection against clinical influenza was found. Overall, these data and the current study findings do not support a differential response by vaccine type among smokers and nonsmokers.

Regarding excessive alcohol use, resultant negative cellular and innate immune system effects, including weakened antiviral defense mechanisms, have been described [2–4,6–9]. The antigen-presenting function of innate immune cells (eg, monocytes and macrophages) may be inhibited by alcohol exposure, and both T-cell proliferation and the distribution and functions of memory T cells and natural killer cells altered. Despite these potential immunologic changes, we did not find a differential response by vaccine type among problem drinkers.

Transient immunosuppression has been documented following intense and/or prolonged physical activity, though baseline disease rates have not been shown to differ between athletes and nonathletes [19–21], and athletes typically report decreased rates of infection on surveys [19]. Specific immune system effects of exercise such as low salivary IgA associated with intense exercise in elite athletes have been documented and may vary according to an individual's conditioning [20,21]. However, studies have found that 2–4 weeks after prolonged intensive exercise, individuals mount a normal antibody response to vaccination (tetanus, diphtheria, pneumococcus) [22–24]. It seems plausible that altered immunity could also appear with a sedentary lifestyle. Boosting of immunity and reduction in the number of days reporting upper respiratory symptoms among those engaging in exercise compared with sedentary controls have been described [19,27]. Although, a difference in efficacy conferred by LAIV compared with TIV might be hypothesized among groups with minimal or high exercise levels, we found no differences in ILI by vaccine type.

Overall, no difference in risk of ILI between LAIV and TIV recipients by each of the health behaviors of interest was found,

Table 3. Univariable Hazard Risk Ratios for ILI Among US Service Members, 18–49 Years of Age, During 2006/2007 and 2008/2009 Influenza Seasons.

Characteristic	ILI Events	
	No. (%)	HR (95% CI)
Vaccine type		
TIV	787 (12.7)	1.00 (Ref)
LAIV	3149 (13.9)	1.02 (0.95–1.11)
Recent smoking history		
Yes	1123 (14.1)	1.09 (1.02–1.17)[a]
No	2813 (13.4)	1.00 (Ref)
Potential alcohol problem		
Yes	267 (12.0)	0.90 (0.79–1.02)
No	3669 (13.7)	1.00 (Ref)
Exercise level		
Minimal	439 (14.4)	1.05 (0.94–1.16)
Moderate	2782 (13.7)	1.00 (Ref)
High	133 (10.4)	0.79 (0.66–0.95)
Unknown	582 (13.7)	1.00 (0.91–1.09)
Age, y		0.99 (0.98–0.99)[a]
Sex		
Male	2339 (11.1)	1.00 (Ref)
Female	1597 (20.1)	1.84 (1.72–1.96)[a]
Race/ethnicity		
White	2823 (13.4)	1.00 (Ref)
Black	486 (13.4)	1.00 (0.91–1.10)
Hispanic	290 (14.0)	1.08 (0.95–1.22)
Other/unknown	337 (15.7)	1.17 (1.04–1.32)[a]
Marital status		
Married	2420 (13.6)	1.00 (Ref)
Other	1516 (13.7)	1.02 (0.96–1.09)
Service branch		
Air Force	2363 (16.5)	1.00 (Ref)
Army	1047 (11.1)	0.74 (0.68–0.79)[a]
Marine Corps	197 (6.6)	0.43 (0.37–0.50)[a]
Navy	329 (14.6)	0.90 (0.80–1.02)
Military rank		
Enlisted	3140 (14.3)	1.00 (Ref)
Officer	796 (11.4)	0.77 (0.71–0.84)[a]
Occupation		
Combat	531 (10.2)	0.76 (0.69–0.84)[a]
Health care	783 (18.3)	1.28 (1.18–1.39)[a]
Other	2622 (13.5)	1.00 (Ref)
US geographic area		
Southwest	1203 (13.8)	1.00 (Ref)
Southeast	1192 (13.3)	0.98 (0.90–1.06)
Northeast	832 (13.1)	0.92 (0.84–1.00)
Northwest	709 (14.7)	1.04 (0.95–1.15)
Influenza season		
2006–2007	1860 (14.1)	1.00 (Ref)
2008–2009	2076 (13.2)	1.07 (1.00–1.14)[a]

Abbreviations: CI, confidence interval; HR, hazard ratio; ILI, influenza-like illness; LAIV, live, attenuated influenza vaccine; TIV, trivalent inactivated influenza vaccine.
[a]$p < 0.05$.

Table 4. Risk of ILI by Vaccine Type and Health Behavior During Two Influenza Seasons (2006/2007, 2008/2009).

	Total Study Population			Vaccine Type							
				LAIV			TIV				
				All	ILI Diagnosis		All	ILI Diagnosis			
	N	ILI	%	N	N	%	N	N	%	*p*	HR (95% CI)[a]
Overall	28,929	3936	13.61	22,734	3149	13.85	6195	787	12.70		0.98 (0.90–1.06)
Recent smoking history										0.099	
Nonsmoker	20,974	2813	13.41	16,496	2228	13.51	4478	585	13.06		0.94 (0.85–1.03)
Smoking history	7955	1,123	14.12	6238	921	14.76	1717	202	11.76		1.09 (0.94–1.27)
Possible alcohol problems										0.209	
No drinking problem	26,708	3669	13.74	21,079	2933	13.91	5629	736	13.08		0.96 (0.89–1.05)
Possible drinking problem	2221	267	12.02	1655	216	13.05	566	51	9.01		1.19 (0.86–1.63)
Exercise level										0.114	
Moderate	20,345	2782	13.67	16,032	2209	13.78	4313	573	13.29		0.92 (0.84–1.01)
Minimal	3039	439	14.45	2334	348	14.91	705	91	12.91		1.08 (0.85–1.36)
High	1283	133	10.37	1007	108	10.72	276	25	9.06		1.12 (0.71–1.76)
Unknown	4262	582	13.66	3361	484	14.40	901	98	10.88		1.19 (0.96–1.48)

Abbreviations: CI, confidence interval; HR, hazard ratio; ILI, influenza-like illness; LAIV, live, attenuated influenza vaccine; TIV, trivalent inactivated influenza vaccine.
[a]Hazard ratio for each health behavior stratum is evaluated at the average level of other behaviors in the study population and adjusted for all other demographic covariates.

likely reflecting the lack of effect on vaccine responses. It is also possible that the behavior categorization did not adequately separate those more likely to experience immune system effects due to their behavior from those at low risk of such effects; however, the military does contain sufficient numbers of persons with varying health behaviors, and the evaluation of more extreme behaviors may be less generalizable to the overall population.

One methodological limitation of this study is that the outcomes measured were based on ICD-9 codes rather than laboratory-confirmed influenza diagnosis; however, the codes used have been previously shown to correlate with viral culture or polymerase chain reaction-confirmed influenza events [38,39,46]. Also, illnesses that did not result in a health care visit within the military system could not be captured. Health behavior data were self-reported on a questionnaire and may not reflect the actual behaviors at the time of vaccine receipt. Since this study examined the potential associations between exposures and the effectiveness of the different vaccine types, by design it was only able to evaluate the apparent relative effectiveness of each vaccine. Lastly, this study included only a subset of adults serving in the US military; hence, data may not be representative of the entire military population. Further, although service members reflect a fairly broad spectrum of socioeconomic status and geographic distribution, additional research may be warranted to examine differential vaccine type effects on influenza outcomes among civilian groups with other health behavior profiles.

To the authors' knowledge, this is the first study to examine the effects of particular health behaviors on the relationship between vaccine type and influenza outcome. Strengths of this study include its robust size with nearly 30,000 vaccination events evaluated. In addition, the study utilized self-reported health behavior data proximate to vaccine receipt in a large population with reliable health care encounter capture. Further, military vaccine records used were comprehensive and highly reliable. Finally, the ILI rate (13.6%, n>3,000) allowed for robust measurement of the effects of health behavior factors.

In summary, LAIV and TIV have similar effectiveness in preventing ILI events among healthy 18- to 49-year-olds who are smokers, have potential alcohol problems, or endorse minimal or high exercise levels. These data suggest that clinicians and public health practitioners need not tailor vaccine regimens according to the particular health behavior groups studied here, and instead should focus vaccination efforts on simply ensuring widespread vaccination.

Acknowledgments

The views expressed in this article are those of the authors and do not reflect the official policy or position of the Department of the Navy, Department of Defense, or the US Government. Approved for public release; distribution is unlimited. This research has been conducted in compliance with all applicable federal regulations governing the protection of human subjects in research (Protocol NHRC.2010.0027). The authors are grateful to the many military personnel who participated in and to the researchers who support the Millennium Cohort Study, all of whom made this work possible.

Author Contributions

Conceived and designed the experiments: TW CP NC CS PB DF. Performed the experiments: CP CS. Analyzed the data: CP CS NC. Contributed to the writing of the manuscript: TW CP CS NC. Manuscript review: PB DF.

References

1. Edwards D (2009) Immunological effects of tobacco smoking in "healthy" smokers. COPD 6: 48–58.
2. Cook RT (1998) Alcohol abuse, alcoholism, and damage to the immune system–a review. Alcohol Clin Exp Res 22: 1927–1942.
3. Szabo G, Chavan S, Mandrekar P, Catalano D (1999) Acute alcohol consumption attenuates interleukin-8 (IL-8) and monocyte chemoattractant peptide-1 (MCP-1) induction in response to ex vivo stimulation. J Clin Immunol 19: 67–76.
4. Szabo G (1999) Consequences of alcohol consumption on host defence. Alcohol Alcohol 34: 830–841.
5. Szabo G, Mandrekar P (2009) A recent perspective on alcohol, immunity, and host defense. Alcohol Clin Exp Res 33: 220–232.
6. Pavia CS, La Mothe M, Kavanagh M (2004) Influence of alcohol on antimicrobial immunity. Biomed Pharmacother 58: 84–89.
7. Brown LA, Cook RT, Jerrells TR, Kolls JK, Nagy LE, et al. (2006) Acute and chronic alcohol abuse modulate immunity. Alcohol Clin Exp Res 30: 1624–1631.
8. Mandrekar P, Catalano D, White B, Szabo G (2006) Moderate alcohol intake in humans attenuates monocyte inflammatory responses: inhibition of nuclear regulatory factor kappa B and induction of interleukin 10. Alcohol Clin Exp Res 30: 135–139.
9. Lau AH, Szabo G, Thomson AW (2009) Antigen-presenting cells under the influence of alcohol. Trends Immunol 30: 13–22.
10. Roseman C, Truedsson L, Kapetanovic MC (2012) The effect of smoking and alcohol consumption on markers of systemic inflammation, immunoglobulin levels and immune response following pneumococcal vaccination in patients with arthritis. Arthritis Res Ther 14: R170.
11. Meyerholz DK, Edsen-Moore M, McGill J, Coleman RA, Cook RT, et al. (2008) Chronic alcohol consumption increases the severity of murine influenza virus infections. J Immunol 181: 641–648.
12. Arcavi L, Benowitz NL (2004) Cigarette smoking and infection. Arch Intern Med 164: 2206–2216.
13. Finklea JF, Sandifer SH, Smith DD (1969) Cigarette smoking and epidemic influenza. Am J Epidemiol 90: 390–399.
14. Stanley WM (1945) The Preparation and Properties of Influenza Virus Vaccines Concentrated and Purified by Differential Centrifugation. J Exp Med 81: 193–218.
15. Jefferson T, Di Pietrantonj C, Rivetti A, Bawazeer GA, Al-Ansary LA, et al. (2010) Vaccines for preventing influenza in healthy adults. Cochrane Database Syst Rev: CD001269.
16. Cox NJ, Subbarao K (1999) Influenza. Lancet 354: 1277–1282.
17. Fiore AE, Uyeki TM, Broder K, Finelli L, Euler GL, et al. (2010) Prevention and control of influenza with vaccines: recommendations of the Advisory Committee on Immunization Practices (ACIP), 2010. MMWR Recomm Rep 59: 1–62.
18. Cox RJ, Brokstad KA, Ogra P (2004) Influenza virus: immunity and vaccination strategies. Comparison of the immune response to inactivated and live, attenuated influenza vaccines. Scand J Immunol 59: 1–15.
19. Nieman DC, Pedersen BK (1999) Exercise and immune function. Recent developments. Sports Med 27: 73–80.
20. Gleeson M, McDonald WA, Pyne DB, Cripps AW, Francis JL, et al. (1999) Salivary IgA levels and infection risk in elite swimmers. Med Sci Sports Exerc 31: 67–73.
21. Mackinnon LT, Ginn EM, Gj S (1993) Temporal relationship between decreased salivary IgA and upper respiratory tract infection in elite athletes. Aust J Sci Med Sport 25: 94–99.
22. Bruunsgaard H, Hartkopp A, Mohr T, Konradsen H, Heron I, et al. (1997) In vivo cell-mediated immunity and vaccination response following prolonged, intense exercise. Med Sci Sports Exerc 29: 1176–1181.
23. Gleeson M, Pyne DB, McDonald WA, Clancy RL, Cripps AW, et al. (1996) Pneumococcal antibody responses in elite swimmers. Clin Exp Immunol 105: 238–244.
24. Eskola J, Ruuskanen O, Soppi E, Viljanen MK, Jarvinen M, et al. (1978) Effect of sport stress on lymphocyte transformation and antibody formation. Clin Exp Immunol 32: 339–345.
25. McGinnis JM, Foege WH (1993) Actual causes of death in the United States. JAMA 270: 2207–2212.
26. Hahn RA, Teutsch SM, Rothenberg RB, Marks JS (1990) Excess deaths from nine chronic diseases in the United States, 1986. JAMA 264: 2654–2659.
27. Venjatraman JT, Fernandes G (1997) Exercise, immunity and aging. Aging (Milano) 9: 42–56.
28. U. S. Department of Health and Human S (2004) The health consequences of smoking: a report of the Surgeon General. Atlanta, GA: US Department of Health and Human Services.
29. Ryan MA, Smith TC, Smith B, Amoroso P, Boyko EJ, et al. (2007) Millennium Cohort: enrollment begins a 21-year contribution to understanding the impact of military service. J Clin Epidemiol 60: 181–191.
30. Centers for Disease Control and P (2007) Update: Influenza Activity — United States and Worldwide, 2006–07 Season, and Composition of the 2007–08 Influenza Vaccine. Available: http://www.cdc.gov/mmwr/preview/mmwrhtml/mm5631a2.htm. 789–794 p. Accessed 20 Mar 2013.

31. Centers for Disease Control and P (2008) Influenza Activity — United States and Worldwide, 2007–08 Season. Available: http://www.cdc.gov/mmwr/preview/mmwrhtml/mm5725a5.htm. 692–697 p. Accessed 20 Mar 2013.
32. Centers for Disease Control and P (2009) 2008–2009 Influenza Season Week 12 ending March 28, 2009. Available: http://www.cdc.gov/flu/weekly/weeklyarchives2008-2009/weekly12.htm. Accessed 20 Mar 2013.
33. Centers for Disease Control and P (2008) 2007–2008 Influenza (Flu) Season. Centers for Disease Control and Prevention. Available: http://www.cdc.gov/flu/pastseasons/0708season.htm. Accessed 2013 Mar 20.
34. Dudding BA, Top FH Jr, Winter PE, Buescher EL, Lamson TH, et al. (1973) Acute respiratory disease in military trainees: the adenovirus surveillance program, 1966–1971. Am J Epidemiol 97: 187–198.
35. Gaydos CA, Gaydos JC (1995) Adenovirus vaccines in the U.S. military. Mil Med 160: 300–304.
36. Gray GC, Callahan JD, Hawksworth AW, Fisher CA, Gaydos JC (1999) Respiratory diseases among U.S. military personnel: countering emerging threats. Emerg Infect Dis 5: 379–385.
37. Russell KL (2006) Recruit Medicine. In: Lenhart MK, editor. Textbooks of Military Medicine. pp. 227–253.
38. Eick AA, Wang Z, Hughes H, Ford SM, Tobler SK (2009) Comparison of the trivalent live attenuated vs. inactivated influenza vaccines among U.S. military service members. Vaccine 27: 3568–3575.
39. Marsden-Haug N, Foster VB, Gould PL, Elbert E, Wang H, et al. (2007) Code-based syndromic surveillance for influenzalike illness by International Classification of Diseases, Ninth Revision. Emerg Infect Dis 13: 207–216.
40. Dawood FS, Jain S, Finelli L, Shaw MW, Lindstrom S, et al. (2009) Emergence of a novel swine-origin influenza A (H1N1) virus in humans. N Engl J Med 360: 2605–2615.
41. Jacobson IG, Ryan MA, Hooper TI, Smith TC, Amoroso PJ, et al. (2008) Alcohol use and alcohol-related problems before and after military combat deployment. Jama 300: 663–675.
42. Spitzer RL, Kroenke K, Williams JB (1999) Validation and utility of a self-report version of PRIME-MD: the PHQ primary care study. Primary Care Evaluation of Mental Disorders. Patient Health Questionnaire. JAMA 282: 1737–1744.
43. Centers for Disease Control and P (2011) How much physical activity do adults need? Available: http://www.cdc.gov/physicalactivity/everyone/guidelines/adults.html. Accessed 3 Jun 2013.
44. Centers for Disease Control and P (2013) Prevention and control of seasonal influenza with vaccines. Recommendations of the Advisory Committee on Immunization Practices–United States, 2013–2014. MMWR Recommendations and reports: Morbidity and mortality weekly report Recommendations and reports/Centers for Disease Control 62: 1.
45. Cruijff M, Thijs C, Govaert T, Aretz K, Dinant GJ, et al. (1999) The effect of smoking on influenza, influenza vaccination efficacy and on the antibody response to influenza vaccination. Vaccine 17: 426–432.
46. Wang Z, Tobler S, Roayaei J, Eick A (2009) Live attenuated or inactivated influenza vaccines and medical encounters for respiratory illnesses among US military personnel. JAMA 301: 945–953.

The Associations of Objectively Measured Physical Activity and Sedentary Time with Cognitive Functions in School-Aged Children

Heidi J. Syväoja[1,2]*, Tuija H. Tammelin[1], Timo Ahonen[2], Anna Kankaanpää[1], Marko T. Kantomaa[1,3]

1 LIKES - Research Center for Sport and Health Sciences, Jyväskylä, Finland, **2** Department of Psychology, University of Jyväskylä, Jyväskylä, Finland, **3** Department of Epidemiology and Biostatistics, MRC–HPA Centre for Environment and Health, Imperial College London, London, United Kingdom

Abstract

Low levels of physical activity among children have raised concerns over the effects of a physically inactive lifestyle, not only on physical health but also on cognitive prerequisites of learning. This study examined how objectively measured and self-reported physical activity and sedentary behavior are associated with cognitive functions in school-aged children. The study population consisted of 224 children from five schools in the Jyväskylä school district in Finland (mean age 12.2 years; 56% girls), who participated in the study in the spring of 2011. Physical activity and sedentary time were measured objectively for seven consecutive days using the ActiGraph GT1M/GT3X accelerometer. Self-reported moderate to vigorous physical activity (MVPA) and screen time were evaluated with the questions used in the "WHO Health Behavior in School-aged Children" study. Cognitive functions including visual memory, executive functions and attention were evaluated with a computerized Cambridge Neuropsychological Test Automated Battery by using five different tests. Structural equation modeling was applied to examine how objectively measured and self-reported MVPA and sedentary behavior were associated with cognitive functions. High levels of objectively measured MVPA were associated with good performance in the reaction time test. High levels of objectively measured sedentary time were associated with good performance in the sustained attention test. Objectively measured MVPA and sedentary time were not associated with other measures of cognitive functions. High amount of self-reported computer/video game play was associated with weaker performance in working memory test, whereas high amount of computer use was associated with weaker performance in test measuring shifting and flexibility of attention. Self-reported physical activity and total screen time were not associated with any measures of cognitive functions. The results of the present study propose that physical activity may benefit attentional processes. However, excessive video game play and computer use may have unfavorable influence on cognitive functions.

Editor: Yoko Hoshi, Tokyo Metropolitan Institute of Medical Science, Japan

Funding: This study was funded by Finnish Ministry of Education and Culture (101/627/2010, http://www.minedu.fi/OPM/?lang = en) and the Academy of Finland (grant 273971). The funders had no role in study design, data collection and analysis, decision to publish, or preparation of the manuscript.

Competing Interests: The authors have declared that no competing interests exist.

* Email: heidi.syvaoja@likes.fi

Introduction

In past decades, our lifestyles have become increasingly inactive [1]; only one-third of children are sufficiently active according to current physical activity recommendations [2]. Low levels of physical activity have raised concerns over the effects of a physically inactive lifestyle on children's physical health and, recently, also on children's learning, especially on cognitive prerequisites of learning [3].

Previous studies have shown that physical activity enhances neurocognitive function and protects against neurodegenerative diseases in elderly [4–6]. During past few years, physical activity has been linked to enhanced cognition also in children. The meta-analytic study of Sibley & Etnier [7], showed the significant overall positive association between physical activity and cognition in children. In addition, in the study of Ruiz et al. [8] leisure time physical activity was associated with better cognitive performance in adolescents. Moreover, Ardoy et al. [9] reported that children participating in high intensity physical education intervention improved their cognitive performance compared to control children.

Regular physical activity has been especially linked to executive functions [10]. Executive functions (also called executive control/cognitive control) are the collection of higher-order cognitive processes controlling goal-directed actions. Core executive functions are inhibitory control (including selective attention and the inhibition of inappropriate or interfering responses), working memory and mental flexibility [11]. School-based interventions has shown that increased physical activity may improve children's inhibitory control [12], planning ability [13] and working memory performance [14,15]. In addition, in recent studies, children with high aerobic fitness have demonstrated better inhibitory control [16–18] as well as better working memory performance [19] than less-fit children.

However, evidence of the favorable effects of physical activity on cognitive functions in healthy children and adolescents is still somewhat inconsistent [20–22] and based on scarce research data [10]. Significantly, physical fitness has often been used as a proxy indicator of regular physical activity, without direct measurement

Table 1. Summary of the CANTAB tests used to measure different dimensions of cognitive function.

Dimension of cognitive function	Test	Abbreviation
Visual memory	1. Pattern Recognition Memory	PRM
Executive function	2. Spatial Span	SSP
	3. Intra-Extra Dimensional Set Shift	IED
Attention	4. Reaction Time	RTI
	5. Rapid Visual Information Processing	RVP

of physical activity levels. This is particularly important, because in childhood, habitual physical activity is rarely intensive and lengthy enough to enhance aerobic fitness, and therefore, the relationship between physical activity and fitness may not be meaningful [23]. Moreover, few studies have measured a broad range of cognitive functions, highlighting the need for new studies to clarify the benefits of physical activity on different dimensions of cognitive functions.

Besides physical activity, sedentary behavior and excessive media use may be associated with cognitive function in children and youth. Extensive screen time has been linked to elevated risk of attention and learning difficulties [24–27] and decreased verbal memory performance [28]. However, in other recent studies, screen time had no association with visuospatial cognition [29], and even had a positive association with enhanced attentional skills [30] and higher-developed language skills [31] in children and adolescents. Diverging research results indicates that the association of sedentary behavior and cognition is more complicated than previously believed and needs clarification.

To our knowledge, no previous studies have examined the associations of objectively measured overall physical activity and sedentary time on cognitive functions in children. However, as the rates of childhood physical inactivity are increasing worldwide, it is important to better understand the potential effects of lack of physical activity and excessive sedentary time on cognitive prerequisites of learning. The purpose of this study was to examine how objectively measured and self-reported physical activity are associated with cognitive functions in school-aged children. In addition, this study aimed to determine how objectively measured sedentary time and self-reported screen time are associated with children's cognitive functions. We hypothesized that physical activity is positively, and both sedentary time and screen time are inversely, associated with cognitive functions.

Method

Ethics Statement

The study was approved by the Ethics Committee of the University of Jyväskylä, and followed the principles of the Declaration of Helsinki and the Finnish legislation. Participation in the study was voluntary, and all participants had the right to drop out of the study at any time without a specific reason. Only children with a fully completed consent form (Certificate of Consent signed by a parent/guardian and the child) on the day of the first measurements were included in the study.

Participants

During spring 2011, 475 fifth and sixth graders were invited to participate in the study. 277 children (participation rate 58%) from five schools in the Jyväskylä school district in Central Finland participated in the study. 230 of the 277 children were selected to participate in cognitive tests according to successful objective measurement of physical activity. If a child's measurement did not succeed because of technical problems or the child did not remember to wear the accelerometer, they were not invited to the cognitive tests. Seven children (3 boys, 4 girls) were excluded from analysis because, according to their parents' survey, they had physical disabilities, chronic diseases or severe learning disabilities. The final sample size used in the analyses was 224.

Cognitive functions

Cognitive functions (Table 1) were assessed using the Neuropsychological Test Automated Battery (CANTAB) (a PaceBlade Slimbook P110 tablet PC with a 12-inch touch-screen monitor and Windows XP Professional operating system, CANTABeclipse version 3). The test battery was run individually in a silent location with the guidance of trained research assistants and in accordance with the standard instructions. The execution required about 45 minutes for each individual.

Visual memory was assessed with a Pattern Recognition Memory (PRM) test. PRM measures recognition memory of visual patterns in a two-choice forced discrimination paradigm. In this test, children had to remember the presented geometric patterns and discriminate them from the novel patterns. The score of the task is the number of correct responses.

Executive functions were assessed with Spatial Span (SSP) and Intra-Extra Dimensional Set Shift (IED) tests. SSP measures the length of the visuospatial working memory span based on the Corsi blocks task [32]. In this test, specified number of white boxes changed their color one by one and children had to reproduce the same sequence by touching the boxes in the same order the boxes changed their color. The score of the task is the maximum number of items that the child can successfully remember in the correct order. IED is based on the Wisconsin Card Sorting test [33] and measures sifting and flexibility of attention. Specifically, it measures the ability to maintain attention to different stimuli within a relevant dimension, and shift attention to a previously irrelevant dimension. There are nine stages with increasing difficulty in this task. The children were instructed to choose one of the two different dimensions: one is correct, and the other is incorrect. According to immediate feedback, they were expected to choose the correct pattern and learn the rule. The score in this task is based on the number of stages completed.

The tests assessing attention were Reaction Time (RTI) and Rapid Visual Information Processing (RVP). RTI measures children's reaction time and speed of response to a visual target. In the unpredictable five-choice condition, a yellow spot appeared randomly in one of the five circles on the screen. Children were instructed to hold down the press pad button until they saw the yellow spot and then touch the middle of the correct circle as quickly as possible. The total score of this task is the sum of reaction time (ms) and movement time (ms). RVP is similar to the

Continuous Performance Task measuring sustained attention. In this test, children had to touch the press pad button every time they discriminate the target sequence (digits 3, 5, and 7) from the digits appearing in a pseudo-random order at the rate of 100 digits per minute. The score of this task is RVP A', which measures the child's skill at detecting target sequences (3, 5, 7) from a pseudo-random sequence of numbers (range 0.00 to 1.00; bad to good).

Internal reliability, assessed with Cronbach's alpha reliability coefficients, was 0.49 for the RVP A', 0.65 for the PRM number of correct responses, 0.66 for the RTI five-choice reaction time and 0.87 for the RTI five-choice movement time. For hampering tests (SSP and IED), Cronbach's alpha could not be determined.

Objectively measured physical activity and sedentary time

The ActiGraph GT1M/GT3X accelerometers with vertical axel were used to measure children's moderate to vigorous physical activity (MVPA) and sedentary time. The accelerometer was worn on the right hip with an elastic waistband during waking hours for seven consecutive days. During bathing, swimming, and other water activities, the monitor was requested to be removed because it was not water-resistant. The ActiLife accelerometer software (ActiLife version 5; http://support.theactigraph.com/dl/ActiLife-software) was used to collect the data. Epoch length was 10 seconds and non-wearing time 30 minutes. Customized software was used for data reduction and analysis. A cut-off value of 2,296 counts per minute was used for MVPA [34], and 100 counts per minute for sedentary time. Children were included in the analysis if they had valid data for at least 500 minutes per day on two weekdays and on one weekend day. In order to compare children, who had worn the accelerometers for different amounts of time per day, objectively measured sedentary time was expressed as percentage of daily registration time.

Self-reported physical activity and screen time

Physical activity and screen time were assessed with a self-reported questionnaire used earlier in the WHO Health Behavior in School-aged Children (HBSC) study [35]. Self-reported MVPA was measured with the following question: "Over the past 7 days, on how many days were you physically active for a total of at least 60 minutes per day?" The response categories were as follows: 0 days, 1 day, 2 days, ... 7 days. There was a short description about what kind of physical activity should be taken into account when answering the question: "In the next question, physical activity is defined as any activity that increases your heart rate and makes you get out of breath some of the time." Examples included running, walking quickly, rollerblading, biking, dancing, skate-boarding, swimming, snowboarding, cross-country skiing, soccer, basketball, and Finnish baseball. Test-retest agreement for self-reported MVPA has been very good (ICC = 0.82) [36,37]. Self-reported screen time was evaluated with the question: "About how many hours a day do you usually a) watch television (including videos), b) play computer or video games, or c) use a computer (for purposes other than playing games, for example, emailing, chatting, or surfing the Internet or doing homework) in your free time?" The response options were as follows: not at all, about half an hour per day, about an hour a day, about two hours per day, ... about five hours per day or more. Children responded separately for both weekdays and weekends. Test-retest agreement for watching television (ICC = 0.72–0.74) and for playing computer or video games (ICC = 0.54–0.69) has been substantial, and fair to moderate (ICC = 0.33–0.50) for using the computer [37]. Total daily screen time averages were calculated by adding these three questions, including weekdays and weekends, together.

Potential confounders

The parent or the child's main caregiver filled in a questionnaire including the mother and father's education, family income, marital status, and children's learning difficulties and need for remedial education. The highest level of parental education, which was calculated from the mother's and father's education, was categorized as tertiary level education (1) and basic or upper secondary education (0). Marital status of the main caregiver was categorized as married or cohabiting (1) and divorced or single/widow (0). Children's learning difficulties and need for remedial education were categorizes as yes (1) and no or don't know (0).

Statistical analysis

The SPSS 19.0 for Windows statistical package (SPSS (2010) IBM SPSS Statistics 19 Core System User's Guide (SPSS Inc., Chicago, IL)) and the Mplus statistical package (Version 7; Muthèn & Muthèn, 1998–2012) [38] were used for the statistical analyses. Pearson's correlation coefficients were calculated to estimate preliminary associations between objectively and subjectively measured physical activity, sedentary behavior, cognitive tests and potential confounders. Structural equation modeling was applied to examine physical activity and sedentary time in association with cognitive function. Structural equation modeling was used because it enables to estimate the measurement errors away and, therefore, increases the reliability of cognitive tests. Single scores of every problem or level of the tests were applied instead of the total score. Item parcels [39] were constructed to combine the large number of these single scores for each latent factor. These parcels were then used as indicators for latent variables. Multiple logistic regression was used to examine physical activity and sedentary time in association with cognitive function, when the outcome was dichotomous. Full information maximum likelihood (FIML) estimation with robust standard errors (MLR) was used under the assumption of data missing at random. Gender, the highest level of parental education and child's need for remedial education were chosen to represent different aspects of potential confounders and were added to the main analysis. In order to avoid multicollinearity, highly correlated objectively measured MVPA and sedentary time were added to the model using a Cholesky factoring of the predictors [40]. The Satorra–Bentler scaled $\chi 2$-test, the comparative fit index (CFI), the Tucker–Lewis Index (TLI), the root mean square error of approximation (RMSEA) and the standardized root-mean-square residual (SRMR) were used to evaluate the goodness-of-fit of the models. The model fits the data well if the p-value for the χ^2-test is non-significant, CFI and TLI values are close to 0.95, the RMSEA value is below 0.06 and the SRMR value is below 0.08 [41].

Results

The mean age of the children was 12.2 years and 56% of the children were girls (Table 2). 71% of children's mothers and 56% of children's fathers had tertiary level education, and 76% of parents were married or cohabiting. 5% of children had a diagnosed learning difficulty and 13% of children needed remedial education, according to their parent's reports.

Based on objective physical activity measurements, children had, on average, 58 minutes of MVPA per day, with no statistically significant gender difference (Table 2). However, girls spent more of their waking hours sedentary than boys (Table 2). Based on self-reports, children reported at least 60 minutes of MVPA a day for 5 days per week on average, with no significant difference between boys and girls (Table 2). Boys reported more

Table 2. Sample characteristics according to gender and overall participants.

	Boys			Girls			All			p[a]
	Mean	SD	N	Mean	SD	N	Mean	SD	N	
Age (years)	12.2	0.6	97	12.2	0.6	127	12.2	0.6	224	0.984
Measurements of cognitive function										
PRM no. of correct	20.9	2.8	97	20.9	2.2	127	20.9	2.5	224	0.981
SSP span length (scale 0–9)	6.6	1.3	97	6.7	1.4	127	6.6	1.3	224	0.561
RTI five-choice (ms)	623	78	97	680	98	127	655	94	224	<0.001
RVP A′ (scale 0.00–1.00)[b]	0.97	0.02	97	0.97	0.03	127	0.97	0.02	224	0.946
IED no. of children who completed the test (%)	67		97	66		127	67		224	0.891
Measurements of physical activity and sedentary behavior										
Objectively measured MVPA (min/day)[c]	60.3	22.4	89	56.9	16.9	118	58.4	19.5	207	0.231
Objectively measured sedentary time (%/day)[d]	66.1	5.9	89	67.9	5.1	127	67.2	5.5	207	0.013
Self-reported MVPA (d/week with ≥60 min MVPA)	5.0	1.8	95	5.0	1.5	127	5.0	1.6	222	0.923
Self-reported total screen time (h/day)	4.0	2.0	95	3.4	1.8	127	3.7	1.9	222	0.015
TV	1.6	1.0	96	1.6	0.9	127	1.6	0.9	223	0.982
Computer/video games	1.4	0.9	95	0.7	0.8	127	1.0	0.9	222	<0.001
Computer use (other than playing)	1.0	0.8	96	1.1	0.8	127	1.0	0.8	223	0.244

Abbreviations: SD, standard deviation; MVPA, moderate to vigorous physical activity; PRM, Pattern Recognition Memory; SSP, Spatial Span; RTI, Reaction Time; RVP, Rapid Visual Information Processing; IED, Intra-Extra Dimensional Set Shift.

[a]P-values for the gender differences (T-test).

[b]A′ indicates the result in RVP test. The scale is 0.00–1.00, whereas 0.00 indicates a poor result and 1.00 a good result.

[c]MVPA measured with the ActiGraph accelerometer using a cut-off value of 2,296 counts per minute.

[d]Sedentary time measured by the ActiGraph accelerometer using a cut-off value 100 counts per minute and expressed as percentage of daily monitoring time (%/day).

total screen time than girls, especially they spent more time playing computer or videogames than girls (Table 2). In cognitive tests, boys were faster than girls in the RTI test, but no significant gender differences were observed in performance in the PRM, SSP, RVP or IED tests.

For structural equation modeling, three subscales of RTI were formed from 15 individual patterns of the RTI, and each subscale divided by 10. Each subscale loaded on the hypothesized factor. The model for the associations of objectively measured MVPA, sedentary time (SED) and performance in the Reaction Time (RTI) test is presented in Figure 1. The goodness-of-fit statistics of the model were good (χ^2 (10) = 14.52 p = 0.763, CFI = 0.979, TLI = 0.948, RMSEA = 0.045, SRMR = 0.018). Objectively measured MVPA was negatively associated with the RTI five-choice test score (ms), whereas objectively measured sedentary time was not associated with the RTI five-choice test score after adjusting for gender, the highest level of parental education and child's need for remedial education (Table 3).

The RVP A' (multiplied by 10) scores of the three blocks of the test were used as indicator variables in the structural equation modeling. Each block loaded on the hypothesized factor. The model for the associations of objectively measured MVPA, sedentary time (SED) and performance in the Rapid Visual Information Processing (RVP) test is presented in Figure 2. The goodness-of-fit statistics of the model were good (χ^2 (10) = 9.45 p = 0.490, CFI = 1.000, TLI = 1.010, RMSEA = 0.000, SRMR = 0.028). Objectively measured sedentary time was positively associated with RVPA', whereas objectively measured MVPA was not associated with RVPA' after adjusting for gender, the highest level of parental education and child's need for remedial education (Table 3).

Self-reported playing of computer/video games was negatively associated with SSP span length after adjusting for gender, the highest level of parental education and child's need for remedial education (Table 3). The model was fully saturated. Self-reported use of computer for other purposes than playing was negatively associated with IED number of children who completed the test (Table 4).

Discussion

According to the results of this study, a high level of objectively measured MVPA was associated with good performance in the reaction time test (RTI), which measures children's reaction time and the speed of response to a visual target. In addition, a high level of objectively measured sedentary time was associated with good performance in the sustained attention test (RVP). However, objectively measured physical activity or sedentary time were not

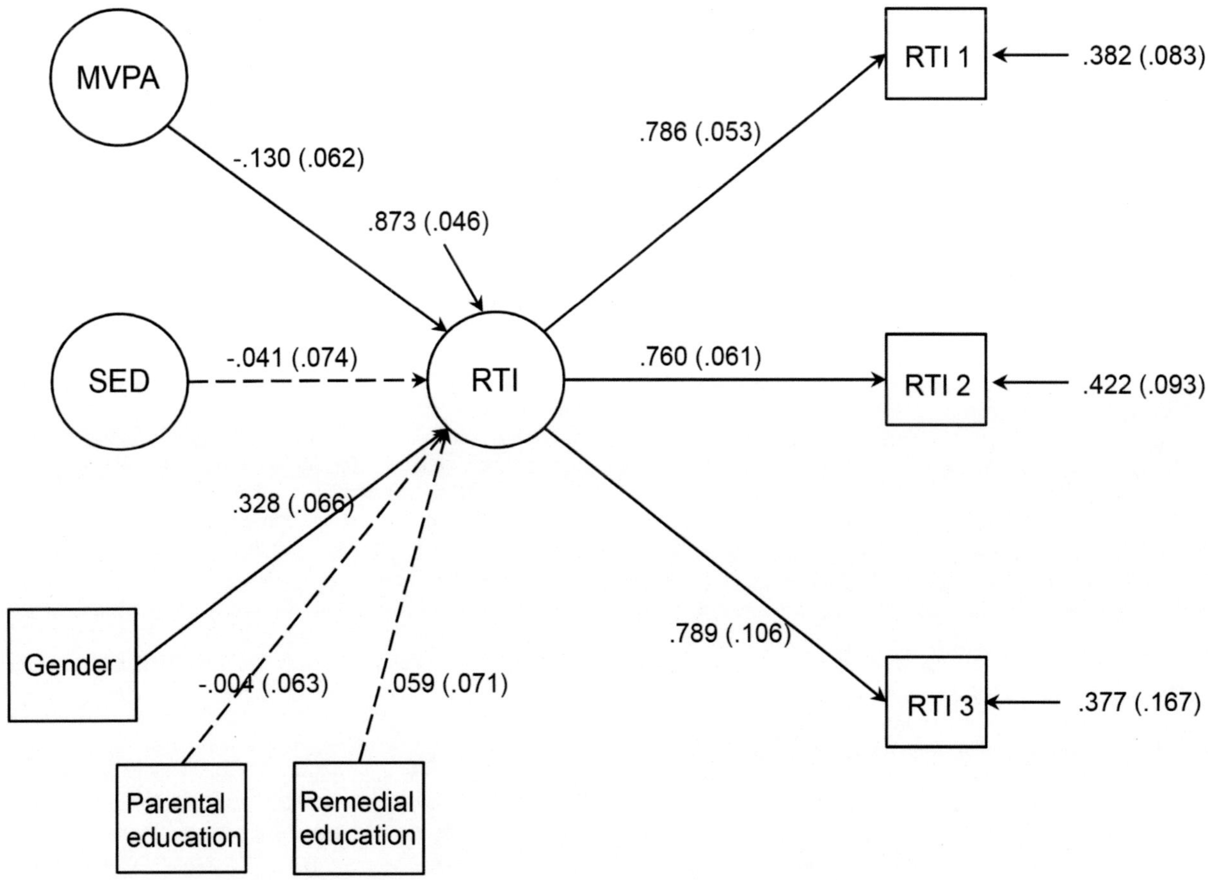

Figure 1. Objectively measured physical activity and performance in attentional reaction time test. This figure presents the estimation results of the model for the associations of objectively measured moderate to vigorous physical activity (MVPA), sedentary time (SED) and the Reaction Time (RTI) test. Standardized parameter estimates and standard errors are presented. For structural equation modeling, three subscales of the RTI (RTI 1, RTI 2, RTI 3) (divided by 10) were formed from 15 patterns of RTI. The RTI test result is in milliseconds, where faster time indicates better performance. Confounding factors, gender (female), the highest level of parental education (tertiary level) and child's need for remedial education (yes) were taken into account. Highly correlated objectively measured MVPA and sedentary time were added to the model as latent variables.

Table 3. The associations between children's cognitive processes and objectively measured physical activity, sedentary time and self-reported screen time.

	B	SE	95% CI	P[g]
Reaction Time (RTI)[a]				
Objectively measured MVPA[b]	−0.130	0.062	−0.253, −0.008	0.037
Objectively measured sedentary time[c]	−0.041	0.074	−0.186, 0.104	0.581
Rapid Visual Information Processing (RVP)[d]				
Objectively measured MVPA	−0.040	0.093	−0.223, 0.143	0.669
Objectively measured sedentary time	0.305	0.078	0.153, 0.457	0.000
Spatial Span (SSP)[e]				
Self-reported viewing of TV[f]	−0.003	0.067	−0.134, 0.129	0.970
Self-reported playing of computer/video game[f]	−0.179	0.079	−0.333, −0.024	0.023
Self-reported use of computer (other than playing)[f]	0.094	0.068	−0.040, 0.227	0.171

Abbreviations: B, estimate; SE, standard error; CI, confidence interval; p, P-value; MVPA, moderate to vigorous physical activity.
[a]RTI measures children's reaction time and speed of response to a visual target in milliseconds, where faster time indicates better performance.
[b]MVPA measured with the ActiGraph accelerometer using a cut-off value of 2,296 counts per minute and expressed as min/day.
[c]Sedentary time measured by the ActiGraph accelerometer using a cut-off value of 100 counts per minute and expressed as percentage of daily monitoring time (%/day).
[d]RVP measures the sustained attention. The score of this task is RVP A', where range is 0.00 to 1.00; bad to good.
[e]SSP measures length of the visuospatial working memory span. The score of this task is the maximum number of items that the child can successfully reproduce.
[f]Self-reported viewing of television, playing of computer/video games and use of computer (other than playing) are expresses as h/day.
[g]P-values for parameter estimates.
Models have been adjusted with gender (female), the highest level of parental education (tertiary level) and child's need for remedial education.

associated with any other assessments of cognitive functions. High amount of self-reported playing of computer or video games was associated with weaker performance in Spatial Span (SSP) test measuring visuospatial working memory. Moreover, self-reported use of computer for other purposes than playing was negatively associated with performance in Intra-Extra Dimensional Set Shift (IED) test, which measures sifting and flexibility of attention. Self-reported physical activity, total screen time or television viewing had no association with any of the cognitive tests measuring visual memory, executive functions or attention.

Physical activity and cognitive functions

In our study, a high level of objectively measured physical activity was associated with better performance in attentional reaction time test. Recent study of Spitzer and Hollmann [42] supports our finding by reporting that implementation of physical activity had positive effects on children's attention. In addition, recent intervention study of Chaddock-Heyman et al. [12] showed that physical activity enhances children's performance in inhibitory control task requiring selective attention and inhibition of interfering responses (e.g. the Eriksen flanker task; [43]). Similarly, according to Castelli et al. [44] engagement in vigorous physical activity was positively associated with performance in inhibitory control task. However, in the studies of Fisher et al. [14], Davis et al. [13] and Puder et al. [20] physical activity intervention had no effect on children's attentional processes. Previous studies have also reported that physically fit children outperform their less fit peers inhibitory control task [17,18,45], but also no differences in inhibitory control performance between physically fit and less fit children [22,44].

Physical activity may enhance attentional processes and other cognitive functions through different mechanisms. It has been suggested that physical activity may improve brain volume in regions supporting executive functions [19,46]; produce specific changes in the activity patterns in the brains [12,13]; increase the levels of brain-derived neurotrophic factor (BDNF) [47,48] and enhance cerebrovascular function [49]; all of which may mediate the effects of physical activity on cognition. In addition, motor function has shown to be closely connected to children's cognitive and academic skills and development [50,51], and may be an important factor driving the effects of physical inactivity on cognitive prerequisites of learning [52]. Furthermore, obesity has been related to poorer academic [52] and cognitive performance [53] and may, thereby, be one factor mediating the association of physical activity and cognition. Moreover, participation in physical activities is often a social phenomenon offering opportunities for interaction with other children and adults, and this interaction may also have a significant impact on children's cognitive development and learning. However, this has rarely been taken into account in research [54]. Finally, physical activity may facilitate cognitive function through the cognitive demands inherent in the structure of goal-directed and engaging exercise [55].

In the present study, neither objectively measured nor self-reported physical activity was associated with visual memory, working memory, sifting and flexibility of attention or sustained attention performance. These results are in line with studies showing that physical activity is not necessary associated with all domains of cognitive functions [13–15,20,21]. These diverging results indicate the importance of future studies to define these associations. Some of the cognitive tests used in the present study were not able to differentiate healthy 12-year-old children. Neuropsychological test batteries have originally been developed to detect neurocognitive deficits, and due to that, the tests may be too easy for healthy children. In the present study, particularly in the tests of visual memory (PRM), sifting and flexibility of attention (IED) and sustained attention (RVP), children, on average, achieved very high results, which may partly explain the lack of association between physical activity and cognitive test results. Additionally, Stroth et al. [22] speculated that one reason behind

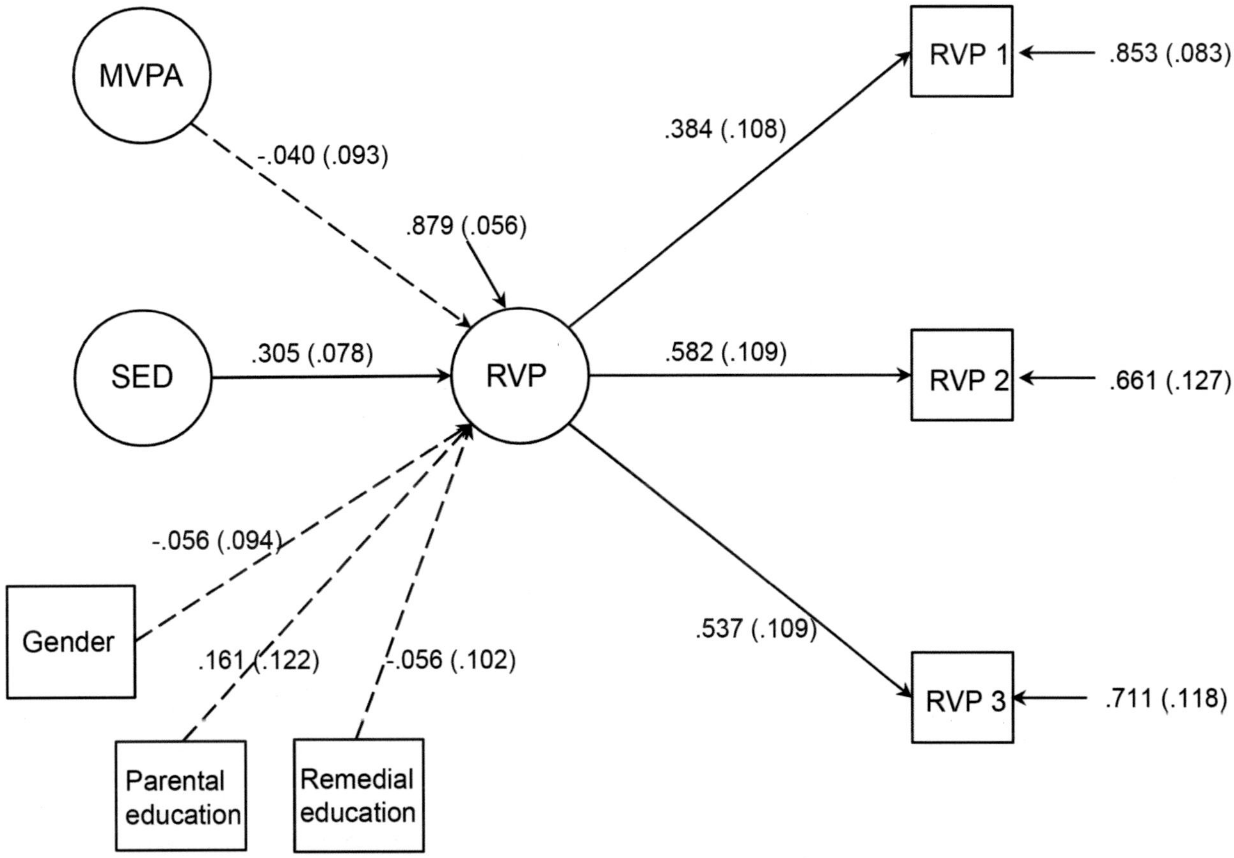

Figure 2. Objectively measured sedentary time and performance in sustained attention test. This figure presents the estimation results of the model for the associations of objectively measured MVPA, sedentary time (SED) and the Rapid Visual Information Processing (RVP) test. Standardized parameter estimates and standard errors are presented. The RVP (multiplied by 10) of the three blocks of the test (RVP 1, RVP 2, RVP 3) were used as indicator variables in the structural equation modeling. The scale for the RVP test result (A') is 0.00–1.00, where 0.00 indicates a poor result and 1.00 a good result. Confounding factors, gender (female), the highest level of parental education (tertiary level) and child's need for remedial education (yes) were taken into account. Highly correlated objectively measured MVPA and sedentary time were added to the model as latent variables.

the result of aerobic fitness not being associated with children's performance in cognitive control tasks may be the ceiling effect.

In previous studies, aerobic fitness has often been used as a proxy measure of regular physical activity, which might contribute to diverging results: physical activity is behavior, which increases energy expenditure and occurs within a cultural context, while physical fitness is an adaptive state of the human body, affected by heritable and environmental factors and physical activity. Especially in childhood, both the levels of physical activity and physical fitness may vary independently of each other due to growth, maturation and aging [23,56]. In addition, aerobic fitness measures are often confounded by adiposity and obesity in childhood [57], which are also potential factors attenuating cognitive and academic performance [53]. Moreover, the definitions, patterns and measurements of cognitive functions and physical activity have varied across different studies. Therefore, it

Table 4. The associations between children's working memory capacity and self-reported screen time.

	OR	95% CI
Intra-Extra Dimensional Set Shift (IED)[a]		
Self-reported viewing of TV[b]	0.868	0.623, 1.210
Self-reported playing of computer/video game[b]	1.321	0.943, 1.850
Self-reported use of computer (other than playing)[b]	0.639	0.421, 0.972

Abbreviations: OR, odds ratio; CI, confidence interval.
[a]IED measures sifting and flexibility of attention and was categorized as 1 children who completed the test and 0 children who did not completed the test.
[b]Self-reported viewing of television, playing of computer/video games and use of computer (other than playing) are expresses as h/day.
Model has been adjusted with gender (female), the highest level of parental education (tertiary level) and child's need for remedial education.

is difficult to directly compare and summarize the results of earlier studies and determine the specific benefits regular physical activity may have on cognitive functions.

Our finding that only objectively measured physical activity was associated with attentional reaction time may reflect the difference between objective and subjective measurements of physical activity. Accelerometer-measured MVPA mainly illustrates cardiovascular activity with increased heart rate and respiratory frequency, while self-reported physical activity may represent different constructs and contexts. Self-reported physical activity may include skill-specific types of physical activities, which require balance and agility but hardly accumulate activity counts [58]. Our results may indicate that moderate to vigorous intensity exercise that increases cardiovascular function has benefits on attentional processes.

Sedentary behavior and cognitive functions

Previous studies have largely suggested that screen-based sedentary behaviors have an unfavorable effect on children's cognition, especially on attention and learning difficulties [24–27]. The results of the present study supports the previous results by showing a negative association between self-reported computer/ video game playing and visuospatial working memory as well as negative association between self-reported use computer and shifting and flexibility of attention. Drowak et al. [28], reported also declines in verbal memory performance after computer game exposure. However, some previous studies have reported that screen-based sedentary behavior, especially videogames, is linked to enhanced cognitive skills [59–61]. According to Dye and Matthew [30], children who used to play video games had faster reaction times in attention control tests (ANT) without a notable loss in accuracy compared to non-players, indicating that action game players made faster correct responses to targets and had more resources to process distractions. Bittman et al. [31] reported that computer use was associated with higher-developed language skills.

In the present study, some children spent excessive amounts of time in front of the screens on their free time: one fifth of the children reported having screen time about 5 or more hours per day. Excessive amounts of screen time may displace activities involving learning opportunities and increase children's impulsive behavior, and eventually decrease academic skills [62].

Disadvantages, but also benefits of screen-based sedentary behavior on cognitive functions may be explained by the content of the screen time: not all screen time has an equal role in benefitting or impairing children's cognitive skills and learning [63,64]. For example, Ennemoser & Schneider [65] reported that educational program viewing was positively, but entertainment program viewing negatively, correlated with reading speed and comprehension in children. In the study of Feng et al. [66], action game training in young adults improved performance and attenuated the gender differences favoring males in spatial attention test, while control subjects who played a non-action game showed no improvements. According to Kuhn et al. [67], video game playing may induce structural brain plasticity in the areas important to spatial navigation, strategic planning, working memory and motor performance. On the other hand, in the study of Drowak et al. [28], interactive computer game play resulted significant declines in verbal memory performance and slow wave sleep, which is important for memory consolidation, whereas viewing exciting films had no effects. Finally, it should be kept in mind that computer-based cognitive assessments may require similar cognitive skills as video and computer games, which would favor children who play a lot of video and computer games.

Most of the previous studies have used self-reported methods assessing sedentary behavior. In the present study, objectively measured sedentary time was positively associated with sustained attention; children who spent more time being sedentary achieved higher scores in sustained attention test. Objectively measured sedentary time is a summary measure of all kinds of sedentary behaviors, including various activities such as screen time, reading, doing homework, interaction with friends, et cetera. During some sedentary activities, such as reading and doing homework, sustained attention and distraction exclusion are needed, which may explain objectively measured sedentary time being associated with good performance in sustained attention test.

In the present study, however, objectively measured sedentary time was not associated with visual memory, working memory, set-sifting/mental flexibility or attentional reaction time. In addition, total screen time or television viewing were not associated with cognition. Neither did Ferguson et al. [29] observe any association between video game playing and visuospatial cognition. Moreover, in two recent studies [31,68], television viewing was not associated with cognitive and language skills after adjusting for the parent's role in monitoring and involvement in the child's media use.

Strength and limitations of the study

To our knowledge, this was the first study examining the association of objectively measured overall physical activity and sedentary time with cognitive functions in children. Conclusions regarding causality of the observed associations cannot be drawn due to the cross-sectional design. In addition, the content of sedentary time and screen-based sedentary behavior was not assessed, which limits the interpretation of the results concerning sedentary behavior. Moreover, some cognitive tests used in the present study may have been too easy for 12-year-old healthy children, and did not optimally discriminate children's performance. Furthermore, pubertal timing, motor skills and fitness were not assessed, which limits the interpretation of the results.

Future direction

Studies with longitudinal designs or randomized controlled trials are needed to clarify the effects of total physical activity and sedentary behavior on cognitive prerequisites of learning. Future studies should assess what kind of physical activity or sedentary behavior affects specific kinds of cognition, as well as the mechanisms behind these associations. In the future, social interaction and context-related factors should be considered to be taken into account. In addition, the cognitive tests should be chosen so as to measure a wide range of cognitive performance.

Conclusion

In this study, objectively measured physical activity and sedentary time were positively associated with attentional processes, but not with other domains of cognitive functions. Self-reported computer/video game play was negatively associated with visuospatial working memory, whereas computer use was negatively associated with shifting and flexibility of attention. Self-reported physical activity and total screen time were not associated with any of the cognitive tests measuring visual memory, executive functions or attention in children. The results of the present study propose that physical activity may benefit attentional processes. However, excessive video game play and computer use may have unfavorable influence on cognitive functions.

Author Contributions

Conceived and designed the experiments: HJS THT TA MTK. Performed the experiments: HJS THT MTK. Analyzed the data: HJS THT AK MTK. Contributed reagents/materials/analysis tools: HJS THT TA AK MTK. Wrote the paper: HJS. Gave critical input on all versions of the manuscript: HJS THT TA AK MTK. Approved the final version of the manuscript: HJS THT TA AK MTK.

References

1. Pate RR, Mitchell JA, Byun W, Dowda M (2011) Sedentary behaviour in youth. Br J Sports Med 45: 906–913. doi: 10.1136/906 bjsports-2011-090192.
2. Ekelund U, Tomkinson G, Armstrong N (2011) What proportion of youth are physically active? Measurement issues, levels and recent time trends. Br J Sports Med 45: 859–865. doi: 10.1136/bjsports-2011-090190.
3. Hillman CH, Kamijo K, Scudder M (2011) A review of chronic and acute physical activity participation on neuroelectric measures of brain health and cognition during childhood. Prev Med 52: S21–S28. doi: 10.1016/j.ypmed.2011.01.024.
4. Erickson KI, Voss MW, Prakash RS, Basak C, Szabo A, et al. (2011) Exercise training increases size of hippocampus and improves memory. Proc Natl Acad Sci U S A 108: 3017–3022. doi: 10.1073/pnas.1015950108.
5. Lautenschlager NT, Cox KL, Flicker L, Foster JK, van Bockxmeer FM, et al. (2008) Effect of physical activity on cognitive function in older adults at risk for alzheimer disease: A randomized trial. JAMA 300: 1027–1037. doi: 10.1001/jama.300.9.1027.
6. Kramer AF, Erickson KI (2007) Effects of physical activity on cognition, well-being, and brain: Human interventions. Alzheimers Dement 3: S45–S51. doi: 10.1016/j.jalz.2007.01.008.
7. Sibley BA, Etnier JL (2003) The relationship between physical activity and cognition in children: A meta-analysis. Pediatr Exerc Sci 15: 243–256.
8. Ruiz JR, Ortega FB, Castillo R, Martín-Matillas M, Kwak L, et al. (2010) Physical activity, fitness, weight status, and cognitive performance in adolescents. J Pediatr 157: 917–922. doi: 10.1016/j.jpeds.2010.06.026.
9. Ardoy D, Fernández-Rodríguez J, Jiménez-Pavón D, Castillo R, Ruiz J, et al. (2014) A physical education trial improves adolescents' cognitive performance and academic achievement: The EDUFIT study. Scand J Med Sci Sports 24: e52–e61. doi: 10.1111/sms.12093.
10. Guiney H, Machado L (2013) Benefits of regular aerobic exercise for executive functioning in healthy populations. Psychon Bull Rev 20: 73–86. doi: 10.3758/s13423-012-0345-4.
11. Diamond A (2013) Executive functions. Annu Rev Psychol 64: 135–168. doi: 10.1146/annurev-psych-113011-143750.
12. Chaddock-Heyman L, Erickson KI, Voss MW, Knecht AM, Pontifex MB, et al. (2013) The effects of physical activity on functional MRI activation associated with cognitive control in children: A randomized controlled intervention. Front Hum Neurosci 7. doi: 10.3389/fnhum.2013.00072.
13. Davis C, Tomporowski P, McDowell J, Austin B, Miller P, et al. (2011) Exercise improves executive function and achievement and alters brain activation in overweight children: A randomized, controlled trial. Health Psychol 30: 91–98. doi: 10.1037/a0021766.
14. Fisher A, Boyle J, Paton J, Tomporowski P, Watson C, et al. (2011) Effects of a physical education intervention on cognitive function in young children: Randomized controlled pilot study. BMC Pediatr 11: 97. doi: 10.1186/1471-2431-1-97.
15. Kamijo K, Pontifex M, O'Leary K, Scudder M, Wu C, et al. (2011) The effects of an afterschool physical activity program on working memory in preadolescent children. Dev Sci: 1–13. doi: 10.1111/j.1467-7687.2011.01054.x.
16. Chaddock L, Hillman CH, Pontifex MB, Johnson CR, Raine LB, et al. (2012) Childhood aerobic fitness predicts cognitive performance one year later. J Sports Sci 30: 421–430. doi: 10.1080/02640414.2011.647706.
17. Chaddock L, Erickson KI, Prakash RS, Voss MW, VanPatter M, et al. (2012) A functional MRI investigation of the association between childhood aerobic fitness and neurocognitive control. Biol Psychol 89: 260–268. doi: 10.1016/j.biopsycho.2011.10.017.
18. Pontifex MB, Raine LB, Johnson CR, Chaddock L, Voss MW, et al. (2011) Cardiorespiratory fitness and the flexible modulation of cognitive control in preadolescent children. J Cogn Neurosci 23: 1332–1345. doi: 10.1162/jocn.2010.21528.
19. Chaddock L, Erickson K, Prakash R, Kim J, Voss M, et al. (2010) A neuroimaging investigation of the association between aerobic fitness, hippocampal volume, and memory performance in preadolescent children. Brain Res 1358: 172–183. doi: 10.1016/j.brainres.2010.08.049.
20. Puder J, Marques-Vidal P, Schindler C, Zahner L, Niederer I, et al. (2011) Effect of multidimensional lifestyle intervention on fitness and adiposity in predominantly migrant preschool children (ballabeina): Cluster randomised controlled trial. BMJ 343: d6195. doi: 10.1136/bmj.d6195.
21. Reed JA, Maslow AL, Long S, Hughey M (2012) Examining the impact of 45 minutes of daily physical education on cognitive ability, fitness performance, and body composition of African American youth. J Phys Act Health 10: 185–197.
22. Stroth S, Kubesch S, Dieterle K, Ruchsow M, Heim R, et al. (2009) Physical fitness, but not acute exercise modulates event-related potential indices for executive control in healthy adolescents. Brain Res 1269: 114–124. doi:10.1016/j.brainres.2009.02.073.
23. Armstrong N, Tomkinson G, Ekelund U (2011) Aerobic fitness and its relationship to sport, exercise training and habitual physical activity during youth. Br J Sports Med 45: 849–858. doi: 10.1136/bjsports-2011-090200.
24. Johnson JG, Cohen P, Kasen S, Brook JS (2007) Extensive television viewing and the development of attention and learning difficulties during adolescence. Arch Pediatr Adolesc Med 161: 480–486.
25. Landhuis CE, Poulton R, Welch D, Hancox RJ (2007) Does childhood television viewing lead to attention problems in adolescence? Results from a prospective longitudinal study. Pediatrics 120: 532–537. doi: 10.1542/peds.2007-0978.
26. Swing EL, Gentile DA, Anderson CA, Walsh DA (2010) Television and video game exposure and the development of attention problems. Pediatrics 126: 214–221. doi: 10.1542/peds.2009-1508.
27. Weis R, Cerankosky BC (2010) Effects of video-game ownership on young boys' academic and behavioral functioning: A randomized, controlled study. Psychol Sci 21: 463–470. doi: 10.1177/0956797610362670.
28. Dworak M, Schierl T, Bruns T, Strüder HK (2007) Impact of singular excessive computer game and television exposure on sleep patterns and memory performance of school-aged children. Pediatrics 120: 978–985. doi: 10.1542/peds.2007-0476.
29. Ferguson CJ, Garza A, Jerabeck J, Ramos R, Galindo M (2012) Not worth the fuss after all? Cross-sectional and prospective data on violent video game influences on aggression, visuospatial cognition and mathematics ability in a sample of youth. J Youth Adolesc: 42: 109–122. doi: 10.1007/s10964-012-9803-6.
30. Dye MW, Green CS, Bavelier D (2009) Increasing speed of processing with action video games. Curr Dir Psychol Sci 18: 321–326. doi: 10.1016/j.neuropsychologia.2009.02.002.
31. Bittman M, Rutherford L, Brown J, Unsworth L (2011) Digital natives? New and old media and children's outcomes. AJE 55: 161–175.
32. Milner B (1971) Interhemispheric differences in the localization of psychological processes in man. Br Med Bull 27: 272–277.
33. Mishkin M, Appenzeller T (1987) The anatomy of memory. Sci Am 256: 80–89. doi: 10.1038/scientificamerican0687-80.
34. Evenson KR, Catellier DJ, Gill K, Ondrak KS, McMurray RG (2006) Calibration of two objective measures of physical activity for children. J Sports Sci 24: 1557–1565. doi: 10.1080/02640410802334196.
35. Currie C, Zanotti C, Morgan A, Currie D, De Looze M, et al. (2012) Social determinants of health and well-being among young people. Health behaviour in school-aged children (HBSC) study. International report from the 2009/2010 survey. Health policy for children and adolescents. Available: http://www.euro.who.int/__data/assets/pdf_file/0003/163857/Social-determinants-of-health-and-well-being-among-young-people.pdf. Assessed 2014 May 6.
36. Booth M, Okely A, Chey T, Bauman A (2001) The reliability and validity of the physical activity questions in the WHO health behaviour in schoolchildren (HBSC) survey: A population study. Br J Sports Med 35: 263–267. doi: 10.1136/bjsm.35.4.263.
37. Liu Y, Wang M, Tynjälä J, Lv Y, Villberg J, et al. (2010) Test-retest reliability of selected items of health behaviour in school-aged children (HBSC) survey questionnaire in Beijing, china. BMC Med Res Methodol 10: 73. doi: 10.1186/1471-2288-10-73.
38. Muthén L, Muthén B, editors (1998–2012) Mplus User's guide. Seventh edition. Los Angeles: CA: Muthén & Muthén.
39. Little TD, Cunningham WA, Shahar G, Widaman KF (2002) To parcel or not to parcel: Exploring the question, weighing the merits. Struct Equ Modeling 9: 151–173. doi:10.1207/S15328007SEM0902_1.
40. de Jong PF (1999) Hierarchical regression analysis in structural equation modeling. Struct Equ Modeling 6: 198–211. doi: 10.1080/10705519909540128.
41. Hu L, Bentler PM (1999) Cutoff criteria for fit indexes in covariance structure analysis: Conventional criteria versus new alternatives. Struct Equ Modeling 6: 1–55. doi: 10.1080/10705519909540118.
42. Spitzer US, Hollmann W (2013) Experimental observations of the effects of physical exercise on attention, academic and prosocial performance in school settings. Trends Neurosci Educ 2: 1–6. doi: 10.1016/j.tine.2013.03.002.
43. Eriksen BA, Eriksen CW (1974) Effects of noise letters upon the identification of a target letter in a nonsearch task. Percept Psychophys 16: 143–149.
44. Castelli D, Hillman C, Hirsch J, Hirsch A, Drollette E (2011) FIT kids: Time in target heart zone and cognitive performance. Prev Med 52: S55–S59. doi: 10.1016/j.ypmed.2011.01.019.
45. Hillman CH, Buck SM, Themanson JR, Pontifex MB, Castelli DM (2009) Aerobic fitness and cognitive development: Event-related brain potential and task performance indices of executive control in preadolescent children. Dev Psychol 45: 114–129. doi: 10.1037/a0014437.
46. Chaddock L, Erickson K, Prakash R, VanPatter M, Voss M, et al. (2010) Basal ganglia volume is associated with aerobic fitness in preadolescent children. Dev Neurosci 32: 249–256. doi: 10.1159/000316648.

47. Gomez-Pinilla F, Hillman C (2013) The influence of exercise on cognitive abilities. Compr Physiol 3: 403–428. doi: 10.1002/cphy.c110063.
48. Hopkins M, Davis F, Vantieghem M, Whalen P, Bucci D (2012) Differential effects of acute and regular physical exercise on cognition and affect. Neuroscience 215: 59–68. doi: 10.1016/j.neuroscience.2012.04.056.
49. Brown AD, McMorris CA, Longman RS, Leigh R, Hill MD, et al. (2010) Effects of cardiorespiratory fitness and cerebral blood flow on cognitive outcomes in older women. Neurobiol Aging 31: 2047–2057. doi:10.1016/j.neurobiolaging.2008.11.002.
50. Haapala EA, Poikkeus A, Tompuri T, Kukkonen-Harjula K, Leppänen P, et al. (2013) Associations of motor and cardiovascular performance with academic skills in children. Med Sci Sports Exerc: In press. doi: 10.1249/MSS.0000000000000186.
51. Iverson JM (2010) Developing language in a developing body: The relationship between motor development and language development*. J Child Lang 37: 229. doi: 10.1017/S0305000909990432.
52. Kantomaa MT, Stamatakis E, Kankaanpää A, Kaakinen M, Rodriguez A, et al. (2013) Physical activity and obesity mediate the association between childhood motor function and adolescents' academic achievement. PNAS 110: 1917–1922. doi:10.1073/pnas.1214574110/−/DCSupplemental.
53. Burkhalter TM, Hillman CH (2011) A narrative review of physical activity, nutrition, and obesity to cognition and scholastic performance across the human lifespan. Adv Nutr 2: 201S–206S. doi: 10.3945/an.111.000331.
54. Hillman CH, Erickson KI, Kramer AF (2008) Be smart, exercise your heart: Exercise effects on brain and cognition. Nat Rev Neurosci 9: 58–65. doi:10.1038/nrn2298.
55. Best JR (2010) Effects of physical activity on children's executive function: Contributions of experimental research on aerobic exercise. Dev Rev 30: 331–351. doi: 10.1016/j.dr.2010.08.001.
56. Malina RM (1996) Tracking of physical activity and physical fitness across the lifespan. Res Q Exerc Sport 67: S48–S57. doi 10.1080/02701367.1996.10608853.
57. Rowland T (2013) Oxygen uptake and endurance fitness in children, revisited. Pediatr Exerc Sci 25: 508–514.
58. Syväoja HJ, Kantomaa MT, Ahonen T, Hakonen H, Kankaanpää A, et al. (2013) Physical activity, sedentary behavior, and academic performance in Finnish children. Med Sci Sports Exerc 45: 2098–2104. doi: 10.1249/MSS.0b013e318296d7b8.
59. Boot WR, Blakely DP, Simons DJ (2011) Do action video games improve perception and cognition? Frontiers in Psychology 2. doi: 10.3389/fpsyg.2011.00226.
60. Spence I, Feng J (2010) Video games and spatial cognition. Rev Gen Psychol 14: 92–104. doi: 10.1037/a0019491.
61. Granic I, Lobel A, Engels RC (2013) The benefits of playing video games. Am Psychol 69: 66–78. doi: 10.1037/a0034857.
62. Shin N (2004) Exploring pathways from television viewing to academic achievement in school age children. J Genet Psychol 165: 367–381. doi: 10.3200/GNTP.165.4.367-382.
63. Kirkorian HL, Wartella EA, Anderson DR (2008) Media and young children's learning. Future Child 18: 39–61. doi: 10.1353/foc.0.0002.
64. Schmidt ME, Vandewater EA (2008) Media and attention, cognition, and school achievement. Future Child18: 63–85. doi: 10.1353/foc.0.0004.
65. Ennemoser M, Schneider W (2007) Relations of television viewing and reading: Findings from a 4-year longitudinal study. J Educ Psychol 99: 349–368. doi: 10.1037/0022-0663.99.2.349.
66. Feng J, Spence I, Pratt J (2007) Playing an action video game reduces gender differences in spatial cognition. Psychol Sci 18: 850–855. doi: 10.1111/j.1467-9280.2007.01990.x.
67. Kühn S, Gleich T, Lorenz R, Lindenberger U, Gallinat J (2013) Playing super mario induces structural brain plasticity: Gray matter changes resulting from training with a commercial video game. Mol Psychiatry 19: 265–271. doi: 10.1038/mp.2013.120.
68. Munasib A, Bhattacharya S (2010) Is the 'Idiot's Box'raising idiocy? Early and middle childhood television watching and child cognitive outcome. Econ Educ Rev 29: 873–883. doi: 10.1016/j.econedurev.2010.03.005.

proposed. Moreover, we offer here a decisional tree for validation in other centers interested in mountain medicine.

Methods

Study design and data collection

A prospective open cohort study involved all subjects who came to the outpatient altitude medicine consultation at Avicenne Hospital (Bobigny, France) between January 1st, 1992 and December 31, 2011 before a stay of at least 3 days above 4000 m with an overnight sleeping above 3500 m. From the previous study [2], 102 subjects were added (10% of the population) to perform the score calculation. The present study is based on a 20-yr experience of evaluating persons before a stay at high altitude. Individual informed consent was collected. For this non-interventional study, no Ethics committee approval was needed according to French law.

For the subjects who came several times during the study period, only the first visit was included in the analysis. Subjects were given a questionnaire based on Hackett's score [7] thus allowing the definition of the clinical outcome (suffering or not from SHAI). None of the subjects spent more than 4 days above 3000 m in the preceding 2 months. Subjects who sent back the questionnaire and did not take acetazolamide or other medication used for altitude sickness (PDE5 inhibitors, calcium blockers or dexamethasone) during the stay at high altitude were finally included in the study.

Baseline examination. Subjects were questioned about their socio-demographic characteristics, personal and familial medical history, treatments, objective of the stay (tourism, mountaineering, trekking or work, precise geographical location), previous history of SHAI, recent stay at high altitude, previous history of migraine (criteria defined by the International Headache Society) [8], regular endurance training activity (at least 40 minutes, 3 times a week) as previously defined in detail [2]. Each subject performed a hypoxic exercise test (inspired fraction of O_2: 0.115, exercise intensity of approximately 30% of maximal aerobic power that allowed the calculation of three main physiological parameters: desaturation induced by hypoxia at exercise, ventilatory response to hypoxia at exercise, and cardiac response to hypoxia at exercise [2,9–11]. These last two parameters are calculated from the ratio of increased ventilation or heart rate over the decrease in arterial oxygen saturation induced by hypoxia during exercise. They are an indirect measurement of the chemosensitivity to a hypoxic challenge [2]. Data were collected from the patient's medical chart containing the clinical observations and the physiological measurements made by the physician who examined the patient at the consultation. Patient gave authorization for using his/her data and data were anonymized before any statistical treatment. The study was declared to French National data protection organization (Commission nationale de l'informatique et des libertés (CNIL)/ registration number 1740068) and data collection and informatics treatments followed the principles of the CNIL.

Follow-up and clinical outcome. Outcome was the occurrence of SHAI. Each subject was asked to fill out a daily questionnaire based on Hackett's score of severe AMS and symptoms of HAPE or HACE during their future stay at high altitude and send it back upon returning home [7]. Moderate AMS was defined by a Hackett's score <6, without significant impact on planned activity. Severe AMS was defined by a Hackett's score ≥6, with incapacitating symptoms leading to a stop or a significant reduction of planned activity. HAPE was defined by the presence of clinical signs of respiratory distress (dyspnea, cyanosis, rales), confirmed by a thorax X-Ray upon descent to low altitude. HACE was defined by clinical signs of neurological deficit (ataxia, mental confusion). The diagnosis of HAPE or HACE was always confirmed by an expert, either on the spot where the disorder occurred or later on when hospitalized. Subjects were asked to note any medication taken during their stay, especially acetazolamide, widely used among trekkers for the prevention of AMS [12]. From the questionnaire, subjects were classified as no or moderate AMS, severe AMS, HAPE or HACE. Severe AMS, HAPE and HACE were pooled as SHAI and considered as being intolerant to high altitude. Information about the ascent characteristics (daily speed of ascent, altitude reached) was collected in the follow-up questionnaire. This questionnaire is part of the usual care as it is systematically given to all patients coming to the consultation in order to have a follow-up in case of health problems during the stay at high altitude.

Statistical analysis

Qualitative variables were expressed in N (%), quantitative variables in mean (standard deviation SD) or median (25th-75th percentiles as appropriate).

History of SHAI is a major risk factor of SHAI [1,2]. However, it can be determined only in subjects with previous exposure to high altitude. Therefore the entire analysis was stratified according to previous history (or not) of high altitude sojourn. The baseline characteristics of subjects were compared according to their previous history (or not) of sojourn at high altitude using Student t-test or Wilcoxon-Mann-Whitney and the Pearson chi square-test or Fisher's exact test, as appropriate. Due to deviation from linearity assumption, physiological variables were expressed in dummy variables defined by tertiles in the group of subjects without SHAI.

Two multivariate models were built for each group (previous sojourn or not), one with the classical risk factors and one with supplemental adjustment for physiological variables. The variables entered in the multivariate model were those previously identified: history of SHAI (only in the group with previous high altitude sojourn), planned rapid ascent, history of migraine, geographical location, age, sex, physical activity for the classical risk factors and hypoxic ventilatory response, hypoxic cardiac response and desaturation in hypoxia at exercise for physiological variables [2]. Two-by-two analyses were performed to assess potential interactions and confounding by fitting. We examined interactions between these variables, and between these variables and the presence of previous high altitude sojourn.

We developed risk prediction scores using established methods in both groups [13–15]. We used a multivariate logistic regression model to estimate the β coefficients for each risk factor. Variables were retained in the final multivariate model if they had an odds ratio (OR) of more than 1.2 (for binary variables) [14] and $p<0.20$. We internally validated the scores by using bootstrap resampling with 1000 replications of both groups to estimate β' shrinkage coefficients [16]. We used the median bootstrapped regression coefficients rounded to the nearest half point as weights, which we combined with the baseline logit function to derive risk prediction scores. We assessed calibration and discrimination of the multivariate models and of the scores in the two groups. Calibration was evaluated by computing the Hosmer-Lemeshow chi-square statistic and discrimination by the C-statistic (Area Under ROC Curve, AUC) with 95% confidence intervals: the usual thresholds were considered: ≥0.7 = good discrimination; ≥ 0.8: very good and ≥0.9 = excellent. Discrimination was also quantified by calculating the Net Reclassification Improvement index (NRI): NRI indicates the proportion of patients correctly classified (in the group who will and the group who will not

Risk Prediction Score for Severe High Altitude Illness: A Cohort Study

Florence Canouï-Poitrine[1,2]*, Kalaivani Veerabudun[1,2], Philippe Larmignat[3], Murielle Letournel[5], Sylvie Bastuji-Garin[1,2]❡, Jean-Paul Richalet[4,5]❡

1 Université Paris Est, Faculté de Médecine, EA 4393, Laboratoire d'Investigation Clinique, Créteil, France, **2** AP-HP, Groupe Henri Mondor-Albert Chenevier, Service de Santé Publique, Créteil, France, **3** AP-HP, Hôpital Avicenne, Service d'Anesthésie et Réanimation, Bobigny, France, **4** Université Paris 13, Sorbonne Paris Cité, EA2363 « Réponses cellulaires et fonctionnelles à l'hypoxie », U.F.R. SMBH, Bobigny, France, **5** AP-HP, Hôpital Avicenne, Service de Physiologie, Explorations Fonctionnelles et Médecine du Sport, Bobigny, France

Abstract

Background: Risk prediction of acute mountain sickness, high altitude (HA) pulmonary or cerebral edema is currently based on clinical assessment. Our objective was to develop a risk prediction score of Severe High Altitude Illness (SHAI) combining clinical and physiological factors. Study population was 1017 sea-level subjects who performed a hypoxia exercise test before a stay at HA. The outcome was the occurrence of SHAI during HA exposure. Two scores were built, according to the presence (PRE, n = 537) or absence (ABS, n = 480) of previous experience at HA, using multivariate logistic regression. Calibration was evaluated by Hosmer-Lemeshow chisquare test and discrimination by Area Under ROC Curve (AUC) and Net Reclassification Index (NRI).

Results: The score was a linear combination of history of SHAI, ventilatory and cardiac response to hypoxia at exercise, speed of ascent, desaturation during hypoxic exercise, history of migraine, geographical location, female sex, age under 46 and regular physical activity. In the PRE/ABS groups, the score ranged from 0 to 12/10, a cut-off of 5/5.5 gave a sensitivity of 87%/87% and a specificity of 82%/73%. Adding physiological variables via the hypoxic exercise test improved the discrimination ability of the models: AUC increased by 7% to 0.91 (95%CI: 0.87–0.93) and 17% to 0.89 (95%CI: 0.85–0.91), NRI was 30% and 54% in the PRE and ABS groups respectively. A score computed with ten clinical, environmental and physiological factors accurately predicted the risk of SHAI in a large cohort of sea-level residents visiting HA regions.

Editor: Gernot Zissel, University Medical Center Freiburg, Germany

Funding: The Universities of Paris 13 and Paris Est contributed to the financial support of this study. The funders had no role in study design, data collection and analysis, decision to publish, or preparation of the manuscript.

Competing Interests: The authors have declared that no competing interests exist.

* Email: florence.canoui-poitrine@hmn.aphp.fr

❡ These authors contributed equally to this work.

Introduction

An increased number of sea-level residents visit areas above 4000 m of altitude for leisure, sport or work. They may suffer from severe acute mountain sickness, high altitude pulmonary or cerebral edema, especially when they are not yet acclimatized to the hypoxic environment [1]. The above clinical outcomes have been regrouped in a clinical entity called Severe High Altitude Illness (SHAI).

Recently, we assessed several clinical, environmental and physiological independent risk factors of SHAI in a cohort of 1326 sea-level residents who came to an outpatient mountain medicine consultation and underwent a hypoxic exercise test before a stay at altitude above 4000 m [2]. The main risk factors evidenced were previous history of SHAI, low ventilatory and cardiac response to hypoxia at exercise, speed of ascent above 400 m per day in the acclimatization period, high desaturation during exercise in hypoxia, history of migraine, geographical location (Aconcagua, Mont-Blanc, Ladakh), female gender, regular endurance training and age under 46 years old. Some of these factors such as history of SHAI or migraine were already mentioned in the literature [1,3–6]. However this study was the first to demonstrate that adding physiological measurements to clinical evaluation greatly improved the discrimination between susceptible and non-susceptible subjects [2]. As 45% of the subjects coming to the outpatient consultation had no previous experience of sojourn at high altitude, one of the main risk factor (history of SHAI) could not be taken into account in the risk prediction.

The main aim of the present study was to develop and internally validate, in a large cohort of sea-level residents visiting high-altitude regions, a risk prediction score for SHAI occurrence including clinical and physiological factors. The secondary endpoint is to assess and quantify the benefit of performing a hypoxia exercise test to predict the risk of SHAI, especially in subjects without previous experience at high altitude. This score may be useful to detect highly susceptible subjects and improve the prevention of SHAI for newcomers at high altitude. This is a clear added value to our previous work where no prediction score was

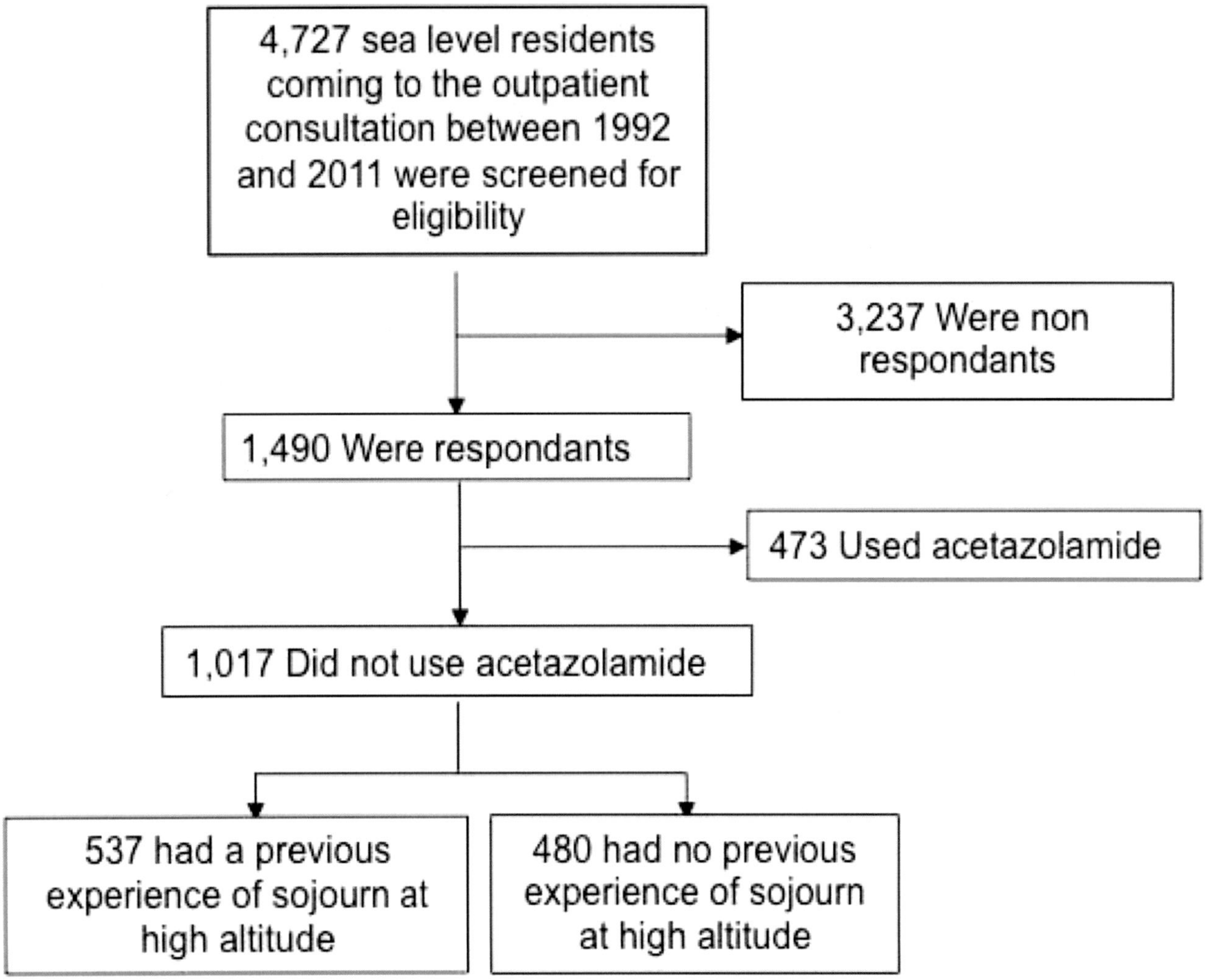

Figure 1. Flow chart of the study.

develop SHAI) when adding physiological markers to the clinical model [17].

We calculated the sensitivity, specificity, predictive values and proportion of correctly classified subjects for each value of the risk prediction score to determine thresholds.

All tests were two-tailed. No imputation of missing data was made. Data were analyzed using STATA software version 12 (Stata Inc., College Station, TX). Reporting of the present study was done using STrengthening the Reporting of OBservational studies in Epidemiology (STROBE) guidelines.

Results

Baseline characteristics

Overall, 4727 subjects came for the first time to the outpatient altitude medicine consultation at Avicenne Hospital between January 1st, 1992 and December 31, 2011. After exclusion of non-respondents and subjects who took acetazolamide, 1017 subjects were included in the study (Figure 1). Baseline characteristics of groups with and without previous high altitude sojourn are shown in Table 1. Subjects with no previous sojourn at high altitude were younger, more frequently women, had higher blood pressure, lower planned rapid ascent, less frequent special geographical locations and regular endurance physical activity. No difference was found regarding physiological variables.

Subjects with previous sojourn at high altitude

The multivariate model included history of SHAI, rapid ascent, geographical location, female sex and regular endurance physical activity had a very good discrimination (AUC = 0.84) and an adequate calibration (p-value Hosmer-Lemeshow chisquare = 0.87) (Table 2). When adding physiological variables, the discrimination significantly increased by 7.5% up to an excellent discrimination (>0.90). The multivariate physio-clinical model showed an adequate calibration (Table 2). A 30% NRI indicates that 30% of subjects were correctly reclassified when adding the physiological variables into the predictive model (toward lower risk category for subjects who will not developed SHAI, and toward high risk category for subjects who will developed SHAI). Desaturation was not included in the physio-clinical model due to close correlation with history of SHAI leading to over-adjustement and default of calibration. We found no significant interaction.

Bootstrapped multivariate regression β' coefficients were almost similar to those of original multivariate regression model [2]. Points rounded to the nearest half point were assigned to the

Table 1. Characteristics of the patients according to history of previous high altitude sojourn.

	Previous high altitude sojourn (N = 537)	No previous high altitude sojourn (N = 480)	P*
Age - yr	45.8 (13.5)	42.6 (15.1)	<0.0004
Female sex - no. (%)	164 (31.4)	214 (45.1)	<0.001
Current smokers – no. (%)	55 (10.5)	49 (10.3)	0.92
Body Mass Index – kg/m² ≥25 kg/m²	93 (17.8)	95 (20.0)	0.37
Systolic Blood Pressure - mmHg	132.3 (14.1)	128.4 (14.1)	<0.001
History of Severe High Altitude Illness – no. (%)	126 (24.1)	-	-
History of migraine – no. (%)	71 (13.6)	51 (10.8)	0.17
Rapid ascent (>400 m/day) – no. (%)	157 (30.54)	112 (24.0)	0.023
Geographical location (Aconcagua, Mont Blanc or Ladakh) - no. (%)	121 (23.1)	56 (11.8)	<0.001
Regular endurance physical activity – no. (%)	216 (41.4)	108 (22.7)	<0.001
Hypoxic ventilatory response at exercise - l/min/kg <0.68	225 (44.0)	207 (44.2)	
(0.68–0.94)	152 (29.7)	136 (29.1)	0.98
≥0.94	135 (26.4)	125 (26.7)	
Hypoxic cardiac response at exercise - b/min/% <0.72	193 (37.6)	160 (34.1)	
(0.72–0.95)	171 (33.3)	159 (33.9)	0.46
≥0.95	149 (29.1)	150 (32.0)	
Desaturation at exercise in hypoxia - % <19	149 (28.5)	147 (31.1)	
(19–24)	178 (34.1)	155 (32.8)	0.67
≥24%	195 (37.4)	170 (36.0)	

Data are expressed as n (%) or means (SD); * Pearson chisquare or Student t-test as appropriate

bootstrapped β' coefficients (Table 2). The score was then computed by means of a linear combination of the rounded coefficients as follows:

SHAI risk prediction score for subjects with previous exposure to high altitude =

2.5* (History of SHAI)

+2* (ascent > 400 m/day)

+1.5* (history of migraine)

+1*(Geographical location = Aconcagua, Mont Blanc or Ladakh)

+0.5* (age<46 years)

+0.5* (regular physical activity)

+3* (hypoxic ventilatory response at exercise <0.68 L/min/kg) or 1*(0.68< hypoxic ventilatory response at exercise <0.94 L/min/kg)

+1* (hypoxic cardiac response at exercise <0.72 b/min/%).

The calibration of the score was adequate (Figure 2, lower panel) and the discrimination was very good (Figure 3). Median SHAI risk prediction score was 3 (1.5–4.5) in patients free of SHAI and 6.5 (5.5–8) in patients with SHAI. A cut-off of 5 gave a sensitivity of 87%, a specificity of 81.8%, a positive likelihood ratio of 4.8 and negative likelihood ratio of 0.16.

Subjects without previous sojourn at high altitude

The multivariate model included history of SHAI, rapid ascent, geographical location, female sex and regular endurance physical activity had adequate calibration (p-value Hosmer-Lemeshow chisquare = 0.91) and good discrimination (AUC = 0.72) (Table 3). When adding physiological variables, the discrimination significantly increased by 17% up to a very good discrimination (AUC>0.80). The multivariate physio-clinical model showed an adequate calibration (p-value Hosmer-Lemeshow chisquare = 0.36) (Table 3). A 54% NRI indicates that 54% of subjects were correctly reclassified when adding the physiological variables into the predictive model. We found no significant interaction.

The score was computed as for the previous group, but with different coefficients (Table 3):

SHAI risk prediction score for subjects without previous exposure to high altitude =

2* (ascent > 400 m/day)

+0.5* (Geographical location = Aconcagua, Mont Blanc or Ladakh)

+0.5* (female sex)

+1* (regular physical activity)

+3* (hypoxic ventilatory response at exercise <0.68 L/min/kg) or 1* (0.68< hypoxic ventilatory response at exercise < 0.94 L/min/kg)

+1* (hypoxic cardiac response at exercise < 0.95 b/min/%)

+2* (desaturation at exercice in hypoxia ≥24%) or 1* (19%< desaturation at exercice in hypoxia <24%).

The calibration of the score was adequate (Figure 2, upper panel) and the discrimination was very good (Figure 3). Median SHAI risk prediction score was 4 (2–5.5) in patients free of SHAI and 6.5 (6–7.5) in patients with SHAI. A cut-off of 5.5 gave a sensitivity of 87.3%, a specificity of 73.1%, a positive likelihood ratio of 3.2 and a negative likelihood ratio of 0.17.

We included female sex and migraine in the two multivariate models (for the groups with and without previous high-altitude sojourn). However, in the multivariate analysis after adjustment for others confounders, the variable female sex in the group with previous experience and the variable migraine in the group without remained not significant leading to a nul weight in the final score.

Table 2. Adjusted Odds Ratios (95% CI) for clinical and physio-clinical multivariate model and scoring system in subjects **with** previous high-altitude sojourn (n = 501, 36 missing).

	Clinical model		Physio-clinical model			
Variables	**Odds Ratio (95% CI) ***	**P Value†**	**Odds Ratio (95% CI) ***	**P value†**	**β′ regression coefficient‡**	**Points ¶**
History of Severe High Altitude Illness	12.35 (7.24–21.08)	<0.001	12.89 (6.78–24.49)	<0.001	2.58	2.5
Rapid ascent (> 400 m/night)	4.69 (2.79–7.90)	<0.001	5.89 (3.19–10.87)	<0.001	1.84	2
History of migraine	2.21 (1.15–4.24)	0.017	4.29 (1.93–9.54)	<0.001	1.27	1.5
Geographical location (Aconcagua, Mt Blanc, Ladakh)	2.7 (1.47–4.88)	0.001	2.43 (1.28–4.61)	0.006	0.79	1
Age < 46 years	1.62 (1.00–2.63	0.05	1.82 (1.00–3.29)	0.049	0.48	0.5
Female sex	1.60 (0.96–2.67)	0.073	1.38 (0.75–2.54)	0.30	0.29	0
Regular endurance physical activity	1.9 (1.09–3.19)	0.53	1.46 (0.80–2.65)	0.12	0.45	0.5
Hypoxic ventilatory response at exercise (l/min/kg)	-	-				
low < 0.68			20.59 (6.76–62.7)	<0.001	3.07	3
moderate (0.68–0.94)	-	-	3.41 (1.10–10.59)	0.034	1.18	1
high ≥0.94	-	-	ref	ref	ref	0
Hypoxic cardiac response at exercise (b/min/%)	-	-				
low <0.72			2.41 (1.16–5.03)	0.019	0.97	1
moderate (0.72–0.95)	-	-	0.94 (0.44–2.01)	0.89	0.07	0
high ≥0.95	-	-	ref	ref	ref	0
C-statistic (Area Under ROC Curve) (CI 95%)‡	0.84 (0.78–0.88)	-	0.91 (0.87–0.93)			
Calibration: Hosmer-Lemeshow chisquare	3.81 (p = 0.87)	-	4.52 (p = 0.81)			
Net Reclassification Index ¥	-	-	30% (p<0.001)			

*Adjusted odds ratio from multivariate logistic regression adjusted for all variables listed in the column; † Wald test; ‡ Estimations obtained after 1000 resampling; ¶ β′ Coefficient rounded to the near half integer; ¥ Net Reclassification Index indicates the proportion of patients correctly classified (in the group who will and the group who will not develop SHAI when adding physiological variables to the clinical model.

Discussion

This is the first study proposing a risk prediction scoring system for SHAI based on a large cohort of sea-level residents visiting high altitude regions. Ten clinical, environmental and physiological variables were used to compute the risk prediction scoring, with a different weight applied to the 10 items according to presence or absence of previous experience at high altitude. It ranged from 0 to 10 points in subjects without previous experience and 0 to 12 in those with. The obtained scoring systems had very good to excellent discrimination ability and adequate calibration. The two groups showed some different characteristics (Table 1): as it might be expected, subjects with previous experience at high altitude were older, more trained, more men, had slightly higher blood pressure and went to higher risk locations. These differences justify the stratification made before performing the multivariate logistic regression. We chose to develop two separate multivariate models leading to two prediction scores, in the group of subjects with previous exposure and in the group of subjects without. Indeed, even if the two multivariate models are very close, some predictors differ, precluding the possibility of using one group as development and the other one as validation datasets. In particular, the weight of history of SHAI (available only in the group with previous exposure to high altitude) modifies the weight of the other variables of the model and therefore modifies the final score.

Previous episodes of SHAI, history of migraine and high speed of ascent are risk factors already mentioned in several studies [4,5,18]. Adding physiological variables linked to the tolerance to hypoxia during moderate exercise increases the accuracy of the prediction and allows a mechanistic approach [2,18–20]. In subjects with previous experience of high altitude exposure, adding physiological variables allowed a reclassification of 30% of the subjects, while in altitude naïve subjects, 54% of the subjects were reclassified. This clearly demonstrates the benefit of performing a hypoxia exercise test in subjects before a sojourn at high altitude, especially when no information is available about their susceptibility to SHAI, which was the case in almost half of our consultants. The fact that regular endurance training is not a protecting factor for SHAI is important to mention; in fact it is rather detrimental, due to a more severe desaturation during exercise in this population compared to sedentary subjects [21]. Including the geographical location in the prediction score allows a personalization of the prevention process. However, as Mont-Blanc is mainly climbed by Europeans, it might be considered as a surrogate for any mountain around 4800 m high, the ascent of which is done without prior acclimatization. It is important to mention that this higher risk is adjusted for speed of ascent, i.e the risk of developing AMS in Mt Blanc, Ladakh or Aconcagua is still higher than other locations independently from the speed of ascent. So that there is something more we do not explain, or because people who climb Mont-Blanc come from the big cities and do not take time to acclimatize before climbing the mountain. No subject was acclimatized (no recent stay above 3000 m) when they travelled to high altitude, so that pre-acclimatization, which is a well known factor reducing the risk of SHAI was not taken into in account in our prediction model.

The strength of the study was the prospective design, the use of validated criterion to assess SHAI, and the large population with systematic measurement of physiological response to hypoxia at

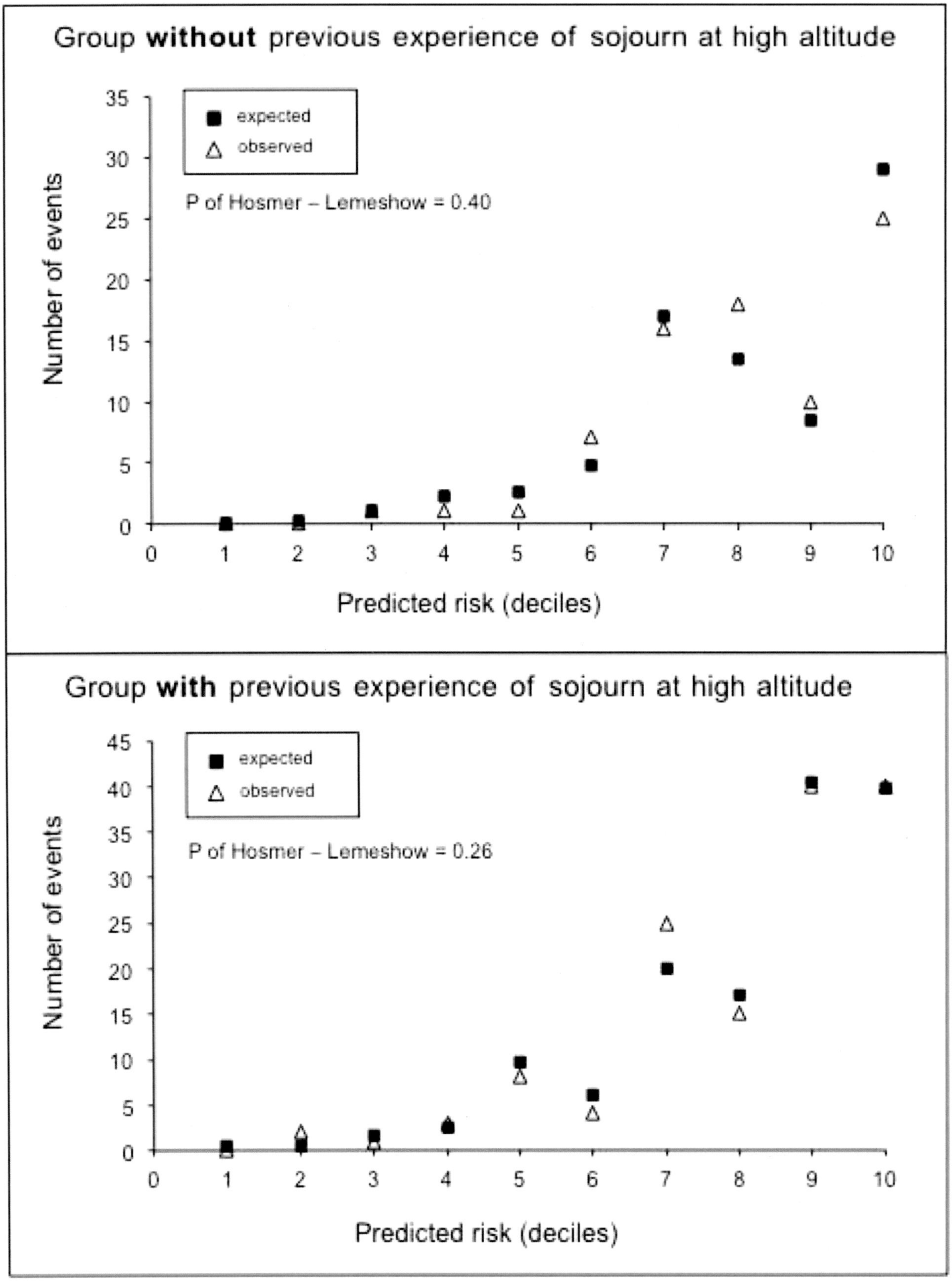

Figure 2. Calibration of the risk prediction score for Severe High Altitude Illness in the group without previous experience of sojourn at high altitude (upper panel, n = 480) and with previous experience of sojourn at high altitude (lower panel, n = 537).

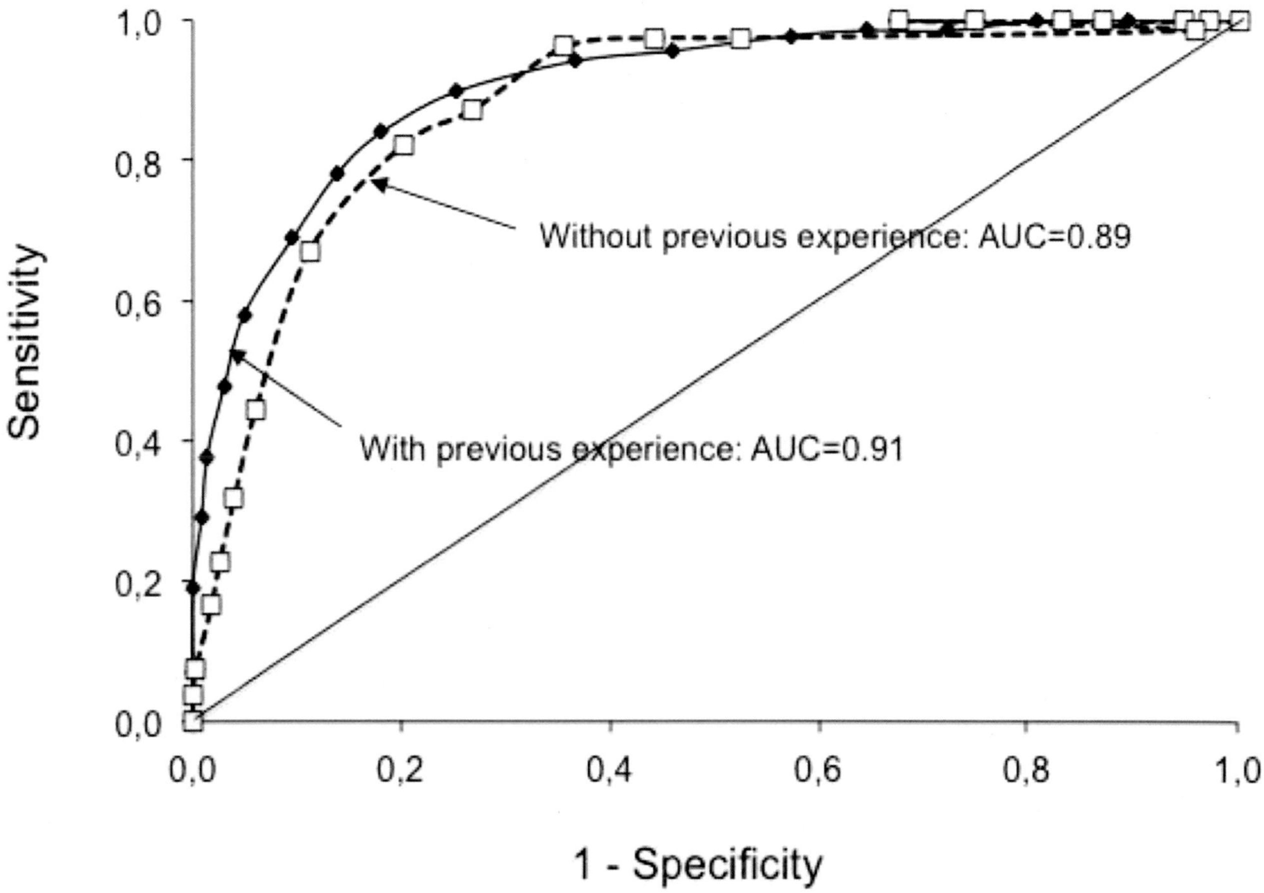

Figure 3. ROC curve of the risk prediction score for Severe High Altitude Illness in the groups without (n = 480) and with (n = 537) previous experience of sojourn at high altitude.

baseline. To develop and validate the score, we used a rigorous procedure for involving internal validation (bootstrap of the β regression coefficient). Shrinkage of the regression coefficients aims to correct for over-optimism in the model and may help to make models more transportable [16]. We used bootstrap resampling with 1000 replications of both groups and not split-sample analyses as it has been shown by Steyerberg et al that the latter methods gave overly pessimistic estimates whereas the former provided stable estimates with low bias [16].

Other tests have been proposed to assess, for example, the specific individual susceptibility to HAPE by measuring the pulmonary vascular reactivity to hypoxia and/or exercise [22]. More usual tests such as ECG or pulmonary function tests have failed to demonstrate any prediction power [1]. Finally, our approach, here, is not mechanistic, looking at the precise physiopathological causes of HAPE or HACE, although we address the basic common reason of all severe manifestations, i.e. severe hypoxemia, whatever the following effects on the lungs or on the brain. Our approach is very practical for a physician in front of a person who wants to know his own level of risk. The common trait of all SHAI manifestations is that the subject has to stop his trip and take urgent measures (such as descent, re-oxygenation, drugs…).

The reported results should be interpreted with some limitations in mind. The response rate was low, leading to a possible selection bias, although no major difference was found in the clinical and physiological characteristics between responders and non-responders (results not shown). However, we cannot discard the possibility that non-respondents had a successful stay at altitude and perhaps felt less compelled to return the questionnaire. Classification of SHAI was based on a self-evaluation without immediate medical control leading to a possible classification bias. However an expert using a validated score made the adjudication. Similarly, information concerning speed of ascent and history of migraine was self-declarative and subject to caution. We used the Hackett's score since when the study was started, in 1991, the Lake Louise score was not yet in use for epidemiological studies of AMS. Besides, the Hackett's score has been highly correlated to the Lake Louise score and the Environmental Symptoms Questionnaire for the clinical evaluation of AMS [23]. Although we included a long list of potential predictor variables and established which factors remain independent after adjustment and their relative importance [2], a residual confounding bias may persist.

Finally, this study was conducted from a single outpatient altitude medicine consultation and its transportability has to be evaluated in other populations, by means of an external validation. However, the recruitment of this consultation comes from all regions of France and surrounding French-speaking countries.

Practical considerations for physicians

For a given set of variables entered in the score, a physician can compute the probability of developing SHAI during a stay at high altitude. This probability depends on intrinsic factors such as sex,

Table 3. Adjusted Odds Ratios (95% CI) for clinical and physio-clinical multivariate model and scoring system in subjects **without** previous high-altitude sojourn (n = 457, 23 missing).

	Clinical model		Physio-clinical model			
Variables	**Odds Ratio (95% CI) ***	**P Value†**	**Odds Ratio (95% CI) ***	**P Value†**	**β′ regression coefficient‡**	**Points ¶**
History of Severe High Altitude Illness	-	-	-	-	-	-
Rapid ascent (>400 m/night)	4.26 (2.54–7.16)	<0.001	7.26 (3.70–14.22)	<0.001	2.09	2
History of migraine	1.18 (0.55–2.55)	0.67	1.31 (0.51–3.33)	0.57	0.26	0
Geographical location (Aconcagua, Mt Blanc, Ladakh)	1.31 (0.63–2.75)	0.47	1.87 (0.76–4.61)	0.18	0.63	0.5
Age < 46 years	1.44 (0.84–2.46)	0.18	1.47 (0.77–2.79)	0.24	0.42	0
Female sex	1.51 (0.90–2.52)	0.12	1.73 (0.94–3.18)	0.08	0.6	0.5
Regular endurance physical activity	1.68 (0.96–2.94)	0.07	2.00 (1.00–3.99)	0.049	0.75	1
Hypoxic ventilatory response at exercise (l/min/kg)	-	-		<0.001		
low <0.68			17.3 (3.62 -82.47)		3.12	3
moderate (0.68–0.94)	-	-	3.28 (0.66–16.4)		1.30	1
high ≥0.94	-	-	ref		ref	0
Hypoxic cardiac response at exercise (b/min/%)	-	-		0.12		
low <0.72			2.19 (0.94–5.06)		0.85	1
moderate (0.72–0.95)	-	-	2.22 (0.97–5.11)		0.85	1
high ≥0.95	-	-	ref		ref	0
Desaturation at exercise in hypoxia - %	-	-		<0.001		
low <19			ref		ref	0
moderate (19–24)	-	-	3.29 (0.86–12.31)		1.23	1
high ≥24		-	9.03 (2.48–32.89)		2.3	2
C-statistic (Area Under ROC Curve) (CI 95%)‡	0.72 (0.66–0.78)		0.89 (0.85–0.91)			
Calibration: Hosmer-Lemeshow chisquare	2.68 (p = 0.91)		8.79 (p = 0.36)			
Net Reclassification Index ¥			54% (p<0.001)			

*Adjusted odds ratio from multivariate logistic regression adjusted for all variables listed in the column; † Wald test; ‡ Estimations obtained after 1000 resampling; ¶ β′ Coefficient rounded to the near half integer; ¥ Net Reclassification Index indicates the proportion of patients correctly classified (in the group who will and the group who will not develop SHAI when adding physiological variables to the clinical model.

history of migraine, physiological response to hypoxia, endurance training status which are fixed for a given individual, but also on extrinsic factors such as the geographical location of the destination or the speed of altitude ascent that can be modified by the individual, following the advice of the physician. There could be a certain degree of uncertainty concerning one of the three most important factors imbedded in the score, i.e. the history of SHAI since about 44% of the population coming to the consultation has never been at high altitude beforehand. To avoid this bias, the physician can compute one of the two versions of the prediction score considering the presence or absence of previous exposure to high altitude. Finally, for a patient with a score above the cut-off value of 4.5 or 5.5, the physician may propose further preventive measures such as alternative routes or preventive medication with acetazolamide which has been shown to reduce by almost 50% the relative risk of SHAI at the dose of 250 mg/day, starting the day before reaching 3,000 m of altitude [2]. In any case, this consultation will be the occasion to inform all the patients about the guidelines of prevention and treatment of severe high-altitude as well as cold-related diseases [1,24]. Based on objective measurements, this score may be a useful tool for physicians practicing High Altitude medicine consultations, allowing a better prevention of the risk of severe medical problems in newcomers to high altitude. More effective prevention could therefore reduce the risk of costly evacuations from remote regions of the world.

In conclusion, we developed a scoring system based on 10 clinical, environmental and physiological factors that accurately predicted the SHAI risk in sea-level residents visiting high altitude regions. The use of a hypoxia exercise test greatly improved the prediction, especially in subjects with no previous experience of high altitude sojourn. The three most robust risk factors of SHAI are previous history of SHAI, excessive speed of ascent and hypoxic ventilatory response at exercise. A validation in an independent cohort undertaken by an independent team is needed to confirm its transportability. These findings may be useful to clinicians for reducing the risk of SHAI.

Author Contributions

Conceived and designed the experiments: JPR PL. Performed the experiments: JPR PL ML. Analyzed the data: KV FCP SBG. Contributed reagents/materials/analysis tools: FCP KV JPR SBG. Wrote the paper: JPR KV FC-P PL. Guarantor of the study: JPR. Designed the study and collected the data: JPR ML PL. Made the statistical analysis: FC-P KV. Made the interpretation of the data: FC-P KV SBG. Revised the manuscript: PL ML.

References

1. Bartsch P, Swenson ER (2013) Acute high-altitude illnesses. N Engl J Med 369:1666–1667.
2. Richalet JP, Larmignat P, Poitrine E, Letournel M, Canoui-Poitrine F (2012) Physiological risk factors for severe high-altitude illness: a prospective cohort study. Am J Respir Crit Care Med 185:192–198.
3. Bloch KE, Turk AJ, Maggiorini M, Hess T, Merz T, et al. (2009) Effect of ascent protocol on acute mountain sickness and success at Muztagh Ata, 7546 m. High Alt Med Biol 10:25–32.
4. Honigman B, Theis MK, Koziol-McLain J, Roach R, Yip R, et al. (1993) Acute mountain sickness in a general tourist population at moderate altitudes. Ann Intern Med 118:587–592.
5. Mairer K, Wille M, Bucher T, Burtscher M (2009) Prevalence of acute mountain sickness in the Eastern Alps. High Alt Med Biol 10:239–245.
6. Schneider M, Bernasch D, Weymann J, Holle R, Bartsch P (2002) Acute mountain sickness: influence of susceptibility, preexposure, and ascent rate. Med Sci Sports Exerc 34:1886–1891.
7. Hackett PH, Rennie D, Levine HD (1976) The incidence, importance, and prophylaxis of acute mountain sickness. Lancet 2(7996):1149–1155.
8. Headache Classification Subcommittee of the International Headache S (2004) The International Classification of Headache Disorders: 2nd edition. Cephalalgia : an international journal of headache 24 Suppl 1:9–160.
9. Lhuissier FJ, Brumm M, Ramier D, Richalet JP (2012) Ventilatory and cardiac responses to hypoxia at submaximal exercise are independent of altitude and exercise intensity. J Appl Physiol 112:566–570.
10. Richalet JP, Gimenez-Roqueplo AP, Peyrard S, Venisse A, Marelle L, et al. (2009) A role for succinate dehydrogenase genes in low chemoresponsiveness to hypoxia? Clin Auton Res 19:335–342.
11. Lhuissier FJ, Canoui-Poitrine F, Richalet JP (2012) Ageing and cardiorespiratory response to hypoxia. The Journal of physiology 590(Pt 21):5461–5474.
12. van Patot MC, Leadbetter G 3rd, Keyes LE, Maakestad KM, Olson S, et al. (2008) Prophylactic low-dose acetazolamide reduces the incidence and severity of acute mountain sickness. High Alt Med Biol 9:289–293.
13. Assmann G, Cullen P, Schulte H (2002) Simple scoring scheme for calculating the risk of acute coronary events based on the 10-year follow-up of the prospective cardiovascular Munster (PROCAM) study. Circulation 105:310–315.
14. Hippisley-Cox J, Coupland C (2011) Development and validation of risk prediction algorithm (QThrombosis) to estimate future risk of venous thromboembolism: prospective cohort study. BMJ 343:d4656.
15. Hippisley-Cox J, Coupland C, Vinogradova Y, Robson J, May M, et al. (2007) Derivation and validation of QRISK, a new cardiovascular disease risk score for the United Kingdom: prospective open cohort study BMJ 335:136.
16. Steyerberg EW, Harrell FE Jr, Borsboom GJ, Eijkemans MJ, Vergouwe Y, et al. (2001) Internal validation of predictive models: efficiency of some procedures for logistic regression analysis. J Clin Epidemiol 54:774–781.
17. Pencina MJ, D'Agostino RB Sr, D'Agostino RB Jr, Vasan RS (2008) Evaluating the added predictive ability of a new marker: from area under the ROC curve to reclassification and beyond. Stat Med 27:157–172; discussion 207–12.
18. Hackett PH, Roach RC (2004) High altitude cerebral edema. High Alt Med Biol 5:136–146.
19. Hackett PH, Roach RC, Schoene RB, Harrison GL, Mills WJ Jr (1988) Abnormal control of ventilation in high-altitude pulmonary edema. J Appl Physiol 64:1268–1272.
20. Matsuzawa Y, Fujimoto K, Kobayashi T, Namushi NR, Harada K, et al. (1989) Blunted hypoxic ventilatory drive in subjects susceptible to high-altitude pulmonary edema. J Appl Physiol 66:1152–1157.
21. Mollard P, Woorons X, Letournel M, Lamberto C, Favret F, et al. (2007) Determinant factors of the decrease in aerobic performance in moderate acute hypoxia in women endurance athletes. Respir Physiol Neurobiol 159:178–186.
22. Dehnert C, Grunig E, Mereles D, von Lennep N, Bartsch P (2005) Identification of individuals susceptible to high-altitude pulmonary oedema at low altitude. Eur Respir J 25:545–551.
23. Savourey G, Guinet A, Besnard Y, Garcia N, Hanniquet AM, et al. (1995) Evaluation of the Lake Louise acute mountain sickness scoring system in a hypobaric chamber. Aviat Space Environ Med 66:963–967.
24. Luks AM, McIntosh SE, Grissom CK, Auerbach PS, Rodway GW, et al. (2010) Wilderness Medical Society consensus guidelines for the prevention and treatment of acute altitude illness. Wilderness Environ Med 21:146–155.

11

The Road to Gold: Training and Peaking Characteristics in the Year Prior to a Gold Medal Endurance Performance

Espen Tønnessen[1]*, Øystein Sylta[2], Thomas A. Haugen[1], Erlend Hem[1], Ida S. Svendsen[3], Stephen Seiler[2]

1 The Norwegian Olympic Federation, Oslo, Norway, **2** Faculty of Health and Sport Sciences, University of Agder, Kristiansand, Norway, **3** School of Sport, Exercise and Health Sciences, Loughborough University, Leicestershire, United Kingdom

Abstract

Purpose: To describe training variations across the annual cycle in Olympic and World Champion endurance athletes, and determine whether these athletes used tapering strategies in line with recommendations in the literature.

Methods: Eleven elite XC skiers and biathletes (4 male; 28±1 yr, 85±5 mL. min^{-1}. kg^{-1} $\dot{V}O_{2max}$, 7 female, 25±4 yr, 73±3 mL. min^{-1}. kg^{-1} $\dot{V}O_{2max}$) reported one year of day-to-day training leading up to the most successful competition of their career. Training data were divided into periodization and peaking phases and distributed into training forms, intensity zones and endurance activity forms.

Results: Athletes trained ~800 h/500 sessions.year^{-1}, including ~500 h. year^{-1} of sport-specific training. Ninety-four percent of all training was executed as aerobic endurance training. Of this, ~90% was low intensity training (LIT, below the first lactate threshold) and 10% high intensity training (HIT, above the first lactate threshold) by time. Categorically, 23% of training sessions were characterized as HIT with primary portions executed at or above the first lactate turn point. Training volume and specificity distribution conformed to a traditional periodization model, but absolute volume of HIT remained stable across phases. However, HIT training patterns tended to become more polarized in the competition phase. Training volume, frequency and intensity remained unchanged from pre-peaking to peaking period, but there was a 32±15% ($P<.01$) volume reduction from the preparation period to peaking phase.

Conclusions: The annual training data for these Olympic and World champion XC skiers and biathletes conforms to previously reported training patterns of elite endurance athletes. During the competition phase, training became more sport-specific, with 92% performed as XC skiing. However, they did not follow suggested tapering practice derived from short-term experimental studies. Only three out of 11 athletes took a rest day during the final 5 days prior to their most successful competition.

Editor: Matjaz Perc, University of Maribor, Slovenia

Funding: The authors received no specific funding for this work.

Competing Interests: The authors have declared that no competing interests exist.

* Email: espen.tonnessen@olympiatoppen.no

Introduction

Winning a gold medal in a major international championship requires not only outstanding athletic ability and long-term training progression, but also that the athlete achieves peak performance at the right time. In recent years, increased attention has been given to quantifying the training characteristics of elite endurance athletes [1–3] and this information has provided a fruitful foundation for hypothesis testing regarding training load and physiological adaptation. At the same time, a strong knowledge base has developed regarding best practice for the tapering and peaking process, based largely on experimental interventions [4–6]. However, studies linking the characteristics of the long-term training process to those of the short term pre-peaking and peaking process are lacking.

Recently, a number of descriptive studies, both retrospective and prospective, have been published on the training characteristics of athletes from endurance sports such as running [7–12], cycling [13–14], XC skiing [15–17], swimming [18–19], rowing [20–21], triathlon [22–23], speed skating [24–25] and kayaking [26]. Training load variables such as volume, frequency and intensity distribution appear to play an interactive role in maximizing physical capacity and performance [27]. Depending on the specific muscular loading characteristics of the sport, athletes typically train 500 h (distance running) [7,8,11,12,28,29] to well in excess of 1000 h per year (rowing, swimming, cycling, triathlon) [13–14,18–23] performed during 400–800 annual training sessions [11–12,15–17,23], in order to reach an internationally elite level. When examining the intensity distribution of this large training volume, a number of studies across a broad range of sports converge on the finding that 75–90% of all endurance training time is performed as low intensity training (LIT, below the first lactate turn point) for athletes training >

500 h per year. The remaining 10–25% is comprised of high intensity training (HIT) performed above the first lactate turn point [7–8,14–15,22–23]. This approximate "80–20" distribution between low and high intensity training among high-level performers is a robust finding [3], even if mechanistic explanations for its ubiquity remain speculative. Furthermore, the "best practice" magnitude and distribution of HIT remains unclear. In addition, the training-dose response relationship has a significant individual variation component, which further complicates the generalizability of the picture. While the influx of descriptive data on the training of elite endurance athletes has informed training practice, and stimulated new experimental studies, methodological compromises are inherent to the challenge of measuring behavior reliably and precisely in highly selected groups. Available descriptive studies typically only present data over a shorter time frame [7–8,12], at a sub-elite level [9,14–15,17,21–22] or as single case studies [11,23,28–29]. Accuracy in training monitoring is also unclear, due to weaknesses in methods such as questionnaires [10] or compilation and analysis of data that are in part or completely based on training plans instead of strict quantification of actual training performed [7–8,20]. Limited data currently exist on the long-term training of highly trained and elite athletes, based on accurate training monitoring [30].

Short-term training manipulations to achieve peaking for optimal sports performance have been investigated for more than 20 years. A synthesis of studies on well-trained athletes from a variety of different sports has shown a performance improvement of up to 3%, providing the final 4–28 days of training are executed correctly [5–6,31–33]. All other things being equal, a well-executed peaking phase can therefore dramatically increase the odds of winning a gold medal at a championship event for an individual athlete with finalist potential. In the research literature, the peaking process is typically divided into two phases: a pre-tapering phase, and the final taper period culminating with the intended competition. The aim of the pre-tapering phase is to stimulate a controlled "over-reaching" state and elicit a super-compensatory adaptive response in the following taper. Experimentally, the optimal duration of the actual taper depends on the training executed in the pre-taper [6,33–34]. The taper is initiated approximately 14 days prior to the desired peak performance, and the aim of this phase is to facilitate regeneration and reduce fatigue, while maintaining or increasing fitness and technical/psychological readiness in order to mobilize maximal performance in competition [4–6,35]. The optimal training volume, frequency and intensity in each phase is debated [4–6,31,35], but a reduction in training load of between 41–60% from pre-taper to taper has been recommended. This reduction appears to be best achieved via reduced training duration per session, while maintaining session frequency [5]. Maintaining training intensity is considered to be a key factor in a successful peaking regime, and it is therefore recommended that the frequency of HIT sessions be maintained during the taper [36–39]. Despite 20 years of research on tapering and peaking for athletic performance, we are unaware of any study that has successfully quantified the "real life" peaking strategies of athletes achieving ultimate success in Olympic Games or World Championship events. It is therefore unclear how the models developed from controlled experimental studies are translated to the actual peaking practices of elite endurance athletes. Furthermore, few studies havelinked peaking strategies to annual training characteristics and the competitive season of elite athletes [30].

The current study therefore aimed to: 1) present highly accurate day-to-day annual training data from a cohort of endurance athletes that all won Olympic or World Championship gold medals and, 2) quantify and examine relationships between annual training and peaking characteristics in these athletes.

Methods

Subjects

Four male and seven female former and current Norwegian elite XC skiers and biathletes were included in the study (Table 1). All athletes had won a least one individual Olympic or World Championship senior gold medal during their career. In total, included males had won 41 (5–26) and females 25 (1–9) gold medals (includes both individual and relays from 1985 through 2011). In addition, included athletes had systematically and accurately recorded their day-to-day training in detail from junior through to senior level. In the current study, we have analyzed and reported the year specifically leading up to their most successful competition at senior level. The regional ethics committee of Southern Norway reviewed the study and concluded that, due to the nature of the investigation, it did not require their approval. The study was therefore submitted to and approved by the Norwegian Social Science Data Services (NSD), and all athletes gave their oral and written informed consent prior to study participation.

Physiological testing

All athletes underwent regular physiological testing during their career. The test values presented in Table 1 represent the highest result achieved during the analyzed year. There were no physiological tests performed during the competition period, and the presented results therefore represent tests from October or November, while Olympic or World Championship events were typically held in February-March. All physiological testing was conducted at the Norwegian Olympic training center. $\dot{V}O_{2max}$ testing was performed as running at 10.5% inclination on a motorized treadmill (Woodway Gmbh, Weil am Rhein, Germany) calibrated for speed and incline. The procedure started with an extensive warm-up sequence, followed by a stepwise increase in running velocity every minute thereafter until volitional exhaustion, normally occurring after 4–6 minutes. Starting velocity for all athletes corresponded to 85–90% of $\dot{V}O_{2max}$. The increase was 1 $km.h^{-1}.min^{-1}$, and the last velocity step was held for at least 1 min. The test was terminated before voluntary exhaustion if the $\dot{V}O_2$values leveled off or decreased despite increasing workload and ventilation, in addition to respiratory exchange ratio (RER) > 1.10. $\dot{V}O_{2max}$ was defined as the highest average of two consecutive 30 s measurements. Oxygen uptake was measured using EOS Sprint (Jaeger-Toennis, Wurtzburg, Germany) until 2002, after which an Oxycon Pro (Jaeger-Toennis, Wurtzburg, Germany) metabolic test system was used. An internal comparison between the two analyzers was conducted during the transition in 2002 and showed identical regression lines for the treadmill running velocity $-\dot{V}O_2$ relationship with both systems. Primarily two exercise physiologists supervised all testing during the entire period.

Training monitoring

Athletes included in the study recorded their day-to-day training during their most successful year in paper diaries designed by the Norwegian Ski Association [40–41], the Norwegian Biathlon Association [42] or, since ~2005, in the digital version developed by the Norwegian Olympic Federation (OLT). The training recorded for each session included total training time distributed across training form (strength, endurance, sprint), activity form

Table 1. General characteristics of athletes included in the study.

Subject	Gender	Age	Height	Weight	$\dot{V}O_{2max}$ (ml·kg^{-1}.min^{-1})	$\dot{V}O_{2max}$ (l.min^{-1})
1	M	28	180	77	92.5	7.13
2	M	26	190	82	81.9	6.73
3	M	29	189	83	84.8	7.07
4	M	28	179	66	81.2	5.25
5	F	23	172	55	72.9	3.90
6	F	23	176	63	73.6	4.64
7	F	29	173	63	76.6	4.81
8	F	20	175	69	70.4	4.83
9	F	28	166	61	69.1	4.24
10	F	22	162	51	76.0	3.93
11	F	30	169	64	71.4	4.60
Mean ± SD, Male		28±1	185±6	77±8	85.1±5.2	6.5±0.9
Mean ± SD, Female		25±4	170±5	61±6	72.9±2.8	4.4±0.4

Values are reported from the analyzed year in the current study.

(skiing, roller-skiing, running, cycling etc.), and intensity zone, as well as specific comments regarding session details. All paper training diaries were transferred session by session to digital format by persons from the current research group. Total training time and frequency of sessions was distributed in line with the structure in Figure 1. Digitized diary data was rigorously cross-checked for internal consistency among different training distribution breakdowns at the individual level. Internal consistency of digitized training records from all included athletes was ≥99%.

All the athletes included in the study used a 5 intensity zone model, where zones 1–2 are classified as LIT and zones 3–5 as HIT. The intensity scale presented in Table 2 represents average self-reported zone-cut offs from 29 elite XC-skiers from a previous study [43]. In the results section we have presented the data either in a binary model (LIT/HIT) or a 5-zone model were zones 1–2 are below the first lactate threshold (LT^1), zone 3 between LT^1 and LT^2, and zones 4–5 above LT^2 [3,44]. The intensity distribution is classified both according to a time in training zone approach and a frequency based session goal approach (SG). These methods and the intensity zones cut-offs have been described in detail recently [43].

Annual periodization phases and peaking model

General training data from the entire year are either presented as annual training characteristics or divided into different periodization phases as presented in Table 3. Peaking characteristics were quantified based on the final 6 weeks of training prior to the gold medal winning performance, as delineated in Table 3.

Statistical analyses

All data in text, tables or figures are presented as mean ± standard deviation (SD) and/or range. Statistical comparisons between different periodization phases are focused on the general preparation period (GP), specific preparation period (SP) and competition period (CP) in addition to comparing the actual peaking phase with pre-peaking phase, GP and SP. Data were not normally distributed. Therefore each variable from the GP, SP and CP (overall, pre-peaking and peaking phase) was tested with a non-parametric Friedman test, followed by a post-hoc test (Wilcoxon Signed Rank) to locate statistical differences. Male and female athlete data are merged, as a Mann-Whitney U Test revealed no significant differences in any relevant variables across gender (data not shown). All figures and statistical analyses were performed using Microsoft Excel or SPSS 18.0 (SPSS Inc, Chicago, IL, USA) and statistical significance was accepted at the $P<.05$ level or Bonferroni adjusted alpha level.

Results

Annual training characteristics

Total training volume was 770±99 h (622–942) distributed across 470±68 sessions (375–585) throughout the gold medal year. Endurance training accounted for 94±3% of all training time with the remaining 5±2% composed of strength training and 1±1% ski sprint training. Time in training zone based intensity distribution showed that 91±1% of all endurance training time was executed as LIT (zone 1–2) and 9±1% as HIT (zone 3–5).

Monthly training distribution of specific and non-specific activity forms during each training phase are presented in Figure 2. Endurance and sprint training was executed with sport-specific movement patterns (ski or roller ski) for 64±3% (465±56 h/min-max: 376–569 h) of total training time, with the remaining 36±3% (265±47 h/min-max: 196–337 h), composed of non-specific activity forms (running, cycling etc.) throughout the year. The proportion of sport-specific training increased significantly from GP (48±6%) to SP (87±8%) and CP (92±4%) ($P<.01$).

The distribution across all five intensity zones was: zone 1: 86.0±3.4%, zone 2: 5.3±3.0%, zone 3: 3.3±0.9%, zone 4: 3.3±1% and zone 5: 2.1±1.0%. When all endurance sessions were nominally categorized using the SG approach, the distribution was 77±2% LIT and 23±2% HIT (Figure 3, A). Weekly training patterns during each training phase are presented in Table 4.

Total annual HIT duration (including competitions) was 63±14 h (46–85 h) distributed across 106±20 sessions (85–147) throughout the year. The relative distribution of HIT duration in intensity zones 3, 4 and 5 was 39±10%, 37±13% and 24±13% respectively, and 32±6%, 38±14% and 30±13% according to a SG distribution. Monthly frequency of HIT sessions increased

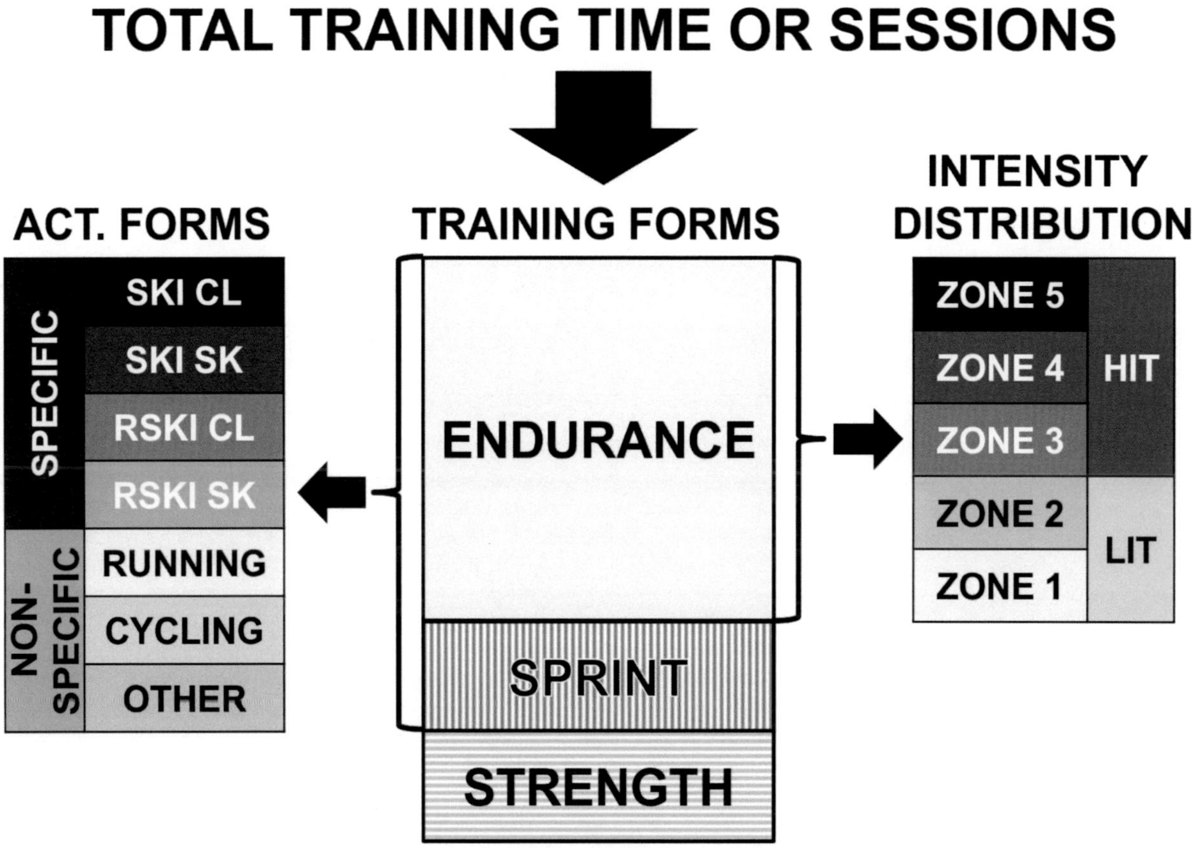

Figure 1. Training distribution methods. Total training time was divided into training forms (endurance, sprint and strength). Endurance time and frequency were further distributed into 5 intensity zones in line with table 2. Zones 1–2 are LIT and zones 3–5 are HIT. Endurance and sprint time together were divided into activity forms. Ski and roller ski were classified as specific, and running, cycling or other as non-specific activity forms.

from GP to SP ($P<.01$). In addition, the monthly frequency of intensity zone 5 sessions increased from GP to SP and then remained unchanged in the CP ($P<.01$) (Figure 3, B). Weekly HIT patterns during each training phase are presented in Table 4.

Peaking characteristics

Total training time ($h.wk^{-1}$) decreased by 9±14% from the pre-peaking to peaking phase, but this did not reach statistical significance. However, the reduction from GP, when training volume was highest, to the peaking phase, was 32±15% ($P<.01$). This decrease in total training volume was entirely due to a reduction in non-sport-specific training. Individual data for each of the 11 athletes are presented in Figure 4. The decrease in training volume from GP and pre-peaking phase to the peaking phase was achieved via a reduction in both endurance and strength training, while sprint training time remained stable, although there was a tendency for sprint training time to increase slightly from the pre-peaking phase to the peaking phase. There were no significant changes in total session frequency per week between the peaking phase and any of the other phases (Figure 5 A and Table 4).

There was non-significant decrease of 9±15% in LIT endurance training ($h.wk^{-1}$) from the pre-peaking phase to the peaking phase. However, LIT training volume decreased by 31±17% ($P<.01$) from GP to the peaking phase. In contrast, HIT time ($h.wk^{-1}$) remained stable from both pre-peaking phase to the

Table 2. The 5-zone, 3-zone, and binary intensity scales used in the current study.

Intensity Zone	Typical Blood lactate[A] (mmol. L^{-1})	Typical Heart Rate (% max)	Three zone model	Binary model
5	>5.8	>94	>LT^2	
4	3.7–5.7	89–93		HIT
3	2.1–3.6	84–88	LT^1–LT^2	
2	1.3–2.0	74–83		LIT
1	<1.2	54–73	<LT^1	

[A]Measured with Lactate Pro LT-1710. Reference values presented are derived from the average self-reported zone-cut offs of 29 elite XC-skiers [43], and individual adjustments are required.

Table 3. Training phases in annual cycle, including peaking phases.

Period in annual training cycle	Duration
Preparation period (PP)	May-December
Transition period	*May*
General preparation period (GP)	*June-October*
Specific preparation period (SP)	*November-December*
Competition Period (CP)	January-March
Pre-peaking phase	*6–3 weeks before championship event*
Peaking phase	*Last 14 days before championship event*
Regeneration period	April

peaking phase and from GP to the peaking phase (Figure 5 A and Table 4).

LIT endurance session frequency decreased from GP to the peaking phase by 21±24% (P=.016) but remained stable from pre-peaking phase to the peaking phase. Weekly HIT session frequency increased by 40±27% (P<.01) from GP to the peaking phase, but remained stable from pre-peaking phase to the peaking phase (Figure 5 B). Training volume and frequency distribution among zones 3, 4 and 5 through the different phases are presented in Figure 5 B and Table 4.

Discussion

To the authors' knowledge, this is the first study to connect accurate annual day-to-day training data to a specific peaking period in a group of athletes achieving ultimate international success in an endurance sport. The main findings of the present study are: 1) The annual training data for these Olympic and World champion XC skiers and biathletes conforms to previously reported training patterns amongst elite endurance athletes. 2) In contrast, peaking characteristics for these gold medalists did not conform to suggested best practice for tapering strategies in elite endurance athletes, as derived from partly experimental studies.

Annual training characteristics

Training volume. High training volume has emerged as a key commonality in successful endurance training [20,1–3,25]. Athletes in the current study trained ~800 h.year^{-1}across ~500 annual training sessions although there were individual differences. This finding is in line with previous studies reporting training volume in elite XC skiers [1,16–17]. Muscular loading differences and stress associated with different activities probably explain why there is large variation in reported annual training volume across sports. For example, top international runners are reported to train "only" 500–600 h.year^{-1} [7–8] while a case study of an international level triathlete reports >1000 h.year^{-1} [23]. The current data show a tendency for developments in training

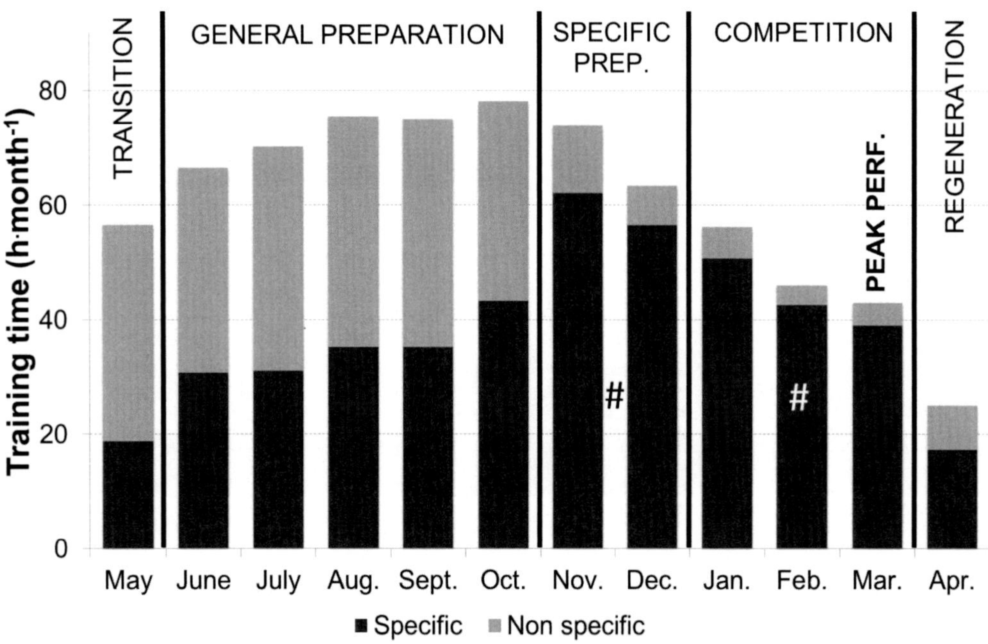

Figure 2. Annual organization of specific and non-specific activity forms. Endurance and sprint training time (h) distributed into specific (ski and roller ski) and non-specific (running, cycling and other) activity forms during each month and divided in phases. # Difference in specific training time vs. GP (P<.01).

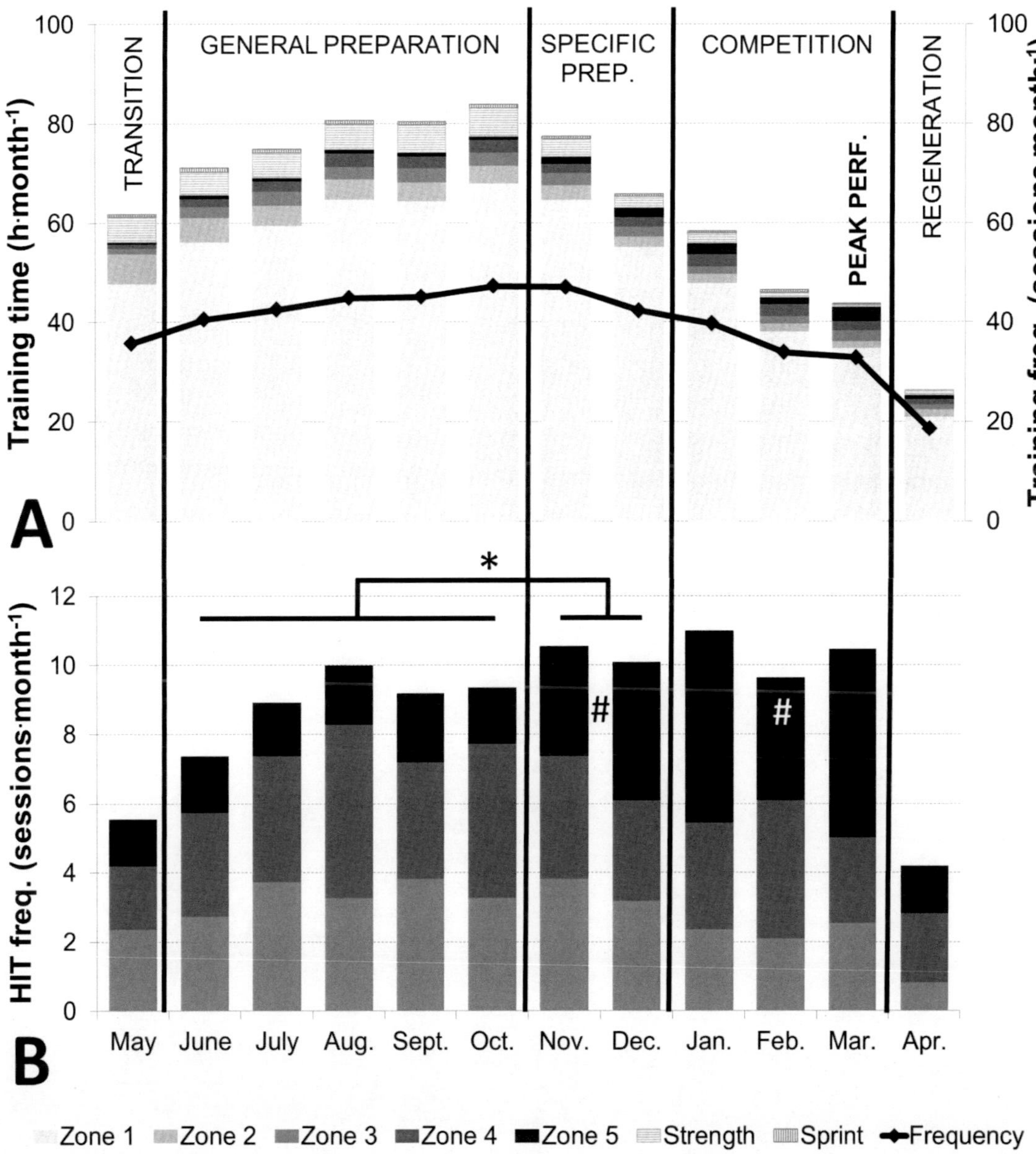

Figure 3. Annual training characteristics. A: Total training time (h) distributed into endurance training (zones 1–5), strength and sprint (bars, y-axis), and total training frequency (sessions) (line, z-axis) during each month and divided into phases. B: HIT frequency (sessions) distributed into zones 3, 4 and 5 (bars, y-axis) during each month and divided in phases. There was a statistically significant difference (P<.05) in total HIT sessions and zones 3, 4 and 5 respectively across the GP, SP and CP. Pairwise post-hoc tests showed: * Difference in total HIT sessions across phases (P<.01). # Difference between zone 5 sessions vs. GP (P<.01).

patterns during the time period from 1985 to 2011, with a positive relationship between total training volume and year of championship title ($r = .59$, $P = .055$). Increased training volume appears to be mainly due to increased frequency of training sessions from 1985 to 2011, while average duration per training session has remained relatively stable at 1.7±0.2 h.

During the entire training year, 94% of all training *time* was executed as endurance training. However, strength and sprint training appear to play an important role in the training of XC skiers [45]. Strength training was carried out as general, specific or maximal, while sprints included both specific ski sprint-related exercises and jumps. Interestingly, ~90% of all strength and sprint training was executed during the preparation period (PP). In practice, this means two to three strength and sprints sessions.-week^{-1} in PP compared to one weekly session during CP, typically conducted at the end of endurance training sessions. The main underlying philosophy for these athletes was to build up a prescribed strength level during PP and then maintain this level during CP. Unfortunately, systematic strength testing documentation was not available for these athletes. We are therefore not able to verify whether strength characteristics of these athletes were stable during CP. However, previous research suggests that one bout of strength training per week is sufficient to maintain strength levels over shorter time frames [46].

Table 4. Weekly training patterns during different phases throughout the season.

				Competition phase			
Weekly training patterns	**Transition phase**	**General preparation phase**	**Specific preparation phase**	**Overall**	**Pre-peaking**	**Peaking**	**Regeneration phase**
Total training:							
Training time (h.wk^{-1})	13.9±5.3	17.9±2.5	16.5±2.4	11.6±2.2 $^{\#\beta}$	13.5±3.1 $^{\#\beta}$	12.1±2.4 $^{\#\beta}$	6.1±3.7
Tr. sessions·wk^{-1}	8.1±2.8	10.1±1.0	10.3±1.7	8.3±2.1 $^{\#\beta}$	8.9±1.9 $^{\#\beta}$	9.2±2.3	4.3±2.3
Training forms:							
Endurance (h·wk^{-1})	12.7±4.9	16.5±2.6	15.7±2.2	11.2±2.0 $^{\#\beta}$	12.9±2.8 $^{\beta}$	11.7±2.3 $^{\#\beta}$	5.9±3.6
Strength (h·wk^{-1})	1.1±1.0	1.2±0.5	0.7±0.4 *	0.3±0.2 $^{\#\beta}$	0.5±0.4 $^{\#}$	0.2±0.2 $^{\#\beta}$	0.2±0.3
Sprint (h·wk^{-1})	0.1±0.1	0.2±0.2	0.1±0.1	0.1±0.1	0.1±0.1	0.2±0.2	0.0±0.0
Intensity distribution:							
Zone 1 (h·wk^{-1})	10.8±4.7	14.3±2.6	13.8±2.1	9.4±2.3 $^{\#\beta}$	11.2±2.8 $^{\beta}$	9.7±2.0 $^{\#\beta}$	4.9±2.9
Zone 2 (h·wk^{-1})	1.3±0.9	0.9±0.6	0.6±0.5 *	0.4±0.3 $^{\#}$	0.4±0.5 $^{\#}$	0.6±0.8	0.3±0.5
Zone 3 (h·wk^{-1})	0.3±0.2	0.6±0.2	0.5±0.2	0.4±0.3	0.4±0.2 $^{\#}$	0.4±0.4	0.2±0.3
Zone 4 (h·wk^{-1})	0.2±0.2	0.5±0.2	0.4±0.3	0.5±0.3	0.5±0.4	0.7±0.4 $^{\beta}$	0.3±0.3
Zone 5 (h·wk^{-1})	0.1±0.1	0.2±0.1	0.4±0.2 *	0.5±0.3	0.4±0.3	0.2±0.3	0.2±0.2
Activity forms:							
Specific (h·wk^{-1})	4.3±3.3	8.1±1.7	13.7±2.3 *	10.3±1.5 $^{\#\beta}$	12.2±2.6 $^{\#}$	10.8±1.8 $^{\#}$	4.1±3.2
Non-Specific (h·wk^{-1})	8.5±4.6	8.6±1.5	2.1±1.2 *	1.0±0.6 $^{\#\beta}$	0.8±0.6 $^{\#\beta}$	1.0±1.0 $^{\#\beta}$	1.8±1.5

Values are mean ± SD and represent training hours per week in different phases. A non-parametric Friedman test indicated that there was a statistically significant difference in all variables across the GP, SP and CP (P<.05 level). A pairwise post-hoc test (Wilcoxon Signed Rank) was used to determine whether there was a statistically significant difference between the GP, SP or CP, as well as pre-peaking and peaking phases (P<.01 level).

*P<.01, GP vs. SP;

$^{\#}$P<.01, GP vs. CP, pre-peaking or peaking;

$^{\beta}$P<.01, SP vs. CP, pre-peaking or peaking;

†P<.01, pre-peaking vs. peaking.

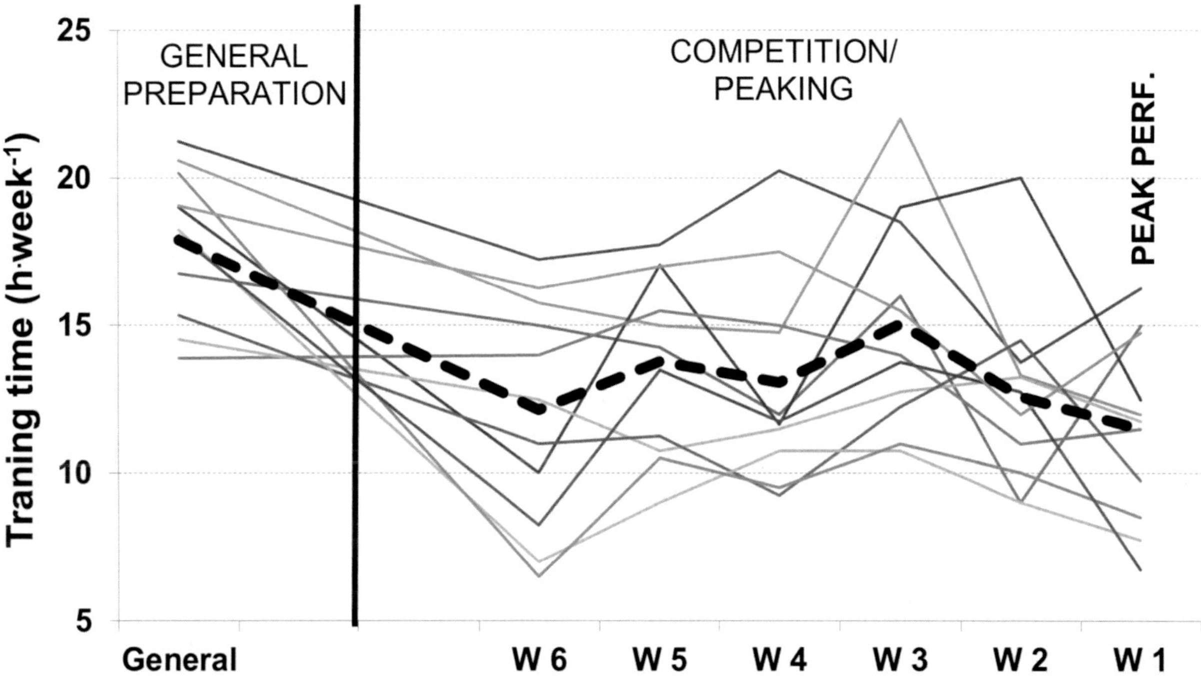

Figure 4. Individual peaking characteristics. Individual (lines) and average (dotted bold line) total weekly training volume during GP, and the last 6 weeks prior to championship title.

Activity forms. During the entire training year, 64% (~500 h) of all training was executed with sport-specific movement patterns (skiing/roller-skiing). However, over the course of the training year the amount of specific training increased from ~50 to 90%. That is, in line with the early periodization models [48], when training load was highest in PP only ~50% of all training was executed as ski or roller-ski. Otherwise, when training load was lowest in CP, >90% was performed as sport-specific training.

Sport-specific training is outlined as a key to improving $\dot{V}O_{2max}$ [51–52]. Hence, a high portion of sport-specific training during the CP for these athletes appears to be essential in order to reach an international performance level. However, we maintain that a large volume of non-specific activity forms during PP serve an important purpose in increasing trainability and improving general aerobic capacity [53–54].

Intensity distribution. Recently there has been some debate regarding findings suggesting that HIT induces superior physiological and performance adaptations compared with LIT [47]. The trend among endurance athletes is to adopt a polarized intensity distribution model integrating both intensity domains [7,9,16,20,25]. The present data consistently demonstrate that these 11 gold medalists executed a large proportion of their total training as LIT throughout the annual cycle. Total LIT time was progressively increased during PP, in line with some key features from the early periodization models of Matwejew [48], before being reduced dramatically during CP. However, it is important to emphasize that the marked intensity shift to more HIT described in Matwejew's models was not observed in this group of elite athletes.

The current study contributes unique knowledge to our understanding of the self-selected duration and distribution of HIT in elite endurance sports. Depending on the quantification methods used [43], results from several other studies suggest that an approximate 80/20% LIT/HIT distribution is optimal, although the percentage of HIT varies from ~10–30% [7–9,14–16,44,49–50] using a time in training zone method [43]. However, in the current study only 9% of annual endurance training time, or ~60 h/~100 sessions were reported to be above LT[1]. This is in contrast to other top Olympic athletes reported to perform a greater amount of HIT in addition to high total training volume [23,28–29]. The total volume of HIT training was evenly distributed throughout the year with an average of 5±2 h or 9±3 sessions·month^{-1}. Interestingly, it was also found that HIT training sessions were distributed virtually equally among zones 3, 4 & 5, with average durations of 0.8/0.6/0.5 h in zones 3/4/5 respectively. However, from the PP to CP, both duration and frequency in zones 3 and 4 were maintained, while the frequency of zone 5 training sessions increased. That is, as the main performance peak came closer, LIT time decreased dramatically while HIT patterns shifted towards a more polarized model, despite virtually constant HIT training time.

Peaking practice

Training volume and specificity. Optimizing the reduction in training load during the peaking phase is believed to be a key to optimal championship performance [6,30]. Training load is described as a combination of training volume, intensity and frequency [27]. A meta-analysis conducted by Bosquet et al [5] concluded that athletes could maximize taper-associated benefits by reducing training volume by ~50%, without reducing training frequency or training intensity.

In line with current best practice [4–6], we defined the peaking phase as the last 14 days prior to the athletes' most successful competition (Olympic/World Championship gold medal), and compared training patterns in this final training phase to the penultimate phase beginning 4 weeks prior to the peaking phase (pre-peaking phase). With regards to training volume, we found

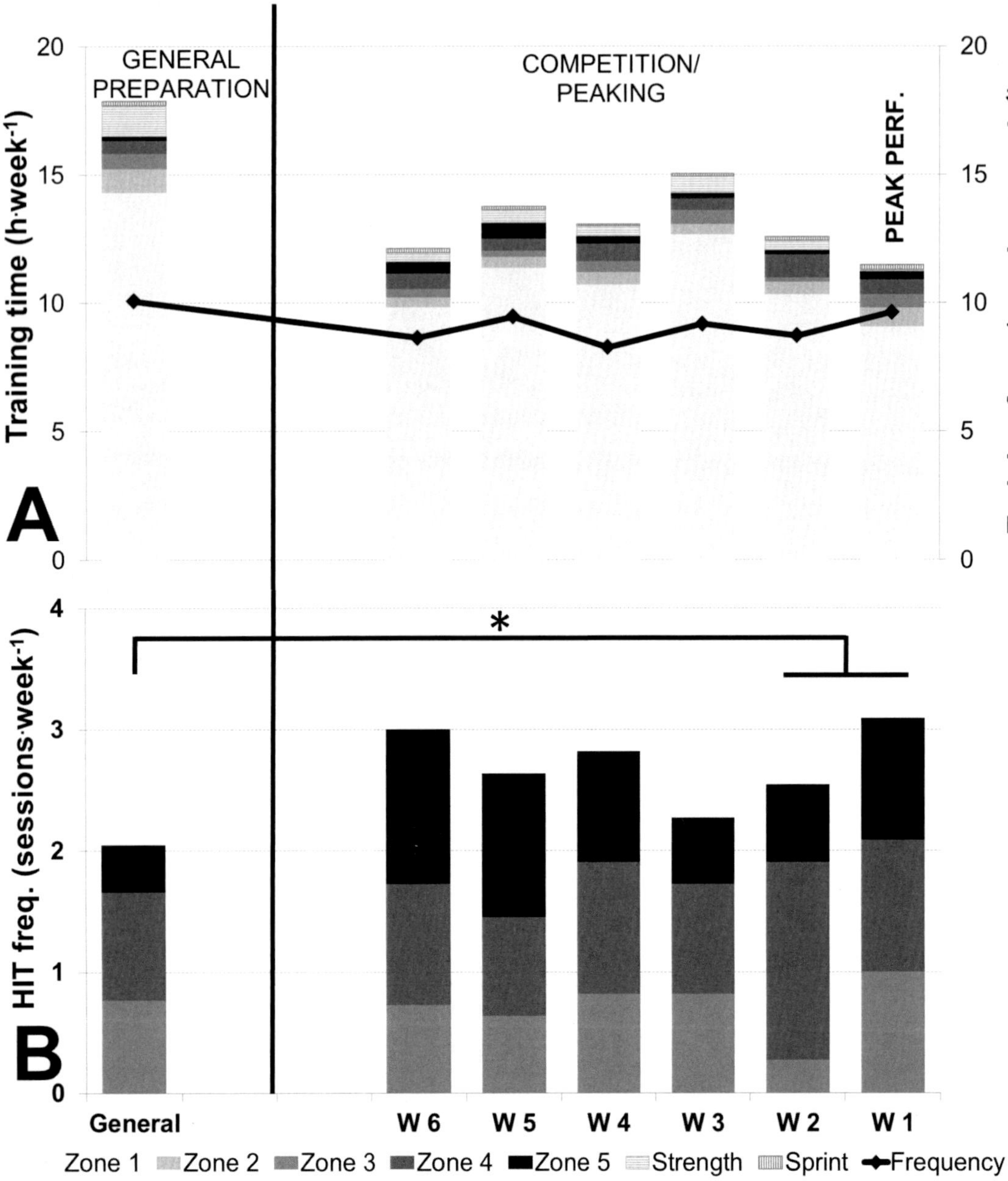

Figure 5. Peaking characteristics. A: Weekly training time (h) distributed into endurance training (zones 1–5), strength and sprints (bars, y-axis), and total training frequency (sessions) (line, z-axis) during GP, and during the last 6 weeks prior championship title. B: HIT frequency (sessions) distributed into zones 3, 4 and 5 (bars, y-axis) during GP, and during the last 6 weeks prior to championship title. There was a statistically significant difference ($P<.05$) in total HIT sessions and zones 3 and 5 respectively across GP, pre-peaking phase and peaking phase. Pairwise post-hoc tests showed: * Difference in total HIT sessions across phases ($P<.01$). There were no statistically significant differences in zones 3, 4 or 5 across phases.

only a 4 and 15% (NS) decrease in training volume during days -14 to -8 and days -7 to-1 respectively, compared to the pre-peaking phase. This is substantially less than the current taper recommendations of a ~50% reduction (Figure 6). It is possible to speculate as to why these champion athletes chose a strategy very different from experimentally derived optimum. Bosquet et al [5] reported no effect on performance if the reduction in training volume was 20% or less. However, there was large individual variation in peaking behavior in the current study, and no clear patterns emerged. In fact, 4 of the 11 athletes increased their training volume during the last seven days. However, existing research has limitations in terms of narrow focus on one single competition [32]. In contrast, our results demonstrate that competitions are frequently integrated into the peaking process in elite sports. The competition schedule, designed by the International Ski Federation, is crucial in planning a taper and must be integrated into the peaking regime. The WC season in these sports typically consists of two competition days per week over up to 14 weeks with a maximum of two to four competition free weeks. Such a schedule may interfere with an optimal tapering process. Rather than incorporating a single tapering phase, such a schedule may rather require the athlete to perform repeated "mini-tapers" prior to each competition.

Since there was minimal decrease (NS) in overall training volume during the four-week pre-peaking period, we chose to compare training performed during the peaking phase to GP, where weekly training volume was highest. Once the athletes started their WC season, in either XC or biathlon, their total training volume was consistently lower than that reported during GP. Relative to GP, training volume was, respectively, 29 and 35% lower during the penultimate and final weeks before each athlete's gold medal race. High competition stress load and frequent travel may dictate the reduced training volume during this phase, rather than a predetermined periodization model. These data indicate that peak training volume for these athletes was markedly dissociated in time from peak performance by up to 4 months, even accepting individual variations. It is unclear whether high training volume executed during PP 4–9 months prior still influences physical capacity during the peaking phase, following an extended period of reduced training volume where competitions themselves become a key source of HIT.

Several decades ago, Hickson et al [55] reported that trained athletes retain most of their physiological and endurance performance adaptations during 15 subsequent weeks of reduced training. However, for an Olympic athlete, even a small performance decrement associated with reduced training could be the difference between a medal and fourth place. Unfortunately, similar to strength performance, we do not have data for endurance tests throughout the year. Our objective testing data for these athletes terminates 3–4 months prior to their gold medal performances. In elite practice, laboratory testing typically ends when the competitive season begins. However, in a similar group of athletes with virtually identical training patterns as in the current study, Losnegaard et al [17] found that aerobic physiological adaptations were maintained, and performance and anaerobic adaptations were even enhanced, several months after peak training volume.

To our knowledge, no data are available providing mechanistic links that span such an extended time period. It is possible to speculate that a prolonged period of high training volume during PP could favorably alter genomic sensitivity to training during the season through epigenetic mechanisms [51]. Such cellular level adaptations to high training volume could be a mechanistic bridge linking PP training characteristics to training effects several months later, when high training volumes are precluded by the competition and travel stress load.

During both the pre-peaking phase and the peaking phase, virtually all (92%) training was conducted as XC skiing. This shift towards more specific movement patterns when competition approaches may explain why peak performance is possible even after several months with reduced training volume [51–52].

Training frequency. The athletes in the current study trained, on average, 8–10 sessions·week^{-1}, with no significant differences in training frequency between the peaking phase and other phases (Table 2). This finding is in line with current taper recommendations [1–6]. Nor were there any significant differences in the number of LIT or HIT sessions from the pre-peaking

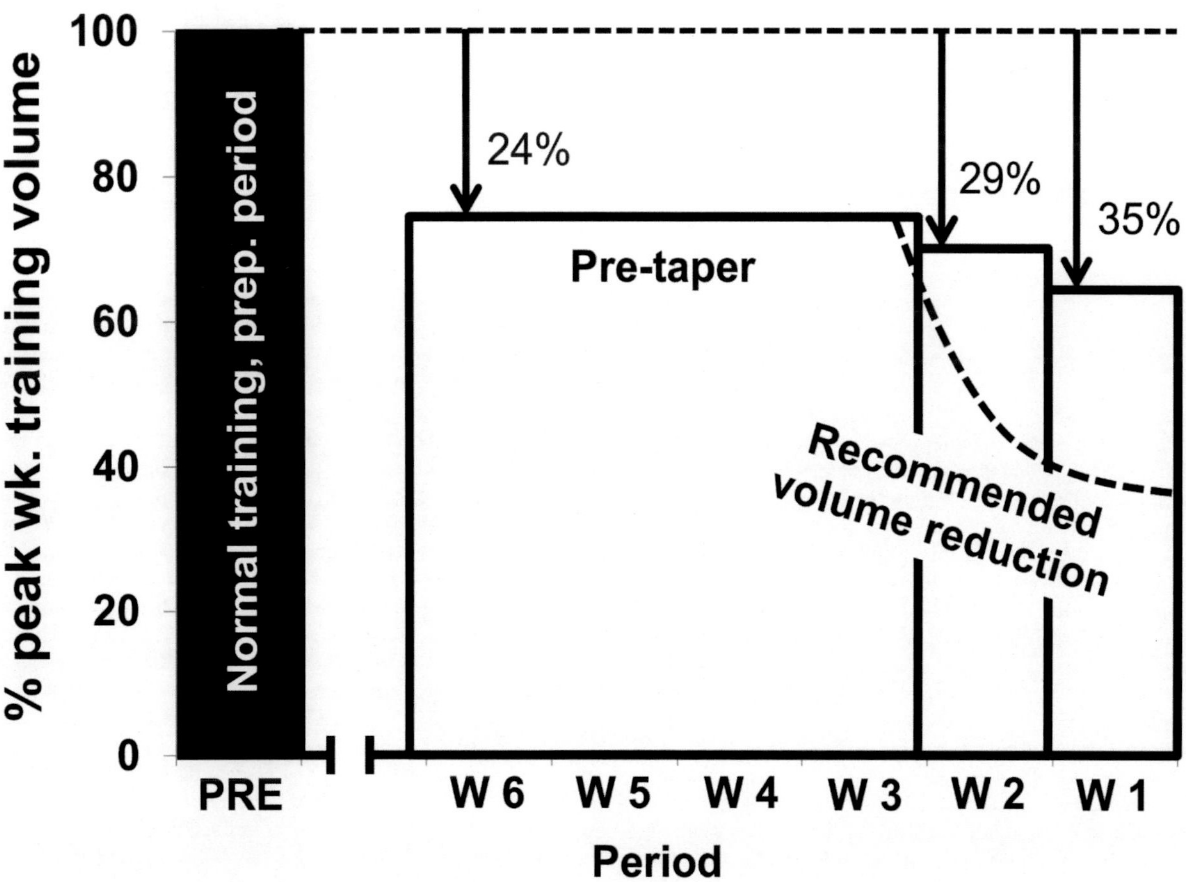

Figure 6. Taper comparison. Schematic representation of the actual taper observed in current study compared to recommended volume reduction. Adapted from Mujika & Padilla [4].

phase to the peaking phase. However, LIT frequency decreased from GP (8 sessions·week^{-1}) to the peaking phase (6 sessions·week^{-1}), indicating that the observed reduction in total LIT time was a result of both reduced session frequency and session duration.

Intensity distribution and rest days. Adaptive stimuli from HIT sessions appear to be a key component in maintaining and enhancing physiological and performance adaptations q during a taper period [36–37,39]. McNeely & Sandler [31] reported that frequent short HIT bouts >90% $\dot{V}O_{2max}$ are more effective than LIT to enhance endurance performance, and that, during a taper, steady-state workouts should be replaced by HIT intervals and short sprints in order to improve performance. Interestingly, we found that HIT duration did not change (1.3 h·week^{-1}) during any of the phases. However, HIT frequency increased from 2 sessions·week^{-1} in GP to 3 sessions·week^{-1} in the peaking phase ($P<.01$). In addition, there was a tendency towards increased sprint training duration from the pre-peaking phase to the peaking phase. Hence, HIT sessions during the peaking phase were typically executed more frequently but with shorter duration than during GP, alongside more frequent bouts of sport-specific "anaerobic sprint training". Examining distribution of training among intensity zones 3, 4 and 5, we observed a tendency toward a decrease in zones 3 and 4 and an increase in zone 5 in both duration and frequency from GP to CP. This suggests that total HIT duration did not change throughout the year, but that the actual executed intensity shifted towards a more polarized model as the major competition approached.

To our knowledge, details regarding best practice models of HIT patterns and recovery strategies during the final days prior to peak performance are lacking in the literature. However, the current data show that short bouts of HIT were performed evenly throughout the final 14 days (~5 sessions in total per athlete) (Figure 7). Interestingly, 10 out of 11 athletes performed a HIT session within 48 h of competition. The exact intensity during these HIT sessions is somewhat inconsistent, but was typically above LT^2. Competitions performed during the final days but not seen as "primary events" were also integrated into the peaking strategy. Whether these contribute to a beneficial peaking regime, or interfere with the optimal strategy is not clear. Eight of 11 athletes in the present study competed in at least one championship final prior to the event in which they won a gold medal. With regard to recovery strategies, rest days were typically concentrated in days 12 to 6. Among all 11 athletes, only 3 athletes took a rest day during the last 5 days, compared with 14 athlete rest days taken in the middle period of the peaking phase. That is, rest days were 3 times more likely to be taken during the middle portion of the peaking phase (days 12–6) compared with the final 5 days. However, it is not clear whether this organization of HIT and rest days during the final 14 days was the result of strategic planning to optimize performance, or merely coincidental. It has been previously reported that runners taking a rest every third day during a six day taper performed worse than those athletes who trained every day [56], and this topic may be a fruitful area for future research.

Altitude training. Altitude training is incorporated into the training of most world-class XC skiers, and is a consistent feature of Norwegian endurance training. For athletes in the current study, precise records are not available regarding all days spent at altitude or the specific altitude at which each training session was performed. For the last 2–3 decades, 4–6 annual training camps of 14–21 d duration living at 1800–2000 m above sea level and training at 1200 to 2800 m above sea level, have been integrated throughout the annual cycle. The aim of these altitude training camps is to stimulate increased hemoglobin mass, and specifically acclimate to competition venues located above 1400 m. The athletes in the current study typically spent 60 to 100 days training at altitude during the season quantified, although this was likely somewhat lower for those athletes winning gold prior to 1992. In addition, where championship events were held at moderate altitude (e.g. in Salt Lake City, 2002) altitude camps were also an important feature of the final weeks of training. Based on a previous study of 29 XC skiers training at altitude [43], objective data suggest that intensity distribution during altitude camps shifts towards lower intensity. Training at the highest aerobic intensities during such camps is essentially absent, unless it is performed at reduced altitudes. The likely impact of this emphasis on altitude training was to somewhat reduce the amount of HIT performed during PP.

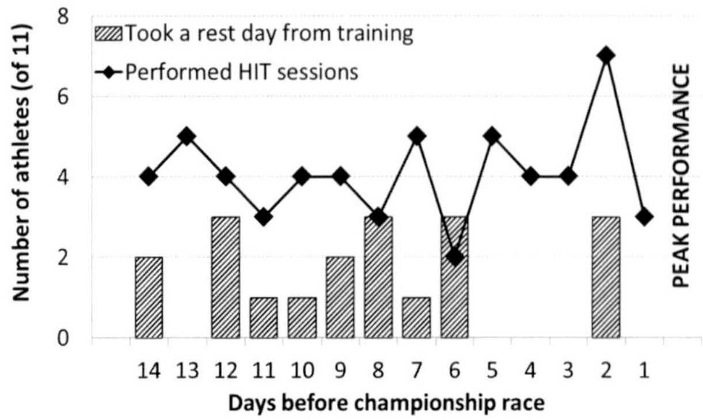

Figure 7. Peaking phase. Number of athletes (of 11) who performed HIT sessions (line) and number of athletes who took a rest day from training (bars) during the final 14 days prior to peak performance.

Winning an international title in endurance sports clearly requires outstanding physiological capacity and performance level. Controlled laboratory trials of world-class elite athletes are challenging, and training literature based on less well-trained individuals may be misleading when linking findings to elite athletes. Our current data outlines unique and accurate day-to-day training data throughout a season that concluded with each athlete winning an Olympic or World championship title. Experimental approaches may in many ways be artificial, while descriptive training studies allow investigation of elite endurance athletes in a real-life situation. This may therefore provide a fruitful foundation from which to generate novel experimental research questions.

We did not find evidence of athletes following the current tapering recommendations regarding training volume reduction. However, when comparing training patterns during the peaking phase to training executed during PP several months earlier, we found a picture more analogous to that derived from experimental studies, although the magnitude of training time reduction was still lower. It is possible to speculate as to whether the medal-winning performances of these athletes was truly representative of their best possible performance, or if they could have skied even faster had they followed recommended tapering strategies specifically for that one event. On the other hand, the more progressive reduction in training time from GP to CP observed in the current study, continued to a lesser degree throughout the CP up until the major competition, may be the ideal strategy in sports where the competition schedule is organized as it is in XC skiing and biathlon. A three month competition phase during which athletes are typically required to compete once or twice every week, precludes the application of the recommended tapering strategy presented in the research literature. Regardless, the performance of these athletes was sufficient to beat the rest of the field on the day, and take home the gold medal.

A central concern in a descriptive study such as this, where training self-report is the key data source, is whether the data are accurate and valid. We have recently demonstrated that elite endurance athletes report their training accurately, although we found some small discrepancies related to intensity distribution [57]. We believe the current data represent the same validity as shown in Sylta et al [57], since both athlete groups used similar monitoring routines, and some of the athletes are, in fact, represented in both papers. In addition, athletes recorded their training on a daily basis, which likely reduced reporting error.

Conclusions

These data show that winning an international title in XC skiing or biathlon requires a training load of ~800 h/500 sessions·year^{-1}, of which ~500 h is executed as sport-specific movement patterns. Endurance training time for these athletes was distributed as approximately 90% LIT and 10% HIT, equal to a ~80/20% SG distribution. Training volume was highest during GP and decreased progressively during SP and CP. Concurrently, the proportion of sport-specific training increased markedly. Total amount of HIT remained stable across all phases, although HIT training patterns tended to become more polarized in CP.

These athletes did not appear to incorporate a taper in the final weeks leading up to competition, with training volume, frequency and intensity remaining unchanged from the pre-peaking phase to the peaking phase. Hence, we did not observe the recommended ~50% training volume reduction that has been proposed as the optimal tapering strategy based on previous experimental studies. However, there was a clear reduction in training volume from GP to the peaking phase. This reduction was almost entirely due to a reduction in non-sport-specific LIT with virtually all training during the pre-peaking phase and the peaking phase composed of ski training. Only three out of 11 athletes incorporated a rest day in the final five days leading up to the best athletic performance of their career, A very large training load during the GP appears to be an important precondition for exceptional athletic performance several months later, although exactly how training loads in June-October are mechanistically connected to performance several months later remains unclear.

Author Contributions

Conceived and designed the experiments: ET SS. Performed the experiments: EH IS ET ØS. Analyzed the data: ET ØS SS IS TH. Contributed reagents/materials/analysis tools: ET EH. Contributed to the writing of the manuscript: ET EH ØS SS IS TH.

References

1. Tønnessen E (2009) Hvorfor ble de beste best? En casestudie av kvinnelige verdensenere i orientering, langrenn og langdistanseløp. Oslo: Norges Idrettshøgskole. 299 p.
2. Seiler S, Tønnessen E (2009) Intervals, Thresholds, and Long Slow Distance: the Role of Intensity and Duration in Endurance Training. Sportscience 13: 1–27.
3. Seiler S (2010) What is Best Practice for Training Intensity and Duration Distribution in Endurance Athletes? Int J Sports Physiol Perform 5: 276–291.
4. Mujika I, Padilla S (2003) Scientific bases for precompetition tapering strategies. Med Sci Sports Exerc 35: 1182–7.
5. Bosquet L, Montpetit J, Arvisais D, Mujika I (2007) Effects of tapering on performance: a meta-analysis. Med Sci Sports Exerc 39: 1358–65.
6. Le Meur Y, Hausswirth C, Mujika I (2012) Tapering for competition: A review. Science & Sports 27: 77–87.
7. Billat V, Demarle A, Slawinski J, Paiva M, Koralsztein JP (2001) Physical and training characteristics of top-class marathon runners. Med Sci Sports Exerc 33: 2089–2097.
8. Billat V, Lepretre PM, Heugas AM, Laurence MH, Salim D, et al. (2003) Training and bioenergetic characteristics in elite male and female Kenyan runners. Med Sci Sports Exerc 35: 297–304.
9. Esteve-Lanao J, San Juan AF, Earnest CP, Foster C, Lucia A (2005) How Do Endurance Runners Actually Train? Relationship with Competition Performance. Med Sci Sports Exerc 37: 496–504.
10. Karp J R (2008) Training characteristics of US Olympic Marathon Trials qualifiers. New Studies in Athletics 23: 31–37.
11. Ingham SA, Fudge BW, Pringle JS (2012) Training Distribution, Physiological Profile, and Performance for a Male International 1500-m Runner. Int J Sports Physiol Perform 7: 193–195.
12. Stellingwerff T (2012) Case study: Nutrition and training periodization in three elite marathon runners. Int J Sport Nutr Exerc Metab 22: 392–400.
13. Schumacher OY, Mueller P (2002) The 4000-m team pursuit cycling world record: Theoretical and practical aspects. Med Sci Sports Exerc 34: 1029–1036.
14. Zapico AG, Calderón FJ, Benito PJ, González CB, Parisi A, et al. (2007) Evolution of physiological and haematological parameters with training load in elite male road cyclists: A longitudinal study. J Sports Med Phys Fitness 47: 191–196.
15. Seiler KS, Kjerland GØ (2006) Quantifying training intensity distribution in elite endurance athletes: is there evidence for an "optimal" distribution? Scand J Med Sci Sports 16: 49–56.
16. Sandbakk O, Holmberg HC, Leirdal S, Ettema G (2011) The physiology of world-class sprint skiers. Scand J Med Sci Sports 21: 9–16.
17. Losnegard T, Myklebust H, Spencer M, Hallén J (2013) Seasonal variations in VO2max, O2-cost, O2-deficit and performance in elite cross-country skiers. J Strength Cond Res 27: 1780–1790.
18. Gao J (2008) A Study on Pre-Game Training Characteristics of Chinese Elite Swimmers. J Beijing Sport Univ 31: 832–834.
19. Siewierski M (2010) Volume and structure of training loads of top swimmers in direct starting preparation phase for main competition. Pol J Sport Tourism 17: 227–232.
20. Fiskerstrand Â, Seiler KS (2004) Training and performance characteristics among Norwegian International Rowers 1970–2001. Scand J Med Sci Sports 14: 303–310.
21. Guellich A, Seiler S, Emrich E (2009) Training Methods and Intensity Distribution of Young World-Class Rowers. Int J Sports Physiol Perform 4: 448–460.
22. Neal CM, Hunter AM, Galloway SD (2011) A 6-month analysis of training-intensity distribution and physiological adaptation in Ironman triathletes. J Sports Sci 29: 1515–23.
23. Mujika I (2013) Olympic Preparation of a World-Class Female Triathlete. Int J Sports Physiol Perform: In press.
24. Hongjun Y, Chen X, Zhu W, Cao C (2012) A Quasi-Experimental Study of Chinese Top-Level Speed Skaters' Training Load: Threshold Versus Polarized Model. Int J Sports Physiol Perform 7: 103–112.
25. Orie J, Hofman N, de Koning JJ, Foster C (2014) Thirty-eight years of training distribution in olympic speed skaters. Int J Sports Physiol Perform 9: 93–9.
26. Garcia-Pallares J, García-Fernández M, Sánchez-Medina L, Izquierdo M (2010) Performance changes in world-class kayakers following two different training periodization models. Eur J Appl Physiol 110: 99–107.
27. Wenger HA, Bell GJ (1986) The Interactions of Intensity, Frequency and Duration of Exercise Training in Altering Cardiorespiratory Fitness. Sports Med 3: 346–356.
28. Tjelta LI (2013) A Longitudinal Case Study of the Training of the 2012 European 1500 m Track Champion. Int J Appl Sports Sci 25: 11–18.
29. Tjelta LI, Tønnessen E, Enoksen E (2014) A case study of the training of nine times New York Marathon winner Grete Waitz. Int J Sports Sci Coach 9: 139–159.
30. Mujika I, Chatard JC, Busso T, Geyssant A, Barale F, et al. (1995) Effects of training on performance in competitive swimming. Can J Appl Physiol 20: 395–406.
31. Mujika I, Padilla S, Pyne D (2002) Swimming performance changes during the final 3 weeks of training leading to the Sydney 2000 Olympic Games. Int J Sports Med 23: 582–7.
32. McNeely E, Sandler D (2007) Tapering for endurance athletes. Strength Cond J 29: 18–24.
33. Pyne D B, Mujika I, Reilly T (2009) Peaking for optimal performance: Research limitations and future directions. J Sports Sci 27: 195–202.
34. Thomas L, Busso T (2005) A theoretical study of taper characteristics to optimize performance. Med Sci Sports Exerc 37: 1615–1621.
35. Mujika I (1998) The influence of training characteristics and tapering on the adaptation in highly trained individuals: a review. Int J Sports Med 19: 439–46.
36. Hickson RC, Foster C, Pollock ML, Galassi TM, Rich S (1985) Reduced Training Intensities and Loss of Aerobic Power, Endurance, and Cardiac Growth. J Appl Physiol 58: 492–499.

37. Shepley B, MacDougall JD, Cipriano N, Sutton JR, Tarnopolsky MA, et al. (1992) Physiological-Effects of Tapering in Highly Trained Athletes. J Appl Physiol 72: 706–711.
38. Houmard JA, Scott BK, Justice CL, Chenier TC (1994) The Effects of Taper on Performance in Distance Runners. Med Sci Sports Exerc 26: 624–631.
39. Mujika I (2010) Intense training: the key to optimal performance before and during the taper. Scand J Med Sci Sports 20: 24–31.
40. NSF (1992) Treningsdagbok – Langrenn. Oslo: Norges Skiforbund.
41. NSF (1985) Treningsdagbok - Langrenn. Oslo: Norges Skiforbund.
42. NSSF (1991) Treningsdagbok - Skiskyting. Oslo: Norges Skiskytterforbund.
43. Sylta O, Tonnessen E, Seiler S (2014) From heart-rate data to training quantification: a comparison of 3 methods of training-intensity analysis. Int J Sports Physiol Perform 9: 100–7.
44. Lucia A, Hoyos J, Carvajal A, Chicharro JL (1999) Heart rate response to professional road cycling: the Tour de France. Int J Sports Med 20: 167–172.
45. Sandbakk O, Holmberg HC (2014) A reappraisal of success factors for olympic cross-country skiing. Int J Sports Physiol Perform 9: 117–121.
46. Rønnestad B, Hansen E, Raastad T (2010) In-season strength maintenance training increases well-trained cyclists' performance. Eur J Appl Physiol 110: 1269–1282.
47. Laursen PB (2010) Training for intense exercise performance: high-intensity or high-volume training? Scand J Med Sci Sports 20: 1–10.
48. Matwejew L (1975) Periodisierung des sportlichen trainings, 2nd ed. Berlin: Bartels & Wernitz.
49. Lucia A, Hoyos J, Santalla A, Earnest C, Chicharro JL (2003) Tour de France versus Vuelta a Espana: which is harder? Med Sci Sports Exerc 35: 872–878.
50. Esteve-Lanao J, Foster C, Seiler S, Lucia A (2007) Impact of training intensity distribution on performance in endurance athletes. J Strength Cond Res 21: 943–949.
51. Tanaka H (1994) Effects of cross-training – transfer of training effects on VO_{2max} between cycling, running and swimming. Sports Med 18: 330–339.
52. Foster C, Hector LL, Welsh R, Schrager M, Green MA, et al. (1995) Effects of specific versus cross-training on running performance. Eur J Appl Physiol 70: 367–372.
53. Steinacker JM, Lormes W, Lehmann M, Altenburg D (1998) Training of rowers before world championships. Med Sci Sports Exerc 30: 1158–1163.
54. Bompa T (1999) Periodization: Theory and methodology of training (4th ed.). Champaign, IL: Human Kinetics.
55. Hickson RC, Kanakis C Jr, Davis JR, Moore AM, Rich S (1982) Reduced Training Duration Effects on Aerobic Power, Endurance, and Cardiac Growth. J Appl Physiol 53: 225–229.
56. Mujika I, Goya A, Ruiz E, Grijalba A, Santisteban J, Padilla S (2002) Physiological and performance responses to a 6-day taper in middle-distance runners: influence of training frequency. Int J Sports Med 23: 367–373.
57. Sylta O, Tonnessen E, Seiler S (2014) Do elite endurance athletes report their training accurately? Int J Sports Physiol Perform 9: 85–92.

12

Loneliness, Social Integration and Consumption of Sugar-Containing Beverages: Testing the Social Baseline Theory

Roger Ekeberg Henriksen[1]*, Torbjørn Torsheim[2], Frode Thuen[1]

1 Centre for Evidence-Based Practice, Bergen University College, Bergen, Norway, **2** Faculty of Psychology, Department of Psychosocial Science, University of Bergen, Bergen, Norway

Abstract

Objective: Social Baseline Theory (SBT) proposes that close relationships aid in metabolic resource management and that individuals without significant relationships may experience more demands on their own neural metabolic resources on a daily basis when solving problems, remaining vigilant against potential threats and regulating emotional responses. This study tests a hypothesised consequence derived from SBT: relative social isolation leads to increased levels of sugar intake.

Methods: Based on cross-sectional, self-reported data from the Norwegian Mother and Child Cohort Study (N = 90 084), information on social integration and the consumption of both sugar-sweetened and artificially sweetened sodas and juices was obtained from a large number of women in early pregnancy. Multiple regression analyses were conducted to assess whether loneliness, marital status, relationship satisfaction, advice from others than partner, and cohesion at work is associated with consumption of sodas and juices.

Results: Perceived loneliness was associated with elevated intake of all sugary beverages, while relationship satisfaction was negatively associated with all sugary beverages. Being married or cohabitating, having supportive friends, and having a sense of togetherness at work were associated with lower intake of two out of three sugar-containing beverages. These associations were significant, even after controlling for factors such as body mass index, weight related self-image, depression, physical activity, educational level, age and income. In comparison, a statistically significant relationship emerged between relationship satisfaction and artificially sweetened cola. No other predictor variables were significantly associated with any type of artificially sweetened beverage.

Conclusions: This study indicates that loneliness and social integration influence the level of consumption of sugary beverages. The results support the hypothesis derived from the Social Baseline Theory that relative social isolation leads to increased levels of sugar intake.

Editor: Marià Alemany, Faculty of Biology, Spain

Funding: The Norwegian Mother and Child Cohort Study is supported by the Norwegian Ministry of Health and the Ministry of Education and Research (National Institutes of Health (NIH)/National Institute of Environmental Health Sciences contract no. NO1-ES-75558, NIH/National Institute of Neurological Disorders and Stroke grant no. 1 UO1 NS 047537-01 and grant no. 2 UO1 NS047537-06A1) and the Norwegian Research Council/FUGE (grant no. 151918/S10). However, the funders had no role in study design, data collection and analysis, decision to publish, or preparation of the manuscript, and the authors received no specific funding for this work.

Competing Interests: The authors have declared that no competing interests exist.

* Email: roger.ekeberg.henriksen@hib.no

Introduction

This study examines whether there is an association between social integration and sugar intake, as proposed by the Social Baseline Theory [1].

The brain is the most metabolically active organ of the human body. Even in a resting state of non-specific neural activity, it counts for as much as 20% of the body's total energy utilization [2]. The adult human brain is almost completely dependent on glucose as a source for energy. Unlike other organs, the brain has very little metabolic reserve because it oxidizes glucose at relatively close to its maximum rate. Because more than 85% of the glucose is utilized by neurons, the rate at which the brain oxidizes glucose is proportional to neuronal activity [2,3]. This implies that specific neural effort must be followed by a rapid supply of glucose from the blood in an amount that corresponds with the metabolic cost of the specific effort [3]. In an illustrative study, Scholey, Harper and Kennedy [4] showed that a cognitively demanding subtraction task was followed by an immediate, significant fall in peripheral blood glucose. Moreover, by offering a glucose-containing drink to one group and a placebo drink to the other, they also demonstrated that glucose intake after a fall in blood glucose level was associated with better performance on a subsequent cognitively demanding task. Similar studies were performed by Gailliot and colleagues [5], who found that different types of mental effort, such as thought suppression, attention control and emotion regulation, were followed by an immediate fall in peripheral blood glucose levels.

Restoring the blood glucose to normal levels after a drop is of high biological priority. Even a few seconds without cerebral glucose oxidation will lead to unconsciousness, and after a few minutes, the death of neurons will occur. In order to counteract a dangerous glucose shortage in the brain, humans possess a highly sophisticated glucose regulatory system [6]. In addition to the role of hepatic glycogen in counter-regulation of hypoglycemia [7], the brain has the ability to rapidly sense a drop in circulating glucose and induce a range of other counter-regulatory responses. These include the secretion of galanin and GABA, which minimizes the chance of glucose deprivation by inhibiting neural activity, as well as stimulating cortisol release, which aims to increase blood sugar through gluconeogenesis in the liver [2,6]. In addition, cortisol has been shown to suppress insulin secretion from pancreatic b-cells and impair insulin initiated translocation of the intracellular glucose transporter, GLUT 4 [8–10]. This leads to decreased insulin-dependent glucose uptake into peripheral cells and makes glucose available to the brain via glucose transporter GLUT 1 [3,10,11]. Another set of regulatory mechanisms involves directed behavior. Naturally, most efficient are behavioral actions that regulate glucose levels by facilitating exogenous supplies of carbohydrates from nutritional sources. Indeed, a substantial body of research has linked different types of demanding mental work to the subsequent intake of food, with a significant preference for foods high in carbohydrates [12–18]. This point is thoroughly discussed by Peters, Kubera, Hubold and Langemann [19] who have developed a model called the Cerebral Supply-Chain Model, which explains how both cortisol-induced and eating-induced supplies of glucose are initiated by the brain during times of energy-demanding psychosocial stress.

During periods of evolutionary pressure, it is likely that individuals with efficient glucose regulatory responses have been evolutionarily favored. Social Baseline Theory (SBT) [1,20,21] argues that in order to conserve metabolic resources, the human brain is phylogenetically designed to benefit from social networks when engaging in demanding mental activities, such as effortful decision making, creative problem solving and emotion regulation. SBT uses the principles of risk distribution and load sharing to explain the brain's metabolic benefit from social interaction. *Risk distribution* refers to how individuals in a group perceive and react to environmental risk, as opposed to how the corresponding risk would be handled by socially isolated individuals. For example, as a group has more eyes and ears than a single individual, effort toward vigilance against possible dangers in the environment are distributed across the group. In this way, fewer neural resources are needed for each group member as compared with the cost of the precautions and worries solitary individuals must engage in to ensure a similar safety level. In close relationships, participants receive benefits beyond those associated with risk distribution. *Load sharing* refers to the energy-conserving effects of trust and interdependence, which are found between, for example, romantic partners, family members and close friends. In close relationships, the members tend to engage in behaviors that facilitate one another's well-being, for example, sharing resources, sharing goals and assisting in problem solving [22]. Central to SBT is the notion that "as an individual becomes accustomed to load sharing, his social system becomes an extension of the way his brain interacts with the world" [1]. The theory proposes that such "outsourcing" of mental work is particularly beneficial in the regulation of emotional responses because self-regulating processes supported by the prefrontal cortex are believed to be more metabolically costly than most other cognitive processes. Thus, socially mediated forms of emotion regulation may have significant energy-conserving advantages [1,23,24]. According to SBT, due to the evolutionary benefits of adjusting to the principles of risk distribution and load sharing, the human brain leans on social resources as a default strategy: "the human brain is designed to assume that it is embedded within a relatively predictable social network characterized by familiarity, joint attention, shared goals, and interdependence" [1]. A violation of this "baseline assumption", however, signals the need for increased threat-related vigilance and reactivity. Thus, socially isolated individuals regulate their emotions at a higher metabolic expense compared with socially integrated individuals. In sum, SBT predicts that relative social isolation requires more neural metabolic resources in order to both manage daily life routines and to regulate emotions. This hypothesis builds on research showing that neural systems that support self-regulatory efforts are less active when social support is provided [20,24]. Furthermore, in a context in which social support is provided, the down-regulation of neural response is a function of relational quality. In an fMRI-study conducted by Coan, Schaefer and Davidson [25], 16 women were confronted with the threat of a mild electric shock while either alone, holding a stranger's hand, or holding their partners' hands. While holding their partners' hands, the women in the highest-quality relationships showed the least threat-related brain activity. When holding a stranger's hand, the level of threat-related activity increased as compared with holding the partners' hands. Finally, when exposed to the threat of shock without the support of handholding, the threat-related brain activity reached its highest level.

Given that socially isolated individuals frequently demand extra supplies of glucose from the blood to maintain optimal brain function, one might expect elevated intake of food and beverages that rapidly elevate blood glucose in this group [19]. This assumption is consistent with findings showing that low levels of emotional support predict the higher intake of carbohydrates [26]. On the basis of these findings and in accordance with the framework of SBT, we expect to find a covariance between loneliness and social connectedness on the one hand and consumption of sugar on the other.

Hypotheses

Sodas and juices contain high amounts of sugar and are highly available in western societies, easy to grab and convenient to drink. The per capita consumption of soda and juice in Norway is among the highest in the world [27]. Therefore, sugar-containing sodas and juices are likely to work well as an indicator of intake of sugar that has the ability to quickly provide glucose to the bloodstream. The main hypothesis (H^1) of the present study is thereby that degree of loneliness and social connectedness are associated with degree of intake of sugar – in the form of sugar-containing sodas and juices. However, sugary beverages consist of more than just sugar. If the null hypothesis of H^1 should be rejected, indicating that less socially connected people consume more soda and juice than their more socially integrated counterparts, sugar may not necessarily be the reason for the higher intake (it could be the sweet taste, the water, the citric acid, or any of the other components that sodas and juices consist of). To clarify the role of sugar in the potential relationship between social connectedness and intake of sugar-containing drinks, an additional hypothesis may be useful (H^2): degree of social connectedness is associated with degree of intake of artificially *sweetened* sodas and juices. If the null hypotheses of both H^1 and H^2 should be rejected, we cannot claim that intake of sugary soda and juice related to social connectedness necessarily is an expression of attractiveness to sugar. If, however, we reject the null hypothesis of H^1 but not the one of H^2, indicating that less socially connected people consume more sugary drinks but not more artificially sweetened drinks, we can conclude that there is a strong indication that sugar is the key-component of these relationships. In this study, we were able to extract these variables from a huge pregnancy cohort.

Methods

The Norwegian Mother and Child Cohort Study (MoBa) is a prospective population-based pregnancy cohort study conducted by the Norwegian Institute of Public Health [28]. In the period 1999–2008, all hospitals in Norway (except two) with more than 100 births per year invited pregnant women to participate in the study provided that they could read Norwegian. They received a postal invitation three weeks before the ultrasound examination routinely offered to all pregnant women in Norway. 38.7% of invited women consented to participate, and the cohort now includes 109 000 children, 91 000 mothers and 71 700 fathers. Blood samples were obtained from both parents during pregnancy and from mothers and children (umbilical cord) at birth. Follow-up is conducted by questionnaires at regular intervals and by linkage to national health registries. Several sub-studies are conducting additional collections of data and biological materials. The current study is based on version 7 of the quality-assured data files released for research on October 17th 2012. Informed consent was obtained from each MoBa participant upon recruitment. The study was approved by The Regional Committee for Medical Research Ethics in Western Norway.

Participants

The present study includes women participating in the MoBa study for the first time. Women who participated multiple times only provided data regarding their first participating pregnancies, and participants with diabetes type 1 were excluded. The included participants ($N = 90\ 084$) had a mean age of 29.2 years (std. deviation 4.40). Among them, 46.5% were married, 50.7% were cohabitating, and 2.8% were single. The average level of education was higher for the sample than for the general population of women aged between 16–49 years (official statistics from 2008 in brackets): compulsory school, 3.3% (28.1%); vocational school/three-year college, 34.9% (34.8%), and university/higher education, 61.7% (34.4%).The full sample has been compared with the general population of pregnant women in Norway and is described in more detail elsewhere [29].

Measures

MoBa collects many diverse variables. Of special interest for this study were sugar-containing beverages and five factors reflecting aspects of social connectedness: loneliness, marital status, couple relationship quality, social support from others than the partner and perceived cohesion at work.

To measure the consumption of sugar-containing sodas and juices, participants were asked three questions. They were asked to report how many glasses of 1) *sugar-containing cola*, 2) *other sugar-containing soda products,* and 3) *sugar-containing juices* they had been drinking daily during the last 17 weeks. To be able to assess whether potential associations between social connectedness and sugar-containing beverages are related to attractiveness to sugar, we also included reports on how many glasses of 1) *artificially sweetened cola*, 2) *other artificially sweetened sodas*, and 3) *artificially sweetened juices* the participants had been drinking daily during the same period. A table for converting bottles and large glasses into the standardized study unit (1 glass ≈ 2cl) was given in brackets next to the questions. For the purpose of this paper, the numbers of reported units of the six groups of beverages were respectively divided into seven categories spanning from '0 units' to '6 or more units'.

Loneliness was measured by a five-point scale spanning from "almost never" to "almost always" based on a single item: "Do you often feel lonesome?"

Marital status was measured via the following categories: "married", "co-habiting", "single" and 'separated/divorced'. To group the participants that were not in a relationship, "single" and "separated/divorced" were collapsed into one category.

The full ten-item version of the *Relationship Satisfaction Scale* was used to assess the quality of the co-habiting or married participants' relationships. The scale was developed for the MoBa and based on core items used in previously developed measures of marital satisfaction and relationship quality [30–32]. The scale has a six-step scoring format spanning from 1, "totally agree", to 6, "don't agree at all". Examples of items are as follows: "My partner and I have problems in our relationship", "I am very happy in my relationship" and "My partner is generally very understanding". In the current sample, the scale had a Cronbach's Alpha of 0.90. This scale has been used in previous studies [33,34].

Social support from other than the partner was measured via one item: "Do you have anyone other than your husband/partner whom you can ask for advice in a difficult situation?" There were three response categories: "no", "yes, one to two people" and "yes, more than two people".

Perceived cohesion at work was measured by one statement: 'There is a great cohesion at work', and four response categories spanning from 'agree' to 'not agree at all'. For the purpose of the present analysis, the scoring scale was reversed.

Control variables

Eight control variables that may influence the level of intake of sodas or juices were included: participation in sports, physical strain at work, body mass index, weight related self-image, depression, age, level of education and income.

Because sport activities and other physical strain increase thirst and energy utilization, they may influence the level of soda or juice consumption. We therefore included measures for engagement in sports and other physical activities, as well as physical strain at work. *Sports* was measured by 14 items covering activities such as, "running", "biking", "horse riding", "dancing", "walking" and "fitness studio". The respondents were asked how often they had exercised during the first 17 weeks of the current pregnancy. There were five response categories: "never", "1–3 times per month", "once per week", "twice per week" and "3 times or more per week". *Physical strain at work* was based on a single item, "My work is physically hard", and was measured on a four-point scale spanning from "correct" to "not correct".

Individuals with high body mass index (BMI) scores tend to have elevated carbohydrate intake in the absence of hunger compared with normal-weight subjects [35]. Thus, specific mechanisms related to overweight may account for some of the variance in the consumption of sugar-containing beverages. We therefore included BMI as a control variable. BMI scores were calculated on the basis of self-reported height and weight at the beginning of pregnancy.

Weight concerns related to self-perceptions, for example, internalization of the "thin ideal", may impact eating behaviors and dieting [36]. We therefore included a single-item variable reflecting weight concerns motivated by self-image: *"Is it important for your self-image that you keep a certain weight?"* There were three response categories: "Yes, very important", "Yes, somewhat important" and "No, not particularly important".

Depression has been linked to a desire for sweet foods [37,38] and may therefore explain a potential association between social interaction and consumption of sweet beverages. Depression was measured based on one item from a checklist covering a wide range of diseases and health problems. The respondents were asked to mark whether they had or had had ongoing depression during the first 17 weeks of the current pregnancy.

Age is associated with the level of soda consumption, with young people consuming more [39,40]. In this study, age was measured as age in years at the point of the study.

Higher educational levels are associated with lower consumption of sugar-containing soda [39]. *Educational level* was measured by six categories, from public school to >4 years of university/college.

A low level of income has been associated with high consumption of sugary drinks [40,41]. Here, we measured *maternal income* by dividing it into seven categories, from 1 = no income to 7 ≥ NOK 500,000 (≈ EUR 66,000).

Statistical analyses

All statistical analyses were conducted using the IBM SPSS Version 21. To determine the bivariate associations between the main predictor variables and the outcome variables, Pearson product moment correlations were computed. The associations between the main predictor variables and consumption of cola, soda and juice (sugar- and artificially sweetened) were tested via six separate linear multiple regression analysis, one for each type of beverage as an outcome variable. The analyses were performed with the simultaneous entry of all predictor variables, including the following control variables: participation in sports, physical strain at work, body mass index, weight related self-image, depression, age, level of education and income. Because the participants did not necessarily report on all questions concerning consumption of beverages, the different models are based on different sample sizes.

Results

First, bivariate correlations were computed between scores for loneliness, relationship satisfaction, advice from others and cohesion at work, and the six outcome variables. Pearson product moment coefficients as well as mean scores and standard deviations of scores for consumption of soda, cola and juice are given in Table 1. The results of the bivariate correlational analysis showed that all social factors were significantly correlated with scores on all sugar-containing beverages in the predicted direction. The social factors were also significantly correlated with scores on most of the artificially sweetened beverages. All correlations were generally weak, but consistently stronger between the predictor variables and the scores for sugar-containing beverages than between the predictor variables and the scores for artificially sweetened beverages. Next, a series of regression analysis was performed (see Table 2) to develop three separate models for predicting scores for the intake of sugar-containing cola, sugar-containing sodas (other than cola) and sugar-containing juices, from scores for loneliness, marital status (co-habiting and married), relationship satisfaction, advice from others and cohesion at work. All models were statistically significant; Model 1: (dependent variable: sugar-containing sodas) $F(14, 28494) = 205.395$, $p<.001$; Model 2: (dependent variable: sugar-containing cola) $F(14, 25655) = 150.331$, $p<.001$; Model 3: (dependent variable: sugar-containing juices) $F(14, 50040) = 71.502$, $p<.001$. The models explained 7.5% (adjusted $R^2 = .075$), 9.1% (adjusted $R^2 = .091$), and 1.9% (adjusted $R^2 = .019$) of the variance in consumption of the beverages, respectively. Results from the regression analysis showed that high levels of perceived loneliness were positively associated with high levels of intake of sugar-containing soda. Significantly negative relationships emerged between both relationship satisfaction and advice from others than partner, and sugar-containing soda. Marital status and cohesion at work were not statistically significantly associated with consumption of sugar-containing soda. As shown in Table 2, all six variables related to social interaction were significantly associated with self-reported levels of intake of sugar-containing cola. A high level of perceived loneliness was associated with high levels of cola intake. Negative associations were found between cola intake and relationship satisfaction, being married (compared with being single), cohabitating (compared with being single), the possibility of seeking advice from others than the partner, and perceived cohesion at work. Table 2 also shows that high levels of perceived loneliness were associated with high levels of consumption of sugar-containing juices. Negative associations were found between relationship satisfaction, being married (compared with being single), cohabitating (compared with being single), and perceived cohesion at work on the one hand, and consumption of sugar-containing juices on the other. In this analysis, the possibility of seeking advice from others than the partner was not significantly associated with consumption of sugar-containing juices.

Finally, three equivalent analyses, with the inclusion of the same control variables as included in the models above, were conducted for artificially sweetened soda (other than cola), cola and juice as outcome variables. The models were statistically significant: Model 4: (dependent variable: artificially sweetened soda) $F(14, 24208) = 74.772$, $p<.001$; Model 5: (dependent variable: artificially sweetened cola) $F(14, 29282) = 177.886$, $p<.001$; Model 6: (dependent variable: artificially sweetened juices) $F(14, 26603) = 62.250$, $p<.001$. The models explained 4.1% (adjusted $R^2 = .041$), 7.8% (adjusted $R^2 = .078$), and 3.1% (adjusted $R^2 = .031$) of the variance in consumption of the three types of artificially sweetened beverages, respectively. Table 2 shows that none social factors were significantly associated with consumption of artificially sweetened soda (other than cola) or juices. A significant negative association was found between relationship satisfaction and consumption of artificially sweetened cola. No other social factors were significantly associated with consumption of artificially sweetened cola.

Discussion

Overall, our results confirmed that perceived loneliness was associated with elevated intake of sugar in the form of soda, cola and juice. High levels of relationship satisfaction, on the other hand, was negatively associated with all three types of sugary beverages. Other aspects of social connectedness such as being married, having supportive friends, and having a sense of togetherness at work were associated with lower intake of two out of three types of sugar-containing beverages. These associations were statistically significant, even after controlling for factors such as body mass index, weight-related self-image, depression, physical activity, educational level, age and income.

Table 1. Mean scores, standard deviations of scores, and Pearson product moment coefficients for inter-correlations of scores for main predictor variables and consumption of soda, cola and juice.

			Sugar-sweetened			Artificially sweetened		
	Mean	**SD**	**Soda**	**Cola**	**Juice**	**Soda**	**Cola**	**Juice**
Loneliness	1.77	0.86	$.095^{**}$	$.107^{**}$	$.047^{**}$	$.021^{**}$	$.025^{**}$	$.033^{**}$
Relationship satisfaction	5.32	0.65	$-.060^{**}$	$-.078^{**}$	$-.023^{**}$	$-.031^{**}$	$-.044^{**}$	$-.015^{**}$
Advise from others	2.49	0.57	$-.078^{**}$	$-.078^{**}$	$-.022^{**}$	$-.035^{**}$	$-.023^{**}$	−.006
Cohesion at work	3.36	0.71	$-.026^{**}$	$-.037^{**}$	$-.016^{**}$	$-.013^{*}$	$-.017^{**}$	$-.014^{*}$

** Correlation is significant at the 0.01 level (2 tailed).
* Correlation is significant at the 0.05 level (2 tailed).
N varies from n = 29010 (lowest) to n = 65693 (highest).

Although the associations were weak, all of the five tested social factors were significantly associated with consumption of at least two types of sugar-sweetened beverages. In the regression analyses, statistically significant relationships did emerge as predicted in 14 out of 18 cases. The systematic structure of these results suggests that the associations found in this sample were not coincidental. Hence, these results support the main hypothesis of the study proposing that perceived social isolation, as well as perceived social integration, influence consumption of sugar-containing sodas and juices. The assumption that sugar is a key component of the relationship between relative social isolation and intake of sugary beverages is supported by the analyses that included artificially sweetened beverages as outcome variables. Most of the variables were significantly correlated in the bivariate analyses. However, in the regression analyses, after isolating the unique contribution of the predictor variables by controlling for scores on BMI, physical activity, weight-related self-image, depression, and demographic variables, a statistically significant association with an artificially sweetened beverage emerged in only one out of 18 cases. These results are in a striking contrast to the number of statistically significant relationships that emerged for scores on sugar-sweetened drinks. This may be interpreted as a strong indication that the associations between social connectedness and sugar-containing beverages in a great part are counted for by the sugar, and to a less extent by any of the other components that soda and juices consist of. However, these findings do not rule out the possibility that other components than sugar may also come into play. One candidate is the caffeine in cola. Caffeine is a central-nervous-system stimulant that has been shown to increase vigilance, alertness, mood, ability to concentrate and ability to solve problems [42]. As the results show, sugar-containing cola is the only variable that was significantly associated with all main predictor variables. In addition, there was a significantly negative association between high levels of relationship satisfaction and artificially sweetened cola. Moreover, the independent variables had a greater effect on sugar-containing cola than on the other dependent study variables. This may be taken as an indication that caffeine might partly count for the associations found between social connectedness and cola. However, the general pattern of the present findings indicates that sugar is the factor mainly responsible for the associations between social connectedness and intake of sugary sodas and juices.

To date, very few studies have focused on the associations between social integration and intake of sugar-sweetened beverages. One exception is a study by Cacioppo and colleagues [43], in which no significant association was found between loneliness and soda consumption. This finding was based on data from a group of 89 participants and might have suffered from insufficient statistical power. A number of studies, however, have found significant associations between social factors and food consumption. For example, in an experimental study by Baumeister and colleagues [44], it was found that social rejection caused participants to eat more sweet food than non-rejected participants. In a population-based cohort study conducted in Finland, it was found that low levels of emotional support (among women) and being single or divorced (among men) were the strongest predictors of elevated levels of high-carbohydrate food consumption [26]. Moreover, researchers have also found significant associations between loneliness and overeating [45,46]. Thus, the present results seem to be consistent with previous research on the links between social factors and nutritional intake.

The dataset used in this study did not include information on brain metabolism or blood glucose levels. Nevertheless, Social Baseline Theory [1] provides a possible explanation for the

Table 2. Multiple regression analyses: predicted scores for consumption of soda (other than cola), cola and juices from scores for loneliness, marital status (co-habiting and married), relationship satisfaction, advice from others, and cohesion at work.

	Sugar-sweetened			Artificially sweetened		
	Soda	Cola	Juice	Soda	Cola	Juice
Loneliness	.02**	.03**	.02**	−.00	−.00	.01
Married	−.05	−.12**	−.09**	−.00	.00	−.05
Cohabitating	−.02	−.09**	−.07*	.03	.02	.01
Relationship satisfaction	−.02*	−.04**	−.01*	−.01	−.03**	−.00
Advice from others	−.03**	−.02**	−.00	−.01	.00	.01
Cohesion at work	−.01	−.02**	−.01*	−.01	−.01	−.01
Mean	0.48	0.65	1.84	0.41	1.22	0.70
SD	1.00	1.22	1.36	1.14	1.84	1.30
N	25670	28509	50055	24223	29297	26618

Results are adjusted for scores on participation in sports, physical strain at work, body mass index, weight related self-image, depression, age, level of education and income.
** Correlation is significant at the 0.01 level (2 tailed).
* Correlation is significant at the 0.05 level (2 tailed).

association between loneliness and intake of sugar-containing beverages that is related to relative neuronal hypoglycemia. The theory proposes that the human brain is phylogenetically designed to utilize support from social networks to save metabolic resources when engaging in demanding mental activities. As a logical consequence, individuals who perceive themselves as socially isolated must spend more neural resources on a daily basis due to the metabolic expenses of solitary strategies for problem-solving, emotion regulation and vigilance against threats. As pointed out previously in this article, when neural metabolic activity and brain glucose utilization is high, then the rapid restoration of glucose supplies is required. Lonely people may have higher neuronal metabolic activity, which requires greater glucose supplies, and hence consume more sugar than their more socially connected counterparts. Because sodas and juices are easily accessible sources of sugar, the observed associations between relative social isolation and intake of sugar-containing beverages may reflect an expression of brain glucose regulatory mechanisms [2]. In contrast, consistent with the hypothesis that individuals profit metabolically from the energy-conserving effects of close relationships, the present results showed that perceiving ones' romantic relationship as satisfying was significantly associated with lower levels of consumption of sugar-containing beverages. This corresponds with an fMRI based study of social regulation of the threat-related brain activity demonstrating that down-regulation of neural response was a function of marital quality [25]. Further support for the hypothesis that individuals profit metabolically from social relationships is provided by the findings that being in a relationship, having supportive friends, and experiencing cohesion at work were associated with lower levels of consumption of two out of three types of sugar-containing beverages.

Some limitations of the present study should be acknowledged. The analyses were conducted based on the expectation that social factors predict the intake of sugar-containing beverages to some degree. However, a cross-sectional design does not make it possible to determine the causal relationships between research variables. On the other hand, the fact that casual directions have been demonstrated in corresponding experimental studies makes it reasonable to interpret the present results as done above. Moreover, it is challenging to see how a weak tendency to consume soda should, for example, cause changes in marital status or cohesion at work. Another concern is that despite the inclusion of several control variables, we cannot rule out the possibility that the present results may be partly explained by confounding variables not taken into account in this study. Another limitation is that this sample consisted of women in early pregnancy. The fact that pregnancy is associated with food craving [47] suggests that the scores for consumption of sweet beverages may differ between pregnant and non-pregnant woman. It should be noted that this is a limitation in terms of the generalizability of the findings, but not a limitation in terms of the assessment of the main hypothesis. However, pregnancy may be a period when women require more social support in terms of emotion regulation and practical preparations for the future. The lack of social support during pregnancy may therefore lead to a higher degree of neural activation than would otherwise occur. The associations between social factors and sugar intake may therefore be lower in the population of non-pregnant women. Gender differences may also come into play because men, in general, report a lower level of craving for sweet foods than women [18,48,49]. Future studies should therefore be based on samples including men and non-pregnant women, and also include consumption of non-sweet carbohydrates as outcome variables. Another limitation is that this study was based on self-report questionnaires and the data may therefore be subject to reporting bias.

Conclusions

The aim of this study was to test a hypothesis derived from the Social Baseline Theory that relative social isolation and social connectedness influence the level of consumption of sugar. The results from a series of regression analyses support the hypothesis by showing that loneliness and social connectedness is associated with degree of sugar consumption in the form of sugar-containing sodas and juices. This is the first time the present hypothesis has been tested in a large-scale study.

Supporting Information Tables S1 to S6 show data from the multiple regression analyses additional to the information given in Table 2. This includes mean scores and standard deviations of the main predictor variables, as well as unstandardized and standardized regression coefficients, t-test values and p-values.

Table S1 Predicted scores for consumption of sugar-containing soda (other than cola) from scores for loneliness, marital status (co-habiting and married), relationship satisfaction, advice from others, and cohesion at work. Results are adjusted for scores on participation in sports, physical strain at work, body mass index, weight related self-image, depression, age, level of education and income.

Table S2 Predicted scores for consumption of sugar-containing cola from scores for loneliness, marital status (co-habiting and married), relationship satisfaction, advice from others, and cohesion at work. Results are adjusted for scores on participation in sports, physical strain at work, body mass index, weight related self-image, depression, age, level of education and income.

Table S3 Predicted scores for consumption of sugar-containing juice from scores for loneliness, marital status (co-habiting and married), relationship satisfaction, advice from others, and cohesion at work. Results are adjusted for scores on participation in sports, physical strain at work, body mass index, weight related self-image, depression, age, level of education and income.

Table S4 Predicted scores for consumption of artificially sweetened soda (other than cola) from scores for loneliness, marital status (co-habiting and married), relationship satisfaction, advice from others, and cohesion at work. Results are adjusted for scores on participation in sports, physical strain at work, body mass index, weight related self-image, depression, age, level of education and income.

Table S5 Predicted scores for consumption of artificially sweetened cola from scores for loneliness, marital status (co-habiting and married), relationship satisfaction, advice from others, and cohesion at work. Results are adjusted for scores on participation in sports, physical strain at work, body mass index, weight related self-image, depression, age, level of education and income.

Table S6 Predicted scores for consumption of artificially sweetened juice from scores for loneliness, marital status (co-habiting and married), relationship satisfaction, advice from others, and cohesion at work. Results are adjusted for scores on participation in sports, physical strain at work, body mass index, weight related self-image, depression, age, level of education and income.

Author Contributions

Conceived and designed the experiments: REH. Performed the experiments: REH. Analyzed the data: REH TT FT. Contributed reagents/materials/analysis tools: REH FT TT. Contributed to the writing of the manuscript: REH.

References

1. Beckes L, Coan JA (2011) Social Baseline Theory: The Role of Social Proximity in Emotion and Economy of Action. Social and Personality Psychology Compass 5: 976–988.
2. Heininger K (2002) The cerebral glucose-fatty acid cycle: Evolutionary roots, regulation, and (patho)physiological importance. In: Donard SD, editor. International Review of Neurobiology: Academic Press. pp. 103–158.
3. Hertz L, Dienel GA (2002) Energy metabolism in the brain. In: Donard SD, editor. International Review of Neurobiology: Academic Press. pp. 1–102.
4. Scholey AB, Harper S, Kennedy DO (2001) Cognitive demand and blood glucose. Physiol Behav 73: 585–592.
5. Gailliot MT, Baumeister RF, DeWall CN, Maner JK, Plant EA, et al. (2007) Self-control relies on glucose as a limited energy source: willpower is more than a metaphor. J Pers Soc Psychol 92: 325–336.
6. Levin BE, Dunn-Meynell AA, Routh VH (2002) CNS sensing and regulation of peripheral glucose levels. In: Donard SD, editor. International Review of Neurobiology: Academic Press. pp. 219–258.
7. Kishore P, Gabriely I, Cui MH, Di Vito J, Gajavelli S, et al. (2006) Role of hepatic glycogen breakdown in defective counterregulation of hypoglycemia in intensively treated type 1 diabetes. Diabetes 55: 659–666.
8. Ahren B (2000) Autonomic regulation of islet hormone secretion - Implications for health and disease. Diabetologia 43: 393–410.
9. Lambillotte C, Gilon P, Henquin JC (1997) Direct glucocorticoid inhibition of insulin secretion - An in vitro study of dexamethasone effects in mouse islets. Journal of Clinical Investigation 99: 414–423.
10. Wilcox G (2005) Insulin and insulin resistance. The Clinical biochemist Reviews/Australian Association of Clinical Biochemists 26: 19–39.
11. Hitze B, Hubold C, van Dyken R, Schlichting K, Lehnert H, et al. (2010) How the selfish brain organizes its supply and demand. Front Neuroenergetics 2: 7.
12. Born JM, Lemmens SG, Rutters F, Nieuwenhuizen AG, Formisano E, et al. (2010) Acute stress and food-related reward activation in the brain during food choice during eating in the absence of hunger. Int J Obes (Lond) 34: 172–181.
13. Christensen L, Pettijohn L (2001) Mood and carbohydrate cravings. Appetite 36: 137–145.
14. Epel E, Lapidus R, McEwen B, Brownell K (2001) Stress may add bite to appetite in women: a laboratory study of stress-induced cortisol and eating behavior. Psychoneuroendocrinology 26: 37–49.
15. Groesz LM, McCoy S, Carl J, Saslow L, Stewart J, et al. (2012) What is eating you? Stress and the drive to eat. Appetite 58: 717–721.
16. Kandiah J, Yake M, Jones J, Meyer M (2006) Stress influences appetite and comfort food preferences in college women. Nutrition Research 26: 118–123.
17. Tomiyama AJ, Dallman MF, Epel ES (2011) Comfort food is comforting to those most stressed: Evidence of the chronic stress response network in high stress women. Psychoneuroendocrinology 36: 1513–1519.
18. Zellner DA, Loaiza S, Gonzalez Z, Pita J, Morales J, et al. (2006) Food selection changes under stress. Physiology & Behavior 87: 789–793.
19. Peters A, Kubera B, Hubold C, Langemann D (2011) The selfish brain: stress and eating behavior. Front Neurosci 5: 74.
20. Coan JA, Kasle S, Jackson A, Schaefer HS, Davidson RJ (2013) Mutuality and the social regulation of neural threat responding. Attach Hum Dev 15: 303–315.
21. Coan JA, Beckes L, Allen JP (2013) Childhood maternal support and social capital moderate the regulatory impact of social relationships in adulthood. International Journal of Psychophysiology 88: 224–231.
22. Smaldino PE, Newson L, Schank JC, Richerson PJ (2013) Simulating the Evolution of the Human Family: Cooperative Breeding Increases in Harsh Environments. PLoS ONE 8: e80753.
23. Coan JA (2010) Adult attachment and the brain. Journal of Social and Personal Relationships 27: 210–217.
24. Gross E, Proffitt D (2013) The economy of social resources and its influence on spatial perceptions. Frontiers in Human Neuroscience 7: 772.
25. Coan JA, Schaefer HS, Davidson RJ (2006) Lending a hand: Social regulation of the neural response to threat. Psychological Science 17: 1032–1039.
26. Laitinen J, Ek E, Sovio U (2002) Stress-Related Eating and Drinking Behavior and Body Mass Index and Predictors of This Behavior. Preventive Medicine 34: 29–39.
27. Bye EK (1999) Bruk av drikkevarer - hvem, hva og hvor? Lysaker: Statens Institutt for Forbruksforskning. 8 8.
28. Magnus P, Irgens LM, Haug K, Nystad W, Skjaerven R, et al. (2006) Cohort profile: The Norwegian Mother and Child Cohort Study (MoBa). International Journal of Epidemiology 35: 1146–1150.
29. Nilsen RM, Vollset SE, Gjessing HK, Skjaerven R, Melve KK, et al. (2009) Self-selection and bias in a large prospective pregnancy cohort in Norway. Paediatric and Perinatal Epidemiology 23: 597–608.
30. Blum J, Mehrabian A (1999) Personality and temperament correlates of marital satisfaction. Journal of Personality 67: 93–125.
31. Snyder DK (1997) Marital Satisfaction Inventory–Revised (MSI-R) manual. Los Angeles: Western Psychological Services.

32. Hendrick SS (1988) A Generic Measure of Relationship Satisfaction. Journal of Marriage and the Family 50: 93.
33. Mortensen O, Torsheim T, Melkevik O, Thuen F (2012) Adding a Baby to the Equation. Married and Cohabiting Women's Relationship Satisfaction in the Transition to Parenthood. Family Process 51: 122–139.
34. Rosand GMB, Slinning K, Eberhard-Gran M, Tambs K (2011) Partner relationship satisfaction and maternal emotional distress in early pregnancy. BMC Public Health 11: 12.
35. Lemmens SG, Rutters F, Born JM, Westerterp-Plantenga MS (2011) Stress augments food 'wanting' and energy intake in visceral overweight subjects in the absence of hunger. Physiol Behav 103: 157–163.
36. Stice E (2001) A prospective test of the dual-pathway model of bulimic pathology: Mediating effects of dieting and negative affect. Journal of Abnormal Psychology 110: 124–135.
37. Fernstrom MH, Krowinski RL, Kupfer DJ (1987) Appetite and food preference in depression: effects of imipramine treatment. Biol Psychiatry 22: 529–539.
38. Macht M (2008) How emotions affect eating: A five-way model. Appetite 50: 1–11.
39. Bugge BB (2010) Forbidden fruit tastes the sweetest – A study of Norwegians eating and drinking pattern of chocolate, sweets, salty snacks, soft drinks and the like. Oslo: National Institute for Consumer Research. 296 p.
40. Ogden CL, Kit BK, Carroll MD, Park S (2011) Consumption of Sugar Drinks in the United States, 2005–2008. Hyattsville.
41. George GC, Milani TJ, Hanss-Nuss H, Freeland-Graves JH (2005) Compliance with dietary guidelines and relationship to psychosocial factors in low-income women in late postpartum. Journal of the American Dietetic Association 105: 916–926.
42. Glade MJ (2010) Caffeine-Not just a stimulant. Nutrition 26: 932–938.
43. Cacioppo JT, Hawkley LC, Crawford LE, Ernst JM, Burleson MH, et al. (2002) Loneliness and health: Potential mechanisms. Psychosomatic Medicine 64: 407–417.
44. Baumeister RF, DeWall CN, Ciarocco NJ, Twenge JM (2005) Social exclusion impairs self-regulation. Journal of Personality and Social Psychology 88: 589–604.
45. Levine MP (2012) Loneliness and eating disorders. J Psychol 146: 243–257.
46. Masheb RM, Grilo CM (2006) Emotional overeating and its associations with eating disorder psychopathology among overweight patients with binge eating disorder. International Journal of Eating Disorders 39: 141–146.
47. Bowen DJ (1992) Taste and food preference changes across the course of pregnancy. Appetite 19: 233–242.
48. Christensen L, Brooks A (2006) Changing food preference as a function of mood. Journal of Psychology 140: 293–306.
49. Lafay L, Thomas F, Mennen L, Charles MA, Eschwege E, et al. (2001) Gender differences in the relation between food cravings and mood in an adult community: Results from the Fleurbaix Laventie Ville Sante study. International Journal of Eating Disorders 29: 195–204.

13

Leisure in Children and Adolescents with Juvenile Idiopathic Arthritis

Sabrina Cavallo[1,2,3,4]*, Karine Toupin April[5,6], Viviane Grandpierre[5,7], Annette Majnemer[2,8], Debbie Ehrmann Feldman[1,3,4,9,10]

1 Département de Médecine Sociale et Préventive, École de Santé Publique, Université de Montréal, Montréal, Québec, Canada, **2** Montreal Children's Hospital, McGill University Health Center, Montréal, Québec, Canada, **3** Institut de Recherche en Santé Publique Université de Montréal, Montréal, Québec, Canada, **4** Centre de Recherche Interdisciplinaire en Réadaptation du Montréal Métropolitain, Institut de Réadaptation de Montréal, Montréal, Québec, Canada, **5** Children's Hospital of Eastern Ontario Research Institute, Ottawa, Ontario, Canada, **6** Department of Pediatrics, Faculty of Medicine, University of Ottawa, Ottawa, Ontario, Canada, **7** School of Rehabilitation Sciences, Faculty of Health Sciences, University of Ottawa, Ottawa, Ontario, Canada, **8** School of Physical and Occupational Therapy, Faculty of Medicine, McGill University, Montréal, Québec, Canada, **9** École de Réadaptation, Faculté de Médecine, Université de Montréal, Montréal, Québec, Canada, **10** Direction de Santé Publique de Montréal, Montréal, Québec, Canada

Abstract

The aim of this systematic review is to describe participation in social and physical leisure activities among children and adolescents with JIA, as well as identify potential determinants of leisure participation.

Methods: Electronic databases were systematically searched for articles published up until June 2013 pertaining to participation in leisure activities among youth with JIA and other rheumatic diseases. Studies were included if they measured involvement in either social or physical leisure activities. Selection and quality appraisal of articles were completed independently by two authors.

Results: Eight hundred and ninety-three articles were found through electronic and reference search. One hundred and nine full articles were reviewed to assess for eligibility. Twelve articles met inclusion criteria and findings were reviewed. Most focused on describing participation in physical rather than social activities. Results suggest that youth with JIA participated less in both social and physical leisure activities as compared to healthy peers, and those with JIA did not meet national recommendations for physical activity. Potential determinants of leisure participation were socio-demographic (age, sex), anthropometric (height, weight) and disease-related (JIA subtype, disease duration, pain, number of swollen or painful joints, stiffness, fatigue, well-being) factors.

Conclusion: Characterization of leisure activity remains limited and mostly focused on physical activity in JIA. Assessment of more comprehensive outcome measures is warranted to obtain a better description of leisure in this population. Evidence of the influence of contextual factors as potential determinants of involvement in leisure among children with pediatric rheumatologic diseases is needed.

Editor: Dominique Heymann, Faculté de médecine de Nantes, France

Funding: The first author benefited from doctoral student bursaries awarded by the Fonds de Recherche Santé Québec and the MENTOR program of the Canadian Institutes of Health Research. Dr. Karine Toupin April would like to acknowledge funding from the Children's Hospital of Eastern Ontario Research Institute. The funders had no role in study design, data collection and analysis, decision to publish, or preparation of the manuscript.

Competing Interests: The authors have declared that no competing interests exist.

* Email: sabrina.cavallo@yahoo.ca

Introduction

Juvenile idiopathic arthritis (JIA), which includes juvenile rheumatoid arthritis (JRA), is one of the most common chronic conditions of childhood [1]. Children and adolescents with JIA are at greater risk for adopting a more sedentary lifestyle compared to their healthy peers in part due to disease related factors such as pain, fatigue, swollen and stiff joints [1,2]. In the past decade there has been a growing interest for the study of leisure participation in children with disabilities. However this concept has been vastly understudied in youth with pediatric rheumatologic diseases.

Leisure participation has been defined as the 'involvement in the formal and informal everyday activities of childhood in all types of non-school environments, including environments for play, sport, entertainment, learning, and religious expression'(King et al., 2003, p. 65) [3]. Participation in leisure activities is of critical importance in childhood and adolescence to maintain a fit lifestyle, develop friendships, engage in focus-oriented activities, as well as acquire cognitive and social skills important for development [4–6]. If participation in leisure activities remains limited on a long-term basis, children and adolescents may not have enough social contacts with peers, may be less able to make friends, experience greater social isolation, and may be at greater risk for depression

[7]. Furthermore, engagement in active physical activities is important for physical and cardiovascular health.

Participation is a key component of the International Classification of Functioning, Disability and Health (ICF) endorsed by the World Health Organization (WHO) [8]. As depicted in the ICF, a child's participation in leisure may be influenced by various factors to include those related to the health condition (e.g. disease severity), as well as personal (e.g. age, sex) and environmental (e.g. accessibility to services) [8,9].

Most of the existing literature in JIA focuses on describing the level of involvement and benefits of exercise or physical activity programs on health outcomes such as quality of life, physical function and fitness, as well as other JIA related disease outcomes (e.g. number of swollen joints and bone mineral density) [10–14], as well as describing the level of involvement. However limited research has been done in the broader area of leisure participation in JIA.

The main purpose of this systematic review was to describe involvement in social (e.g. outings with friends and/or family) and physical (e.g. sports, biking, swimming, etc.) leisure activities among children and adolescents with JIA. It reports on the type and frequency of these activities as compared with either healthy controls, normative data or health guidelines. A secondary objective was to identify potential socio-demographic, disease-related, personal and environmental determinants of leisure activities in children and adolescents with JIA.

Materials and Methods

Literature Search

The first author (SC) devised an electronic search strategy (Appendix S1) in collaboration with a librarian. The librarian also assisted in identifying the appropriate key terms for the systematic review and reviewed the final search strategy to ensure correctness. An example of the detailed search strategy formatted for the MEDLINE database with all key words is provided (Appendix S1). In addition to MEDLINE (1946 to Present), we searched the following electronic databases: CINAHL (1982 to December week 1 2013), Base de Données en Santé Publique (June 2013), ERIC (1965 to April 2013), Health and Psychosocial Instruments (1985 to April 2013), OT Seeker (June 2013), PsycINFO (1806 to May Week 3 2013), EMBASE (1974 to 2013 Week 21), Cochrane Database of Systematic Reviews (2005 to March 2013), ACP Journal Club (1991 to April 2013), Database of Abstracts of Reviews of Effects (2nd Quarter 2013), Cochrane Central Register of Controlled Trials (March 2013) and Cochrane Methodology Register (3rd Quarter 2012). Key term selection was guided by using a PICOS (populations, interventions, comparators, outcomes, study design) framework [15–17]. The search strategy did not restrict on language or design of the study; non pertinent articles were sifted out by authors after the search was completed. Scientific journals, internet browsers and reference lists of reviewed articles were also consulted for any pertinent information and potential articles.

Inclusion and Exclusion Criteria

We included studies related to participation in physical or social leisure-time activities completed by children between the ages of 0 and 21 years diagnosed with juvenile idiopathic arthritis, juvenile chronic arthritis, or juvenile rheumatoid arthritis. All diagnostic classifications provided by the International League of Associations for Rheumatology (ILAR), the European League Against Rheumatism (EULAR) or the American College of Rheumatism (ACR) were accepted. As both social and physical activities are considered leisure pursuits we have focused on including a variety of habitual activities performed for the purpose of having fun. Studies reporting findings exclusively on participation in exercise programs done during school classes or as part of a regimented exercise program in a controlled setting (laboratory) were excluded. Both English and French publications were included in the search. We restricted our search to quantitative studies. Although reviewed for pertinent information and potential references, review papers, abstracts, commentaries or letters to the editor, study protocols, work group or conference proceedings and studies aimed at validating measures were not retained for the systematic review. Results from our search were exported into EndNote X6 and subsequently managed in excel database sheets.

Identification of Studies

After duplicates were removed, two authors from the team (SC and VG) independently screened titles, abstracts and key words for pertinent articles according to the identified eligibility criteria. After initial screening the retained full articles were assessed to ensure that they met inclusion criteria and a list of relevant articles was compiled. A review of these articles was completed by each reviewer who then independently decided which articles met the eligibility criteria and should be included in the systematic review. If consensus could not be reached between reviewers, a third author (KTA) resolved any disagreements.

Data Extraction

Two authors (SC and VG) independently extracted data from the retained articles using a previously pilot-tested extraction table. After thorough review of selected articles information on the studies (study design, geographical location, sample size, participant characteristics [i.e. age and sex distribution, diagnosis], objectives) and the methods of data collection (measure of leisure participation, child or proxy report, psychometric properties) were summarized in a table, as well as information on potential determinants of leisure participation was reported in a separate table. The Preferred Reporting Items for Systematic Reviews and Meta-Analyses (PRISMA) statement was used to inform reporting of this systematic review (see completed PRISMA checklist in Appendix S2) [18].

Study appraisal

Studies meeting the inclusion criteria were systematically appraised using the Quality Assessment Tool for Quantitative Studies [19]. This tool has been deemed suitable for quality assessment of randomised and non-randomised studies [20]. Ratings of strong, moderate or weak were assigned for each of the following six quality components: selection bias, study design, confounders, blinding, data collection methods, withdrawals and dropouts [21]. The tool's test-retest (intra-rater) reliability was assessed for two reviewers and results on agreement were acceptable (Kappa 0.74 and 0.61, respectively for each reviewer) [19]. Adequate content and construct validity were also demonstrated [19].

Synthesis of findings

A narrative summary allowed us to analyse our findings by describing content and highlighting strengths and weaknesses of reviewed studies. Due to the heterogeneous characteristics of the included studies (demographic distributions, leisure outcomes, units of measure) it was not feasible to conduct a meta-analysis [22].

Results

The electronic search yielded 884 unique references (i.e. after duplicates were removed). An additional 9 references were obtained through manual review of reference lists from consulted articles and through internet browser search. A total of 893 titles and abstracts were screened. One hundred and nine full articles were reviewed to assess for eligibility. Of these, 12 articles met inclusion criteria and were included in the qualitative synthesis of results (Figure 1).

The identified studies were rated as to their quality. Using the Quality Assessment Tool for Quantitative Studies, none of the studies met all of the quality criteria [19,21]. All studies exhibited some level of selection bias. Selected participants were deemed to be at most somewhat likely to represent the studied population, appraisal scores ranged from weak (n = 2) [23,24] to moderate (n = 10) [2,25–33]. Retained studies were observational. Half of the studies adequately controlled for important confounders [25,26,30–33], such as age and sex. Only 3 studies collected data on leisure-time activities using outcome measures with known or properly cited validity and reliability [23,28,30]. The descriptive characteristics of study participants and information on leisure participation are included in Table 1. Studies reporting on potential determinants of leisure participation are described in Table 2.

Characteristics of the Studies

Only one study included data from a childhood rheumatic disease database [23], while all others recruited participants from tertiary care centers (hospital and centers). One study included 78 participants with JIA and 17 with other rheumatologic diagnoses [25], whereas all other studies included only participants with JIA. A range of ages were studied (4 to 18 years); certain authors focused their examination of leisure participation on specific age groups: children (n = 3) [24,27,30] and/or adolescents (n = 3) [25,26,30], whereas other studies reported outcomes for all ages combined (e.g. 4 to 18 years) (n = 5) [2,23,28,31,33]. Ten out of the 12 studies used comparison analysis to illustrate differences in leisure participation between groups (within JIA group analysis (n = 4), healthy controls (n = 9) and controls with other medical conditions (n = 1)). Of these, only one study employed matching on age and sex, as well as race and county of residence [31], while others either controlled for covariates such as age, sex and anthropometric factors (weight, height or body mass index) [23,24,26,28,32,33], and others simply reported findings in groups of similar age and sex [25,30].

The main objective of 8 studies hinged on reporting information on the level of participation in leisure activities among those living with JIA, as well as identifying potential determinants and comparing findings on leisure participation between patients with JIA and controls [2,24,25,28–30,32,33]. The remaining 4 studies inquired primarily on overall bone health (geometry, density and strength) and participation in leisure-time physical activity as a secondary outcome [23,26,27,31].

Participation in social activities was assessed through self-report and quantified using various scales (e.g. Likert, interval) [2,25,30]. Physical activity was evaluated subjectively through self-report or proxy activity questionnaires [23,24,26,27,29,31–33] and/or objectively with motion and activity monitors (n = 5) [24,26–29]. Studies described involvement in physical activities in terms of exertion level (light, moderate or vigorous), frequency (hr/day or hr/week) (n = 6) [24,26–28,31,32], duration (months in a year) (n = 3) [24,26,27], energy expenditure (Metabolic equivalent of a task (MET)) (n = 2) [23,33] and movement counts (n = 4) [24,26–28]. Some authors also quantified physical activity using ordinal scales to indicate level of participation (how active) [29,30].

There were 3 studies that focused on social activities [2,25,30], 10 that also reported on physical activities [23,24,26–33], and 5 that explored potential determinants of participation [2,28,29,32,33]. These are summarized below.

Participation in social activities

Schanberg et al. conducted a longitudinal study assessing activity reduction among 41 youth with JIA (aged between 8 to 17 years) and found that 66% had restricted participation in social activities at least one day during the 2 month study [2]. Billings et al. showed that youth (aged ≥10 years) with severe disease reported fewer activities with family members in comparison to those with milder disease, as well as significantly fewer activities with friends compared to healthy controls [25]. Although, participants with mild/inactive disease reported fewer activities with friends compared to healthy controls, they took part in more family activities than healthy controls. Huygen et al.'s investigation into the psychological, behavioural and social adjustment of 47 children and adolescents with JIA revealed that there were no differences among adolescents (ages 12 to 16 years) in terms of the frequency of social interactions between those with JIA and healthy controls [30]. However, children (ages 7 to 11 years) with JIA did not play or visit as frequently with friends as their healthy peers (1 7 (0.1) versus 2.0 (0.0), p = 0.04; 3-point Likert scale) [30].

Participation in physical activities

Results on physical activity measured through self-report in 7 studies were lower in children and adolescents with JIA compared to their healthy controls [23,24,26,30–33]. Specifically participants with JIA participated less in moderate to vigorous physical activities compared to healthy peers [24,32], however no differences were found between groups for participation in light physical activity [24,26,27,32]. Studies examining participation in sports revealed that both children (range 4.6 to 11.0 years) and adolescents (range 11 to 18 years) with JIA took part in sports less frequently than their peers without JIA [24,26,30,32]. Two studies reported fewer weight-bearing physical activities among those with JIA compared to healthy controls [23,31]. However Félin et al. reported that only those with systemic JIA (and not those with polyarticular or oligoarticular JIA) were less involved in weight-bearing activities compared to healthy controls [23].

Significant within group differences for participation in physical activity were found in two studies [23,27]. When exploring disease subtypes, authors reported that patients with systemic JIA (26.0 [3.8, 48.2] METs hours/week) were significantly less involved in weight-bearing PA compared to patients with oligoarticular (45.4 [20.9, 70.9] METs hours/week) or polyarticular (40.7 [23.8, 57.6] METs hours/week) JIA ($p \leq 0.01$) [23]. The other study described how duration of involvement in organized sports was significantly greater in children with normal bone mineral density (1.7 (2.2) months/year) in comparison to those with low bone mineral density (0.2 [0.8] months/year, p = 0.03) [27]. Only one study compared daily average physical activity between boys and girls in 30 patients with JIA and found no statistically significant differences [32].

When measured objectively through accelerometry, most authors reported no statistically significant differences in average daily physical activity (i.e. movement counts) between JIA and healthy groups [24,26,27]. In fact only Maggio et al. found that children and adolescents with JIA participated less in moderate to vigorous physical activity (MVPA) compared to healthy counterparts (JIA, 6.9% of time in MVPA, 54.1±5.7 min/day; healthy

Figure 1. PRISMA 2009 Flow Diagram

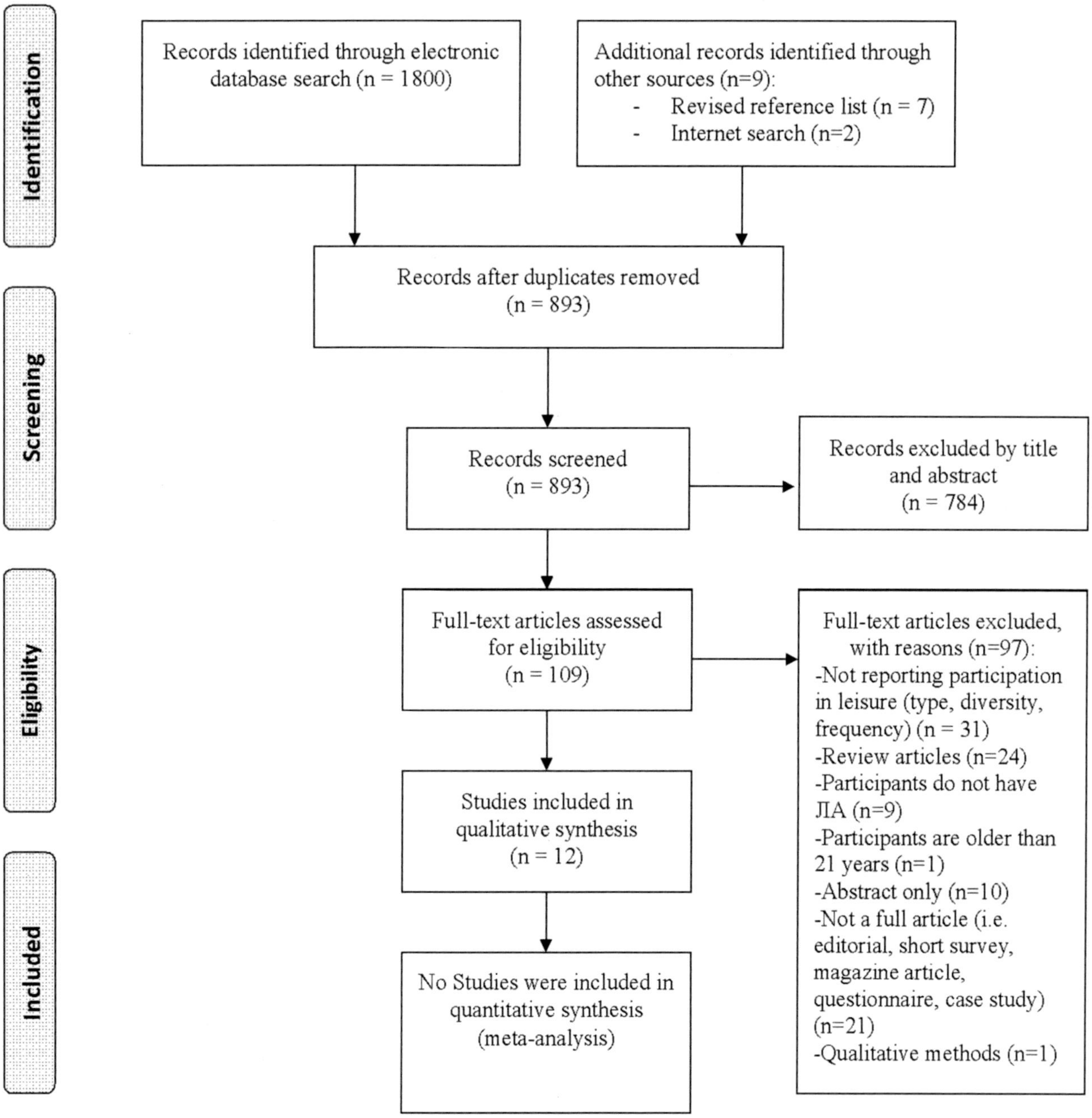

From: Moher D, Liberati A, Tetzlaff J, Altman DG, The PRISMA Group (2009). *P*referred *R*eporting *I*tems for *S*ystematic Reviews and *M*eta-*A*nalyses: The PRISMA Statement. PLoS Med 6(6): e1000097. doi:10.1371/journal.pmed1000097

For more information, visit www.prisma-statement.org.

Figure 1. PRISMA Flow Diagram of Included Articles. Figure 1 presents a PRISMA flow diagram of articles included in the systematic review as well as the main reasons for rejection.

controls, 9.1% of time in MVPA, 71.3±4.5 min/day), p = 0.04 [28]. Furthermore, two studies indicated that fewer children with JIA met international recommendations of 60 minutes of daily MVPA compared to healthy controls [28,32], and the proportion varied between one-third (23% vs. 66%) to two-thirds (38% vs. 60%) than that of healthy controls [28,32].

Potential determinants of leisure

Potential determinants of leisure participation were assessed in 5 studies [2,28,29,32,33], however only 4 reported statistically significant associations with leisure [2,28,29,32] (Table 2). Socio-demographic factors were assessed in two studies [28,29]. Results showed that when adjusted for age boys displayed higher physical activity levels than girls [28]. Also, the younger the child, the higher the level of physical activity [29]. Disease-related factors were assessed in all studies examining potential determinants [2,28,29,32,33]. However in only four studies were disease-related factors associated with lower levels of leisure activity (systemic JRA subtype, lower well-being, pain, larger number of painful joints, stiffness, and fatigue) [2,23,29]. Whereas longer disease duration was associated with more frequent participation in physical activity [32]. Anthropometric measures were also considered as potential determinants of physical activity participation in one study [28] and higher height and weight were associated with increased physical activity among children and adolescents living with JIA [28].

Discussion

Our systematic review revealed that participation in social and physical activities during leisure-time may be decreased in children and adolescents living with JIA as compared to their healthy peers and fewer JIA patients met national physical activity recommendations. Studies to date have methodological weaknesses; therefore results should be interpreted with caution. Furthermore, only a few studies empirically explored the association between potential determinants and participation in leisure-time activities. Authors used various subjective and objective outcome measures with differing measurement units and scales and lack of validity and reliability to assess involvement in leisure-time activities making it difficult to generalise results on leisure participation in JIA.

The self-report assessment of leisure participation was for the most part restricted to a handful of activities, specifically social (e.g. taking part in play with friends, seeing friends, going to ball games, being part of a club, participating in sports, going to parties or dances) and physical (e.g. participating in organized sports or weight-bearing activities), rather than a larger gamut of recreational activities (e.g. playing board games or card games, screen time activities [computer or video games, watching TV], playing with pets), skill-based (e.g. swimming; learning to sing [choir or individual lessons], learning to dance, playing a musical instrument) and self-improvement (e.g. writing a story, reading, doing volunteer work, shopping). A more comprehensive approach to assessment is needed in order to truly capture a complete picture of leisure in this population. Findings would subsequently enable health care professionals to assess the benefits and potential determinants of participation. As our review demonstrates, social and physical activities of children and adolescents with JIA may vary with age, sex, type of activity, social engagement (friends, family) and disease activity/status.

In our review, social participation in young children was characterised as play with friends, whereas for adolescents it included analysis of spontaneous social contact and going on outings with friends. Among children, social interactions are often fostered through informal play time with friends [4,34]. Children with JIA took part in less play than healthy peers possibly due to physical limitations and pain brought on by their disease. Younger children tend to be involved in more active types of play, which may discourage young patients with JIA affected by fluctuating joint pain and swelling to partake in these activities with friends [2,29].

Adolescents with JIA took part in as many spontaneous social interactions as their healthy peers [30], however did not attend as many outings with friends [25]. These results parallel those found among adolescents (12 to 20 years of age) with cerebral palsy, where participants favoured quiet social activities such as hanging out, listening to music and talking on the phone with friends [35] and less in outings [35]. The similarities found between adolescents with and without JIA may reflect the natural progression of social leisure participation [4,34]; as children get older they become less involved in play and more engaged in socially oriented activities which tend to be less physically straining [36,37].

Social engagement in activities (i.e. with whom they engaged in activities) [38] varied across disease status [25]. The more severe the disease activity the less patients participated in activities with friends and family members [25]. During periods of more severe arthritis, parents may limit their child's participation in activities to avoid exacerbating disease symptoms. The fear of pain may influence the parents' and the child's willingness to take part in social activities [39,40]. This avoidance and the need to monitor their child's health closely may also explain why those even with milder or inactive JIA may be less inclined to participate in social activities with friends and more involved in family activities [25]. Similarly, children and adolescents with systemic JIA (a more severe subtype of JIA) were less involved in weight-bearing physical activities compared to those with oligoarticular or polyarticular JIA [23].

The association of age and sex with participation in physical activity is often studied [41]. Our findings support that physical activity in JIA tends to decrease with age [29], which parallels results from the general pediatric population [4,34]. Boys are often found to be more physically active than girls [37,41–43]. Studies included in our review revealed divergent results. When adjusting for age (mean age 10.8±0.5 years; range 4.8 to 17.9) Maggio et al. (2010) reported that boys with JIA were more physically active than their female counterparts [28]. Whereas when comparing physical activity among adolescents with JIA (mean age of 17.0±0.6 years) Lelieveld et al. (2008) reported no significant differences across sexes [32]. In general, participation in sports and other active pursuits is higher throughout middle childhood and drops during adolescence [34]. This may in part explain why no significant differences in physical activity were found among adolescent boys and girls with JIA [32].

Although results varied, most studies showed that children with JIA spent significantly less time pursuing physical activity compared to healthy controls [23,24,26,28,30–33]. In addition to disease-related factors (e.g. disease duration, number of painful and swollen joints), poor physical fitness may also contribute to lower levels of physical activity in JIA [29]. Children living with

Table 1. Findings of systematic review on leisure participation in children and adolescents living with juvenile arthritis.

Author, Country (year)	Participants		Study design	Leisure outcome measure	Variable recorded	Findings
	JIA	Comparator groups				
Billings, USA (1987)	56 (37 girls and 19 boys); mean age 13.7 years (≥10 years)	Within group comparison and 77 HC	Cross-sectional	Youth Health and Daily living form	# of social activities done with family, friends and at school out of 10	Fewer family activities for severe JIA group compared to those with mild/inactive JIA ($p<0.05$). Fewer activities with friends for JIA groups compared to HC ($p<0.05$). More family activities for mild/inactive JIA compared to HC ($p<0.05$).
Félin, USA (2007)	48, age range 4–18 years	Within group comparison and 266 HC	Cross-sectional	PA questionnaire on weight-bearing activities	Average METs hr/wk in the last year	Decreased weight bearing PA for systematic JIA group compared to oligoarthritis, polyarthritis JIA or HC groups ($p\leq0.01$). No significant differences between oligoarthritis or polyarthritis JIA groups and HC.
Henderson, USA (1995)	23 (16 females), mean age 8.1 years (range 5–11 years	23 HC	Cross-sectional	Caltrac accelerometer and UCMS; Parent-report activity record, 3 day; Parent-report questionnaire on organized sports	Average daily movement counts; Daily activities, type (light, strenuous) and intensity (hours/day); Frequency (hours/week) and amount in the last year (months)	No significant differences in daily movement. Decreased time spent in strenuous activities for JIA group ($p<0.01$). No significant differences in low intensity PA between groups. ↓ time spent participating in sports at baseline ($p=0.01$) and in the last year ($p<0.01$) for JIA group.
Henderson, USA (1997)	48 (37 female, 11 male), mean age 8.1±1.9 years (range = 4.6–11.0 years)	Within-group comparisons	Cross-sectional	Caltrac accelerometer and UCMS; Parent-report activity record, 3 day; Parent-report questionnaire on organized sports	Average daily movement counts; Daily PA, type (light, strenuous) and intensity (hours/day); Frequency (hours/week) and amount in the last year (months)	No significant differences in daily movement. No significant differences in daily PA. Decreased time spent in organized sports for JIA group with low TB BMD compared to those with normal TB BMD ($p=0.03$).
Henderson, USA (2000)	Thirty-six females, mean age 16.0±1.8 years (age range 11 to 18 years)	Within-group comparisons and 51 HC	Cross-sectional	Caltrac accelerometer and UCMS; Self-report activity record, 3 day; Self-report questionnaire on organized sports	Average daily movement counts; Daily PA, type (light, strenuous) and intensity (hours/day); Frequency (hours/week) and amount in the last year (months)	No significant differences in daily movement. No significant differences in daily PA. 50% of JIA patients participated in organized sports compared to 65% of HC ($p=0.01$). Decreased time spent in organized sports for JIA group compared to HC ($p=0.005$).
Huygen, Netherlands (2000)	47 (32 girls and 15 boys), age range 7–16 years (child, 7–11 years of age; adolescents, 12–16 years of age)	52 HC	Cross-sectional	Dutch CBCL, parent-report on the child's social functioning; Dutch Youth Self Report, adolescents self-report on social functioning	3-point Likert scale	Decreased participation in play with friends for children with JIA ($p=0.04$). No significant differences between groups for seeing friends. Decreased participation in sports for adolescents with JIA ($p=0.00$).

Table 1. Cont.

Author, Country (year)	Participants		Study design	Leisure outcome measure	Variable recorded	Findings
	JIA	Comparator groups				
Lelieveld, Netherlands (2008)	30 (18 girls, 12 boys), mean age 17.0±0.6 years	106 HC	Cross-sectional	Self-report activity diary, 3 days	Daily average PA (hours/day)	Decreased PA in JIA group ($p<0.01$). Increased time spent in bed for JIA group. No significant differences in PA between boys and girls among JIA or HC groups. No significant differences in low intensity activities between JIA and HC. Decreased time spent in moderate intensity leisure activities ($p<0.01$); high intensity leisure activities ($p<0.05$); and in competitive sports ($p<0.01$) for JIA group. Only 23% of patients with JIA met public health recommendations to perform ≥1 hour daily MVPA (mean of 87 min/day of MVPA) compared with 66% of HC (mean of 133 min/day of MVPA).
Lien, Norway (2005)	108, age range of 6–18 years	108 HC	Longitudinal	Self-report questionnaire on weight-bearing activities outside of school hours	Frequency (number of times per week), ordinal scale (0.5 = less than once a week, 1 = once a week)	Decreased participation in weight-bearing activities at baseline ($p = 0.033$) and at the 2 year follow-up ($p = 0.040$).
Maggio, Switzerland (2010)	31, mean age 10.8±0.5 years (range 4.8 to 17.9 years)	85 HC, 45 obese, 48 type 1 diabetes mellitus	Cross-sectional	Uniaxial Actigraph accelerometer, 7 days	Average daily PA (minutes/day)	When adjusted for age, decreased daily PA for JIA group compared to HC ($p< 0.001$) and compared to patients with obesity ($p = 0.002$). Decreased time spent in MVPA for JIA group versus HC ($p = 0.036$). 38.1% of JIA, 38.5% of type 1 diabetes mellitus, 51.6% with obesity and 60.4% of HC met the daily recommended 60 minutes of MVPA.
Schanberg, USA (2003)	41 (59% were girls), mean age 12.3±2.9 years (range 8–17 years)	None	Longitudinal	Self-report diary on daily social activities	Reduction in activities, 4-point Likert scale (anchored by 'not at all' and 'a lot')	No control data available for comparison
Takken, Netherlands (2003)	45 (10 male, 35 female), mean age 8.9±2.2 years	None	Cross-sectional	Caltrac activity monitor measuring daily PA for 4 consecutive days; Parent-report PAL	Average daily motion counts; Child's usual PAL, 5 point Likert scale (1 = inactive to 5 = very active)	No control data available for comparison
Tarakci, Turkey (2011)	52 (33girls, 19 boys), mean age 12.13±2.92 years (range 8–17 years)	48 HC	Cross-sectional	Self-report diary on PAL, 1-day	METs/day	↓ time spent in PA for JIA group ($p = 0.000$)

JIA, Juvenile idiopathic arthritis; UCMS, University of Cincinnati Motion Sensor; HC, Healthy controls; PA, Physical activity; PAL, Physical activity level; TB BMD, Total body bone mineral density; CBCL, Child Behaviour Checklist.

Table 2. Potential determinants of participation in leisure-time activities in JIA identified in the systematic review.

	Potential determinants	Association with leisure
Socio-demographic		
	Age [29]	Older age was associated with ↓ PA
	Sex [28]	Male sex was associated with ↑ PA level
Anthropometric		
	Weight [28]	↑ weight was associated with ↑ PA
	Height [28]	↑ height was associated with ↑ PA
Disease		
	Disease duration [32]	Longer disease duration was associated with ↑ PA
	Pain [2]	↑ perceived pain and the number of painful locations were associated with ↓ social activity
	Stiffness [2]	↑ daily stiffness was associated with ↓ social activity
	Fatigue [2]	↑ fatigue was associated with ↓ social activity
	Swollen joints [29]	↑ number of swollen joints was associated with ↓ PA
	Physical fitness** [29]	↑ maximal oxygen consumption (absolute, relative) was associated with ↑ PA
	Well-being [32]	↓ perceived well-being was associated with ↓ PA

PA, Physical activity.
**The association between physical fitness and physical activity may be bidirectional, i.e. physical fitness can be both a determinant and an outcome of PA [29].

polyarticular JIA have been found to be less physically fit than healthy and normally active (non-competitive) controls [44]. The lack of physical fitness is not necessarily associated with disease severity but avoidance of exercise by those with JIA is often encouraged by parents and health care professionals to limit exacerbation of disease related symptoms [44].

Osteopenia (or lower than normal bone mineral density) is of particular concern in children and adolescents with JIA as it may lead to decreased bone strength and a subsequent increased risk for fractures [45,46]. Those suffering from JIA are at greater risk of bone density anomalies secondary to greater disease severity, treatment by glucocorticoids and decreased participation in organized sports or other physical activity [26,27]. The more children took part in organized sports the better their bone mineral density [27]. The study's cross-sectional design restricts inference of causality and one can argue that low bone mineral density (a characteristic of more severe disease [26]) is a potential determinant of participation in sports rather than an outcome.

Self-report measures were a popular means of collecting data on social and physical leisure-time activities. Researchers may appreciate the low cost and convenience of using these tools. Activity monitors were also used albeit less frequently to objectively assess physical activity. Electronic data collection is not affected by recall bias and may be more appropriate for assessing physical activity among children and adolescents [47].

Less than 40% of those with JIA met international recommendations to engage in at least 60 minutes of moderate to vigorous physical activity daily, as compared to 60% of healthy controls [28]. Persons with JIA may intentionally avoid more physically strenuous activities to keep from aggravating disease-related symptoms such as swollen joints [29]. However, there is no evidence that activity in fact exacerbates symptoms [48] and current evidence supports that physical activity is beneficial in JIA in helping to reduce pain, the number of swollen joints, as well as improving overall aerobic endurance and bone health [11,49]. Furthermore, there is a potential for exercise to favor immune function and help reduce chronic inflammation [50–53].

The literature on childhood disability supports that involvement in leisure activities may be influenced by intrinsic and extrinsic factors [3,42]. Most studies in pediatric rheumatology explored the effects of disease severity as a function of disease-related factors (e.g. active joint count, pain, fatigue, function/disability), rather than potential effects of contextual factors relating to the child (personal) and his or her environment (family and community). Only one study explored the potential association of anxiety and depression with participation in social activities, however no significant results were found [33]. No studies reported on such aspects as self-esteem, motivation, activity preferences, family functioning and environmental barriers.

Future research determining extent of involvement in a range of leisure activities in children with JIA and their determinants may benefit from a well grounded theoretical framework such as the ICF, which considers how participation in activities is influenced by body structure and function associated with the health condition (e.g. active joint count, perceived pain), activity limitations as well as personal (e.g. age, sex, motivation) and environmental (e.g. family functioning, availability of community services) factors [8,9].

Limitations

Based on the appraisal criteria of the Quality Assessment Tool for Quantitative Studies [19], no study met all quality criteria. All studies retained for review were observational [20]. Most studies recruited children and adolescents with JIA systematically from a convenience sample (i.e. clinic), weakening external validity. Furthermore, sample sizes were all relatively small, which may lead to type 2 errors. We do recognise how challenging recruitment in pediatric rheumatology is, considering the low prevalence of the disease (range of 0.02 to 0.40 percent of children) [54]. Most studies used outcome measures with questionable psychometric properties threatening the quality of data collection [2,24–27,29,31–33].

Conclusions

In general, children and adolescents with JIA display limitations in participation in either social or physical leisure-time activities. Despite the known benefits of leisure participation, no study to date has fully explored the experience of leisure participation in JIA. In order to properly explore leisure participation in JIA, there is a need for high quality observational studies. Future research into the study of leisure participation in pediatric rheumatic diseases may benefit from using a comprehensive, valid and reliable outcome measure exploring a broad range of possible leisure activities from which to draw valid conclusions [55]. Moreover, the assessment of contextual factors may provide researchers with compelling information on potential barriers and facilitators to leisure in JIA.

Supporting Information

Appendix S1 Search strategy. Appendix S1 presents the search strategy used to identify studies on leisure activities in JIA.

Appendix S2 Completed PRISMA checklist. Appendix S2 presents the completed PRISMA checklist for the systematic review.

Acknowledgments

We would like to thank Myrian Grondin, librarian, for her assistance with the search strategy design.

Author Contributions

Conceived and designed the experiments: SC KTA VG AM DF. Performed the experiments: SC KTA VG. Analyzed the data: SC KTA VG. Contributed reagents/materials/analysis tools: SC KTA VG AM DF. Wrote the paper: SC KTA VG AM DF.

References

1. Cassidy JT, Petty RE (2005) Chronic arthritis in childhood. In: Cassidy JT, Petty RE, Laxer RM, Lindsley CB, editors. Textbook of pediatric rheumatology. pp. 206–260.
2. Schanberg LE, Anthony KK, Gil KM, Maurin EC (2003) Daily pain and symptoms in children with polyarticular arthritis. Arthritis and Rheumatism 48: 1390–1397.
3. King G, Law M, King S, Rosenbaum P, Kertoy MK, et al. (2003) A Conceptual Model of the Factors Affecting the Recreation and Leisure Participation of Children with Disabilities. Physical & Occupational Therapy in Pediatrics 23: 63–90.
4. Larson R (2000) Toward a psychology of positive youth development. American Psychologist 55: 170–183
5. Masten A, Coatsworth J (1998) The development of competence in favorable and unfavorable environments lessons from research on successful children. American Psychologist 53: 205–220.
6. Booth FW, Chakravarthy MV, Gordon SE, Spangenburg EE (2002) Waging war on physical inactivity: using modern molecular ammunition against an ancient enemy. J Appl Physiol 93: 3–30.
7. Reiter-Purtill J, Gerhardt CA, Vannatta K, Passo MH, Noll RB (2003) A controlled longitudinal study of the social functioning of children with juvenile rheumatoid arthritis. J Pediatr Psychol 28: 17–28.
8. World Health Organization (2001) International classification of functioning, disability and health. Geneva: WHO.
9. Guell C (2007) Painful childhood: Children living with juvenile arthritis. Qualitative Health Research 17: 884–892.
10. Singh-Grewal D, Wright V, Bar-Or O, Feldman BM (2006) Pilot study of fitness training and exercise testing in polyarticular childhood arthritis. Arthritis & Rheumatism: Arthritis Care & Research 55: 364–372.
11. Singh-Grewal D, Schneiderman-Walker J, Wright V, Bar-Or O, Beyene J, et al. (2007) The effects of vigorous exercise training on physical function in children with arthritis: a randomized, controlled, single-blinded trial. Arthritis & Rheumatism: Arthritis Care & Research 57: 1202–1210.
12. Takken T, van der Net J, Helders PJ (2001) Do junvenile idiopathic arthritis patients benefit from an exercise program? A pilot study. Arthritis & Rheumatism 45: 81–85.
13. Takken T, Van Der Net J, Kuis W, Helders PJ (2003) Aquatic fitness training for children with juvenile idiopathic arthritis. Rheumatology (Oxford, England) 42: 1408–1414.
14. Sandstedt E, Fasth A, Fors H, Beckung E (2012) Bone health in children and adolescents with juvenile idiopathic arthritis and the influence of short-term physical exercise. Pediatric physical therapy: the official publication of the Section on Pediatrics of the American Physical Therapy Association 24: 155–161; discussion 162.
15. Furlan AD, Irvin E, Bombardier C (2006) Limited search strategies were effective in finding relevant nonrandomized studies. J Clin Epidemiol 59: 1303–1311.
16. Wilczynski NL, Haynes RB (2005) Optimal search strategies for detecting clinically sound prognostic studies in EMBase: an analytic survey. J Am Med Inform Assoc 12: 481–485.
17. Wilczynski NL, Haynes RB, Team tH (2004) Developing optimal search strategies for detecting clinically sound prognostic studies in Medline: an analytic survey. BMC Med 2: 23.
18. Moher D, Liberati A, Tetzlaff J, Altman DG (2009) Preferred reporting items for systematic reviews and meta-analyses: the PRISMA statement. Br Med J 339: 332–336.
19. Thomas BH, Ciliska D, Dobbins M, Micucci S (2004) A process for systematically reviewing the literature: Providing the research evidence for public health nursing interventions. Worldviews on Evidence-Based Nursing 1: 176–184.
20. Deeks JJ, Dinnes J, D'Amico R, Sowden AJ, Sakarovitch C, et al. (2003; Vol. 7: No. 27) Evaluating non-randomised intervention studies. Bury St Edmunds, Suffolk, UK.
21. Effective Public Health Practice Project (1998) Quality Assessment Tool For Quantitative Studies. In: Effective Public Health Practice Project, editor. Hamilton, ON.
22. (2011) Cochrane handbook for systematic reviews of interventions version 5.1.0 Higgins JP, Green S, editors.
23. Felin EMO, Prahalad S, Askew EW, Moyer-Mileur LJ (2007) Musculoskeletal abnormalities of the tibia in juvenile rheumatoid arthritis. Arthritis Rheumatism 56: 984–994.
24. Henderson CJ, Lovell DJ, Specker BL, Campaigne BN (1995) Physical activity in children with juvenile rheumatoid arthritis: quantification and evaluation. Arthritis Care & Research 8: 114–119.
25. Billings AG, Moos RH, Miller JJ, 3rd, Gottlieb JE (1987) Psychosocial adaptation in juvenile rheumatic disease: a controlled evaluation. Health Psychology 6: 343–359.
26. Henderson CJ, Specker BL, Sierra RI, Campaigne BN, Lovell DJ (2000) Total-body bone mineral content in non-corticosteroid-treated postpubertal females with juvenile rheumatoid arthritis: frequency of osteopenia and contributing factors. Arthritis & Rheumatism 43: 531–540.
27. Henderson CJ, Cawkwell GD, Specker BL, Sierra RI, Wilmott RW, et al. (1997) Predictors of total body bone mineral density in non-corticosteroid-treated prepubertal children with juvenile rheumatoid arthritis. Arthritis & Rheumatism 40: 1967–1975.
28. Maggio ABR, Hofer MF, Martin XE, Marchand LM, Beghetti M, et al. (2010) Reduced physical activity level and cardiorespiratory fitness in children with chronic diseases. European Journal of Pediatrics 169: 1187–1193.
29. Takken T, van der Net J, Kuis W, Helders PJM (2003) Physical activity and health related physical fitness in children with juvenile idiopathic arthritis. Annals of the Rheumatic Diseases 62: 885–889.
30. Huygen ACJ, Kuis W, Sinnema G (2000) Psychological, behavioural, and social adjustment in children and adolescents with juvenile chronic arthritis. Annals of the Rheumatic Diseases 59: 276–282.
31. Lien G, Selvaag AM, Flato B, Haugen M, Vinje O, et al. (2005) A two-year prospective controlled study of bone mass and bone turnover in children with early juvenile idiopathic arthritis Arthritis & Rheumatism 52: 833–840.
32. Lelieveld OTHM, Armbrust W, Van Leeuwen MA, Duppen N, Geertzen JHB, et al. (2008) Physical activity in adolescents with juvenile idiopathic arthritis. Arthritis Care and Research 59: 1379–1384.
33. Tarakci E, Yeldan I, Kaya ME, Baydogan SN, Kasapcopur O (2011) The relationship between physical activity level, anxiety, depression, and functional ability in children and adolescents with juvenile idiopathic arthritis. Clinical Rheumatology 30: 1415–1420.
34. Larson RW, Verma S (1999) How Children and Adolescents Spend Time Across the World: Work, Play, and Developmental Opportunities. Psychological Bulletin 125: 703–736.
35. Shikako-Thomas K, Shevell M, Lach L, Law M, Schmitz N, et al. (2013) Picture me playing—A portrait of participation and enjoyment of leisure activities in adolescents with cerebral palsy. Research in Developmental Disabilities 34: 1001–1010.

36. Orlin MN, Palisano RJ, Chiarello L, Kang L-J, Polansky M, et al. (2010) Participation in home, extracurricular, and community activities among children and young people with cerebral palsy. Developmental Medicine and Child Neurology 52: 160–166.
37. King GA, Law M, King S, Hurley P, Hanna S, et al. (2006) Measuring children's participation in recreation and leisure activities: construct validation of the CAPE and PAC. Child: care, health and development 33: 28–39.
38. King G, Law M, King S, Hurley P, Rosenbaum P, et al. (2004) Children's assessment of participation and enjoyment (CAPE) and preferences for activities of children (PAC). San Antonio, TX: Harcourt Assessment Inc.
39. Connelly M, Anthony KK, Sarniak R, Bromberg MH, Gil KM, et al. (2010) Parent pain responses as predictors of daily activities and mood in children with juvenile idiopathic arthritis: the utility of electronic diaries. Journal of Pain & Symptom Management 39: 579–590.
40. Reid GJ, McGrath PJ, Lang BA (2005) Parent-child interactions among children with juvenile fibromyalgia, arthritis, and healthy controls. Pain (03043959) 113: 201–210.
41. Sallis JF, Prochaska JJ, Taylor WC (2000) A review of correlates of physical activity of children and adolescents. Medicine & Science in Sports & Exercise 32: 963–975.
42. Law M, King G, King S, Kertoy M, Hurley P, et al. (2006) Patterns of participation in recreational and leisure activities among children with complex physical disabilities. Developmental Medicine & Child Neurology 48: 337–342.
43. Garton AF, Pratt C (1991) Leisure activities of adolescent school students: Predictors of participation and interest. Journal of Adolescence 14: 305–321.
44. Klepper SE, Darbee J, Effgen SK, Singsen BH (1992) Physical fitness levels in children with polyarticular juvenile rheumatoid arthritis. Arthritis Care & Research 5: 93–100.
45. NTH Consensus Development Panel on Optimal Calcium Intake (1994) Optimal calcium intake. JAMA 272: 1942–1948.
46. Nevitt M (1994) Epidemiology of osteoporosis. 20:535–558, 1994. Rheum Dis Clin North Am 20: 535–558.
47. Rowlands AV, Ingledew DK, Eston RG (2000) The effect of type of activity measure on the relationship between body fatness and habitual physical activity in children: a meta-analysis. Ann Hum Biol 27: 479–497.
48. Takken T, Van Brussel M, Engelbert RHH, Van Der Net J, Kuis W, et al. (2008) Exercise therapy in juvenile idiopathic arthritis: A Cochrane Review. European Journal of Physical and Rehabilitation Medicine 44: 287–297.
49. Klepper SE (1999) Effects of an eight-week physical conditioning program on disease signs and symptoms in children with chronic arthritis. Arthritis Care & Research 12: 52–60.
50. Bruunsgaard H (2005) Physical activity and modulation of systemic low-level inflammation. J Leukoc Biol 78: 819–835.
51. Kasapis C, Thompson PD (2005) The effects of physical activity on serum C-reactive protein and inflammatory markers: a systematic review. J Am Coll Cardiol 45: 1563–1569.
52. Kohut ML, Senchina DS (2004) Reversing age-associated immunosenescence via exercise. Exerc Immunol Rev 10: 6–41.
53. Woods JA, Vieira VJ, Keylock KT (2006) Exercise, Inflammation, and Innate Immunity. Neurol Clin 24: 585–599.
54. Manners PJ, Bower C (2002) Worldwide prevalence of juvenile arthritis why does it vary so much? J Rheumatol 29: 1520–1530.
55. Streiner DL, Norman GR (2008) Validity. Health measurement scales A practival guide to their development and uses. Unites States: Oxford University Press Inc. pp. 247–276.

Alternatives to the Six-Minute Walk Test in Pulmonary Arterial Hypertension

Vincent Mainguy, Simon Malenfant, Anne-Sophie Neyron, Didier Saey, François Maltais, Sébastien Bonnet, Steeve Provencher*

Pulmonary Hypertension Research Group, Centre de recherche de l'Institut universitaire de cardiologie et de pneumologie de Québec, Université Laval, Québec (Québec), Canada

Abstract

Introduction: The physiological response during the endurance shuttle walk test (ESWT), the cycle endurance test (CET) and the incremental shuttle walk test (ISWT) remains unknown in PAH. We tested the hypothesis that endurance tests induce a near-maximal physiological demand comparable to incremental tests. We also hypothesized that differences in respiratory response during exercise would be related to the characteristics of the exercise tests.

Methods: Within two weeks, twenty-one PAH patients (mean age: 54(15) years; mean pulmonary arterial pressure: 42(12) mmHg) completed two cycling exercise tests (incremental cardiopulmonary cycling exercise test (CPET) and CET) and three field tests (ISWT, ESWT and six-minute walk test (6MWT)). Physiological parameters were continuously monitored using the same portable telemetric device.

Results: Peak oxygen consumption (VO_{2peak}) was similar amongst the five exercise tests ($p = 0.90$ by ANOVA). Walking distance correlated markedly with the VO_{2peak} reached during field tests, especially when weight was taken into account. At 100% exercise, most physiological parameters were similar between incremental and endurance tests. However, the trends overtime differed. In the incremental tests, slopes for these parameters rose steadily over the entire duration of the tests, whereas in the endurance tests, slopes rose sharply from baseline to 25% of maximum exercise at which point they appeared far less steep until test end. Moreover, cycling exercise tests induced higher respiratory exchange ratio, ventilatory demand and enhanced leg fatigue measured subjectively and objectively.

Conclusion: Endurance tests induce a maximal physiological demand in PAH. Differences in peak respiratory response during exercise are related to the modality (cycling vs. walking) rather than the progression (endurance vs. incremental) of the exercise tests.

Editor: James West, Vanderbilt University Medical Center, United States of America

Funding: Financial support was provided by Fonds de recherche du Québec-Santé (FRQS). The FRQS was not otherwise involved in study design, data collection and analysis, decision to publish, or preparation of the manuscript.

Competing Interests: The authors have declared that no competing interests exist.

* Email: steve.provencher@criucpq.ulaval.ca

Introduction

Pulmonary arterial hypertension (PAH) is characterized by a progressive increase in pulmonary vascular resistance leading to altered gas exchange, right heart failure and ultimately to patients' death [1]. Numerous exercise abnormalities have been described in PAH. These include considerable reduction of peak oxygen consumption (VO_{2peak}), oxygen pulse (VO_2/HR) and end-tidal carbon dioxide partial pressure ($P_{ET}CO_2$), abnormal increase in the ventilatory equivalent for carbon dioxide (V_E/VCO_2), exercise-induced hypoxemia and early anaerobic threshold [2–4]. These abnormalities have been attributed to decreased cardiac output, underperfused alveoli caused by the remodeled and constricted small pulmonary arteries, hyperventilation as well as respiratory and peripheral muscle dysfunction [4–7].

Exercise capacity is very meaningful in PAH as it correlates with survival and functional status [8–9]. As a result, exercise capacity has been the primary outcome measure in the majority of the recent clinical trials in PAH [10]. While incremental cardiopulmonary cycling exercise test (CPET) provides comprehensive assessment of the cardiac and respiratory adaptation during exercise [9,11], exercise capacity in PAH is most commonly assessed using the six-minute walk test (6MWT). Following the paradigm set by other chronic conditions such as chronic obstructive pulmonary disease (COPD) in which endurance tests are more sensitive to clinical changes following therapeutic intervention than the CPET and 6MWT [12–15], endurance tests including the endurance shuttle walk test (ESWT) and the cycle endurance test (CET) have been proposed in PAH. Whether these tests induce clinically relevant and similar cardiorespiratory response compared to exercise tests currently used in PAH remains unknown.

The objective of this study was to compare the physiological response during endurance (ESWT and CET) and incremental (incremental shuttle walk test (ISWT) and CPET) exercise tests.

We tested the hypothesis that endurance tests would induce a near-maximal physiological demand comparable to incremental tests. We also hypothesized that differences in respiratory and skeletal muscle responses during exercise would be related to the modality (cycling vs. walking) rather than the progression (endurance vs. incremental) of the exercise test.

Methods

Ethics statement

The institutional ethics committee (Comité d'éthique de la recherche de l'Institut universitaire de cardiologie et de pneumologie de Québec, protocol number: CÉR 20414) approved the research protocol and all patients gave written consent prior to study enrolment.

Subjects

PAH patients were recruited at the Institut universitaire de cardiologie et de pneumologie de Québec. The PAH diagnosis was made according to recent guidelines [16]. Only patients with no change in their PAH therapies and in stable clinical condition over the last 4 months were eligible. Exclusion criteria were as follow: (1) recent syncope or World Health Organization (WHO) functional class IV [17]; (2) left ventricular ejection fraction <40%; (3) significant restrictive (more than minimal lung fibrosis on CT scan or total lung capacity <70% of predicted) or obstructive ($FEV_1/FVC<70\%$) lung disease.

Study design

These measures were obtained as part of a controlled trial evaluating the test-retest reliability of the CET, ESWT and 6MWT [18]. Within two weeks, PAH patients performed two different incremental exercise tests (CPET and ISWT), two constant work rate exercise tests (CET and ESWT) and a 6MWT. Oxygen therapy was not required for any patient during any exercise test.

Incremental exercise tests

Incremental exercise tests were performed on two different days. Standardized instructions asking patients to exercise up to symptom limitation were given prior each exercise test and standardized encouragements were provided throughout the tests.

At visit 1, a **CPET** was performed on an electrically braked ergocycle (Corival, Lode B.V., Groningen, The Netherlands) [19]. After 3 minutes of rest and 1 minute of unloaded pedaling, patients exercised using a progressive RAMP protocol until exhaustion. Patients were asked to pedal at a minimum rate of 60 rpm and increments varied from 5 to 20 watts/min for target exercise duration between 8 to 12 minutes. After one hour of rest, a practice CET was performed.

At visit 2, an **ISWT** was performed in an enclosed corridor on a flat 10 meter-long course delimited by two cones positioned 0.5 meters from either end [20]. Patients had to follow the rhythm dictated by an audio signal. The initial walking speed was set at $0.5\ m{\cdot}s^{-1}$ for all patients independently from their age or functional class. Subsequently, the walking speed automatically increased every minute by $0.17\ m{\cdot}s^{-1}$ until exhaustion. After one hour of rest, a practice ESWT was also performed on the same flat 10 meter-long course [21].

Constant work rate exercise tests and 6MWT

At visit 3, patients performed two constant work rate exercise tests and a 6MWT, with a resting period of two hours between the tests. To minimize any confounding effect based on test sequence, the order of the tests was randomized using the Latin Square design. While standardized instructions asking the patients to exercise as long as possible during the constant work rate exercises or to cover the longest distance possible during the 6MWT were given prior to each exercise test, no verbal encouragements were made during these exercises [22]. After 5 min of rest, the **CET** was initiated with 1 min of unloaded pedaling before the workload was set at 80% of peak workload achieved during the CPET. Patients were told to pedal at a minimum rate of 60 rpm. The CET time was defined as the total exercise duration until exhaustion excluding unloaded pedaling. The **ESWT** was performed on the same flat 10 meter-long course as for the ISWT. This test included a 1.5 min warm-up period. The walking speed was then set at 85% of the peak walking speed achieved during the ISWT [21]. The rhythm was dictated by an audio signal at constant intervals. The ESWT time was defined as the total exercise duration until exhaustion excluding the warm-up period. The **6MWT** was performed according to the *American Thoracic Society* recommendations [23], and individual results were compared to predicted values [24].

Physiological monitoring and measurements

Cardiac 12-lead ECG, breath-by-breath respiratory parameters and pulse O_2 saturation (SpO_2) were continuously monitored using the same portable telemetric device (Oxycon Mobile, Viasys Healthcare, Hoechberg, Germany) for all exercise tests. The patients were wearing a facemask. The system had a dead space of 30 ml. The transmitting device was composed of two units equipped with O_2 and CO_2 analysers. Altogether, the system weighted 950 grams including the lithium battery. Patients wore a shoulder belt system to carry the telemetric device while walking or cycling. The receiving unit was connected to a portable computer. Both volume and gas calibration were made systematically before each exercise test. Cardiac and respiratory parameters were analyzed averaging five of seven breaths for every relative time. The ratio of inspiratory time to total breath duration (Ti/Ttot) and the ratio of tidal volume on inspiratory time (V_T/Ti) were used as measurements of respiratory timing and inspiratory drive respectively. The anaerobic threshold was assessed using the V-slope method [19]. The V_E/VCO_2 slope from rest to the anaerobic threshold was assessed for CPET and ISWT.

Dyspnea and leg fatigue were assessed at the end of each test using a 10-point modified Borg scale [25]. The reasons for stopping exercise were categorized into leg fatigue, dyspnea, general fatigue and inability to maintain the imposed cadence. For field exercise tests, the work of walking was also estimated using the product of the walking distance by body weight [26], assuming a constant velocity during the 6MWT [27–28]. In order to assess the objective fatigue of the *vastus lateralis*, both nonvolitional and volitional strengths of the quadriceps were evaluated before and after each constant work rate tests, as previously described [5]. A minimum of 3 sets of maximal voluntary contraction (MVC) and potentiated twitches (TWq) measurements were performed separated by a 1-minute resting period. Reported values for the MVC and TWq were the mean of the three strongest contractions with less than 5% variability. Muscle fatigue was defined as a post-exercise drop in TWq≥15% from baseline [29].

Statistical analysis

A longitudinal mixed model was used to compare the time course of the various exercise parameters during exercise. For getting a general idea of the trend among the five metabolic levels including baseline, 25%, 50%, 75% and 100% of the total exercise duration, separate smooth fitted curves for each exercise test were done. The data exploration and graphical representation of each subject suggested a piece-wise linear model with a linear increase over the first 25% of the total exercise and then a change in slope with a lower increase afterwards, especially for the CET, the ESWT and the 6MWT. For each outcome variable, two experimental factors were designed including the exercise test (random order) and the relative of the total exercise duration (baseline, 25%, 50%, 75% and 100%). The latter was analyzed as a repeated-measure factor with the use of an autoregressive covariance matrix as correlation decreases as exercise duration between observations increases. A random intercept and random slopes for exercise duration from baseline to 25% and 25% to 100% were considered as subjects have higher or lower intercepts and steeper or shallower slopes over exercise duration. The empirical best linear unbiased predictors (EBLUPs) fulfilled the normality assumption. The interactions between "Exercise test" and the slopes were considered. Missing values were not imputed. The residual maximum likelihood was used as the method of estimation and the Kenward–Roger method was used to estimate denominator degrees of freedom for the test of fixed effect. The univariate normality assumption was verified with the Shapiro-Wilk tests on the error distribution from the Cholesky factorization of the statistical model. The Brown and Forsythe's variation of Levene's test statistic was used to verify the homogeneity of variances. All variables were log-transformed to stabilize variances. The results were considered significant with p-values≤0.05. End-exercise parameters for each exercise modality were compared using ANOVA. Pearson correlation was performed to examine the relationship between workload (cycling tests), as well as distance and work of walking (field tests) and VO_{2peak} reached during each test. Data are presented as mean (SD) or mean (SE) when specified. All analyses were conducted using the statistical packages R v3.0.2 (R Foundation for Statistical Computing, Vienna, Austria.) and SAS v9.4 (SAS Institute Inc, Cary, NC, U.S.A.).

Results

Patients' characteristics

Twenty-one PAH patients completed all exercise tests without complication. Baseline characteristics are shown in **Table 1**. No adverse events were observed during exercise tests.

Overall physiological response induced by the various exercise testing modalities

Cardiac and ventilatory responses for each exercise test are described in **Table 2** and **Figures 1–3**, respectively. At 100% exercise, VO_{2peak} was similar for all exercise modalities ($p = 0.90$ by ANOVA). As expected, the slope of the physiological parameters during the tests significantly differed between exercise modalities (**Figure 1**). In the incremental tests, slopes for oxygen consumption, heart rate (HR), minute ventilation (V_E), respiratory exchange ratio (RER), as well as carbon dioxide output and V_E/VCO_2 (data not shown) rose steadily over the entire duration of the tests. Conversely, in the endurance tests, slopes rose sharply from baseline to 25% of maximum exercise (all $p \leq 0.001$ compared to the slopes of incremental tests using the longitudinal mixed model), at which point they appeared far less steep until test end (all $p < 0.05$ compared to the slopes of incremental tests using the longitudinal mixed model). The work rate achieved during CPET and CET significantly correlated with VO_{2peak} reached during these tests ($R^2 = 0.62$ and 0.74, respectively, both $p < 0.01$). The mean 6MWT distance was 447(96) meters, as compared to 384(87) and 460(258) meters for the ISWT and ESWT respectively. While the distance walked during the 6MWT, ISWT and ESWT correlated with the VO_{2peak} reached during these tests

Table 1. Patients' characteristics (n = 21).

PAH Type	
IPAH	n = 9
PAH-Her	n = 1
PAH-CTD	n = 9
PAH-CHD*	n = 2
Sex (F/M)	(17/4)
Age (years)	54 (15)
BMI ($kg \cdot m^{-2}$)	27 (5)
WHO Functional Class (II/III)	(15/6)
Pulmonary Hemodynamics**	
RAP (mmHg)	6.6 (3.5)
mPAP (mmHg)	42 (12)
PCWP (mmHg)	11 (3)
CI ($l/min \cdot m^2$)	3.0 (0.6)
PVR ($WU \cdot m^2$)	6.6 (3.1)
6MWD (m)	447 (96)
6MWD (% predicted)	83 (17)

Values are n or mean (SD).
* Includes two patients with Eisenmenger physiology related to persistent arterial canal and ventricular septal defect.
** Right heart catheterization performed <6 months was used to describe hemodynamic severity.
Table legend: PAH, Pulmonary arterial hypertension; IPAH, Idiopathic PAH; PAH-Her, Heritable PAH; PAH-CTD, PAH associated with connective tissue disease; PAH-CHD, PAH associated with congenital heat disease; BMI, Body mass index; WHO, World Health Organization; RAP, Right atrial pressure; mPAP, Mean pulmonary artery pressure; PCWP, Pre-capillary wedge pressure; CI, Cardiac index; PVRi, Pulmonary vascular resistance index; 6MWD, six-minute walk distance.

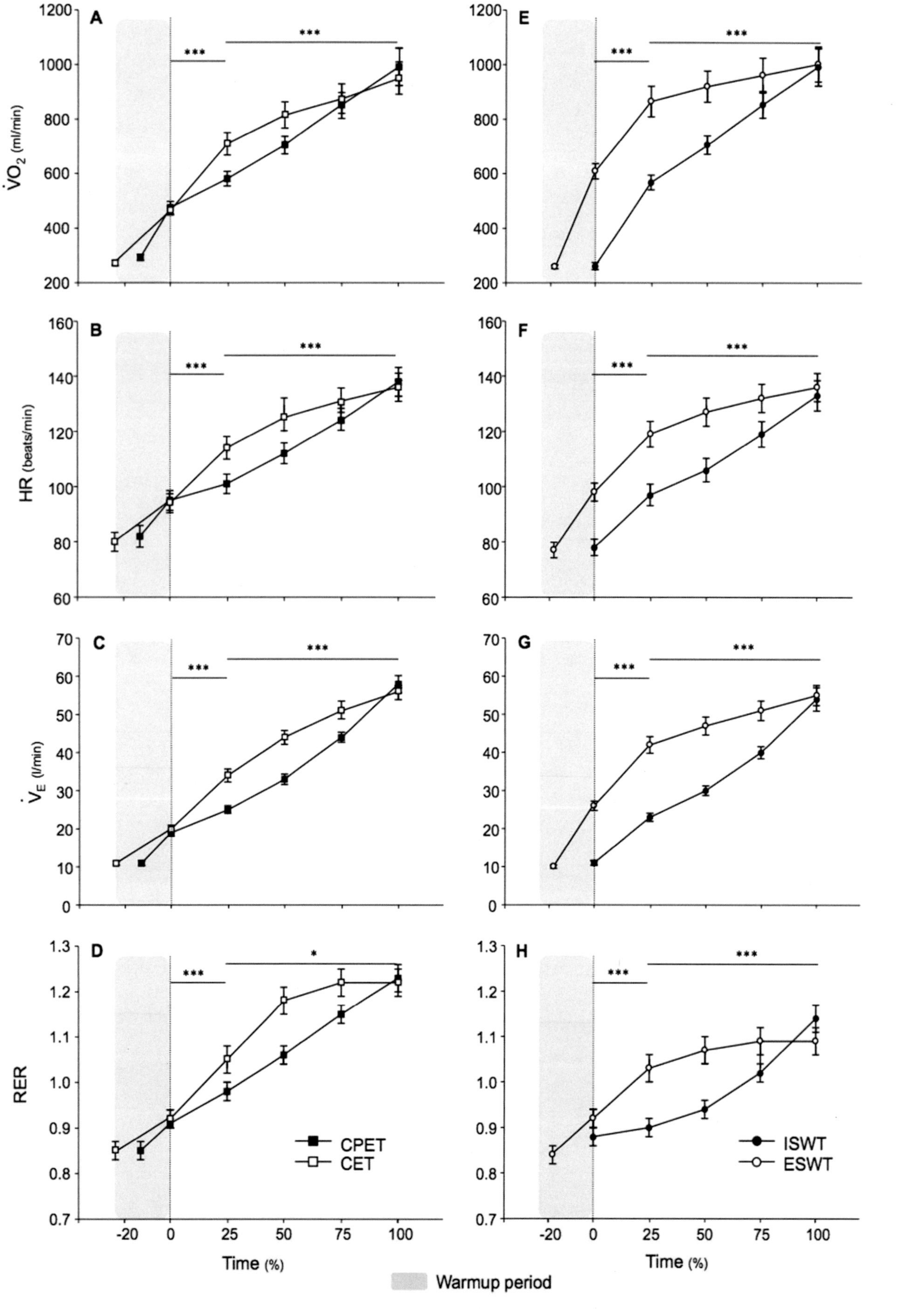
A
B
C
D
E
F
G
H
$\dot{V}O_2$ (ml/min)
HR (beats/min)
$\dot{V}_E$ (l/min)
RER
***
*
CPET
CET
ISWT
ESWT
Time (%)
Warmup period

Figure 1. Comparison of the physiological parameters between incremental and constant work rate exercise tests. At 100% exercise, Oxygen consumption (VO_2), heart rate (HR), minute ventilation (V_E) and respiratory exchange ratio (RER) were similar between incremental and endurance tests. However, slopes for these parameters rose steadily over the entire duration of the incremental cardiopulmonary exercise test (CPET) and the incremental shuttle walk test (ISWT), whereas their slopes rose sharply from baseline to 25% of maximum exercise at which point they appeared far less steep until test end for the cycle endurance test (CET) and the endurance shuttle walk test (ESWT). Mean (SE) values of physiological parameters are expressed at the same relative time (e.g. 0%, 25%, 50%, 75% and 100%) from the maximal exercise duration. The shaded zone represents the initial warm-up period of the CPET, the CET and the ESWT. *p<0.05; **p<0.01; ***p<0.001 for the comparison of the slopes of each parameter from baseline to 25% of exercise duration, and from 25% to 100% (test end).

($R^2=0.25$, 0.41 and 0.33, all $p<0.01$), this correlation was markedly increased when the work of walking was taken into account ($R^2=0.75$, 0.75 and 0.47, all $p<0.01$) or when the distance walked during the 6MWT and the ISWT was correlated with the VO_{2peak}/kg reached during these tests ($R^2=0.67$ and 0.75, all $p<0.01$). Note that these adjustments minimally influenced these correlations for the ESWT (0.47 and 0.20, $p<0.01$, for the work of walking and the VO_{2peak}/kg).

Cycling (CPET) versus field walking (ISWT) incremental exercise tests (Table 2, Figure 2)

The maximal workload achieved during CPET was 69(25) watts, with mean increments of 9(2) watts·min^{-1}, whereas the maximal walking velocity during ISWT was 1.42(0.28) m·sec^{-1}. The mean CPET duration was significantly longer than that of the ISWT (465(124) vs. 370(85) sec, $p\leq0.01$). The slopes and peak values for VO_2, V_E, VCO_2, HR, RER, VO_2/HR, V_T/Ti, Ti/Ttot and $P_{ET}CO_2$ were similar during CPET and ISWT. Nevertheless, RER was higher during CPET. Exercise-induced desaturation was not significantly different during walking ($p=0.08$ at end-exercise). Finally, leg fatigue Borg scores were higher following CPET as compared to ISWT, and the most common reason for stopping exercise was different between the two tests as leg fatigue (n = 10/21) was the main limiting factor for CPET as compared to 4/21 for ISWT ($p=0.01$).

Cycling (CET) versus field walking (ESWT) constant work rate exercise tests (Table 2 and Figure 3)

The ESWT duration was longer than CET duration (399(207) versus 248(123) sec, $p=0.01$). Although differences in the slopes for VO_2, V_E, VCO_2, HR, RER and VO_2/HR were statistically significant between CET and ESWT, clinically relevant differences were only observed for end-exercise VO_2 and RER. Exercise-induced desaturation was also comparable during CET and ESWT ($p=0.13$ at end-exercise). Conversely, quadriceps fatigue was enhanced following the CET compared to ESWT (**Figure 4**). Leg fatigue was the main limiting factor in 9/21 and 5/21 patients for the CET and ISWT ($p=0.57$).

Externally paced (ESWT) versus self-paced (6MWT) constant work rate exercise tests

The mean walking velocity (1.24(0.27) vs 1.16(0.23) m·sec^{-1}, $p=0.28$) and VO_2 (1002 (296) vs 953 (258) ml·min^{-1}, $p=0.11$) were similar for the ESWT and the 6MWT. Nevertheless, ESWT was associated with higher peak VCO_2 (1092 (364) vs 996 (281) ml·min^{-1}, $p<0.01$), HR (136 (23) vs 128 (21) beat·min^{-1}, $p<0.01$), V_E (55 (12) vs 48 (9) L·min^{-1}, $p<0.01$) and breathing frequency (40 (7) vs 37 (8), $p<0.01$).

Discussion

The present study assessed and compared, for the first time, the cardiopulmonary responses of five different exercise testing modalities in patients with PAH. VO_{2peak} were essentially the same amongst the different exercise modalities. The distance walked during field walking exercise tests correlated with the VO_{2peak} achieved during these tests, especially when patients' weight was taken into account. While the pattern of work rate imposition (incremental versus constant work rate) dictated the slopes of the physiological response, the modality of exercise (cycling versus walking) was mainly responsible for differences in end-exercise values for RER, locus of symptom limitation and the degree of quadriceps fatigue.

In this study, VO_{2peak} differed by less than 50 ml among the five different exercise tests. In a previous study, Valli *et al.* [30] described a higher VO_{2peak} during CPET as compared to ISWT in 13 idiopathic PAH patients, although this difference was small in magnitude. Conversely, Deboeck *et al.* [28] documented a higher VO_2 during the 6MWT compared to CPET in 20 PAH patients. The authors carefully acknowledged that this was possibly related to an underestimation of the aerobic capacity by the CPET as patients were unable to achieve their maximal physiological parameters during this test due to premature lactic acidosis and leg fatigue. Taken together, these results demonstrate that endurance tests are associated with clinically relevant metabolic demand in PAH. Therefore, they may constitute an alternative to incremental cycling test to assess the functional status of patients with PAH.

A major physiological difference between walking and cycling is that the amount of muscles involved is markedly different between these two exercise modalities. In PAH, as in heart failure, the maximum muscle O_2 extraction is decreased [31] potentially due to muscle capillary rarefaction [7], making VO_{2peak} relatively more muscle-mass dependent than in healthy active subjects. Given the comparable VO_{2peak} for all exercise test, the VO_2 per muscle unit was likely lower during walking, potentially at a level below the anaerobic threshold. Therefore, the larger muscle mass engaged during walking as compared to cycling could account for lower RER during walking tests. The muscle mecanoreceptors are also more driven by the velocity than by the force deployed [32–34]. The differences between cycling speed and walking cadence might thus cause a different ventilatory response. This is also supported by the lower level of quadriceps fatigability and leg fatigue perception during walking than during cycling. These results are also in keeping with previous reports of later onset and less severe lactic acidosis at the same level of load during walking, compared with cycling exercise in other chronic conditions [35–36]. These results suggest that the respiratory response during exercise is more related to the exercise modality (cycling vs walking) than its progression (incremental vs. constant). To our knowledge, only one study evaluated the responsiveness of the walking versus cycling tests following a therapeutic intervention in PAH [18]. The responsiveness of CET was lower than the 6MWT and ESWT. Cycling tests might be less susceptible to track a beneficial effect on pulmonary hemodynamics following PAH therapy because of the important drop in non-volitional quadriceps strength as seen in our study.

As the distance walked correlates with the VO_{2peak} of PAH patients, it suggests that field walking exercise tests are representative of the maximal exercise capacity achievable by PAH

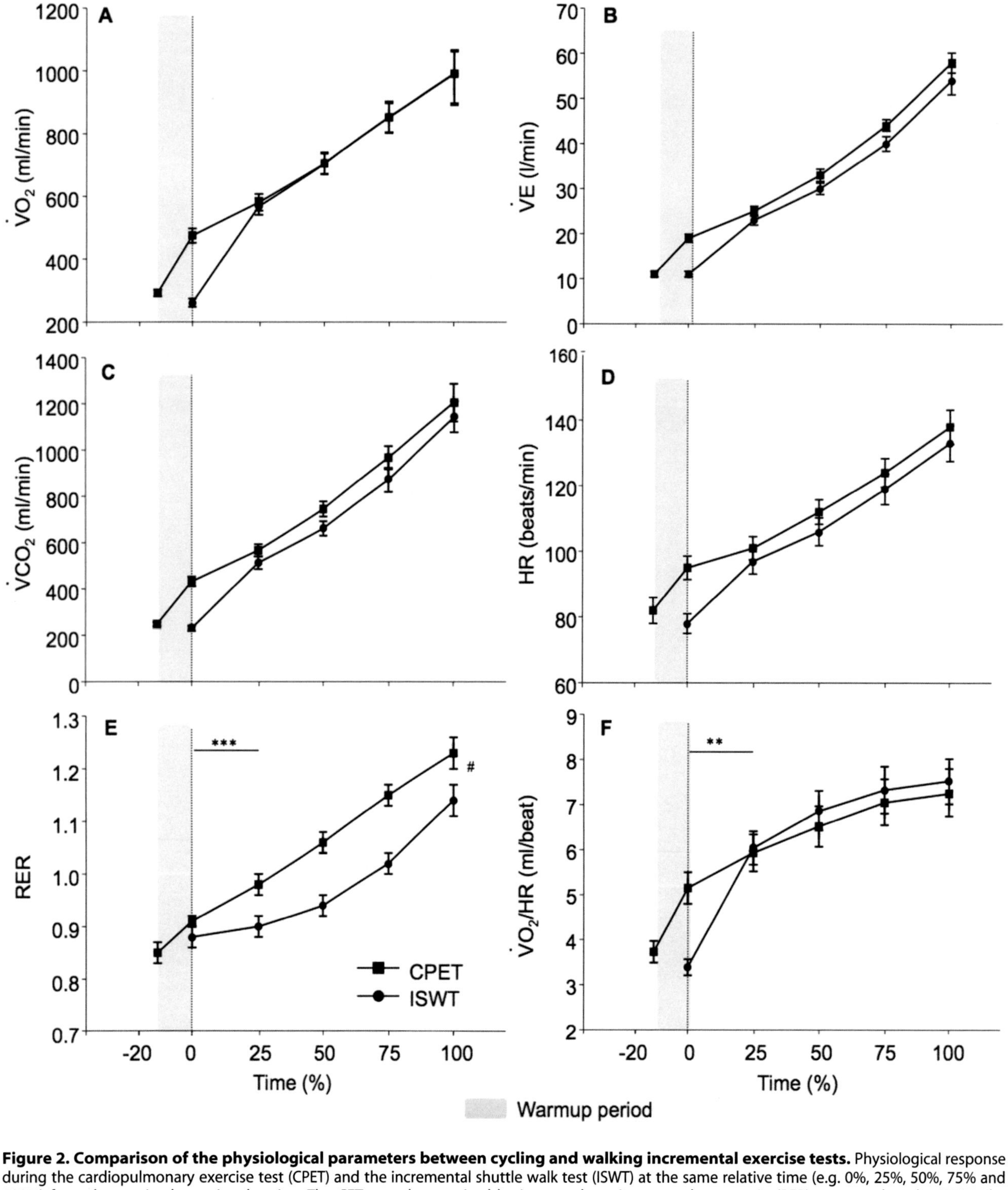

Figure 2. Comparison of the physiological parameters between cycling and walking incremental exercise tests. Physiological response during the cardiopulmonary exercise test (CPET) and the incremental shuttle walk test (ISWT) at the same relative time (e.g. 0%, 25%, 50%, 75% and 100%) from the maximal exercise duration. The CET was characterized by increased respiratory exchange ratio (RER) compared to the ISWT. The shaded zone represents the initial warm-up period of the CPET. Values are means (SE). $^{*}p<0.05$; $^{**}p<0.01$; $^{***}p<0.001$ for the comparison of the slopes of each parameter from baseline to 25% of exercise duration, and from 25% to 100% (test end). $^{\#}p<0.05$ for end-exercise value compared by ANOVA. *Figure legend:* VO_2, *Oxygen consumption;* VCO_2, *Carbon dioxide output; RER, Respiratory exchange ratio;* V_E, *Minute ventilation; HR, Heart rate;* VO_2*/HR, Oxygen pulse; CPET, Cardiopulmonary exercise test; ISWT, Incremental shuttle walk test.*

patients. Interestingly, this correlation between the walking distance and the VO_{2peak} was markedly improved when the work of walking was taken into account, especially for the 6MWT and the ISWT for which the walking distance is directly influenced by the walking velocity. As suggested by Chuang *et al.* [26], the work of walking on a flat course equals the product of distance and weight, assuming a constant walking velocity. However, this estimation does not consider the accelerations and decelerations

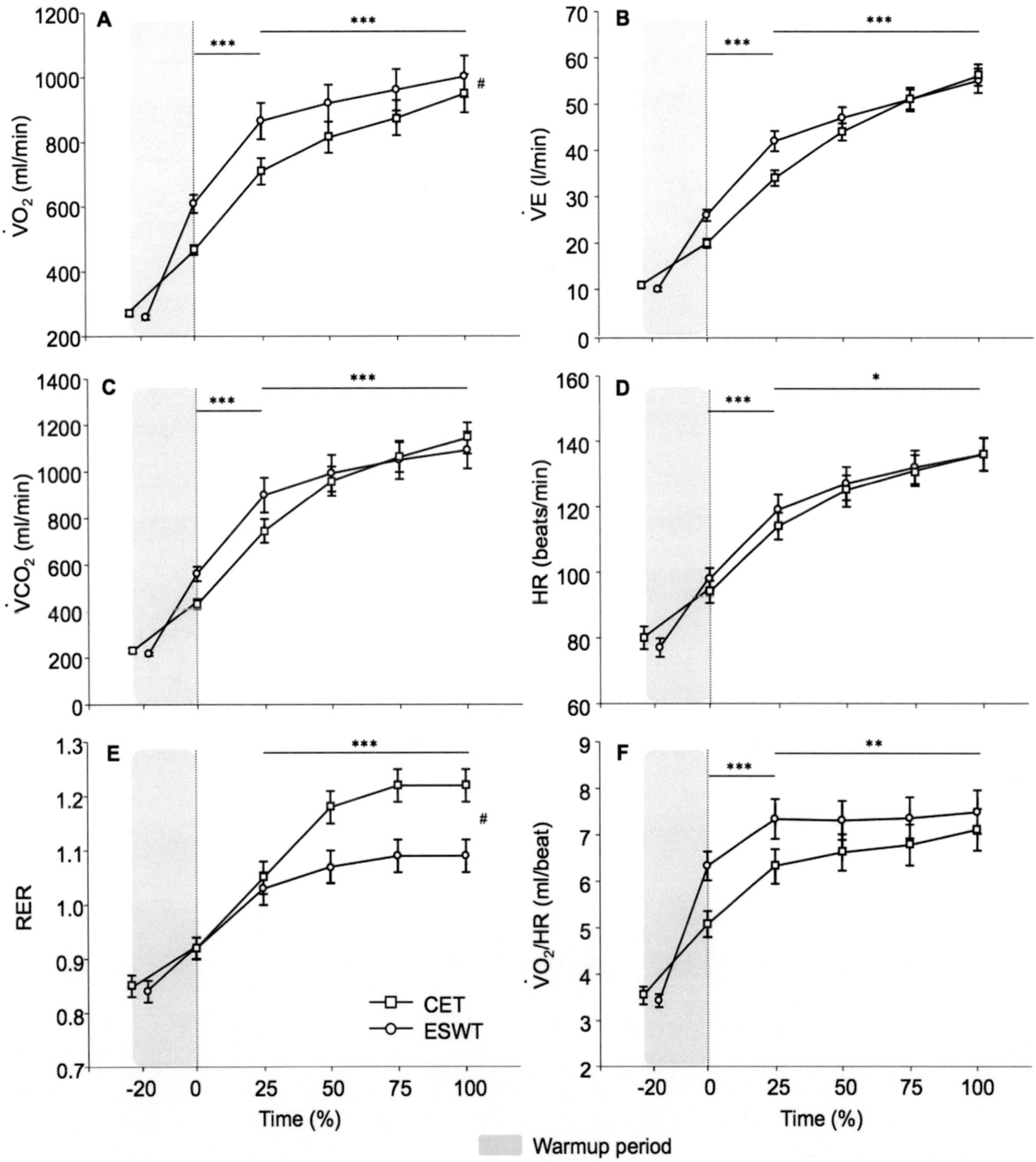

Figure 3. Comparison of the physiological parameters between cycling and walking constant work rate exercise tests. Physiological response during the cycle endurance test (CET) and the endurance shuttle walk test (ESWT) at the same relative time (e.g. 0%, 25%, 50%, 75% and 100%) from maximal exercise duration. The ESWT was characterized by a higher oxygen consumption (VO_2) and a lower respiratory exchange ratio (RER) throughout the exercise. Conversely, carbon dioxide output (VCO_2), minute ventilation (V_E) and oxygen pulse (VO_2/HR) slopes were slightly steeper in the early phase of the CET (from baseline to 25% of exercise duration), to end up with similar end-exercise values. Similarly, heart rate (HR) slopes, although statistically significant, were virtually the same during the CET and the ESWT. The shaded zone represents the initial warm-up period of the ESWT. $^{\#}p \leq 0.01$ between CET and ESWT. Values are means (SE). *$p<0.05$; **$p<0.01$; ***$p<0.001$ for the comparison of the slopes of each parameter from baseline to 25% of exercise duration, and from 25% to 100% (test end).

occurring during the walking tests. This may have led to an underestimation of the work of walking during shuttle walking tests where the 10 meter-long course imposes more acceleration/deceleration than the 30 meter-long course of the 6MWT, and may explain the differences in the physiological response observed between the 6MWT and the ESWT. Whether the work of walking

Table 2. Ventilatory parameters measured at the same relative time during incremental and constant work rate exercise tests as well as the 6MWT (n = 21).

	Incremental exercise tests		Constant work rate exercise tests		6MWT
	CPET	ISWT	CET	ESWT	
BF					
Baseline	19 (4)	19 (5)	19 (5)	20 (4)	20 (5)
25%	25 (7)	25 (6)	27 (3)	33 (6)	29 (5)
50%	29 (7)	29 (6)	32 (8)	37 (7)	33 (6)
75%	33 (6)	32 (6)	37 (7)	38 (6)	35 (6)
100%	40 (7)	39 (7)	40 (7)	40 (7)	37 (8)
V_T					
Baseline	0.6 (0.1)	0.6 (0.1)	0.6 (0.1)	0.6 (0.1)	0.6 (0.2)
25%	1.1 (0.3)	1.0 (0.2)	1.2 (0.4)	1.3 (0.3)	1.3 (0.3)
50%	1.2 (0.3)	1.1 (0.2)	1.4 (0.4)	1.4 (0.3)	1.3 (0.3)
75%	1.4 (0.3)	1.3 (0.3)	1.4 (0.4)	1.4 (0.3)	1.4 (0.3)
100%	1.5 (0.3)	1.4 (0.3)*	1.4 (0.3)	1.4 (0.3)	1.4 (0.3)
V_T/Ti (L·sec^1)					
Baseline	0.53 (0.13)	0.52 (0.16)	0.58 (0.18)	0.51 (0.10)	0.53 (0.15)
25%	1.09 (0.17)	0.95 (0.19)	1.34 (0.29)	1.59 (0.37)	1.38 (0.32)
50%	1.37 (0.22)	1.19 (0.19)	1.66 (0.30)	1.78 (0.39)	1.58 (0.36)
75%	1.68 (0.26)	1.55 (0.26)	1.87 (0.36)	1.85 (0.46)	1.67 (0.35)
100%	2.06 (0.34)	1.91 (0.41)	2.01 (0.38)	1.92 (0.42)	1.80 (0.29)
Ti/Ttot (%)					
Baseline	38 (5)	36 (8)	36 (6)	39 (7)	38 (9)
25%	40 (5)	42 (4)	43 (5)	45 (5)	46 (3)
50%	42 (5)	44 (4)	45 (3)	46 (3)	45 (5)
75%	44 (4)	44 (5)	45 (5)	46 (4)	46 (4)
100%	45 (4)	47 (4)	44 (5)	45 (5)	45 (4)
V_E/VCO_2					
Baseline	45 (9)	48 (9)	47 (9)	49 (8)	47 (9)
25%	45 (9)	46 (10)	47 (11)	49 (13)	49 (14)
50%	46 (11)	47 (12)	49 (12)	51 (15)	49 (15)
75%	48 (12)	48 (14)	50 (13)	52 (16)	51 (16)
100%	51 (13)	50 (15)	52 (13)	53 (17)	51 (16)
$P_{ET}CO_2$ (kPa)					
Baseline	3.83 (0.57)	3.82 (0.53)	3.74 (0.55)	3.77 (0.61)	3.71 (0.56)
25%	3.72 (0.66)	3.59 (0.63)	3.49 (0.74)	3.32 (0.76)	3.34 (0.81)
50%	3.60 (0.77)	3.52 (0.71)	3.34 (0.80)	3.21 (0.75)	3.30 (0.82)
75%	3.45 (0.81)	3.44 (0.80)	3.25 (0.83)	3.14 (0.76)	3.25 (0.83)
100%	3.24 (0.82)	3.23 (0.85)	3.23 (0.80)	3.08 (0.72)	3.17 (0.80)
SpO_2 (%)					
Baseline	95 (4)	95 (4)	94 (5)	95 (4)	94 (4)
25%	92 (5)	91 (5)	89 (7)	88 (6)	89 (5)
50%	92 (5)	89 (5)	89 (8)	87 (6)	87 (6)
75%	90 (5)	88 (5)	88 (8)	86 (7)	87 (6)
100%	89 (6)	87 (6)	87 (8)	85 (7)	85 (7)
Borg (Leg fatigue)	6 (2)	4 (3)*	6 (2)	5 (2)	5 (2)
Borg (dyspnea)	7 (2)	6 (2)	6 (2)	6 (2)	5 (2)

Values are mean (SD).
*$p \leq 0.05$ vs. CPET.
Table legend: *CPET, Cardiopulmonary exercise test; ISWT, Incremental shuttle walk test; CET, Cycle endurance test; ESWT, Endurance shuttle walk test; 6MWT, Six-minute walk test;* V_E, *Minute ventilation; BF, Breath frequency;* V_T, *Tidal volume; Ti, Inspiratory duration; Ttot, Total breath duration;* V_E/VCO_2, *Ventilatory equivalent for carbon dioxide;* $P_{ET}CO_2$, *End-tidal carbon dioxide partial pressure;* SpO_2, *Oxygen saturation by pulse oximetry.*

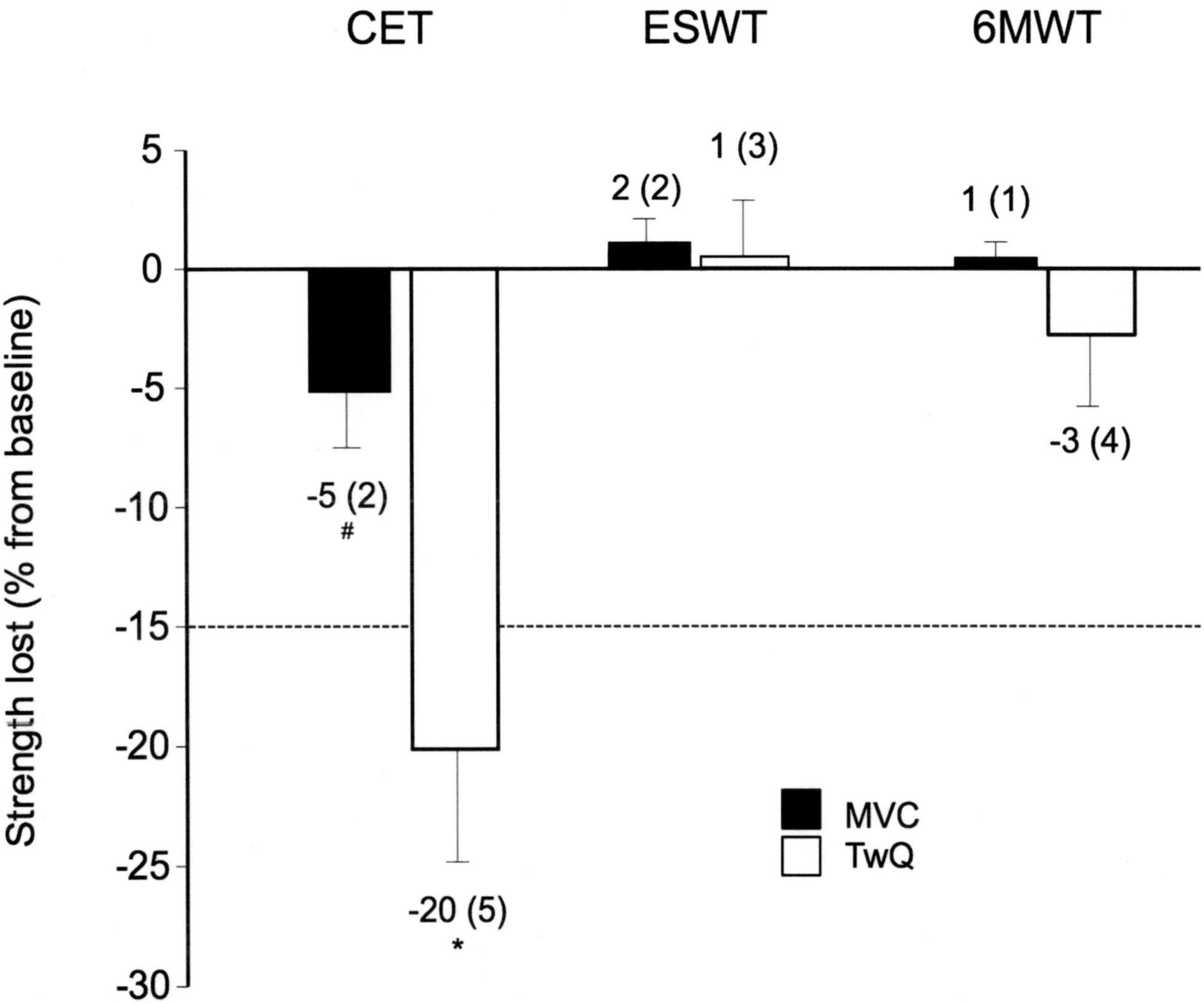

Figure 4. Quadriceps muscle fatigue induced by the constant work rate exercise tests. Relative voluntary and non-volitional quadriceps strengths lost from baseline as assessed by maximal voluntary contraction (MVC) and potentiated twitch (TWq) following the cycle endurance test (CET), the endurance shuttle walk test (ESWT) and the six-minute walk test (6MWT). The CET induced significant quadriceps muscle fatigue defined as a 15% decrease in TWq following exercise (dotted line). Indeed, 12 (57%), 2 (10%) and 3 (14%) patients developed significant quadriceps fatigue following CET, ESWT and 6MWT, respectively. *p≤0.01; # p≤0.05. Values are mean (SE). *Figure legend: CET, Cycle endurance test; ESWT, Endurance shuttle walk test; 6MWT, Six-minute walk test; MVC, Maximal voluntary contraction; TWq: Potentiated twitches.*

would increase the discriminative capacity of the walking tests in PAH compared to the distance alone also remains to be confirmed.

Potential limitations of our study should be discussed. First, patients had to complete three exercise tests during the same day. This was done to minimize the number of study visits and to accommodate patients coming from remote areas. This could have precluded the achievement of maximal capacity in some tests due to patients' fatigue. Nevertheless, the VO_{2peak} achieved during the two constant work rate exercise tests and the 6MWT were not different than the one achieved during the incremental tests while patients had not previously participated to any forms of exercise. Moreover, the exercise tests were separated by 2 hours and the order of the tests for each subject was randomly determined using the Latin Square design to minimize any confounding effect based on test sequence. Because of technical difficulties in arterial sampling during walking exercise tests, blood gases were not measured. This would have been of interest to accurately quantify dead-space ventilation and to provide indirect information (through blood lactate) about muscle metabolism during exercise tests. Finally, the effect of carrying the telemetric device during walking compared to cycling tests was likely to be trivial given its low weight.

The 6MWT is typically considered as a safe procedure even when performed without detailed cardiopulmonary monitoring. Here, we show that the peak VO_2 and heart rate responses achieved during a 6MWT represent ≈95% of that of an incremental cycling exercise test, suggesting that this test may induce more physiological stress than previously thought. Despite this, no adverse effects were noted in the present investigation in which a total of 105 exercise tests were performed. This is consistent with previous studies [4,18,37] in showing that exercise testing procedure are generally safe in class II/III PAH patients. Our findings may have implications for the choice of exercise tests to be used to assess the efficacy of a given intervention. Considering that cycling tests are more demanding on the lower limb muscle and quadriceps fatigue is more common during cycling, this exercise modality may be preferable to assess interventions such as exercise training whose aim is to improve muscle function. Conversely, cycling tests might be less susceptible to track a beneficial effect on pulmonary hemodynamics following PAH specific therapy, as previously suggested [18]. Similarly, walking tests may be more useful to assess the potential exercise-enhancing effect of oxygen therapy because exercise-induced O_2 desaturation is more common with this exercise testing modality.

Conclusions

Despite a similar physiological demand in terms of VO_{2peak}, the modality of exercise test was mainly responsible for the different RER, locus of symptom limitation and quadriceps fatigability. The distance reached during field walking tests correlates with the VO_{2peak} achieved during cycling tests and therefore reflects individual exercise capacity in PAH. As it was proposed in COPD, field walking exercise tests might be of clinical interest in PAH. Whether they might be used as an alternative to the 6MWT for tracking beneficial clinical changes following therapy and to assess exercise-induced desaturation remains to be confirmed in PAH.

Acknowledgments

The authors acknowledge Serge Simard for statistical analysis, and Luce Bouffard for technical assistance.

Author Contributions

Conceived and designed the experiments: SP FM DS VM. Performed the experiments: VM ASN SM SP DS. Analyzed the data: VM SP FM. Contributed reagents/materials/analysis tools: SP SB FM DS. Wrote the paper: VM SP. Read, corrected and approved the manuscript: SM ASN DS FM SB SP VM.

References

1. Rubin LJ (1997) Primary pulmonary hypertension. NEnglJMed 336: 111–117.
2. D'Alonzo GE, Gianotti LA, Pohil RL, Reagle RR, DuRee SL, et al. (1987) Comparison of progressive exercise performance of normal subjects and patients with primary pulmonary hypertension. Chest 92: 57–62.
3. Riley MS, Porszasz J, Engelen MP, Brundage BH, Wasserman K (2000) Gas exchange responses to continuous incremental cycle ergometry exercise in primary pulmonary hypertension in humans. EurJApplPhysiol 83: 63–70.
4. Sun XG, Hansen JE, Oudiz RJ, Wasserman K (2001) Exercise pathophysiology in patients with primary pulmonary hypertension. Circulation 104: 429–435.
5. Mainguy V, Maltais F, Saey D, Gagnon P, Martel S, et al. (2010) Peripheral muscle dysfunction in idiopathic pulmonary arterial hypertension. Thorax 65: 113–117.
6. Meyer FJ, Lossnitzer D, Kristen AV, Schoene AM, Kubler W, et al. (2005) Respiratory muscle dysfunction in idiopathic pulmonary arterial hypertension. EurRespirJ 25: 125–130.
7. Potus F, Malenfant S, Graydon C, Mainguy V, Tremblay E, et al. (2014) Impaired Angiogenesis and Peripheral Muscle Microcirculation Loss Contributes to Exercise Intolerance in Pulmonary Arterial Hypertension. Am J Respir Crit Care Med Epub ahead of print.
8. Miyamoto S, Nagaya N, Satoh T, Kyotani S, Sakamaki F, et al. (2000) Clinical correlates and prognostic significance of six-minute walk test in patients with primary pulmonary hypertension. Comparison with cardiopulmonary exercise testing. AmJRespirCrit Care Med 161: 487–492.
9. Wensel R, Opitz CF, Anker SD, Winkler J, Hoffken G, et al. (2002) Assessment of survival in patients with primary pulmonary hypertension: importance of cardiopulmonary exercise testing. Circulation 106: 319–324.
10. Galie N, Manes A, Negro L, Palazzini M, Bacchi-Reggiani ML, et al. (2009) A meta-analysis of randomized controlled trials in pulmonary arterial hypertension. EurHeart J 30: 394–403.
11. McGoon M, Gutterman D, Steen V, Barst R, McCrory DC, et al. (2004) Screening, early detection, and diagnosis of pulmonary arterial hypertension: ACCP evidence-based clinical practice guidelines. Chest 126: 14S–34S.
12. Dyer CA, Singh SJ, Stockley RA, Sinclair AJ, Hill SL (2002) The incremental shuttle walking test in elderly people with chronic airflow limitation. Thorax 57: 34–38.
13. Eiser N, Willsher D, Dore CJ (2003) Reliability, repeatability and sensitivity to change of externally and self-paced walking tests in COPD patients. Respiratory medicine 97: 407–414.
14. Verkindre C, Bart F, Aguilaniu B, Fortin F, Guerin JC, et al. (2006) The effect of tiotropium on hyperinflation and exercise capacity in chronic obstructive pulmonary disease. Respiration; international review of thoracic diseases 73: 420–427.
15. Eaton T, Young P, Nicol K, Kolbe J (2006) The endurance shuttle walking test: a responsive measure in pulmonary rehabilitation for COPD patients. ChronRespirDis 3: 3–9.
16. Simonneau G, Gatzoulis MA, Adatia I, Celermajer D, Denton C, et al. (2013) Updated clinical classification of pulmonary hypertension. J Am Coll Cardiol 62: D34–41.
17. Humbert M, Sitbon O, Simonneau G (2004) Treatment of pulmonary arterial hypertension. NEnglJMed 351: 1425–1436.
18. Mainguy V, Malenfant S, Neyron AS, Bonnet S, Maltais F, et al. (2013) Repeatability and responsiveness of exercise tests in pulmonary arterial hypertension. Eur Respir J 42: 425–434.
19. (2003) ATS/ACCP Statement on cardiopulmonary exercise testing. AmJRespirCrit Care Med 167: 211–277.
20. Singh SJ, Morgan MD, Scott S, Walters D, Hardman AE (1992) Development of a shuttle walking test of disability in patients with chronic airways obstruction. Thorax 47: 1019–1024.
21. Revill SM, Morgan MD, Singh SJ, Williams J, Hardman AE (1999) The endurance shuttle walk: a new field test for the assessment of endurance capacity in chronic obstructive pulmonary disease. Thorax 54: 213–222.
22. Guyatt GH, Pugsley SO, Sullivan MJ, Thompson PJ, Berman L, et al. (1984) Effect of encouragement on walking test performance. Thorax 39: 818–822.
23. ATS (2002) ATS statement: guidelines for the six-minute walk test. AmJRespirCrit Care Med 166: 111–117.
24. Enright PL, Sherrill DL (1998) Reference equations for the six-minute walk in healthy adults. Am J RespirCrit Care Med 158: 1384–1387.
25. Borg GA (1982) Psychophysical bases of perceived exertion. MedSciSports Exerc 14: 377–381.
26. Chuang ML, Lin IF, Wasserman K (2001) The body weight-walking distance product as related to lung function, anaerobic threshold and peak VO2 in COPD patients. RespirMed 95: 618–626.
27. Casas A, Vilaro J, Rabinovich R, Mayer A, Barbera JA, et al. (2005) Encouraged 6-min walking test indicates maximum sustainable exercise in COPD patients. Chest 128: 55–61.
28. Deboeck G, Niset G, Vachiery JL, Moraine JJ, Naeije R (2005) Physiological response to the six-minute walk test in pulmonary arterial hypertension. EurRespirJ 26: 667–672.
29. Saey D, Debigare R, LeBlanc P, Mador MJ, Cote CH, et al. (2003) Contractile leg fatigue after cycle exercise: a factor limiting exercise in patients with chronic obstructive pulmonary disease. AmJRespirCrit Care Med 168: 425–430.
30. Valli G, Vizza CD, Onorati P, Badagliacca R, Ciuffa R, et al. (2007) Pathophysiological adaptations to walking and cycling in primary pulmonary hypertension. EurJApplPhysiol.
31. Tolle J, Waxman A, Systrom D (2008) Impaired systemic oxygen extraction at maximum exercise in pulmonary hypertension. MedSciSports Exerc 40: 3–8.
32. Casey K, Duffin J, Kelsey CJ, McAvoy GV (1987) The effect of treadmill speed on ventilation at the start of exercise in man. The Journal of physiology 391: 13–24.
33. Kelsey CJ, Duffin J (1992) Changes in ventilation in response to ramp changes in treadmill exercise load. European journal of applied physiology and occupational physiology 65: 480–484.
34. Takano N (1988) Effects of pedal rate on respiratory responses to incremental bicycle work. The Journal of physiology 396: 389–397.
35. Palange P, Forte S, Onorati P, Manfredi F, Serra P, et al. (2000) Ventilatory and metabolic adaptations to walking and cycling in patients with COPD. JApplPhysiol 88: 1715–1720.
36. Page E, Cohen-Solal A, Jondeau G, Douard H, Roul G, et al. (1994) Comparison of treadmill and bicycle exercise in patients with chronic heart failure. Chest 106: 1002–1006.
37. Groepenhoff H, Vonk-Noordegraaf A, Boonstra A, Spreeuwenberg MD, Postmus PE, et al. (2008) Exercise testing to estimate survival in pulmonary hypertension. Med Sci Sports Exerc 40: 1725–1732.

15

A Post-Hospital Home Exercise Program Improved Mobility but Increased Falls in Older People: A Randomised Controlled Trial

Catherine Sherrington[1]*, Stephen R. Lord[2], Constance M. Vogler[3,4], Jacqueline C. T. Close[2,5], Kirsten Howard[6], Catherine M. Dean[7], Gillian Z. Heller[8], Lindy Clemson[9], Sandra D. O'Rourke[2], Elisabeth Ramsay[2], Elizabeth Barraclough[2], Robert D. Herbert[2], Robert G. Cumming[6]

1 The George Institute for Global Health, The University of Sydney, Sydney, New South Wales, Australia, **2** Neuroscience Research Australia, University of New South Wales, Randwick, New South Wales, Australia, **3** Northern Clinical School, The University of Sydney, Sydney, New South Wales, Australia, **4** Department of Aged Care and Rehabilitation, Royal North Shore Hospital, St Leonards, New South Wales, Australia, **5** Prince of Wales Clinical School, University of New South Wales, Randwick, New South Wales, Australia, **6** School of Public Health, The University of Sydney, Sydney, New South Wales, Australia, **7** Department of Health Professions, Faculty of Human Sciences, Macquarie University, Macquarie Park, NSW, Australia, **8** Department of Statistics, Macquarie University, Macquarie Park, New South Wales, Australia, **9** Discipline of Occupational Therapy, Faculty of Health Sciences, The University of Sydney, Lidcombe, New South Wales, Australia

Abstract

Background: Home exercise can prevent falls in the general older community but its impact in people recently discharged from hospital is not known. The study aimed to investigate the effects of a home-based exercise program on falls and mobility among people recently discharged from hospital.

Methods and Findings: This randomised controlled trial (ACTRN12607000563460) was conducted among 340 older people. Intervention group participants (n = 171) were asked to exercise at home for 15–20 minutes up to 6 times weekly for 12 months. The control group (n = 169) received usual care. Primary outcomes were rate of falls (assessed over 12 months using monthly calendars), performance-based mobility (Lower Extremity Summary Performance Score, range 0–3, at baseline and 12 months, assessor unaware of group allocation) and self-reported ease of mobility task performance (range 0–40, assessed with 12 monthly questionaries). Participants had an average age of 81.2 years (SD 8.0) and 70% had fallen in the past year. Complete primary outcome data were obtained for at least 92% of randomised participants. Participants in the intervention group reported more falls than the control group (177 falls versus 123 falls) during the 12-month study period and this difference was statistically significant (incidence rate ratio 1.43, 95% CI 1.07 to 1.93, $p = 0.017$). At 12-months, performance-based mobility had improved significantly more in the intervention group than in the control group (between-group difference adjusted for baseline performance 0.13, 95% CI 0.04 to 0.21, $p = 0.004$). Self-reported ease in undertaking mobility tasks over the 12-month period was not significantly different between the groups (0.49, 95% CI −0.91 to 1.90, $p = 0.488$).

Conclusions: An individualised home exercise prescription significantly improved performance-based mobility but significantly increased the rate of falls in older people recently discharged from hospital.

Trial Registration: Australian New Zealand Clinical Trials Registry ACTRN12607000563460

Editor: Terence J. Quinn, University of Glasgow, United Kingdom

Funding: This trial received project grant funding from the Australian National Health and Medical Research Council (NHMRC ID: 457464). Authors Sherrington, Clemson and Lord receive salary funding from Australian National Health and Medical Research Council Research Fellowships. The funders had no role in study design, data collection and analysis, decision to publish, or preparation of the manuscript.

Competing Interests: The authors have declared that no competing interests exist.

* Email: csherrington@georgeinstitute.org.au

Introduction

The development and widespread implementation of effective strategies to minimise disability and falls among older people is an urgent public health challenge due to the increasing proportion of older people in the global population. Older people recently discharged from hospital are at a particularly high risk of falls [1] and disability [2]. Previous studies have reported that 14% of older people fall in the first month after discharge from hospital [3] and 34% fall within three months of discharge from rehabilitation care [4].

It is well known that group- and home-based exercise programs can prevent falls in community-dwelling older people [5] but one previous trial found that a home exercise program of seated resisted knee extension exercises did not prevent falls in people who had recently been hospitalised [6]. Certain exercise programs have also been found to enhance balance and/or mobility in community-dwelling older people [7] and in those who have been in hospital [8–10]. As our previous meta-analysis [11] found greater effects on falls of exercise programs that challenge balance, a home exercise program that targets balance may prevent falls in people who have been in hospital. However, this has not been previously investigated.

We designed a simple exercise program that can be taught to older people, performed independently at home and individualised to ensure safety yet be sufficiently challenging. The program aimed to enhance balance and mobility and prevent falls by repetition of movements that are similar to daily activities such as standing up, walking, and stair climbing. We have previously found this program to improve mobility when used in a group-setting by stroke survivors [12] and in frail older people when used as part of a multi-disciplinary intervention [13,14]. In this study, we sought to investigate the effects of this home-based exercise program on falls and mobility among older people who have had a recent hospital stay.

Methods

Trial design

A parallel pragmatic randomised controlled trial with equal allocation to intervention and control groups was conducted among 340 older people recently discharged from hospital. The protocol for this trial and supporting CONSORT checklist are available as supporting information; see Checklist S1 and Protocol S1.

Ethical statement and trial registration

Ethical approval was obtained from the relevant human research ethics committees (University of Sydney, Northern Sydney Area Health Service, South Eastern Sydney Area Health Service and Hope Healthcare). When we commenced the trial we were aware of the importance of trial registration but not of the importance of registration prior to recruitment. Thus we recruited four trial participants prior to completing the trial registration process. The trial protocol was published [15].

Participants

Participants were aged 60 years and over and had been admitted to and subsequently discharged from nine aged care, rehabilitation and orthopaedic wards at four public hospitals in Sydney, Australia. Potential participants were excluded if they: resided in a high-care residential facility (nursing home); had cognitive impairment (a Mini-Mental State Examination [16] score of less than 24); had insufficient English language to understand procedures; were unable to walk more than one metre even with an assistive device or the help of one person; or had a medical condition precluding a 12-month home exercise program (e.g. unstable cardiac disease or progressive neurological disease). Potential participants were approached about the study during their inpatient stay and their permission to be contacted after discharge from hospital was sought. Baseline assessments were conducted after participants had returned home, were medically fit to exercise, had completed hospital-initiated rehabilitation and provided written informed consent to study participation.

Randomisation

Randomisation was stratified by hospital site and falls history (0–1 versus 2+ falls in the previous 12 months) using a computer-generated random number schedule with randomly ordered blocks of two, four and six. To ensure concealed randomisation to groups, the randomisation schedule was generated in advance by and only accessible to the first author who was not involved in participant recruitment, interviews or assessments. After completing the baseline assessment, and gaining informed consent and approval for trial participation from individual local medical officers, research staff contacted the first author by email to receive the group allocation for individual participants.

Interventions

Three experienced physiotherapists delivered the intervention in participants' homes. Ten visits were scheduled over the 12-month study period, with more frequent visits at the beginning of the program to ensure safety and enable tailoring and progression of the program. Participants were asked to undertake a 20 to 30 minute program of lower limb balance and strengthening exercises up to six times per week for 12 months. The exercises were primarily conducted while standing and were based on the Weight-bearing Exercise for Better Balance program, which is available at www.webb.org.au. The physiotherapist prescribed the level of difficulty and number of repetitions for each exercise after an assessment of the participant's abilities. The Physical Activity Stage of Change model [17] was also used by the study physiotherapists to guide their approach to encouraging ongoing home-based exercise participation. Exercises that primarily targeted postural control (balance) included standing with a narrower base (aiming for tandem or single leg stance), forwards and sideways stepping/walking, and graded reaching activities in standing. The lower limb extensor muscle groups (i.e. hip and knee extensors and ankle plantar flexors), which act to prevent collapse of the lower limb, were targeted with exercises aiming to enhance muscle strength and control. Strengthening exercises included sit-to-stand, forward and lateral step-ups onto a small block, and heel raises in standing. Where appropriate, resistance for strengthening exercises was added by the use of weight-belts worn around the waist or weighted vests. The use of upper limbs to support the body while exercising was minimised but was advised where necessary to ensure safety. Participants were instructed on how to perform exercises with stable supports (such as a table) located nearby to hold onto if needed and, where appropriate, family members and/or carers were encouraged to assist with supervision of the exercise program. If a participant became unwell or had another admission to hospital, the program was resumed when the participant and the relevant professionals considered him/her well enough to participate again. The optimal intensity and type of exercises for each participant was re-assessed and adjusted by the study physiotherapists to ensure that the intervention remained challenging. Participants were not given any specific advice about general physical activity levels. Participants were provided with a booklet of safety precautions, instructions and photographs of exercises for use in exercise sessions at home. In addition, participants were provided with a logbook for recording exercises completed and effects of exercise (e.g. muscle soreness). The physiotherapists were asked to give their impression of the percentage of prescribed exercise that had actually been undertaken by each participant in the first, third, eighth and twelfth month of the intervention period. This rating was based on review of the exercise logs as well as discussion with the participant and carers present during the visit.

Participants in both groups received a 32-page education booklet about fall prevention. It included information about risk factors for falls, environmental modification for falls risk reduction and what to do after a fall but did not offer any specific advice about exercise. The control group did not receive any additional intervention as part of the study. Participants in both groups received usual care from health and community services. Participants did not commence in the study until they had completed all care from the admission during which they were recruited for the study. Thus usual care involved ongoing management of chronic conditions and routine management for any new conditions. This involved hospitalisation, visits to general practitioners, medical specialists, other health practitioners and Emergency Departments and home visits from community service providers to assist with daily tasks such as showering, dressing, meals and housework. Full details of health and community services used by trial participants will be published elsewhere (manuscript under review).

Data collection

Data were collected from medical records, postal questionnaires, calendars, interviews and physical assessments. Information on medical history, diagnoses and medications at the time of recruitment were collected from medical records while participants were in hospital. Baseline assessments were conducted in participants' homes prior to randomisation. Further assessments were conducted three and 12 months after randomisation by physiotherapists and trained research assistants masked to group allocation. Participants were given 12 calendars and questionnaires about mobility at the baseline assessment and asked to record falls on the calendars and complete the questionnaires each month and return them in pre-paid envelopes to the research centre. Participants who did not return calendars or questionnaires were telephoned by a research assistant masked to group allocation to obtain the information. Participants who reported falling were also telephoned to obtain more information about the circumstances and consequences of such falls.

Blinding

Staff who conducted interviews and assessments, received calendars and questionnaires, made phone calls and entered data were unaware of group allocation.

Primary outcomes

The three primary outcome measures were fall rate, performance-based mobility and self-reported mobility [18].

1. Fall rate was calculated using the information provided on the monthly calendars described above. A fall was defined as an event in which the person unintentionally came to rest on the ground or other lower level which was not as a result of a violent blow, loss of consciousness, sudden onset of paralysis as in a stroke or an epileptic seizure [19].
2. Performance-based mobility was measured at 12 months after randomisation using the performance-based Short Physical Performance Battery [20], which involves the timed performance of three mobility tasks: the ability to stand for up to 10 sec with feet position in three different positions (together side by side, semi-tandem and tandem), 4-metre walk and time to rise from a chair five times. The primary analysis was conducted using the continuously scored lower extremity Summary Performance Score version [21] of this tool.
3. Self-reported level of ease in performing eight mobility tasks was measured monthly on a five-point scale and the scores summed. The eight mobility tasks were; getting in and out of bed, sitting up in bed, walking in the home, bending, walking half a mile and walking up and down stairs, walking 1 mile and undertaking moderate physical activity [18].

Secondary outcomes

Secondary outcome measures were: additional measures of mobility; falls and risk of falling; strength; flexibility; quality of life; falls self-efficacy; health system and community service contact; assistance required from others; difficulty with daily tasks; community participation; and physical activity levels. These measures aimed to enhance understanding of the effects of the exercise program on multiple factors that contribute to an older person's functioning and quality of life.

Additional measures of mobility included: the Maximal Balance Range test (participants' ability to lean as far forward and backwards as possible); the Coordinated Stability test (participants' ability to adjust the body position in a steady and coordinated manner when near the limits of their base of support) [23]; the Step Test (stepping onto and off a 15 cm block as many times as possible in 15 seconds); and the time the participant could stand unsupported in single leg stance; the number of steps required to make a 180 degree turn. Falls were further assessed by comparing the proportion of people experiencing one or more falls over the 12-month follow-up period in the intervention and control groups. Risk of falling was assessed using the Physiological Profile Assessment [22] and choice stepping reaction time tests. The Physiological Profile Assessment provides a composite measure of risk of falling and includes measures of knee extension strength (measured with a spring balance with the participant sitting with the hip and knee at 90 degrees of flexion), postural sway, lower limb proprioception, reaction time and visual contrast sensitivity. Choice stepping reaction time has been found to be a composite measure of risk of falling when assessed with an electronic device [24]. In a modified version of the test, participants stood on a nonslip black mat (0.8 m×1.2 m) marked with four rectangular panels (32 cm×13 cm), one in front of each foot and one to the side of each foot. Participants were instructed to step onto specific rectangle panels in sequence as quickly as possible, using the left foot only for the two left panels (front and side) and the right foot only for the two right panels. The time for the entire routine was recorded in seconds. Grip strength was assessed using a portable dynamometer (JAMAR Hydraulic Hand Dynamometer manufactured by Sammons Prestons). Ankle range of motion was measured in a torque-controlled manner using a modification of the Lidcombe template procedure [25] in which the participant is seated and an inclinometer is used to assess changes in ankle angle. Quality of life was assessed using the physical and mental components of the SF 12 Version 2 and the EQ-5D [26] and a utility score was calculated using the SF6D and the EQ-5D. Fall-related self-efficacy was assessed using the Falls Efficacy Scale-International [27] in which level of concern about falling when carrying out a range of activities is rated on a 4-point scale. Participants were also asked about the need for assistance from others and community participation. Physical activity levels were assessed with the Incidental and Planned Exercise Questionnaire [28].

Adverse events

Adverse effects of the exercise program were monitored using exercise diaries kept by participants. Participants in the intervention group were also advised to telephone study staff if they experienced any major adverse effects of the exercise program (defined as chest pain or muscle soreness lasting for more than 48 hours and interfering with daily activities or requiring medical attention).

Sample size

We anticipated that the intervention would reduce the rate of falling. Sample size calculations indicated that 350 participants (175 per group) would be required for 80% power to detect as significant a 30% reduction in the rate of falling (i.e. an IRR of 0.70 using negative binomial regression analysis) in the 12-month follow-up period (alpha = 5%, two-sided). An 11-month average follow up period was used in the sample size calculation to account for loss to follow-up. This sample size would also be sufficient to detect clinically- and statistically- significant 10% between-group differences in lower extremity Summary Performance Scores and the self-reported mobility measure (power = 80%, p = 0.05, dropouts = 15%, alpha = 5%, two-sided).

Statistical methods

Analyses were conducted according to the pre-defined statistical analysis plan on an intention-to-treat basis and were adjusted only for baseline score except where otherwise indicated. All statistical tests were two-sided and p-values were considered significant when their values were less than 0.05. All analyses were undertaken using Stata software (StataCorp LP, College Station, Texas, versions 12 and 13). The number of falls per person-year was analysed using negative binomial regression to estimate the difference in fall rates between the two groups (primary outcome). Length of follow-up was included as an exposure term in these models, i.e. the logarithm of the days of follow-up was added as an offset. A blind review by the statistician (GH) prior to analysis revealed that the negative binomial model was appropriate. Secondary analyses were also conducted to compare the proportion of fallers in the two groups (using modified Poisson regression models) and to compare the group rates of indoor falls, falls requiring health care intervention, falls in the four 3-month periods of the study. For the performance-based mobility measure (lower extremity Summary Performance Score) linear regression models were used to compare the groups on three-month (secondary outcome) and 12-month (primary outcome) assessment scores adjusted for baseline scores. This approach was also used for the continuously scored secondary outcome measures. Where outcome variables were markedly skewed the difference between initial and final scores was used in the models instead of the final scores. For the self-reported mobility measure, analyses were conducted by comparing the average of the 12 monthly scores between the groups (primary outcome). Negative binomial regression was also used for other count variables such as the numbers of health service contacts and social outings. Ordinal regression was used for the health status question from the EQ-5D. In cases where individuals were unable to carry out a test due to physical impairments, a score of 0 was given for variables where low score indicates poor performances and a score of the mean plus three standard deviations was allocated for variables where high score indicates poor performances.

Pre-planned subgroup analyses were conducted using interaction terms in the models to assess whether the intervention had differential effects in those with 2 or more falls in the year prior to study recruitment (versus 0 or 1 falls), those with poorer cognition (above and below the pre-specified cut-point of the median MMSE score, which was 28) and slower baseline walking speed (as a continuous interaction term). The interaction between group and baseline walking speed for the falls outcome was graphed using R software. Further exploratory analyses were undertaken to investigate whether any differential effects of the intervention on falls were evident on the basis of other baseline characteristics. Secondary analyses tested the impact of adjusting for the stratification variables. Secondary per protocol analyses were also conducted and included only those participants who completed (i) at least 50% and (ii) at least 80% of prescribed interventions. In order to lessen the risk of "confounding by indication" (i.e., the likely tendency for people who are able to do more exercise to have better outcomes) in this analysis, outcomes in intervention group participants who undertook more than 50% and 80% of prescribed sessions were then compared with outcomes in the control group after adjusting for likely predictors of outcome (baseline mobility, age, fear of falling, co-morbidity, past falls, PPA fall risk score and cognition).

Additional secondary analyses used instrumental variable regression to estimate the complier average causal effect [29],[30]. Participants in the intervention group were considered to have adhered to the exercise program if they completed at least 80% of the exercise program, and it was assumed that participants in the control group could not access the intervention. This analysis was conducted on the two primary mobility outcomes, but not on the falls outcome because the exclusion restriction assumption made in instrumental variable regression [29] was considered less tenable for the falls outcome.

Results

Participant flow

Figure 1 shows the flow of participants through the study. Three hundred and forty people were randomised to one of the two groups; 171 to the intervention group and 169 to the control group. Baseline assessments were conducted a median of 62 days (IQR 53) days after hospital discharge. All participants provided at least one month of falls data so were included in the falls analysis. Twelve months of falls data were available for 320 people (94% of those randomised; 159 from the control group and 161 from the intervention group). The average length of falls follow up was 355 (SD 47) days in the exercise group and 354 (SD 51) days in the control group. The 12-month assessment was completed by 312 participants (92% of those randomised) and was undertaken an average of 374 (SD 12) days after the baseline assessment. Twelve months of monthly self-reported mobility data were available for 315 participants (93% of those randomised).

Recruitment

Participant recruitment was undertaken between November 2007 and February 2011. Recruitment was stopped ten participants prior to the original target due to exhaustion of study funds. Follow up was completed in February 2012.

Baseline data

Participants had an average age of 81.2 years (SD 8.0), an average of 6.8 health conditions (SD 2.7), and were prescribed an average of 7.5 medications (SD 3.3). Seventy-four per cent were women and 70% had fallen in the past year. Table 1 provides a summary of the baseline demographics of the study sample and describes the primary diagnoses at hospital admission. Table 2 outlines participant answers to interview questions and performance in the physical assessments at baseline. As the tables show, there were no marked differences between the groups at baseline.

Intervention delivery

The intervention was offered to all 171 participants randomised to the intervention group but nine did not commence a home exercise program due to new health problems (n = 6) or refusal to exercise (n = 3). Participants who commenced the program received an average of 9.2 (SD 1.7) home visits. At the start of the study, participants agreed to undertake an average of 6

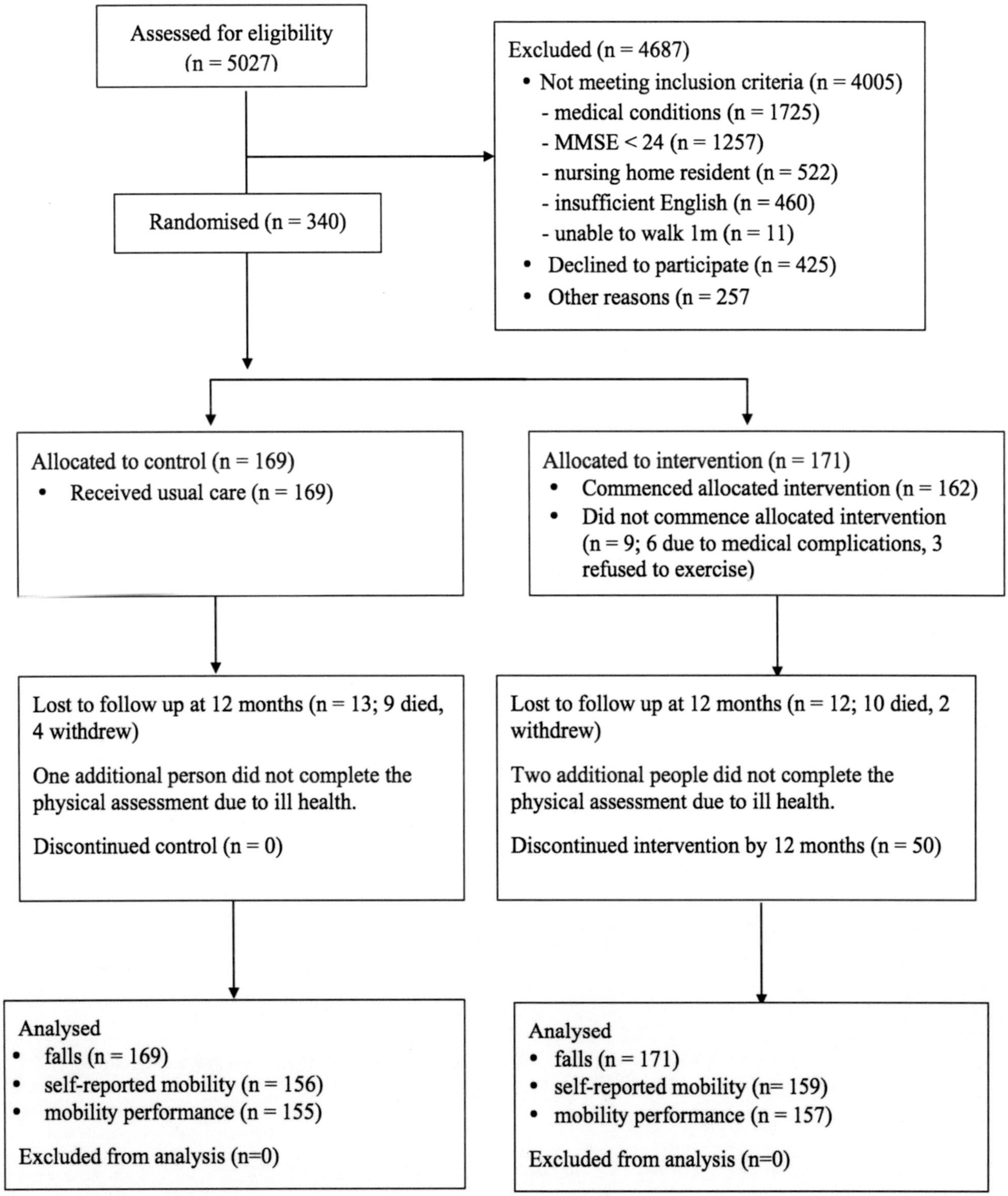

Figure 1. Participant flow.

exercise sessions (range 3 to 7) involving an average of 5 different exercises (range 2 to 8) and an average of 59 exercise repetitions per week (SD 39). In the first month, participants reported completing an average of 5 sessions (range 1 to 7) and study physiotherapists estimated that 77% of prescribed repetitions were completed (SD 34). At the end of 12 months, 103 people (61% of the intervention group) continued to exercise and, among exercisers, the average number of exercise sessions completed was 4 (range 1 to 7). Table 3 provides further details of intervention dose and adherence.

Table 1. Baseline characteristics of participants.

Characteristic	Control (n = 169)	Intervention (n = 171)
Age, mean (SD) years	80.8 (8.2)	81.6 (7.8)
Hospital length of stay, mean (SD) days	15.6 (15.7)	17.0 (19.3)
Mini Mental State Examination score, mean (SD)/30	28.0 (1.8)	27.9 (2.0)
Females, n (%)	128 (76)	123 (72)
1 or more falls in previous 12 months, n (%)	117 (69)	123 (72)
Medications, mean (SD) number	7.5 (3.3)	7.5 (3.3)
Psychotropic medication, n (%)	30 (18)	17 (10)
Benzodiazepine medication, n (%)	31 (18)	20 (12)
Living in low-care residential facility (hostel), n (%)	12 (7)	8 (5)
Co-morbidities, mean (SD) number	6.9 (2.7)	7.2 (2.9)
Primary diagnosis on admission (from medical file) n (%)		
Lower limb fracture	24 (14)	26 (15)
Upper limb fracture	7 (4)	7 (4)
Vertebral fracture	9 (5)	12 (7)
Respiratory illness	13 (8)	11 (6)
Infection	13 (8)	13 (8)
Fall and soft tissue damage	15 (9)	19 (11)
Neurological condition	2 (1)	4 (2)
Musculoskeletal condition	21 (12)	19 (11)
Cerebrovascular disease	4 (2)	4 (2)
Ischaemic heart disease	3 (2)	2 (1)
General medical conditions	11 (7)	12 (7)
General symptoms	14 (8)	12 (7)

Falls

During the 12-month study period, 168 people (49% of participants) reported 300 falls (Table 4). The intervention group reported a higher fall rate (177 falls, 1.0 fall per person, SD 1.23) than the control group (123 falls, 0.73 falls per person, SD 1.22) and this difference (primary outcome) was statistically significant (incidence rate ratio 1.43, 95% CI 1.07 to 1.93, p = 0.017, n = 340). The estimate of effect of the intervention on rate of falls was not changed by adjustment for the stratification variables i.e., study site and past falls (IRR 1.40, 95% CI 1.05 to 1.87, p = 0.021). There was also a higher proportion of fallers in the exercise group (98 people, 57%) than the control group (70 people, 41%) and this difference was statistically significant (RR 1.38, 95% CI 1.11 to 1.73, p = 0.004). Indoor falls were more frequent in the intervention group than in the control group (IRR 1.62, 95% CI 1.13 to 2.33, p = 0.009) but there was no significant difference in outdoor falls (IRR 1.10, 95% CI 0.71 to 1.69, p = 0.670), falls requiring health care intervention (IRR 1.14, 95% CI 0.76 to 1.73, p = 0.524) or fall-related fractures (15 in control group, 14 in intervention group). The increase in falls in the intervention group was particularly evident in the first and second 3-month periods of the study and was statistically significant in the second 3-month period. A loss of balance was the most common participant reported reason for falling (127 falls) followed by a trip (93 falls). No falls were reported while undertaking the home exercise program.

Mobility (primary outcomes)

At 12 months, performance-based mobility (Lower Extremity Summary Performance Score, range 0–3) improved significantly more in the intervention group (mean 2.06, SD 0.52) than in the control group (mean 1.94, SD 0.56, between group difference in change score after adjusting for baseline performance 0.13, 95% CI 0.04 to 0.21, p = 0.004). Self-reported ease in undertaking mobility tasks over the 12-month period (range 0–40) was not significantly different between the groups (0.49, 95% CI −0.91 to 1.90, p = 0.488, Table 2).

Sub-group analyses for the primary outcomes

Pre-planned subgroup analyses found that the increase in falls was greater in participants who walked more quickly at baseline (mean gait speed at baseline 0.73 m/sec, interaction term p = 0.014, see Figure 2 for the graph of the interaction) but there was no evidence of differential effects on falls among those with two or more past falls or lower MMSE scores (<28). Given the unexpected finding for the falls outcome, further exploratory sub-group analyses were undertaken. These did not indicate differential intervention impacts on the basis of gender (p for interaction = 0.86), age (p = 0.88), co-morbidity (p = 0.69), falls efficacy (p = 0.26), walking aid use (p = 0.33), recruitment source (rehabilitation versus acute hospital, p = 0.23), PPA risk of falling score (p = 0.52), or postural sway (p = 0.24) but found trends towards a greater increase in falls among people with better knee extensor strength (p = 0.08) in those with falls as a presenting

Table 2. Primary mobility outcomes and secondary outcomes.

	Control			Intervention			Difference between groups (baseline adjusted)	
	Baseline, n = 169	**3 month, n = 137**	**12 month, n = 155**	**Baseline, n = 171**	**3 month, n = 156**	**12 month, n = 157**	**3month mean (95% CI), p**	**12 month mean (95% CI), p**
Mobility								
Summary Performance Score (primary outcome), 0–3, mean (SD)[a, c]	1.92 (0.48)	1.98(0.53)	1.94(0.56)	1.92 (0.46)	2.05(0.48)	2.06(0.52)	*0.07 (−0.006 to 0.15), p = 0.070*	**0.13 (0.04 to 0.21), p = 0.004**
Mobility task ease over 12 months (primary outcome), 0–40, mean (SD)[a, d]	28.2 (7.2)		27.7 (6.7), n = 156	27.6 (6.7)		28.2 (6.0), n = 159		0.49, 95% CI −0.91 to 1.90, p = 0.488
Short Physical Performance Battery, 0–12, mean (SD)[a, d]	6.73 (2.84)	7.14 (2.96)	6.89 (1.92)	6.72 (2.73)	7.48(2.94)	7.41(2.02)	*0.39 (−0.02 to 0.80), p = 0.065*	**0.50 (0.11 to 0.90), p = 0.013**
Sit to stand, stands/sec, mean (SD)[a, c]	0.22(0.16)	0.23 (0.16)	0.22 (0.2)	0.22 (0.16)	0.26(0.17)	0.28 (0.2)	0.02 (−0.009 to 0.04), p = 0.211	**0.05 (0.02 to 0.84), p = 0.000**
Gait speed, m/sec, mean (SD)[a, d]	0.72 (0.3)	0.74 (0.32)	0.76(0.32)	0.74 (0.3)	0.75(0.30)	0.77(0.31)	−0.007 (−0.05 to 0.049), p = 0.978	−0.011 (−0.06 to 0.04), p = 0.662
Standing Balance, sec, 0–30, mean (SD)[a, c]	23.3 (7.1)	24.1 (7.7)	23.4 (8.3)	22.9(7.4)	24.9 (7.0)	24.4 (7.5)	1.04 (−0.36 to 2.44), p = 0.144	1.18 (−0.30 to 2.7), p = 0.117
Single leg stance time, sec, 0–10, mean (SD)[a, c]	2.2 (3.7)	3.0 (4.1)	3.0 (4.1)	2.2 (3.8)	3.5 (4.2)	3.2 (4.3)	0.32 (−0.42 to 1.07), p = 0.389	0.15 (−0.56 to 0.87), p = 0.677
Maximum Balance Range, mm, mean (SD)[a, d]	115.49(40.91)	114.94(47.3)	115.8(47.6)	111.19(41.87)	120.7(47.0)	122.5(50.3)	**10.16 (1.84 to 18.47), p = 0.017**	*8.06 (−0.46 to 16.6), p = 0.064*
Coordinated Stability, score, mean (SD)[b, c]	21.77(12.64)	19.9 (13.2)	21.7 (15.3)	24.44 (13.82)	22.78(13.7)	22.8 (13.6)	0.76 (−1.44 to 2.95), p = 0.498	−0.395 (−2.81 to 2.02), p = 0.747
Step Test, steps, mean (SD)[a, c]	7.4 (4.9)	8.5 (5.4)	7.9 (5.9)	7.4 (4.8)	8.9 (5.3)	8.7 (6.0)	0.36 (−0.36 to 1.09), p = 0.329	0.69 (−0.14 to 1.51), p = 0.101
Steps required to turn 180 degrees, mean (SD)[b, d]	5.6(1.8)	5.5(1.9)	5.6(2.2)	5.9(2.6)	5.3(1.7)	5.3(2.3)	−0.29 (−0.64 to 0.06) p = 0.110	**−0.43 (−0.82 to −0.05), p = 0.026**
Fall risk								
PPA Score, mean (SD)[b, d]	1.20 (1.41)	1.41 (1.59)	1.59 (1.64)	1.37 (1.49)	1.42 (1.50)	1.61 (1.75)	−0.14 (−0.40 to 0.11), p = 0.269	− 0.45 (−0.32 to 0.23), p = 0.745
Postural sway on foam total length, mean (SD)[b, c]	157.5(99.5)	168.6(101.1)	180.1(107.9)	170.4 (99.5)	161.9(93.7)	167.3(100.0)	**−20.36 (−38.03 to −2.68), p = 0.024**	*−18.03 (−36.58 to 0.52), p = 0.057*
Knee extension strength, kg, mean (SD)[a, d, g]	14.6 (6.1)	13.2 (6.1)	13.3(5.8)	14.6 (6.4)	13.8 (7.0)	14.0(6.8)	0.20 (−1.00 to 1.39), p = 0. 745	0.61 (−0.49 to 1.72), p = 0.275
Hand Reaction time, msec, mean (SD)[b, c]	310.9 (104.6)	333.7(146.1)	334.3(132.7)	307.5 (108.1)	313.3(122.2)	346.9(149.3)	−11.82 (−38.82 to 15.17), p = 0.389	17.48 (−11.25 to 46.20), p = 0.232
Choice Stepping reaction time, step/sec, mean (SD)[a, c]	0.20 (0.13)	0.22 (0.14)	0.21 (0.2)	0.20 (0.13)	0.23 (0.15)	0.22 (0.2)	0.01 (−0.02 to 0.03), p = 0.591	0.01 (−0.02 to 0.03), p = 0.585
Grip strength, kg, mean (SD)[a, d]	20.4 (8.2)	19.99 (8.83)	19.05(7.99)	20.8 (8.9)	20.32 (8.91)	19.61(8.67)	0.48 (−5.07 to 1.40), p = 0.337	0.37 (−0.58 to 1.33), p = 0.444

Table 2. Cont.

	Control			Intervention			Difference between groups (baseline adjusted)	
	Baseline, n = 169	3 month, n = 137	12 month, n = 155	Baseline, n = 171	3 month, n = 156	12 month, n = 157	3month mean (95% CI), p	12 month mean (95% CI), p
Ankle flexibility, score, mean (SD)[a, d]	24.53 (9.54)	26.15(10.68)	24.98(9.62)	25.09 (10.49)	25.21(11.26)	25.08(10.99)	−1.19 (−3.74 to 1.36), p = 0.359	0.014 (−2.29 to 2.33), p = 0.991
Quality of life								
Health compared with past 12 months, n (%)[e]							OR 1.11, (0.72 to 1.72), p = 0.642	**OR 1.81 (1.19 to 2.76), p = 0.006**
Better	46 (27)	38 (28)	37 (24)	30 (18)	44 (29)	60 (38)		
Much the same	69 (41)	48 (35)	69 (45)	59 (35)	50 (33)	60 (38)		
Worse	54 (32)	50 (37)	49 (32)	82 (48)	59 (39)	37 (24)		
EQ5D utility score, mean (SD)[a, c]	0.62(0.23)		0.60(0.33)	0.63(0.23)		0.66(0.27)		0.04, −0.02 to 0.10 p = 0.229
SF12 Physical Component, mean (SD)[a, d]	38.17 (8.36)	40.32 (9.04)	39.27 (9.26)	37.44 (8.90)	40.10 (8.53)	40.37 (8.29)	−0.10 (−1.83 to 1.64), p = 0.914	*1.45 (−0.24 to 3.14), p = 0.093*
SF12 Mental Component, mean (SD)[a, d]	54.70 (6.79)	54.18 (7.01)	55.19 (7.09)	54.71 (6.49)	55.31 (6.37)	55.87 (5.02)	1.06 (−0.38 to 2.5), p = 0.149	0.70 (−0.59 to 1.99), p = 0.288
SF6D utility score, mean (SD)[a, d]	0.67 (0.10)	0.69 (0.12)	0.70 (0.12)	0.66 (0.10)	0.70 (0.11)	0.71 (0.11)	0.01 (−0.01 to 0.03), p = 0.346	*0.02 (−0.004 to 0.04), p = 0.096*
Falls efficacy scale, 7–28, mean (SD)[b, c]	11.56 (4.18)	11.97 (3.82)	13.14(4.87)	11.70 (4.09)	11.69 (3.94)	12.57 (4.22)	−0.31 (−1.03 to 0.41), p = 0.393	−0.52 (−1.40 to 0.36), p = 0.243
Health and community services, mean/month (SD)[b, f]	5.5 (6.7)		3.6 (6.1)	4.5 (5.0)		3.1 (7.4)		IRR 1.09 (0.85 to 1.40), p = 0.482
Assistance occasions/month, mean (SD)[b, f]	37.3 (43.2)		24.7 (37.5)	40.2(42.9)		25.3 (36.9)		IRR 0.91 (0.62 to 1.33), p = 0.631
Ease of personal care tasks, 0–50, mean (SD)[a, c]	41.4 (7.4)		38.7 (10.3)	41.5 (7.3)		40.5 (8.6)		*1.5 (−0.26 to 3.33), p = 0.094*
Community participation outings/month, mean (SD)[a, f]	5.9(7.3)	7.6 (10.3)	6.0(8.2)	5.8 (8.3)	6.2 (8.0)	7.5 (9.7)	0.91 (0.69 to 1.18), p = 0.459	**IRR 1.35 (1.05 to 1.75), p = 0.024**
Physical activity								
Total Physical Activity Score, hours/week[a, c]	18.13 (11.56)	26.26(15.74)	29.29(21.07)	18.5 (12.98)	27.34(16.34)	30.89(20.11)	0.59 (−2.46 to 3.64), p = 0.703	1.05 (−2.89 to 4.99), p = 0.600
Home Exercise, hours/week[a, c]	0.15 (0.33)	0.71 (1.30)	0.45 (0.98)	0.22 (0.47)	0.87 (1.51)	0.81 (1.40)	0.10 (−0.22 to 0.42), p = 0.521	**0.30 (0.03 to 0.58), p = 0.029**

[a]Higher scores reflect better performance.
[b]Lower scores reflect better performance.
[c]Between group differences are from linear regression models with change score (final minus initial) score as the dependent variable and group allocation and baseline performance on that item as independent variables.
[d]Between group differences are from linear regression models with follow-up score as the dependent variable and group allocation and baseline performance on that item as independent variables.
[e]Between group differences are from ordinal regression models with follow-up score as the dependent variable and group allocation and baseline performance on that item as independent variables.
[f]Between group differences are from negative binomial regression models with the total number of events as the dependent variable and group allocation and number of events at baseline as independent variables.
[g]some participants unable to be assessed due to knee pain or skin problems; data available for 168 per group at baseline; 3 months 131 control, 152 intervention;12 months 151 control, 156 intervention.
Bold indicates $p<0.05$ for between group differences. Italics indicate $p<0.1$ for between group differences.

Table 3. Intervention dose prescribed and adherence over the 12 month study period.

Time point	Participants who agreed to exercise, number (% of 171)	Exercise sessions agreed to, median (range)	Different exercises prescribed, median (range)	Exercise repetitions agreed to per session, mean (SD)	Participants who actually exercised, number (% of 171)	Exercise sessions completed, median (range)	Physiotherapist's estimate of % prescribed exercise completed, mean (SD)	Physiotherapist's estimate of number of exercise repetitions completed, mean (SD)
Month 1	162 (95%)	6 (0 to 7)	5 (0 to 8)	59 (39)	153 (90%)	5 (0 to 7)	77 (34)	266 (227)
Month 3	151 (88%)	5 (0 to 7)	6 (0 to 9)	93 (65)	138 (81%)	4 (0 to 7)	64 (38)	391 (396)
Month 8	130 (76%)	3 (0 to 7)	6 (0 to 9)	77 (70)	113 (66%)	3 (0 to 7)	51 (43)	289 (352)
Month 12	121 (71%)	3 (0 to 7)	5 (0 to 10)	72 (71)	103 (60%)	3 (0 to 7)	47 (43)	250 (335)

condition on admission to hospital ($p = 0.12$) and in those with a self-reported current or previous neurological condition ($p = 0.18$).

There was a greater impact on performance-based mobility for those with better MMSE scores (p for interaction = 0.037; between-group difference in those with MMSE scores less than 28 −0.001, 95% CI −0.16 to 0.16, $p = 0.995$, $n = 111$; between-group difference in those with MMSE scores 28 to 30 0.19, 95% CI 0.09 to 0.29, $p < 0.001$, $n = 201$). There was no evidence for differential effects on the performance-based mobility outcome on the basis of baseline gait speed (p for interaction = 0.626) or past falls (p for interaction = 0.274). There was no evidence for differential effects of the intervention on the self-reported mobility outcome on the basis of baseline gait speed (p for interaction = 0.254), MMSE score (p for interaction = 0.589) or past falls (p for interaction = 0.256).

Secondary outcomes

Secondary outcome results are shown in Table 2. The three-month assessment was completed by 292 participants (86% of those randomised) and was undertaken an average of 103 (SD 14) days after the baseline assessment. At 3 months after randomisation, there were significant between group differences for standing balance (maximal balance range and postural sway on foam) that favoured the exercise group after adjustment for baseline performance. There were no significant between-group differences for any other secondary outcomes at 3 months.

At 12 months after randomisation, there were significant between group differences in the 12-item version of the Short Physical Performance Battery, sit-to-stand ability, turning ability, reported health status (from the EQ-5D), social outings and reported home exercise that favoured the exercise group after adjustment for baseline performance. There were no significant between-group differences for any other secondary outcomes at 12 months. There were trends ($p < 0.1$) for better outcomes in the intervention group in measures of balance (maximal balance range and postural sway), quality of life (physical component), ease of daily task performance and community participation.

Adverse events

Twelve intervention group participants reported adverse events that may have been associated with the physical assessment or exercise program that resulted in limitations of activity of daily living for at least 48 hours or required medical attention. These included finger pain following the grip strength assessment in two people, thigh pain after the assessment in one person, low back pain in five people, calf pain in one person, knee pain in one person and exacerbation of hernia symptoms in two people. For 27 other people pre-existing conditions (mainly musculoskeletal) limited progression of the exercises.

Associations between intervention adherence and outcomes

The complier average causal effects of intervention estimated with instrumental variable regression were, inevitably, larger than the intention to treat-based estimates of effect. In compliant participants, exercise increased performance-based mobility by a mean of 0.27 points (95% CI 0.09 to 0.45) and increased self-reported ease of mobility by a mean of 1.1 points (95% CI −2.0 to 4. 2). As with the primary analysis, the effect on performance-based mobility was statistically significant ($p = 0.003$) but the effect on self-reported ease of mobility was not ($p = 0.485$).

Table 4. Falls outcomes.

	Control (n = 169)	Intervention (n = 171)	Difference between groups
Falls per participant, n (%)			
0	99 (59)	73 (43)	1.38 (1.11 to 1.73), p = 0.004[a]
1	45 (27)	58 (34)	
2	12 (7)	16 (9)	
3	4 (2)	13 (8)	
≥4	9 (5)	11 (6)	
All falls (primary outcome)	123	177	1.43 (1.07 to 1.93), p = 0.017[b]
Fall location			
Indoors	79	128	1.62 (1.13 to 2.33), p = 0.009[b]
Outdoors	44	49	1.10 (0.71 to 1.69), p = 0.670[b]
Falls with injuries			
Received health care	53	61	1.14 (0.76 to 1.73), p = 0.524[b]
Fractures	15	14	n/a[c]
Falls by time period			
Months 0–3	27	44	1.61 (0.98 to 2.65), p = 0.061, n = 340[b]
Months 4–6	19	49	2.56 (1.42 to 4.62), p = 0.002, n = 337
Months 7–9	27	25	0.92 (0.52 to 1.62), p = 0.774, n = 327
Months 9–12	50	59	1.16 (0.75 to 1.78), p = 0.503, n = 323
Participant reported cause of fall			
Lost balance	50	77	
Legs gave way	11	14	
Trip	35	58	
Slip	14	17	
Other	13	11	
Falls by gait subgroup			
≥ 0.73 m/s at baseline	80	85	1.95 (1.28 to 2.99), p = 0.002, n = 167
<0.73 m/s at baseline	43	92	1.15 (0.76 to 1.75), p = 0.498, n = 173

[a]Relative risk, 95% confidence interval and p value from modified Poisson regression model for the proportion of participants who had one or more falls in the 12 month follow up period in the intervention group compared to the control group.
[b]Incidence rate ratio, 95% confidence interval and p value from negative binomial regression model comparing the number of falls in the 12 month follow up period in the intervention group compared to the control group.
[c]Incidence rate ratio not calculated due to small numbers.

Discussion

This study found that a physiotherapist-prescribed tailored home exercise program enhanced performance-based mobility but significantly increased falls in older people recently discharged from hospital. Planned sub-group analyses revealed a greater increase in falls in those who walked more quickly at baseline and a greater improvement on performance-based mobility in those with better MMSE scores. The impact on mobility was greater in those who adhered well to the intervention.

The impact of the intervention on the continuously-scored primary measure of performance-based mobility was approximately 7% of baseline values (i.e., less than the 10% between-group difference we considered to be clinically meaningful prior to undertaking the study) yet represented a 0.5 point between-group difference in the 12-point version of the Short Physical Performance Battery a difference previously suggested to be "meaningful" [31]. This positive impact on mobility needs to be interpreted in the context of the increase in falls, which at 40% would probably be considered to be clinically meaningful by most.

The strengths of this study are its relatively large sample size, pragmatic design using a program that could be delivered as part of routine care, broad inclusion criteria and use of methods designed to reduce the risk of bias such as concealed random allocation to groups, blinded outcome assessment, small loss to follow up and pre-planned statistical analyses. The study's primary limitations are the commonly-reported sub-optimal adherence to the home exercise intervention (29% of those randomised to the intervention group no longer exercising at 12 months), the (unavoidable) reliance on self-reported falls data and the large number (93%) of screened participants who did not participate in the study which means that the sample may not be representative of older people recently discharged from hospital. The intention to treat approach used for the primary analyses probably underestimates the impact of the intervention in those who undertake a higher dose of ongoing exercise. A more supervised exercise program may have had different impact as it would have enabled ongoing encouragement and tailoring of exercise as well as the safe delivery of more challenging exercise.

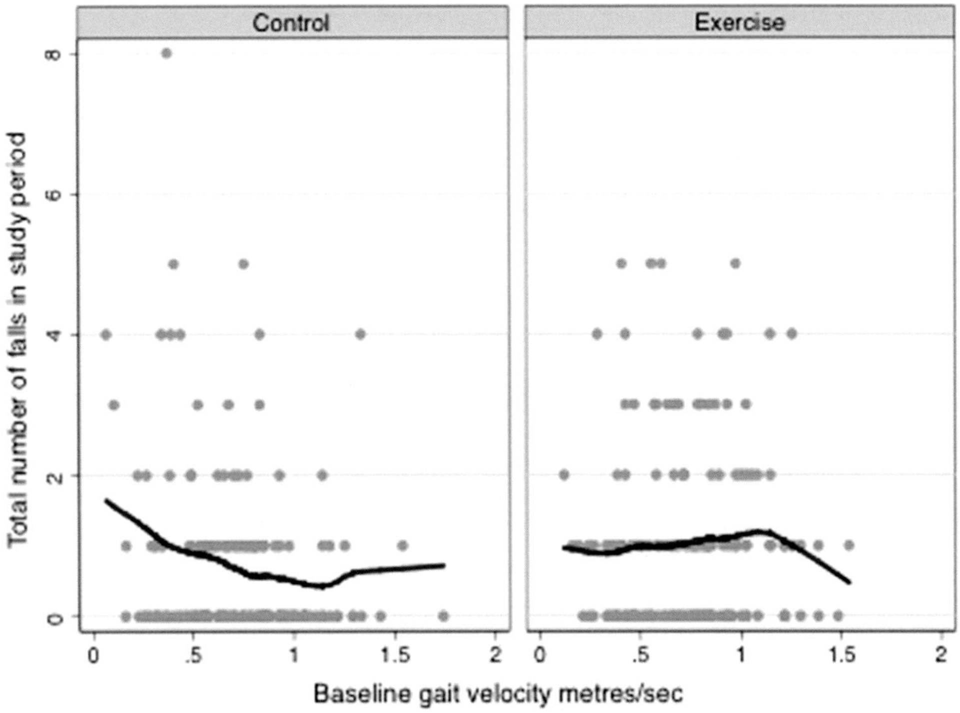

Figure 2. Number of falls in the 12-month study period by baseline walking velocity and group. The lines shown are locally weighted regression lines using Stata's "lowess" command.

These results differ from previous trials and meta-analyses showing fall prevention effects from home exercise interventions [5]. However, previous studies showing home exercise to prevent falls have been conducted in healthier older people than our sample. For example, the studies of the Otago Exercise Programme were conducted in people recruited from general practice records rather than those seeking health care [32]. Participants in the two Otago trials [33,34] were prescribed an average of 2–3 medications whereas participants in our trial were prescribed an average of 7 medications. As the WEBB program used in the present study included several exercises that also form part of the Otago Exercise Programme it seems unlikely that the use of a different program explains the different result in this study. Rather these results suggest that home exercise is not an appropriate single fall prevention intervention for people who have been recently hospitalised and this finding may apply to other high-risk populations. Our meta-analysis found trials of exercise conducted in higher risk samples to have smaller fall prevention effects than those conducted in the general population [11,35]. For example, one trial found a non-significant increase in falls from the Otago Exercise Programme in people with visual impairment [36] and another found a non-significant increase in falls from a group exercise program, especially in frail older people [37]. Conversely a highly supervised group exercise intervention did prevent falls in people with multiple previous falls [38] indicating uncertainty in this field.

Possible explanations for the greater number of falls in the intervention group include; i) harmful impact of exercise due to fatigue, exercise-induced muscle soreness or other pain exacerbated by exercise; ii) increased confidence or exposure to physical activity due to enhanced mobility; iii) harmful impact of partial adherence to the intervention (as outcomes were better in adherers after adjusting for other factors); iv) different time course of improvements in mobility and falls in this population (as the increase in falls was most evident in the first six months of the intervention period but the increase in mobility was greater at 12 months than 3 month assessments); v) over-reporting by the intervention group due to an increased awareness of falls; and vi) chance. Further research in high-risk populations is needed to explore these possibilities. The significant subgroup finding that the increase in falls was primarily among intervention group participants who walked more quickly at baseline should be treated with caution but warrants further investigation. It is possible that the faster walkers were actually walking "too quickly" to be safe given their recent illnesses and that this was somehow exacerbated by the intervention. The differential impact of the intervention on the mobility outcomes suggests that the more cognitively able and those with fewer past falls benefit more from this home exercise intervention in terms of mobility.

The impact of interventions specifically targeting safety (such as occupational therapy interventions), multifactorial programs and supervised exercise programs in people after recent hospital stays warrants investigation. Self-efficacy fall prevention interventions (such as the Stepping On program) [39] have been found to prevent falls in the general older population and also warrant investigation in older people following a hospital stay. Further research could also further investigate the interaction between increased mobility, physical activity, cognition, behaviour, and falls in high-risk people.

In conclusion, this approach to home exercise prescription significantly improved performance-based mobility but significantly increased the rate of falls in people after recent hospital stays. These findings suggest, therefore, that this form of home exercise cannot be recommended as a fall-prevention intervention for this group. Further studies, including the evaluation of the impact of multifactorial programs, are required to identify effective programs for preventing falls in this high-risk population.

Acknowledgments

Catherine Kirkham provided invaluable assistance with intervention delivery, assessments and data checking.

Author Contributions

Conceived and designed the experiments: CS SRL CMV RGC JCTC LC KH CMD. Performed the experiments: SDO EB ER. Analyzed the data: CS SDO GZH. Wrote the paper: CS SRL CMV RGC JCTC LC KH CMD EB ER SDO GZH.

References

1. Mahoney J, Sager M, Dunham NC, Johnson J (1994) Risk of falls after hospital discharge. J Am Geriatr Soc 42: 269–274.
2. Gill TM, Allore HG, Holford TR, Guo Z (2004) Hospitalization, restricted activity, and the development of disability among older persons. JAMA 292: 2115–2124.
3. Mahoney JE, Palta M, Johnson J, Jalaluddin M, Gray S, et al. (2000) Temporal association between hospitalization and rate of falls after discharge. Arch Intern Med 160: 2788–2795.
4. Sherrington C, Lord SR, Close JC, Barraclough E, Taylor M, et al. (2011) A simple tool predicted probability of falling after aged care inpatient rehabilitation. J Clin Epidemiol 64: 779–786.
5. Gillespie LD, Robertson MC, Gillespie WJ, Sherrington C, Gates S, et al. (2012) Interventions for preventing falls in older people living in the community. Cochrane Database Syst Rev 9: Cd007146.
6. Latham NK, Anderson CS, Lee A, Bennett DA, Moseley A, et al. (2003) A randomized, controlled trial of quadriceps resistance exercise and vitamin D in frail older people: the Frailty Interventions Trial in Elderly Subjects (FITNESS). J Am Geriatr Soc 51: 291–299.
7. Pahor M, Blair SN, Espeland M, Fielding R, Gill TM, et al. (2006) Effects of a physical activity intervention on measures of physical performance: Results of the lifestyle interventions and independence for Elders Pilot (LIFE-P) study. J Gerontol A Biol Sci Med Sci 61: 1157–1165.
8. Hauer K, Rost B, Rutschle K, Opitz H, Specht N, et al. (2001) Exercise training for rehabilitation and secondary prevention of falls in geriatric patients with a history of injurious falls. J Am Geriatr Soc 49: 10–20.
9. Timonen L, Rantanen T, Ryynanen OP, Taimela S, Timonen TE, et al. (2002) A randomized controlled trial of rehabilitation after hospitalization in frail older women: effects on strength, balance and mobility. Scand J Med Sci Sports 12: 186–192.
10. Vogler CM, Sherrington C, Ogle SJ, Lord SR (2009) Reducing risk of falling in older people discharged from hospital: a randomized controlled trial comparing seated exercises, weight-bearing exercises, and social visits. Arch Phys Med Rehabil 90: 1317–1324.
11. Sherrington C, Tiedemann A, Fairhall N, Close JC, Lord SR (2011) Exercise to prevent falls in older adults: an updated meta-analysis and best practice recommendations. N S W Public Health Bull 22: 78–83.
12. Dean CM, Rissel C, Sherrington C, Sharkey M, Cumming RG, et al. (2012) Exercise to enhance mobility and prevent falls after stroke: the community stroke club randomized trial. Neurorehabil Neural Repair 26: 1046–1057.
13. Cameron ID, Fairhall N, Langron C, Lockwood K, Monaghan N, et al. (2013) A multifactorial interdisciplinary intervention reduces frailty in older people: randomized trial. BMC Med 11: 65.
14. Fairhall N, Sherrington C, Kurrle SE, Lord SR, Lockwood K, et al. (2012) Effect of a multifactorial interdisciplinary intervention on mobility-related disability in frail older people: randomised controlled trial. BMC Med 10: 120.
15. Sherrington C, Lord SR, Vogler CM, Close JC, Howard K, et al. (2009) Minimising disability and falls in older people through a post-hospital exercise program: a protocol for a randomised controlled trial and economic evaluation. BMC Geriatr 9: 8.
16. Folstein MF, Folstein SE, McHugh PR (1975) "Mini-mental state". A practical method for grading the cognitive state of patients for the clinician. J Psychiatr Res 12: 189–198.
17. Marcus BH, Banspach SW, Lefebvre RC, Rossi JS, Carleton RA, et al. (1992) Using the stages of change model to increase the adoption of physical activity among community participants. Am J Health Promot 6: 424–429.
18. Haley SM, Andres PL, Coster WJ, Kosinski M, Ni P, et al. (2004) Short-form activity measure for post-acute care. Arch Phys Med Rehabil 85: 649–660.
19. Gibson MJ AR, Isaacs B, Radebaugh T, Worm-Petersen J. (1987) The prevention of falls in later life. A report of the Kellogg International Work Group on the Prevention of Falls by the Elderly. Dan Med Bull 34 Suppl 4: 1–24.
20. Guralnik JM, Simonsick EM, Ferrucci L, Glynn RJ, Berkman LF, et al. (1994) A short physical performance battery assessing lower extremity function: association with self-reported disability and prediction of mortality and nursing home admission. J Gerontol 49: M85–94.
21. Onder G, Penninx BW, Lapuerta P, Fried LP, Ostir GV, et al. (2002) Change in physical performance over time in older women: the Women's Health and Aging Study. J Gerontol A Biol Sci Med Sci 57: M289–293.
22. Lord SR, Menz HB, Tiedemann A (2003) A physiological profile approach to falls risk assessment and prevention. Phys Ther 83: 237–252.
23. Lord SR, Ward JA, Williams P (1996) Exercise effect on dynamic stability in older women: a randomized controlled trial. Arch Phys Med Rehabil 77: 232–236.
24. Lord SR, Fitzpatrick RC (2001) Choice stepping reaction time: a composite measure of falls risk in older people. J Gerontol A Biol Sci Med Sci 56: M627–632.
25. Moseley A, Adams R (1991) Measurement of passive ankle dorsiflexion: Procedure and reliability. Aust J Physiother 37: 175–181.
26. Brooks R, Rabin R, F dC (2003) The measurement and valuation of health status using EQ-5D: A European perspective. Dordrecht/Boston/London: Kluwer Academic Publishers.
27. Yardley L, Beyer N, Hauer K, Kempen G, Piot-Ziegler C, et al. (2005) Development and initial validation of the Falls Efficacy Scale-International (FES-I). Age Ageing 34: 614–619.
28. Delbaere K, Hauer K, Lord S (2010) Evaluation of the Incidental and Planned Exercise Questionnaire (IPEQ) for older people. Br J Sports Med 44: 1029–1034.
29. Angrist J, Imbens G, Rubin D (1996) Identification of causal effects using instrumental variables. Journal of the American Statistical Association 91: 444–455.
30. Shrier I, Steele R, Verhagen E, Herbert R, Riddell C, et al. (2014) Beyond intention to treat: What is the right question? Clinical Trials 11: 28–37.
31. Perera S, Mody SH, Woodman RC, Studenski SA (2006) Meaningful change and responsiveness in common physical performance measures in older adults. J Am Geriatr Soc 54: 743–749.
32. Robertson MC, Campbell AJ, Gardner MM, Devlin N (2002) Preventing injuries in older people by preventing falls: a meta-analysis of individual-level data. J Am Geriatr Soc 50: 905–911.
33. Campbell AJ, Robertson MC, Gardner MM, Norton RN, Tilyard MW, et al. (1997) Randomised controlled trial of a general practice programme of home based exercise to prevent falls in elderly women. BMJ 315: 1065–1069.
34. Robertson MC, Devlin N, Gardner MM, Campbell AJ (2001) Effectiveness and economic evaluation of a nurse delivered home exercise programme to prevent falls. 1: Randomised controlled trial. BMJ 322: 697–701.
35. Sherrington C, Whitney JC, Lord SR, Herbert RD, Cumming RG, et al. (2008) Effective exercise for the prevention of falls: a systematic review and meta-analysis. J Am Geriatr Soc 56: 2234–2243.
36. Campbell AJ, Robertson MC, La Grow SJ, Kerse NM, Sanderson GF, et al. (2005) Randomised controlled trial of prevention of falls in people aged > or = 75 with severe visual impairment: the VIP trial. BMJ 331: 817.
37. Faber MJ, Bosscher RJ, Chin APMJ, van Wieringen PC (2006) Effects of exercise programs on falls and mobility in frail and pre-frail older adults: A multicenter randomized controlled trial. Arch Phys Med Rehabil 87: 885–896.
38. Skelton D, Dinan S, Campbell M, Rutherford O (2005) Tailored group exercise (Falls Management Exercise – FaME) reduces falls in community-dwelling older frequent fallers (an RCT). Age Ageing 34: 636–639.
39. Clemson L, Cumming RG, Kendig H, Swann M, Heard R, et al. (2004) The effectiveness of a community-based program for reducing the incidence of falls in the elderly: a randomized trial. J Am Geriatr Soc 52: 1487–1494.

16

Difference in the Recruitment of Hip and Knee Muscles between Back Squat and Plyometric Squat Jump

Norihide Sugisaki[1,2]*, Sadao Kurokawa[3], Junichi Okada[4], Hiroaki Kanehisa[5]

1 Center for Environment, Health and Field Sciences, Chiba University, Kashiwa, Chiba, Japan, **2** Waseda Institute for Sport Sciences, Waseda University, Tokorozawa, Saitama, Japan, **3** Center for Liberal Arts, Meiji Gakuin University, Yokohama, Kanagawa, Japan, **4** Faculty of Sport Sciences, Waseda University, Tokorozawa, Saitama, Japan, **5** National Institute of Fitness and Sports in Kanoya, Kanoya, Kagoshima, Japan

Abstract

Athletes who aim to improve both muscular endurance and power often perform exercises that involve similar joint actions under different lifting conditions, such as changes in the load or speed, which are implemented at different times during a periodized exercise program or simultaneously. The prescribed exercises are considered to recruit the same muscles even if the lifting conditions differ to each other. The present study aimed to clarify this by examining whether the recruitment of individual hip and knee muscles during the squat exercise differs between lifting conditions adopted for muscular endurance and power training regimens. Moderately trained men performed back squats (BS), with a load of approximately 60% of one repetition maximum, as a muscular endurance training exercise, and they performed plyometric squat jumping (PSJ) for power training. During each exercise, the lower limb joint torques and the recruitment of five hip and knee muscles were determined with inverse-dynamics and T2-weighted magnetic resonance imaging, respectively. While the maximal and mean knee joint torques were greater during PSJ than during BS ($p<0.01$), the T2 values for the quadriceps femoris muscle did not differ between the exercises. In contrast, the T2 values of the gluteus maximus and hip adductor muscles were higher during PSJ ($p<0.05$) than during BS, although there was no significant difference in the mean hip extension torque between the two exercises. The current results indicate that the individual use of the agonist muscles differs between BS and PSJ, and it does not always correspond with the joint kinetics during the exercises. Therefore, in addition to the exercise type, the lifting condition should also be taken into consideration as a determinant of the major muscles trained during a resistance exercise.

Editor: Amir A. Zadpoor, Delft University of Technology (TUDelft), Netherlands

Funding: This study was supported by JSPS Grant-in-Aid for Scientific Research (24700667), (http://www.jsps.go.jp/j-grantsinaid/index.html). The funders had no role in study design, data collection and analysis, decision to publish, or preparation of the manuscript.

Competing Interests: The authors have declared that no competing interests exist.

* Email: sugisaki@chiba-u.jp

Introduction

The muscular endurance and power generation capabilities of the lower body are essential factors of fitness in not only athletes but also in the untrained populations. In general, exercises aimed to improve muscular endurance are performed at a relatively slow speed with a load corresponding to 15−20 repetitions maximum (RM) or 50−65% of one repetition maximum (1 RM) [1–5]. Exercises aimed at improving muscular power are generally performed at a high speed (explosive motion) with a relatively low load (e.g., 30–60% of 1 RM) [6–8] or without load (i.e., body weight plyometric exercise) [1,9]. Depending on the circumstances, athletes who aim to improve both muscular endurance and power often perform exercises that involve similar joint actions such as hip and knee extension and flexion, with different lifting conditions as mentioned above, in different training periods of a periodized program or simultaneously [1,2,10,11]. Both lifting conditions are considered to recruit (i.e. train) the same muscles because the major muscles involved are usually designated according to the event of exercise without regard to the lifting conditions, e.g., the gluteus maximus (GM), hamstrings (Ham), and quadriceps femoris muscles for squat exercises [12]. However, no study has examined whether the same muscles are recruited during an exercise performed under different lifting conditions. Clarifying this will be useful for designing an effective training program that aims to improve both muscular endurance and power.

Physical movements are usually achieved by forces produced by more than one muscle (i.e., synergist muscles). Synergist muscles differ in several ways, including the fiber type distribution [13], muscle architecture [14], and recruitment patterns [15]. Voigt et al. [15] reported that the soleus muscle dominated the plantar flexion movement in slow motion, while the activity of the gastrocnemius muscle increased in rapid motion. Considering these findings, it is natural to assume that the differences in lifting conditions between the muscular endurance and power training regimens produce a different synergist muscle use, even when exercises with almost similar joint involvement and motions are adopted.

The standard approach to evaluating muscular recruitment during exercise involves the use of surface electromyography (EMG). However, surface EMG has several disadvantages. For example, the detectable region is limited to a small part of the muscle, and it is difficult to detect deep muscle activity. In addition, the surface EMG signal of a small muscle could be affected by crosstalk from nearby muscles [16]. Furthermore, there are problems with surface EMG recordings during dynamic movements, such as a shift of the muscle relative to the electrode position and greater signal variability due to the rapid recruitment of motor units [17]. Several studies have provided evidence to support the use of transverse relaxation time (T2) measurements from magnetic resonance (MR) images of muscles as an alternative approach to assessing the recruitment of exercised muscles. It has been established that the increase in signal intensity and T2 of the muscles is associated with the exercise intensity [18] and osmotically driven shifts of fluid into an intracellular compartment (i.e., metabolic response) [19]. Furthermore, recent studies have revealed that regional increases in T2 after exercise training corresponded with the hypertrophic changes induced after chronic resistance training [20]. These findings indicate that the quantification of the exercise-induced increase in T2 is useful to evaluate the recruitment of individual muscles during an exercise with relation to the differences in the lifting conditions.

In the present study, we performed two experiments, which aimed to clarify the differences in the joint torque (Experiment 1) and recruitment of the thigh and hip muscles (Experiment 2) between the back squat (BS), with a load programmed for improving muscular endurance, and plyometric repeated squat jumping (PSJ) as a power training exercise. BS and PSJ are the most popular exercises for strengthening lower limb muscles and are characterized as multi-joint exercises involving hip, knee, and ankle joint extension, which require the use of various lower limb muscles. We hypothesized that the recruitment of the individual muscles involved in an exercise differs between BS and PSJ, even when the difference in the developed joint torque is taken into consideration.

Materials and Methods

Ethics Statement

This study was approved by the Ethics Committee on Human Research of Waseda University, and all procedures were conducted in accordance with the Declaration of Helsinki. Prior to the experiments, all subjects were fully informed of the purpose and risks of the experiment and gave their written consent.

Subjects

Ten healthy men (age 28±4 years, height 173±5 cm, weight 69±6 kg, PSJ jump height 44±6 cm, mean ± SD) voluntarily participated in Experiment 1, and 8 healthy men (age 24±2 years, height 172±8 cm, weight 69±6 kg, PSJ jump height 43±6 cm) in Experiment 2. Seven of the subjects in Experiment 2 were also involved in Experiment 1, and they completed all procedures in both experiments. The subjects had practiced squat training for at least 1 year and were familiar with the proper technique for executing the BS and PSJ tasks, which was confirmed by a certified strength and conditioning coach.

Procedures

Experiment 1. Joint kinematics and the ground reaction forces were determined during BS and PSJ. Prior to the test, the subjects performed at least 5 min of warm-up exercises, including static and less intensive dynamic stretching. The subjects were allowed to perform warm-up exercises of their choice except that they were required to perform static and dynamic stretching exercises for the triceps surae, the quadriceps femoris, the Ham, and the gluteus muscles. At the end of the warm-up session, the subjects performed one or two repetitions of BS and PSJ with the same conditions as the test trials to get familiar with the tasks. Following at least 5 min of rest after the completion of the warm-up session, the subjects performed barbell BS with a load equivalent to their body weight, which was determined using 5 kg increments. PSJ was performed without an external load. The BS load corresponded to 60±6% of 1 RM. BS and PSJ were performed using the techniques proposed by the National Strength and Conditioning Association [9,21]. Specifically, in BS, the subjects stood erect, grasping the bar with a closed pronated grip and holding the barbell on the upper back and shoulders with their feet shoulder-width apart and parallel to each other (starting position). For the downward movement, they flexed their hips and knees until the posterior surface of the thigh was parallel to the floor. For the upward movement, they extended the hips and knees until they reached the starting position. Throughout the movement, they maintained a flat back, with their elbows high and chest up and out. The number of repetitions was set to three. The subjects performed each repetition every 4 s at a steady speed following a verbal cue from an examiner. In the PSJ trials, the subjects performed six rebound jumps preceded by a counter movement jump. In other words, the subjects jumped explosively from the squatting position (the posterior surface of the thigh was parallel to the floor) using a counter movement with their feet shoulder-width apart, landed in the squat position, and immediately repeated the rebound jump six times. The subjects were instructed to jump as fast and as high as possible. Throughout the movement, they maintained a flat back and placed their hands behind their head. In both exercises, the depth of the descent was confirmed by an examiner and with a high-speed video camera. The number of repetitions was selected as three and six for BS and PSJ, respectively, to minimize the chances of fatigue and to obtain data from stable repetitions of each exercise. The number of repetitions for PSJ was set to six because the jump height in PSJ reached a plateau after the third or fourth jump, which was confirmed in a pilot experiment. The order of the conditions was randomized for each subject. The subjects had a rest period of at least 5 min between the different conditions.

Experiment 2. T2 weighted cross-sectional MR images were obtained before and after the completion of BS and PSJ. The subjects performed BS and PSJ under the same conditions used in Experiment 1. The load for BS was set to 59±5% of 1 RM. The measurements for BS and PSJ were performed on separate days, with a minimum interval of 1 wk. The order of the conditions was randomized for each subject. The subjects performed three sets of 15 repetitions, with a 90 s rest interval between sets, for both the BS and PSJ tasks. Although it is recommended that power-training exercise should be performed without fatigue [9,22], the same number of repetitions and sets and rest intervals, as in BS, were adopted in PSJ to ensure T2 changed and reached a plateau [23].

Data collection and analysis

Experiment 1. The positions of reflective markers placed on six body landmarks (i.e., costa XII, the greater trochanter, the center of rotation of the knee joint, the lateral malleolus, the great toe, and the calcaneal tuber) on the right side were recorded using a high-speed video camera (EX-F1; Casio, Japan) with a sampling frequency of 300 fps. The camera was positioned perpendicular to the sagittal plane of motion at a distance of 15 m from the subject. Simultaneously, vertical and horizontal ground reaction forces on the right foot were recorded using a force platform (Model 6012–15; Bertec, USA). The reflective markers were digitized in each field using a motion analysis software (Frame-DIAS IV; DKH, Japan) to obtain the coordinates in the sagittal plane, and the data were smoothed using a fourth-order zero-lag Butterworth low pass filter with a cut-off of 8 Hz based on residual analysis [24]. The torques at the hip, knee, and ankle were determined from the body landmark coordinates and the ground reaction forces using two-dimensional inverse dynamics analysis [24]. The joint power was calculated by multiplying the joint torque by the joint angular velocity. Subsequently, the maximal and mean extension torques, extension and flexion angular velocity, and positive and negative joint power were calculated. The analyses were performed for the phase from the start to the end of lower limb joint movement for BS, and from touch-down to take-off for PSJ. Data processing was performed using the MATLAB software (MATLAB 7.10; MathWorks, USA). For BS, the average value of three repetitions, and for PSJ, the average value of the last three jumps was used as representative data.

Experiment 2. Before and after the execution of the exercise tasks, 15 consecutive 10-mm thick T2 weighted cross-sectional MR images were obtained at 20 mm intervals using an MR imaging system (Signa HDxt 1.5T; GE, USA) (Figure 1). The MR images were obtained in an order so that the position of the third slice corresponded with the greater trochanter. During imaging, the subject lay prone on the test bench of the MR imaging system and was fixed at the waist and knee with straps. The image sequence for T2 measurement was as follows: echo time, 25, 50, 75, and 100 ms; repetition time, 2500 ms; field of view, 48 cm; matrix, 256 × 192. The MR imaging started within 2 min from the completion of exercise.

The MR images were transferred to a computer, and the cross-sectional areas of the GM, the rectus femoris (RF), the vasti (Vas; including the vastus medialis, vastus lateralis, and vastus intermedius), the hip adductors (Add; including the adductor magnus, adductor brevis, and adductor longus), and the Ham of both legs were determined from each image using an open source image processing software (OsiriX v.2.4; Pixmeo, Switzerland). Care was taken to exclude non-contractile tissues such as intramuscular fat, nerves, and blood vessels. For each muscle, a T2 analysis was performed for the images with a cross-sectional area greater than 1000 mm^2 because the reproducibility of T2 measurement was poor in the images with a cross-sectional area less than 1000 mm^2, i.e., the coefficient of variance and intraclass correlation coefficient for repeated measures were more than 10% and less than 0.8, respectively. The number of slices used for the T2 measurements were 6, 6, 12, 7, and 6 for the GM, RF, Vas, Add, and Ham, respectively. For the pre-exercise images, the T2 for each pixel within each muscle was calculated, and the mean value was computed. In the post-exercise images, the pixels with a T2 value greater than the pre-exercise mean +1 SD were regarded as activated, and the proportion of the total number of pixels in the muscle cross-sectional area was expressed as a percent of the activated area (% activated area) [20,25]. The T2 measurement was performed on both sides, and the mean value was used.

Statistical Analyses

Descriptive data are expressed as mean ± SEM. For the data obtained in Experiment 1, a paired t-test was used to examine the differences between exercises. For the data obtained in Experiment 2, a repeated measures two-way ANOVA was used to test the interaction between the region and exercise for each muscle. Additionally, a repeated measures two-way ANOVA with Bonferroni post-hoc test was used to examine the main effects of muscle (5 muscles) and exercise (2 exercises), as well as their interaction. Cohen's *d* and the partial eta squared (η^2_p) were calculated to demonstrate the effect sizes. The Greenhouse–Geisser statistic was applied when the sphericity assumption was violated. For all statistics, the significance level was set at $p<0.05$.

Results

Experiment 1

Figure 2 shows an example of the time course of torques and angles of the ankle, knee, and hip joints during BS and PSJ. Descriptive data on the maximal and mean joint torques for each of the BS and PSJ are shown in Table 1. The plantar flexion

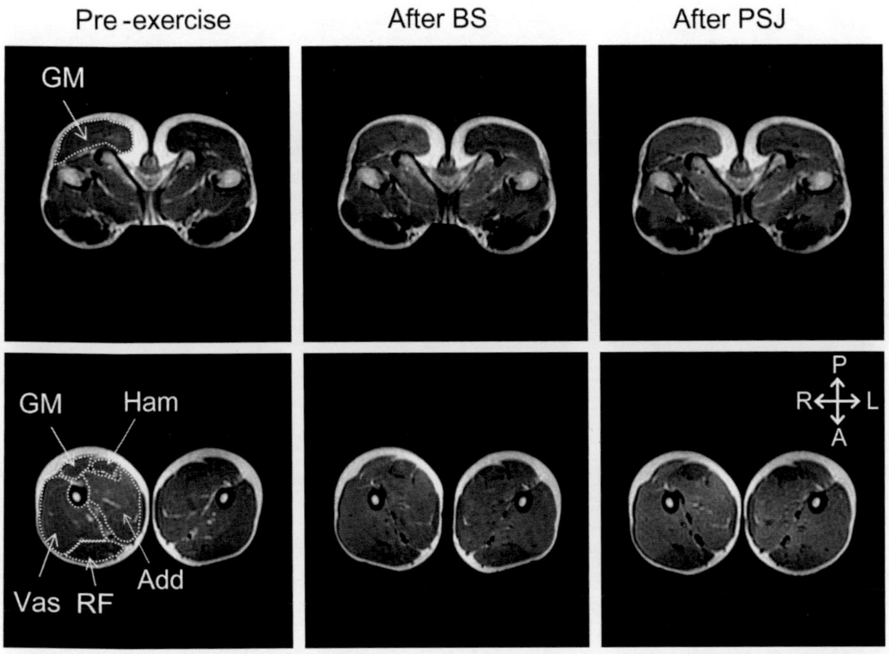

Figure 1. Examples of T2-weighted magnetic resonance images of hip (upper) and thigh (lower) regions at pre-exercise (left), after BS (middle), and after PSJ (right). GM, the gluteus maximus; Vas, the vasti muscles; RF, the rectus femoris muscle; Add, the hip adductors; Ham, the hamstrings. A, anterior; P, posterior; R, right; L, left.

torque in PSJ rapidly increased after foot contact and peaked at 33±8% contact time and decreased immediately before take-off, while that in BS was almost constant over the time course. The maximal and mean plantar flexion torques were significantly greater in PSJ than in BS ($p<0.01$). For the knee joint, an impulsive extension torque was found immediately after foot contact (4±0% contact time) and the torque was greater through the foot contact, especially in the downward phase, i.e., eccentric phase. The maximal and mean knee extension torques were significantly greater in PSJ than in BS ($p<0.01$). In contrast, there was no significant difference in the mean hip extension torque between the two tasks, while the maximal hip extension torque associated with an impulsive hip extension torque after foot contact (12±1% contact time) was significantly greater in PSJ than in BS ($p<0.01$). At all joints, the extension and flexion angular velocities (Table 2) and positive and negative power values (Table 3) were significantly ($p<0.01$) greater in PSJ than in BS.

Experiment 2

Figure 3 shows the % activated area of each muscle along its length. A two-way ANOVA revealed no significant interactions between the exercise and region for all muscles (GM, $F[5,35]=1.520$, $p=0.209$, $\eta^2_p=0.178$; RF, $F[5,35]=1.409$, $p=0.245$, $\eta^2_p=0.168$; Vas, $F[11, 77]=1.599$, $p=0.116$, $\eta^2_p=0.186$; Add, $F[2.3, 16.3]=0.264$, $p=0.802$, $\eta^2_p=0.036$; Ham, $F[5,35]=1.273$, $p=0.298$, $\eta^2_p=0.154$). On the other hand, a 2-way ANOVA for % activated area value averaged for all slices revealed a significant interaction between exercise and muscle ($F[4,28]=3.183$, $p=0.028$, $\eta^2_p=0.313$). Paired comparisons (Table 4) showed that the % activated areas of the GM and Add were significantly larger in PSJ than in BS ($p<0.05$). In addition, in both exercises, the % activated area of the Ham was smaller than that of other muscles except for the RF ($p<0.05$).

Discussion

The joint power output was much greater in PSJ than in BS, which confirms that the PSJ was an appropriate exercise for improving muscular power. The % activated areas of the Vas and RF were similar between BS and PSJ, while the maximal and mean knee extension torques were much greater during PSJ. In contrast, the % activated areas of the GM and Add were greater (16% and 18%, respectively) during PSJ, whereas the mean hip extension torque did not differ between the two exercises. The observed differences had a large effect size. According to Adams et al. [26], a 1% increase in an electrically evoked isometric knee extension torque corresponded with a 0.7% increase in the % activated area of the quadriceps femoris muscle, i.e., a 1% difference in the % activated area corresponded with a 1.4% difference in the joint torque. In addition, a previous study reported that a ~10% difference in the % activated area during a resistance training exercise induced a difference in the magnitude of hypertrophy after a long-term training period [20]. Thus, we may say that the observed differences in muscle recruitment have a practical significance in the designing of a training program that includes BS and PSJ. As noted earlier, it has been established that the changes in T2 reflect the recruitment of individual muscles [18,26]. Therefore, the present findings indicate that the individual muscle recruitment differs between BS and PSJ, which does not necessarily correspond with the joint kinetics. In other words, the current results imply that the lifting condition affects individual muscle recruitment and joint kinetics differently.

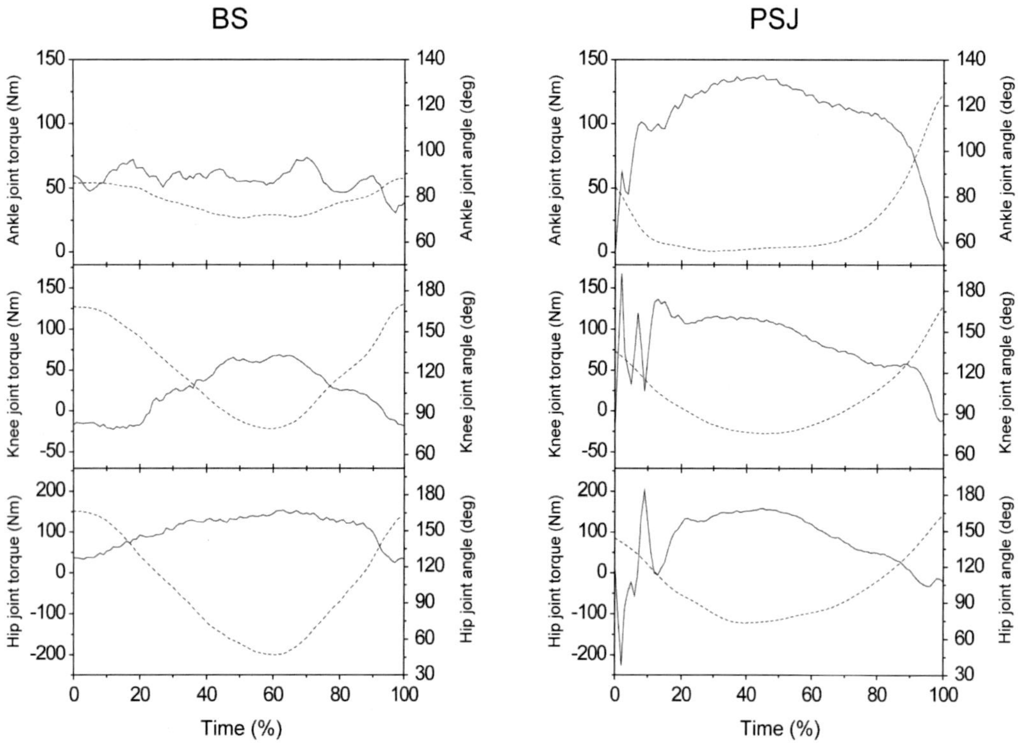

Figure 2. Time course of each joint torque and angle during back squat and plyometric squat jumping. BS, back squat; PSJ squat jumping. Data from 1 subject are presented. The solid and dashed lines indicate the torque and angle, respectively. Positive values indicate extension. Time is represented as percentage of analysis time, i.e., from start to end of repetition in BS and from touch down to take off in PSJ.

Table 1. Comparison of the joint torque between BS and PSJ (N · m).

		BS	PSJ	*d*
Plantar flexion	Maximum	78±3	125±8*	1.87
	Mean	48±2	81±6*	1.70
Knee extension	Maximum	82±3	186±21*	1.70
	Mean	55±2	76±5*	1.61
Hip extension	Maximum	149±5	272±32*	1.27
	Mean	95±4	97±7	0.09

Values are mean ± SEM. PSJ, plyometric squat jumping, BS, back squat.
*indicates that PSJ is greater than BS ($p<0.01$).

The results of the % activated area of the quadriceps femoris muscle (Table 4) indicate that the recruitment of this muscle group was similar between the two exercise tasks, although the maximal and mean knee extension torques were greater during PSJ than during BS (Table 1). This may be due to the difference in the type of muscle contraction between the two lifting conditions. It is well known that during a stretch-shortening cycle type of muscle action, the skeletal muscles can exert greater force than that during pure concentric muscle action [27]. Therefore, it seems that the quadriceps femoris muscle could generate greater knee extension torque during PSJ with the same recruitment level as BS. In addition, EMG studies have shown lower activation levels in isometric contractions compared to dynamic contractions [28]. Similarly, the change in the MR-based signal intensity has been shown to be less during isometric contraction than during dynamic contraction [29], indicating that the signal intensity depends on the type of contraction. During squat exercises with a stretch-shortening cycle, the vastus lateralis muscle fibers contract quasi-isometrically due to tendon elongation [30]. Based on these findings, it may be assumed that the quadriceps muscle fibers could generate a force with a smaller length change during PSJ, which might have contributed to a similar % activated area between PSJ and BS, in spite of the significant difference in the knee extension torque.

Another explanation for the knee extension torque being greater in PSJ with a similar recruitment of the quadriceps muscle is that the passive knee extension force of non-contractile elements such as tendon or connective tissue would be greater in PSJ. In PSJ, the hip was in a more extended position (Figure 2). Therefore, there is a possibility that the RF, which crosses the knee and hip joints, is longer, and consequently, the passive knee extension force would be greater in PSJ. This would result in a greater musculo-tendon force, or joint torque, which is the sum of the forces generated by contractile (active) and non-contractile (passive) elements.

The contraction levels of antagonist muscles can affect the net joint torque and should therefore be considered when discussing the discrepancy in the use of the knee joint and the quadriceps muscles between the two lifting conditions. The net joint torque is the sum of torques produced by the agonist and antagonist muscles. During knee extension, the Ham and gastrocnemius muscles operate as major antagonistic muscles. Thus, there is a possibility that the lower contraction levels of antagonist knee flexors could be associated with greater knee joint torque with the same recruitment level of the quadriceps muscles during PSJ than during BS. However, the % activated area of the Ham did not differ between the two conditions (Table 4). In addition, it is quite unlikely that the recruitment of gastrocnemius muscles was lower during PSJ than during BS because the plantar flexion torque was much greater during PSJ than during BS (Figure 2, Table 1).

Table 2. Comparison of the joint angular velocity between BS and PSJ (deg/s).

			BS	PSJ	*d*
Ankle	Plantar flexion	Maximum	51±5	743±29*	8.02
		Mean	19±2	246±14*	5.19
	Dorsiflexion	Maximum	42±3	679±36*	5.63
		Mean	15±1	208±22*	2.84
Knee	Extension	Maximum	153±13	828±25*	7.01
		Mean	74±5	348±13*	8.61
	Flexion	Maximum	113±7	522±28*	4.32
		Mean	54±3	264±11*	6.21
Hip	Extension	Maximum	150±11	504±25*	4.83
		Mean	74±5	248±10*	5.08
	Flexion	Maximum	117±5	461±34*	3.28
		Mean	60±4	260±22*	2.93

Values are mean ± SEM. PSJ, plyometric squat jumping, BS, back squat.
* indicates that PSJ is greater than BS ($p<0.01$).

Table 3. Comparison of the joint power between BS and PSJ (Watt).

			BS	PSJ	*d*
Plantar flexion	Positive	Maximum	44±6	940±81*	3.50
		Mean	18±3	314±36*	2.60
	Negative	Maximum	29±2	900±81*	3.38
		Mean	10±1	239±36*	2.03
Knee extension	Positive	Maximum	95±7	545±47*	3.00
		Mean	40±3	294±27*	3.14
	Negative	Maximum	97±10	1418±137*	3.05
		Mean	46±5	413±36*	3.29
Hip extension	Positive	Maximum	244±24	664±76*	1.65
		Mean	128±12	289±27*	1.69
	Negative	Maximum	184±15	1948±248*	2.28
		Mean	91±7	442±51*	2.22

Values are mean ± SEM. PSJ, plyometric squat jumping, BS, back squat.
* indicates that PSJ is greater than BS ($p<0.01$).

These aspects suggest that the recruitment of antagonists is unlikely to be the reason for the discrepancy between the knee joint kinetics and the recruitment of the quadriceps muscle.

The influence of the lifting conditions on the joint kinetics and recruitment of muscles at the hip joint differed from that at the knee joint. That is, the % activated area of the GM and Add was greater in PSJ than in BS (Table 4), although there was no significant difference in the mean hip extension torque between the two conditions (Table 1). This indicates that during PSJ, the recruitment of hip extensor was greater so as to generate the same mean joint torque as during BS. Four possibilities might explain these findings. First, the hip angular velocity in PSJ was much greater than that in BS (Table 2). In contrast to the quadriceps femoris muscle, GM and Add do not have long tendons [31], and thus, the contraction velocity of muscle fibers in PSJ would be greater than in BS. Based on the force-velocity characteristic of muscle fibers, the concentric force is greatly affected by the contraction velocity, while the eccentric force is less influenced by it [32]. Thus, it seems that, for GM and Add, force production during the upward (concentric) phase of PSJ would be performed in a disadvantageous condition as compared to that in BS. Second, there could be a difference in the contraction level of the antagonistic muscles between the two conditions. That is, the activities of the hip flexors and/or abductors could be greater during PSJ than during BS. Considering that the % activated area of the RF did not differ between the exercise conditions, it might be assumed that the activities of muscles such as the psoas major and gluteus medius, (a major hip flexor and a major hip abductor, respectively) could be greater during PSJ. For the Add muscles, it is also possible that a greater hip adduction torque would be exerted during PSJ, probably for stabilizing the pelvis during dynamic movement. Third, the difference in the hip joint angle between the two conditions might have affected the present results. During PSJ, the hip joint was in a more extended position than during BS (Figure 2). According to their joint angle and moment arm length relationships [33], the GM and Add can exert a greater hip extension torque in a more flexed position of the hip. Therefore, it seems that during PSJ, the GM and Add would be highly activated to generate the same hip extension torque as during BS. Lastly, a decreased hip flexion angle in PSJ would cause an increase in passive hip flexion force and a decrease in passive hip extension force resulting in increased muscular contribution for developing a given hip extension torque.

Previous studies have reported that during a squat, the EMG activity of the Ham is relatively high (30–80% maximal isometric contraction level) [34–36]. However, regardless of exercise conditions, the % activated area of the Ham was much lower than that of other muscles, except for the RF (Table 4). It seems that 60% of the 1 RM load or body weight was not large enough to elicit a strong co-contraction response of the Ham. However, Ploutz-Snyder et al. [37] reported that there was no MR contrast shift in the Ham following a 10 RM barbell squat. Enocson et al. [38] also reported that the change in the Ham MR signal intensity following the leg press exercise was negligible, regardless of the load. The present results support these findings and indicate that the change in the muscle MR signal intensity does not always correspond with the electromyographic activity. While EMG represents the neural input to a muscle, MR signal intensity is thought to reflect metabolites produced as a result of muscle contraction [19]. We therefore believe that the Ham were used lesser, in the presence of neural drive, during squat exercises, regardless of the load and/or speed conditions. This idea is supported by the evidence of lack of Ham hypertrophy after a 7-week, 3–25 RM BS training program, regardless of the load [39].

The lower % activated area of the Ham during a squat may also be due to the limited length change of these muscles during squat exercises. As described earlier, the change in the MR signal intensity is less during isometric contraction than during dynamic contraction [29]. The Ham cross the hip and knee joints, and flexion of these joints induces elongation and shortening of the Ham, respectively, and vice versa. Therefore, during squat exercises, there would be no change in the length of the Ham, and these muscles would contract almost isometrically resulting in a lower % activated area. In addition, it should be taken into consideration that the T2 change is more prominent in fast twitch fibers than in slow fibers [19]. The percentage of fast twitch fibers of the Ham (33.1% for the biceps femoris) has been reported to be relatively lower than those of the other muscles tested in the present study (GM, 47.6%; RF, 57.2–70.5%; Vas, 38.5–67.3%; Add, 36.7–46.5%) [40]. Therefore, we cannot rule out that the recruitment level of the Ham, assessed with the change in T2,

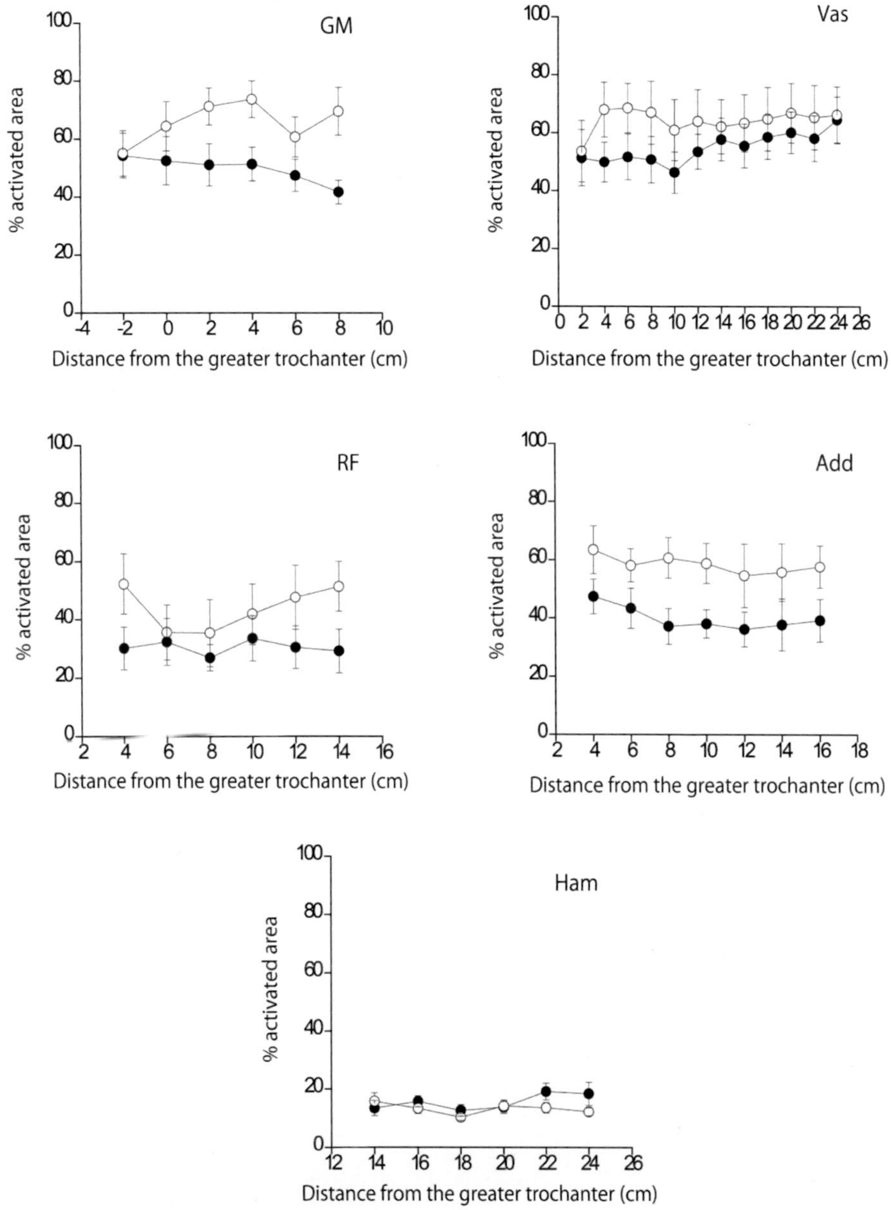

Figure 3. The % activated area of each muscle along its length as a function of the distance from the greater trochanter. The closed and open circles indicate back squat and plyometric squat jumping, respectively. GM, the gluteus maximus; Vas, the vasti muscles; RF, the rectus femoris muscle; Add, the hip adductors; Ham, the hamstrings. There was no significant interaction between the region and exercise condition.

Table 4. % activated area value averaged for all slices.

	BS	**PSJ**	***d***
Gluteus maximus	50±5	66±7*	0.92
Vasti	55±8	64±10	0.35
Rectus femoris	36±10	44±7	0.23
Adductors	40±6	58±7*	1.11
Hamstrings	16±2†	13±1†	0.40

Values are mean ± SEM. PSJ, plyometric squat jumping, BS, back squat.
*indicates that PSJ is greater than BS ($p<0.05$).
†indicates that Hamstrings was smaller than Gluteus maximus, and Adductors ($p<0.01$).

could be affected by the muscle fiber type and consequently might have been underestimated to some degree.

The present results indicated that in a multi-joint exercise, synergist muscle recruitment differs between the two lifting conditions, even though the exercises used are similar in terms of joints involved and their motions (i.e., hip and knee extension and flexion). For designing an effective and efficient training program, however, knowledge of how each of the load and speed conditions affects the synergist muscle use is essential. If the observed differences in individual muscle use between the lifting conditions were caused by differences in the type of muscle action, co-contraction levels, hip joint angular position, and/or velocity, as mentioned above, it seems that the speed of movement (slow constant speed vs. dynamic) rather than the load would be a major factor producing it; this should be clarified in future studies.

In addition, it should be noted that in the T2 measurement adopted here, the time course of muscle recruitment during an exercise cannot be determined. Therefore, we cannot identify the timing or phase of the exercise during which the difference in synergist muscle recruitment between BS and PSJ was yielded. When devising a training program on the basis of specificity (i.e., specific adaptation to imposed demand), information on the recruitment pattern during an exercise is important and should be investigated in future studies. The combined use of EMG and T2 MRI could provide more insight into this issue. Furthermore, the approach to this issue should include limiting the range of motion (i.e., depth of dip) or the phase (i.e., only the descending phase).

Lastly, we would like to comment on the accuracy and repeatability of T2 measurements. The present study used T2 measurements and compared two extremely different lifting conditions and revealed the differences in the synergist muscle use with a large effect size. However, more elaborate studies with higher accuracy and repeatability of T2 measurements would be needed for a more complete understanding of the effect of the lifting conditions on synergist muscle recruitment. It is therefore essential to improve the imaging resolution and examiner's skill required for identification of non-contractile tissue such as intramuscular fat, nerve, tendinous tissue, and blood vessels in MR images. In addition, the subjects should be highly skilled in the tasks used to examine whether muscular recruitment differs between the tasks in spite of the similarity in joints involved and action mode adopted. Furthermore, the observer of T2-weighted MR images in the present study was not blinded to the subjects and pre-/post-exercise images. The post-exercise T2-weighted MR images clearly differed from the pre-exercise images in that some of the muscles appeared lighter on the images. However, the fact that the observer of the images was not blind to the subjects and pre-/post-exercise images raises the possibility of an unintended bias on the observer's part that would affect the results. In future studies, these issues should be improved upon to take advantage of the T2 technique for identifying muscle recruitment during various resistance exercises.

In conclusion, the present study shows that the individual use of hip and knee muscles, assessed based on the T2 measurements from MR images, differs between BS as a muscular endurance training exercise and PSJ as a power training exercise. This difference did not necessarily correspond with the joint kinetics. The current results indicate that the difference in lifting conditions produces a different synergist muscle use, even when an exercise with similar movements of the body segments is adopted. Thus, not only the exercise type but also the lifting condition should be taken into consideration as a determinant of the major muscles trained in a resistance exercise.

Author Contributions

Conceived and designed the experiments: NS JO HK. Performed the experiments: NS. Analyzed the data: NS SK HK. Wrote the paper: NS SK JO HK.

References

1. Ratamess A (2011) Resistance training program design. In: Ratamess A, editor. ACSM's foundation of strength training and conditioning. Philadelphia, PA: Lippincott Williams &Wilkins. 192–228.
2. Wathen D, Baechle TR, Earle RW (2008) Periodization. In: Baechle TR, Earle RW, editors. Essentials of strength training and conditioning 3rd ed. Champaign, IL: Human Kinetics. 507–522.
3. Rhea MR, Phillips WT, Burkett LN, Stone WJ, Ball SD, et al. (2003) A comparison of linear and daily undulating periodized programs with equated volume and intensity for local muscular endurance. J Strength Cond Res 17: 82–87.
4. Smilios I, Hakkinen K, Tokmakidis SP (2010) Power output and electromyographic activity during and after a moderate load muscular endurance session. J Strength Cond Res 24: 2122–2131.
5. Willardson JM, Burkett LN (2006) The effect of rest interval length on the sustainability of squat and bench press repetitions. J Strength Cond Res 20: 400–403.
6. Baker D, Nance S, Moore M (2001) The load that maximizes the average mechanical power output during jump squats in power-trained athletes. J Strength Cond Res 15: 92–97.
7. Kaneko M, Fuchimoto T, Toji H, Suei K (1983) Training effect of different loads on the force-velocity relationship and mechanical power output in human muscle. Scandinavian Journal of Sports Sciences 5: 50–55.
8. Newton RU, Murphy AJ, Humphries BJ, Wilson GJ, Kraemer WJ, et al. (1997) Influence of load and stretch shortening cycle on the kinematics, kinetics and muscle activation that occurs during explosive upper-body movements. Eur J Appl Physiol Occup Physiol 75: 333–342.
9. Potach DH, Chu DA (2008) Plyometric training. In: Baechle TR, Earle RW, editors. Essentials of strength training and conditioning. 3rd ed. Champaign, IL: Human Kinetics. 413–456.
10. Sedano S, Marin PJ, Cuadrado G, Redondo JC (2013) Concurrent training in elite male runners: the influence of strength versus muscular endurance training on performance outcomes. J Strength Cond Res 27: 2433–2443.
11. Taipale RS, Mikkola J, Vesterinen V, Nummela A, Hakkinen K (2013) Neuromuscular adaptations during combined strength and endurance training in endurance runners: maximal versus explosive strength training or a mix of both. Eur J Appl Physiol 113: 325–335.
12. Earle RW, Baechle TR (2008) Resistance training and spotting techniques. In: Baechle TR, Earle RW, editors. Essentials of Strength Training and Conditioning. 3rd ed. Champaign, IL: Human Kinetics. 325–376.
13. Elder GC, Bradbury K, Roberts R (1982) Variability of fiber type distributions within human muscles. Journal of Applied Physiology 53: 1473–1480.
14. Kawakami Y, Abe T, Kanehisa H, Fukunaga T (2006) Human skeletal muscle size and architecture: variability and interdependence. Am J Hum Biol 18: 845–848.
15. Voigt M, Dyhre-Poulsen P, Simonsen EB (1998) Modulation of short latency stretch reflexes during human hopping. Acta Physiol Scand 163: 181–194.
16. Farina D, Merletti R, Enoka RM (2004) The extraction of neural strategies from the surface EMG. J Appl Physiol 96: 1486–1495.
17. Farina D (2006) Interpretation of the surface electromyogram in dynamic contractions. Exerc Sport Sci Rev 34: 121–127.
18. Fisher MJ, Meyer RA, Adams GR, Foley JM, Potchen EJ (1990) Direct relationship between proton T2 and exercise intensity in skeletal muscle MR images. Investigative Radiology 25: 480–485.
19. Prior BM, Ploutz-Snyder LL, Cooper TG, Meyer RA (2001) Fiber type and metabolic dependence of T2 increases in stimulated rat muscles. Journal of Applied Physiology 90: 615–623.
20. Wakahara T, Miyamoto N, Sugisaki N, Murata K, Kanehisa H, et al. (2012) Association between regional differences in muscle activation in one session of resistance exercise and in muscle hypertrophy after resistance training. Eur J Appl Physiol 112: 1569–1576.
21. Baechle TR, Earle RW, Wathen D (2008) Resistance training. In: Baechle TR, Earle RW, editors. Essentials of strength training and conditioning 3rd ed. Champaign, IL: Human Kinetics. 414–456.
22. Ratamess A (2011) Plyometric training. In: Ratamess A, editor. ACSM's foundation of strength training and conditioning. Philadelphia, PA: Lippincott Williams &Wilkins. 331–379.
23. Fleckenstein JL, Watumull D, McIntire DD, Bertocci LA, Chason DP, et al. (1993) Muscle proton T2 relaxation times and work during repetitive maximal voluntary exercise. Journal of Applied Physiology 74: 2855–2859.

24. Winter DA (2009) Biomechanics and motor control of human movement 4th ed. Hoboken, NJ: John Wiley & Sons. 370 p.
25. Adams GR, Harris RT, Woodard D, Dudley GA (1993) Mapping of electrical muscle stimulation using MRI. Journal of Applied Physiology 74: 532–537.
26. Adams GR, Duvoisin MR, Dudley GA (1992) Magnetic resonance imaging and electromyography as indexes of muscle function. Journal of Applied Physiology 73: 1578–1583.
27. Cavagna GA, Dusman B, Margaria R (1968) Positive work done by a previously stretched muscle. J Appl Physiol 24: 21–32.
28. Ball N, Scurr JC (2011) Efficacy of current and novel electromyographic normalization methods for lower limb high-speed muscle actions. European Journal of Sport Science 11: 447–456.
29. Price TB, Kennan RP, Gore JC (1998) Isometric and dynamic exercise studied with echo planar magnetic resonance imaging (MRI). Medicine and Science in Sports and Exercise 30: 1374–1380.
30. Ishikawa M, Finni T, Komi PV (2003) Behaviour of vastus lateralis muscle-tendon during high intensity SSC exercises in vivo. Acta Physiologica Scandinavica 178: 205–213.
31. Yamaguchi GT, Sawa AGU, Moran DW, Fessler MJ, Winters JM (1990) A survey of human musculotendon actuator parameters. In: Winters JM, Woo SL-Y, editors. Multiple muscle system: Biomechanics and movement organization. New York: Springer. 717–773.
32. Edman KA (1979) The velocity of unloaded shortening and its relation to sarcomere length and isometric force in vertebrate muscle fibres. J Physiol 291: 143–159.
33. Dostal WF, Soderberg GL, Andrews JG (1986) Actions of hip muscles. Physical Therapy 66: 351–361.
34. Escamilla RF, Fleisig GS, Zheng N, Barrentine SW, Wilk KE, et al. (1998) Biomechanics of the knee during closed kinetic chain and open kinetic chain exercises. Med Sci Sports Exerc 30: 556–569.
35. Escamilla RF, Fleisig GS, Zheng N, Lander JE, Barrentine SW, et al. (2001) Effects of technique variations on knee biomechanics during the squat and leg press. Med Sci Sports Exerc 33: 1552–1566.
36. Wilk KE, Escamilla RF, Fleisig GS, Barrentine SW, Andrews JR, et al. (1996) A comparison of tibiofemoral joint forces and electromyographic activity during open and closed kinetic chain exercises. Am J Sports Med 24: 518–527.
37. Ploutz-Snyder LL, Convertino VA, Dudley GA (1995) Resistance exercise-induced fluid shifts: change in active muscle size and plasma volume. Am J Physiol 269: R536–543.
38. Enocson AG, Berg HE, Vargas R, Jenner G, Tesch PA (2005) Signal intensity of MR-images of thigh muscles following acute open- and closed chain kinetic knee extensor exercise - index of muscle use. European Journal of Applied Physiology 94: 357–363.
39. Weiss LW, Coney HD, Clark FC (2000) Gross measures of exercise-induced muscular hypertrophy. J Orthop Sports Phys Ther 30: 143–148.
40. Johnson MA, Polgar J, Weightman D, Appleton D (1973) Data on the distribution of fibre types in thirty-six human muscles. An autopsy study. J Neurol Sci 18: 111–129.

17

Low Physical Activity Level and Short Sleep Duration Are Associated with an Increased Cardio-Metabolic Risk Profile: A Longitudinal Study in 8-11 Year Old Danish Children

Mads F. Hjorth[1]*, Jean-Philippe Chaput[2], Camilla T. Damsgaard[1], Stine-Mathilde Dalskov[1], Rikke Andersen[3], Arne Astrup[1], Kim F. Michaelsen[1], Inge Tetens[3], Christian Ritz[1], Anders Sjödin[1]

1 Department of Nutrition, Exercise and Sports, Faculty of Science, University of Copenhagen, Copenhagen, Denmark, **2** Healthy Active Living and Obesity Research Group, Children's Hospital of Eastern Ontario Research Institute, Ottawa, Ontario, Canada, **3** National Food Institute, Division of Nutrition, Technical University of Denmark, Søborg, Denmark

Abstract

Background: As cardio-metabolic risk tracks from childhood to adulthood, a better understanding of the relationship between movement behaviors (physical activity, sedentary behavior and sleep) and cardio-metabolic risk in childhood may aid in preventing metabolic syndrome (MetS) in adulthood.

Objective: To examine independent and combined cross-sectional and longitudinal associations between movement behaviors and the MetS score in 8-11 year old Danish children.

Design: Physical activity, sedentary time and sleep duration (seven days and eight nights) were assessed by accelerometer and fat mass index (fat mass/height^2) was assessed using Dual-energy X-ray absorptiometry. The MetS-score was based on z-scores of waist circumference, mean arterial blood pressure, homeostatic model assessment of insulin resistance, triglycerides and high density lipoprotein cholesterol. All measurements were taken at three time points separated by 100 days. Average of the three measurements was used as habitual behavior in the cross-sectional analysis and changes from first to third measurement was used in the longitudinal analysis.

Results: 723 children were included. In the cross-sectional analysis, physical activity was negatively associated with the MetS-score ($P<0.03$). In the longitudinal analysis, low physical activity and high sedentary time were associated with an increased MetS-score (all $P<0.005$); however, after mutual adjustments for movement behaviors, physical activity and sleep duration, but not sedentary time, were associated with the MetS-score (all $P<0.03$). Further adjusting for fat mass index while removing waist circumference from the MetS-score rendered the associations no longer statistically significant (all $P>0.17$). Children in the most favorable tertiles of changes in moderate-to-vigorous physical activity, sleep duration and sedentary time during the 200-day follow-up period had an improved MetS-score relative to children in the opposite tertiles ($P=0.005$).

Conclusion: The present findings indicate that physical activity, sedentary time and sleep duration should all be targeted to improve cardio-metabolic risk markers in childhood; this is possibly mediated by adiposity.

Editor: Yinglin Xia, University of Rochester, United States of America

Funding: The study is part of the OPUS project 'Optimal well-being, development and health for Danish children through a healthy New Nordic Diet' which is supported by a grant from the Nordea Foundation. The funders had no role in study design, data collection and analysis, decision to publish, or preparation of the manuscript.

Competing Interests: The authors have declared that no competing interests exist.

* Email: madsfiil@life.ku.dk

Introduction

Accelerometer-derived movement behaviors, such as moderate-to-vigorous physical activity (MVPA), sedentary time and sleep duration, have all been associated with cardio-metabolic risk in children [1–3]. Existing evidence in children linking these accelerometer-derived movement behaviors to cardio-metabolic risk is primarily cross-sectional, and combined associations have only recently been investigated between MVPA and sedentary time [4,5], but not with sleep duration, despite its influence on cardio-metabolic risk [1]. Most studies use single cardio-metabolic risk markers as their outcome; however, a clustering of cardio-metabolic risk markers, producing a metabolic syndrome (MetS) score, is a more sensitive approach to identifying children with increased cardio-metabolic risk [6].

To our knowledge, no study to date has investigated independent and combined associations between accelerometer determined PA, sedentary time and sleep duration with several cardio-metabolic risk markers or a MetS-score in a cross-sectional or longitudinal study. As both objectively measured PA and MetS appear to track from childhood to adolescence and adulthood [7,8], a better understanding of the relationships between movement behaviors (PA, sedentary time and sleep duration) and cardio-metabolic risk in childhood may aid in developing lifestyle interventions and public health policies to prevent the MetS in adulthood.

The aim of this paper was to examine independent and combined cross-sectional and longitudinal associations between objectively measured movement behaviors and cardio-metabolic risk markers, including the MetS-score, in a sample of Danish children. We hypothesized that high PA level, low sedentary time and long sleep duration would be independently associated with a lower MetS-score. Furthermore, we hypothesized that children in the most favorable tertiles of changes in MVPA, sedentary time and sleep duration during the follow-up period would have a more favorable development in the MetS-score than children in the opposite tertiles.

Subjects and Methods

The initial sample comprised 834 of the 1,021 invited third and fourth grade students (8–11 years old) from nine Danish municipal schools enrolled in the OPUS (Optimal well-being, development and health for Danish children through a healthy New Nordic Diet) school meal study. The main aim of this cluster-randomized crossover study was to investigate the potential health effects of a New Nordic Diet served at school versus usual packed lunch (control) [9]. Measurements were performed at baseline (August to November 2011), before the end of the first dietary period (approximately 100 days later) and before the end of the second dietary period (after another 100 days). As the school meal intervention did not affect physical activity, sedentary time and sleep duration [10] all participants were used in the present paper regardless of randomization status. Average of the three measurements was used as habitual behavior in the cross-sectional analysis and changes from first to third measurement was used in the longitudinal analysis. Due to missing data [one or more of the five components of the MetS-score at baseline ($n = 87$), during the last visit ($n = 91$) and no measure of pubertal status ($n = 24$)], our cross-sectional and longitudinal samples comprised data from 723 and 632 children, respectively.

Questionnaire data were first collected, followed by simultaneous registrations of movement behaviors and dietary intake within the following two weeks, after which anthropometry, blood pressure and blood samples were collected the following week.

Ethics Statement

The study was approved by the Committees on Biomedical Research Ethics for the Capital Region of Denmark (J.nr. H-1-2010-123). Child assent and written informed parental consent of both custody holders were obtained for all participants. The study was registered in the www.clinicaltrials.gov database (no. NCT01457794).

Movement behaviors

The children were asked to wear an ActiGraph™ tri-axis accelerometer monitor (GT3X+ or GT3X, Pensacola, FL, USA) tightly on the right hip using an elastic belt for seven consecutive days and eight nights (entire 24-hour period); they were only allowed to remove it during water activities (i.e. showering or swimming). At the end of the observation period, data were reintegrated to 60-second epochs and analyzed using ActiLife6 (the ActiGraph 2012, ActiLife version 6). Before analysis of physical activity and sedentary time, we removed 1) data between midnight and six am, as this was expected to be non-awake time; 2) periods of at least 15 minutes of consecutive zero counts using tri-axial vector magnitudes to remove non-wear time and non-awake time; and 3) consecutive wear time periods of less than 60 minutes to remove non-awake time, as sleep for most children is characterized by minor periods of movement that we did not want to include in our analysis of physical activity and sedentary time. Total PA (counts/minute; cpm) was expressed as total vertical counts from monitor wear time divided by monitor wear time. As a secondary variable, total tri-axial PA (cpm) was expressed as a vector magnitude of the total tri-axial counts from monitor wear time, divided by monitor wear time. Time spent in a sedentary state was defined as all minutes showing 100 vertical cpm or less, which is a widely used cut-off point [11]. MVPA was defined as ≥ 2296 vertical cpm, which is a recently suggested pediatric cut-off point [11]. The percentage of time spent in a sedentary state was calculated by dividing sedentary time with monitor wear time and multiplying by 100. The number of children fulfilling the World Health Organization's recommendation of an average of ≥60 minutes MVPA/day [12] was also calculated. The weekly averages of total PA, MVPA and sedentary time were calculated in the proportion of five to two between weekdays (Monday to Friday) and weekend days (Saturday and Sunday). Total PA, MVPA and sedentary time were only considered valid if monitor wear time was at least 10 hours/day for a minimum of three weekdays and one weekend day.

The parents and children were instructed to keep logs for bedtime ("lights off" and trying to sleep) and waking time ("lights on") during the week in which the monitor was worn. Based on these self-reports, we calculated the proportion of children meeting the recommended sleep duration according to the guidelines of the National Sleep Foundation in the USA (≥10 hours/night) [13]. To estimate accelerometer determined sleep duration, the self-reported bedtimes and waking times were used as the possible window of sleep and accelerometer data within this window were scored in ActiLife6 using the algorithm by Sadeh *et al.* [14]. Self-reported sleep logs were missing for some children (98 sleep logs missing out of 1,638); in these cases, sleep was scored visually from the individual actograms as the difference between time when activity stopped and time when activity resumed. In a random subsample of 105 individuals, we found that the mean difference in sleep duration between these two approaches was small (3.8 minutes, $P<0.001$). The weekly average of sleep duration was calculated in the proportion of five to two between weekdays (Sunday to Thursday) and weekend days (Friday and Saturday). Sleep duration was only considered valid if it was measured for a minimum of three weekdays and one weekend day. On any of the three measurement occasions, ≥85% of individuals had valid activity and sleep registrations for seven days and nights.

Anthropometry and cardio-metabolic risk markers

Clinical measurements and venous blood sampling from the antecubital vein were performed in the morning after an overnight fast in a mobile laboratory. Whole-blood glucose was analyzed immediately after sampling using a Hemocue Glucose 201 analyzer (Hemocue Danmark) and serum insulin, plasma triglycerides and plasma high density lipoprotein cholesterol (HDL-C) were analyzed according to a standard protocol described elsewhere [15]. Homeostatic model assessment of insulin resis-

Table 1. Baseline descriptive characteristics of the study population stratified by sex.

Variable	n	Boys (n = 374)	Girls (n = 349)	All (n = 723)
Demographics				
Age (years)	723	10.1±0.6	9.9±0.6 **	10.0±0.6
3rd grade/4th grade (%)	723	46/54	48/52	47/53
Tanner stage (% 1/2/≥3)	723	75.4/20.9/3.7	53.6/37.0/9.5 **	64.9/28.6/6.5
Parents born in Denmark (% 0/1/2)	723	8.6/13.1/78.3	8.3/12.3/79.4	8.4/12.7/78.8
Highest education of parents (%)[1]	721	4.6/32.7/39.7/23.1	5.8/36.2/38.5/19.5	5.1/34.4/39.1/21.4
Anthropometrics				
Weight (kg)	722	35.4±7.2	34.7±6.9	35.1±7.1
Height (cm)	723	142.8±7.1	142.1±7.0	142.4±7.1
Body mass index z-score[2]	722	0.21±1.11	0.06±1.04	0.14±1.08
Weight status (% uw/nw/ow/ob)[3]	722	9.1/77.5/11.2/2.1	11.8/74.7/11.8/1.7	10.4/76.2/11.5/1.9
Fat mass index (kg/height^2)	720	3.1 (2.2;4.8)	4.1 (2.9;5.7) **	3.7 (2.5;5.3)
MetS-score markers				
Waist circumference (cm)	723	62.4 (59.3;68.2)	62.5 (58.9;68.1)	62.4 (59.3;68.2)
MAP (mm Hg)	723	80.9±6.0	81.5±6.6	81.2±6.3
$HOMA_{IR}$	723	1.34 (0.98;1.89)	1.50 (1.09;2.09) *	1.40 (1.02;1.96)
Triglycerides (mmol/L)	723	0.57 (0.48;0.70)	0.66 (0.54;0.83) **	0.61 (0.50;0.77)
HDL-C (mmol/L)	723	1.49±0.32	1.39±0.29 **	1.44±0.31
Movement behaviors				
Total physical activity (cpm)[4]	697	520±138	453±118 **	487±133
Sedentary time (%)[5]	697	52.6±7.0	52.5±6.4	52.5±6.7
Screen time (min/day)	702	154 (114;210)	136 (94;183) **	148 (103;194)
MVPA (min/day)	697	57±24	38±16 **	48±23
Sleep duration (min/night)	679	553±27	556±28	554±27
CSHQ	719	42 (39;45)	42 (39;46)	42 (39;46)
Diet				
Energy intake (kJ/day)	708	8156±1721	7028±1456 **	7613±1694
SFA/Total fat	708	0.39±0.04	0.40±0.04	0.39±0.04

Abbreviations: MVPA, moderate-to-vigorous physical activity; CSHQ, Children's Sleep Habits Questionnaire; MAP, mean arterial blood pressure; $HOMA_{IR}$, homeostatic model assessment of insulin resistance; HDL-C, high density lipoprotein cholesterol; SFA, saturated fatty acid.

Data are presented as mean ± standard deviation, median (interquartile range) or proportions. Sex differences were tested using a two-sample t-test or Pearson's chi-squared test: *, P<0.05; **, P<0.001.

[1]Highest education of parents: ≤10 years/11–12 years/13–16 years/≥17 years.

[2]Based on the World Health Organization Growth Reference from 2007 [18].

[3]Based on age- and sex-specific cut-offs defined to pass through body mass index at 18.5, 25 and 30 kg/m^2 at age 18 years [19,20]; uw/nw/ow/ob, underweight/normal weight/overweight/obese. Data are presented as mean ± standard deviation or proportion.

[4]Total tri-axial physical activity (cpm): Boys, 1052±232; Girls, 928±195 (P<0.001); All, 992±223.

[5]Sedentary time (hh:mm/day): Boys, 7:56±1:07; Girls, 7:51±1:01 (P = 0.25); All, 7:54±1:04.

tance ($HOMA_{IR}$) was calculated as plasma glucose (mmol/l) × serum insulin (mmol/l)/22.5 [16].

After 10 minutes of rest, blood pressure was measured three times in the supine position with an automated device (UA-787 Plus; A&D Medical) using two different cuff sizes (18–22 cm or 22–32 cm). A second device (ProBP 3400 Sure BP, Welch Allyn Inc., NY, USA) was used for children with arm circumferences < 22 cm using three different cuff sizes (12–16 cm; 15–21 cm; and 20–26 cm). The mean of the last two measurements was used in the data analyses. The mean arterial blood pressure (MAP) was calculated as: 1/3 x systolic blood pressure +2/3 x diastolic blood pressure. Height (CMS Weighing Equipment LTD, London, UK) and waist circumference (position of the umbilicus) were measured three times to the nearest millimeter and the average was used. The children were weighed to the nearest 0.1 kg (Tanita BWB-800S, Tanita, Europe) while barefoot and wearing light clothing. Finally, whole-body composition was determined by Dual-energy X-ray absorptiometry (Lunar Prodigy; GE Medical Systems, Madison, Wisconsin, USA) using Encore software version 13.5 (Encore, Madison, WI, USA), and fat mass index (FMI) was calculated as fat mass divided by height squared. As FMI is relatively independent of fat-free mass [17], it was chosen over, for example, percentage of body fat.

The body mass index z-score was calculated based on the World Health Organization Growth Reference data from 2007 [18]. The prevalence of underweight, normal weight, overweight and obese children was calculated based on age- and sex-specific cut-offs defined to pass through a body mass index of 18.5, 25 and 30 kg/m^2 at 18 years of age [19,20]. The prevalence of non-normal triglycerides (>1.7 mmol/L) [21], $HOMA_{IR}$ (>3.0) [22], blood

Table 2. Cross-sectional associations between movement behaviors and cardio-metabolic risk markers in Danish children.

	n	WC, cm	MAP, mm Hg[1]	$HOMA_{IR}$[2]	Triglycerides, mmol/L[2]	HDL-C, mmol/L	MetS-score[3]
Total PA	564	−1.14 (−1.64;−0.64)** ¥	0.05 (−0.32;0.41)	−0.070 (−0.099;−0.042)* ¥ £	−0.035 (−0.057;−0.015)* ¥	0.034 (0.015;0.053)* ¥ £	−0.10 (−0.19;−0.01)*
MVPA	564	−0.93 (−1.23;−0.63)** ¥£	0.00 (−0.22;0.22)	−0.051 (−0.069;−0.034)** ¥	−0.023 (−0.042;−0.016)** ¥	0.023 (0.011;0.035)** ¥	−0.07 (−0.12;−0.01)*
Sedentary time	564	0.07 (−0.03;0.18)	−0.01 (−0.09;0.07)	0.007 (0.001;0.013)*	0.006 (0.002;0.010)*	−0.004 (−0.008;0.0005)	0.01 (−0.01;0.03)
Screen time	702	0.33 (−0.07;0.73)	0.22 (−0.12;0.56)	0.026 (0.000;0.053)*	0.012 (−0.008;0.031)	−0.002 (−0.019;0.014)	0.02 (−0.10;0.15)
Sleep duration	473	−2.21 (−3.79;−0.62)* ¥	−0.58 (−1.74;0.58)	−0.080 (−0.174;0.014) ¥	−0.022 (−0.089;0.046)	0.001 (−0.063;0.066)	−0.12 (−0.43;0.18)
CSHQ	719	0.16 (0.08;0.25)**	0.10 (0.02;0.17)*	0.007 (−0.002;0.013) *	0.006 (0.002;0.010)* £	−0.001 (−0.005;0.002)	0.02 (−0.01;0.05)

Abbreviations: PA, physical activity; MVPA, moderate-to-vigorous physical activity; CSHQ, Children's Sleep Habits Questionnaire; WC, waist circumference; MAP, mean arterial blood pressure; $HOMA_{IR}$, homeostatic model assessment of central insulin resistance; HDL-C, high density lipoprotein cholesterol; MetS-score, metabolic syndrome score.
Data are presented as unstandardized regression coefficients (β) with 95% confidence intervals (CI) using a linear mixed model with school and subject as random effects. The five cardio-metabolic risk markers were adjusted for baseline age, sex, pubertal status, and sex-pubertal status interaction (**Model 1**).
Coefficients represent the change in the outcome for a 100-cpm change in total PA, a 10-minute change in time spent in MVPA, a 1% change in sedentary time, a 60-minute change in screen time and sleep duration and a 1-point change in CSHQ. *, $P<0.05$; **, $P<0.001$.
¥P<0.05 in **Model 2**: Model 1+ mutual adjustments between MVPA, sedentary time and sleep duration. Total PA was only adjusted for sleep duration.
£P<0.05 in **Model 3**: Model 2+ fat mass index.
[1]MAP was also adjusted for height.
[2]$HOMA_{IR}$ and triglycerides were log transformed.
[3]MetS-score = (z-scores by baseline age, sex, pubertal status and sex-pubertal status interaction of) WC + MAP + $HOMA_{IR}$ + triglycerides − HDL-C.

pressure (>95th age-, sex- and height-specific percentile of systolic and/or diastolic pressure) [23] and HDL-C (<1.0) [21] were also calculated.

Questionnaire data

A baseline questionnaire ascertained age, sex, school grade, highest education of the household (divided into four groups according to years of education: ≤10 years, 11–12 years, 13–16 years, ≥17 years), number of parents born in Denmark and screen time. Screen time was computed based on the parent-reported time that the child spent watching television, playing passive video games or using the computer for leisure activities on weekdays and weekend days. Time spent playing the Nintendo Wii or similar active video game devices was not included in screen time. The weekly average of screen time was calculated in the proportion of five to two between weekdays and weekend days. The number of children fulfilling the Canadian recommendation of less than two hours of screen time/day [24] was also calculated. Pubertal status was self-reported (parent and child) based on breast development among girls and pubic hair growth among boys on a scale from 1 to 5 [25]. A dichotomous variable indicating whether or not the child had entered puberty was used in the statistical analyses (1 or ≥2). Finally, the parents were asked to fill out the 33-item Children's Sleep Habits Questionnaire (CSHQ) that screens for common sleep disturbances. On a three-point scale, parents reported the frequency of their child's habits. Items were then summed, and higher scores denote the presence of sleep disturbances. The scale has previously demonstrated test-retest reliability and validity in school-aged children [26].

Dietary assessment

Daily food and beverage intake was recorded over seven consecutive days using a Web-based Dietary Assessment Software for Children (WebDASC) tool that has been validated for fruits and vegetables [27]. Dietary intake was recorded at the end of each day using pictures of different portion sizes. Further description of the WebDASC is available elsewhere [28]. Changes in fat quality of the diet was used as a covariate in the analyses between movement behaviors and the MetS-score, as it has been proposed to be important in the etiology of cardiovascular diseases [29]. This was calculated as the ratio between saturated fatty acids (g/day) and total fatty acids (g/day). No individuals were excluded from the analytical sample due to a low (<1.05) or high (>2.29) reported energy intake, defined as energy intake divided by calculated basal metabolic rate [30].

Statistical analysis

Cross-sectional analysis. Descriptive characteristics of the study sample were presented as mean and standard deviation (SD), median (interquartile range [IQR]) or as proportions. Sex differences were assessed using two-sample t-tests (variables were logarithmically transformed if they were not normally distributed) or Pearson's chi-squared tests.

A linear mixed model with school and subject as random effects was used to test the association between habitual movement behaviors (average of baseline, day 100 and day 200) and cardio-metabolic risk markers (waist circumference, MAP, $HOMA_{IR}$, triglycerides and HDL-C) on all three occasions (except for screen time and CSHQ, which were only obtained at baseline). $HOMA_{IR}$ and triglycerides were positively skewed and were thus log-transformed. These analyses were adjusted for baseline age, sex, pubertal status, and sex-pubertal status interaction (Model 1). Model 2: as in Model 1+ mutual adjustments between MVPA, sedentary time and sleep duration; Model 3: as in Model 2+ fat

Table 3. Associations between changes in movement behaviors and changes in cardio-metabolic risk markers over a 200-day follow-up period in Danish children.

	n	WC, cm	MAP, mm Hg[1]	$HOMA_{IR}$	Triglycerides, mmol/L	HDL-C, mmol/L
Total PA	554	−0.15 (−0.31;0.01)	0.03 (−0.26;0.33)	−0.07 (−0.13;−0.02)* ¥	−0.02 (−0.04;0.004)	0.029 (0.019;0.039)** ¥ £
MVPA	554	−0.12 (−0.23;0.0003)	−0.001 (−0.23;0.21)	−0.07 (−0.11;−0.03)** ¥	−0.02 (−0.04;−0.004)*	0.019 (0.012;0.026)** ¥ £
Sedentary time	554	0.01(−0.03;0.05)	0.0002 (−0.08;0.08)	0.02 (0.003;0.03)*	0.003 (−0.003;0.009)	−0.006 (−0.009;−0.004)** ¥ £
Sleep duration	486	−0.10 (−0.67;0.46)	−0.51 (−1.49;0.47)	−0.18 (−0.36;0.01) ¥ £	−0.03 (−0.11;0.06)	0.003 (−0.034;0.039)

Abbreviations: PA, physical activity; MVPA, moderate-to-vigorous physical activity; WC, waist circumference; MAP, mean arterial blood pressure; $HOMA_{IR}$, homeostatic model assessment of central insulin resistance; HDL-C, high density lipoprotein cholesterol.
Data are presented as unstandardized regression coefficients (β) with 95% confidence intervals (CI) using a linear mixed model with school as random effect. **Model 1:** Adjusted for baseline age, sex, pubertal status, sex-pubertal status interaction, days of follow up, and the particular baseline movement behavior and baseline cardio-metabolic risk component of interest. Coefficients represent the change in the outcome for a 100-cpm change in total PA, a 10-minute change in time spent in MVPA, a 1% change in sedentary time and a 60-minute change in sleep duration.*, $P<0.05$; **, $P<0.001$.
¥P<0.05 in **Model 2**: Model 1+ mutual adjustments between MVPA, sedentary time and sleep duration. Total PA was only adjusted for sleep duration.
£P<0.05 in **Model 3**: Model 2+ baseline and change in fat mass index.
[1]MAP was also adjusted for baseline and change in height.

mass index. The analysis of MAP was additionally adjusted for height.

The MetS-score variables (waist circumference, MAP, $HOMA_{IR}$, triglycerides and HDL-C) were standardized one by one, using linear mixed models with school and subject as random effects, by regressing them onto age, sex, pubertal status and sex-pubertal status interactions, and the standardized residuals (z-scores) from all five risk markers were summed to obtain the corresponding MetS-score. The above mentioned Models 2 and 3 also apply to the MetS-score. Since HDL-C is inversely related to cardio-metabolic risk, it was multiplied by −1. A higher MetS-score indicates a less favorable cardio-metabolic risk profile. The selected MetS-score variables and demographic standardization was suggested by Eisenmann [6].

Longitudinal analysis. A linear regression model was used to evaluate associations between changes in movement behaviors and changes in cardio-metabolic risk markers during the 200-day period. These analyses were adjusted for baseline age, sex, pubertal status, sex-pubertal status interaction, days of follow-up, and the particular baseline movement behavior and baseline cardio-metabolic risk marker of interest (Model 1) [baseline MVPA and MAP is adjusted for in a model, including change in MVPA and MAP etc.]. Model 2: as in Model 1+ mutual adjustments between MVPA, sedentary time and sleep duration; Model 3: as in Model 2+ baseline and change in fat mass index.

Changes in MetS-score and movement behaviors were calculated as the value at day 200 minus the baseline value. The multiple linear regression analyses of the change in MetS-score were adjusted for a number of covariates (Model 1: days of follow-up, the particular baseline movement behavior of interest [baseline MVPA is adjusted for in a model including change in MVPA, etc.] and baseline MetS-score; Model 2: as in Model 1+ exposures mutually adjusted for each other [total PA, MVPA, sedentary time and sleep duration] where total PA was not adjusted for MVPA/sedentary time and vice versa; Model 3: as in Model 2+ waist circumference was removed from the MetS-score and baseline and changes in fat mass index were adjusted for). Removing waist circumference from the MetS-score and adjusting for adiposity is a recommended way to calculate a MetS-score excluding adiposity [31].

To assess whether combining movement behaviors provides synergistic associations, movement behavior variables were divided into tertiles using the first and third tertiles as the reference group and risk groups and presented as the differences in delta MetS-score (adjusted for days of follow-up) using a linear mixed model.

Results from the analyses were reported as partial correlation coefficients, unstandardized regression coefficients and 95% confidence intervals (CI). Linearity between residuals and the dependent variables in the model was visually checked, as were the assumptions of normality and variance homogeneity. Since there was no statistically significant sex interaction between baseline and changes in movement behaviors with the MetS-score, data for both sexes were pooled. The level of significance was set at $P<0.05$ and statistical analyses were conducted using STATA/IC 11.2 (Houston, USA).

Results

Cross-sectional analysis

The children's baseline characteristics are shown in **Table 1**. Overall, 13% of the children were classified as overweight or obese and a total of 8% (n = 57), 6% (n = 46), 4% (n = 26) and 2% (n = 13) had non-normal blood pressure, $HOMA_{IR}$, HDL-C and triglyceride levels, respectively. Only 27% (n = 190) of children accumulated at least 60 min of MVPA/day on average, 34% (n = 241) reported screen time to be no more than two hours/day and 45% (n = 303) reported sleep duration to be 10 hours/night or more.

As shown in **Table 2**, all movement behaviors were associated with at least one of the five cardio-metabolic risk markers, but only total PA and MVPA were negatively associated with the MetS-score (all $P<0.03$) although not after mutual adjustment for movement behaviors and FMI (all $P>0.72$).

Longitudinal analysis

As shown in **Table 3**, changes in total PA, MVPA and sedentary time during the 200 days were all associated with changes in HDL-C ($P<0.001$) and $HOMA_{IR}$ (all $P<0.02$). Additionally, the change in MVPA was negatively associated with the change in triglycerides ($P = 0.01$), and changes in sleep duration was negatively associated with changes in $HOMA_{IR}$ only after adjusting for PA and sedentary time ($P = 0.02$).

As reported in **Table 4**, low total PA, low MVPA and high sedentary time were associated with an increased MetS-score (all $P<0.005$) (*Model 1*). After mutual adjustment for the other movement behaviors, low total PA, low MVPA and short sleep duration were associated with an increased MetS-score (all P<

Table 4. Associations between changes in movement behaviors and changes in the metabolic syndrome (MetS) score[1] over a 200-day follow-up period in Danish children.

		Model 1 (n=486–554)			Model 2 (n=469)			Model 3 (n=465)		
Variable	**N**	**r**	**β (95% CI)**	**P**	**r**	**β (95% CI)**	**P**	**r**	**β (95% CI)**	**P**
Total PA[2]	554	−0.13	−0.18 (−0.29;−0.07)	**0.002**	−0.11	−0.14 (−0.25;−0.02)	**0.02**	−0.03	−0.03 (−0.14;0.07)	0.51
MVPA	554	−0.18	−0.18 (−0.27;0.10)	**<0.001**	−0.10	−0.12 (−0.22;−0.01)	**0.03**	−0.03	−0.03 (−0.13;0.06)	0.48
Sedentary time	549	0.12	0.04 (0.01;0.07)	**0.005**	0.04	0.02 (−0.02;0.06)	0.39	0.04	0.02 (−0.02;0.05)	0.39
Sleep duration	486	−0.06	−0.25 (−0.64;0.15)	0.22	−0.10	−0.46 (−0.87;−0.04)	**0.03**	−0.07	−0.26 (−0.63;0.11)	0.17

Abbreviations: PA, physical activity; MVPA, moderate-to-vigorous physical activity.
Data are presented as partial correlation coefficients (*r*), unstandardized regression coefficients (β) and 95% confidence intervals (CI) using a linear mixed model with school as random effect. Coefficients represent the change in MetS-score for a 100-cpm change in total PA, a 10-minute change in time spent in MVPA, a 1% change in sedentary time and a 60-minute change in sleep duration. **Model 1**: The MetS variables were standardized by age, sex, pubertal status and sex-pubertal status interaction and the MetS-score was adjusted for days of follow up, the particular baseline movement behavior of interest and baseline MetS-score. **Model 2**: Model 1+ mutual adjustments between MVPA, sedentary time and sleep duration. Total PA was only adjusted for sleep duration. **Model 3**: Model 2+ waist circumference was removed from the MetS-score and baseline and changes in fat mass index was adjusted for.
[1]MetS-score = (z-scores by baseline age, sex, pubertal status and sex-pubertal status interaction of) waist circumference + MAP + $HOMA_{IR}$ + triglycerides − HDL-C.
[2]Total tri-axial physical activity (100-cpm), Model 1: [r = −0.15, β = −0.14, P<0.001], Model 2: [r = −0.12, β = −0.11, P = 0.01], Model 3: [r = −0.04, β = −0.03, P = 0.41].

0.03) (*Model 2*). Adjusting for saturated-to-total fatty acids attenuated these prospective associations and were no longer significant (P = 0.054 to 0.07). Adjusting for FMI while removing waist circumference from the MetS-score rendered the associations no longer significant (all P>0.17) (*Model 3*).

The combined associations between tertiles of changes in movement behaviors and the MetS-score during the follow-up period are shown in **Figure 1**. Children in the most favorable tertiles of changes in MVPA, sleep duration and sedentary time had a decrease in the MetS-score of 3.31 (95% CI 1.02;5.61, P = 0.005) relative to children in the opposite tertiles. Mean (SD) change in the MetS-score was −0.04 (3.82). The change in MetS-score between the most favorable and least favorable tertile of movement behavior was due to a difference of 0.54 (95% CI 0.001;1.08; P = 0.049) in $HOMA_{IR}$ and −0.14 mmol/L (95% CI −0.24;−0.04, P = 0.008) in HDL-C but no differences in waist circumference [1.0 cm (95% CI −0.5;2.4, P = 0.19)], triglycerides [0.15 mmol/L (95% CI −0.08;0.37, P = 0.20)] and MAP [0.52 mm Hg (95% CI −2.86;3.89, P = 0.76)].

Of interest, all significant findings between movement behaviors and the MetS-score remained significant (and insignificant associations remained insignificant) if not standardized according to baseline age, sex, pubertal status and their interaction or after further adjusting for the number of parents born in Denmark and highest education of the household.

Discussion

Collectively, we observed that low habitual total PA and MVPA were associated with a higher MetS-score in our cross-sectional sample. In the longitudinal analysis, low total PA, low MVPA and short sleep duration were associated with an increased MetS-score after mutual adjustment for other movement behaviors; however, after adjustment for FMI, the associations became non-significant, suggesting that adiposity could be a mediator of these relationships. Although sedentary time was not independent of MVPA, synergistic effects between movement behaviors and the MetS-score were observed in combined associations. The present findings are interesting and suggest that multiple movement behaviors should be targeted to reduce cardio-metabolic risk in childhood. They also suggest that this is possibly mediated by adiposity.

Results from this study support previous cross-sectional observations showing that higher total PA and MVPA are associated with a healthier cardio-metabolic profile in children and adolescents [2,4,5,31] and that higher sedentary time and/or screen time are associated with a less healthy cardio-metabolic profile [3–5,32–34], at least in subgroups of the population [35]. When mutually adjusting PA and sedentary time for each other, associations between cardio-metabolic risk and PA often remain but attenuate between cardio-metabolic risk and sedentary time [4,5,31], although accelerometer-determined sedentary time has been positively associated with clustered cardio-metabolic risk independent of total PA [36]. Studies tend to find stronger associations between screen time and cardio-metabolic risk markers than between accelerometer-determined sedentary time and cardio-metabolic risk markers [4,32], suggesting screen time to be more detrimental than non-screen sedentary behaviours in relation to cardio-metabolic risk. Reasons for this could be that children tend to eat in the absence of hunger while engaged in such activities [37] and possibly also decrease sleep duration.

In the present study, the only cardio-metabolic risk marker associated with sleep duration was waist circumference as well as $HOMA_{IR}$ after adjusting for PA and sedentary time, whereas self-

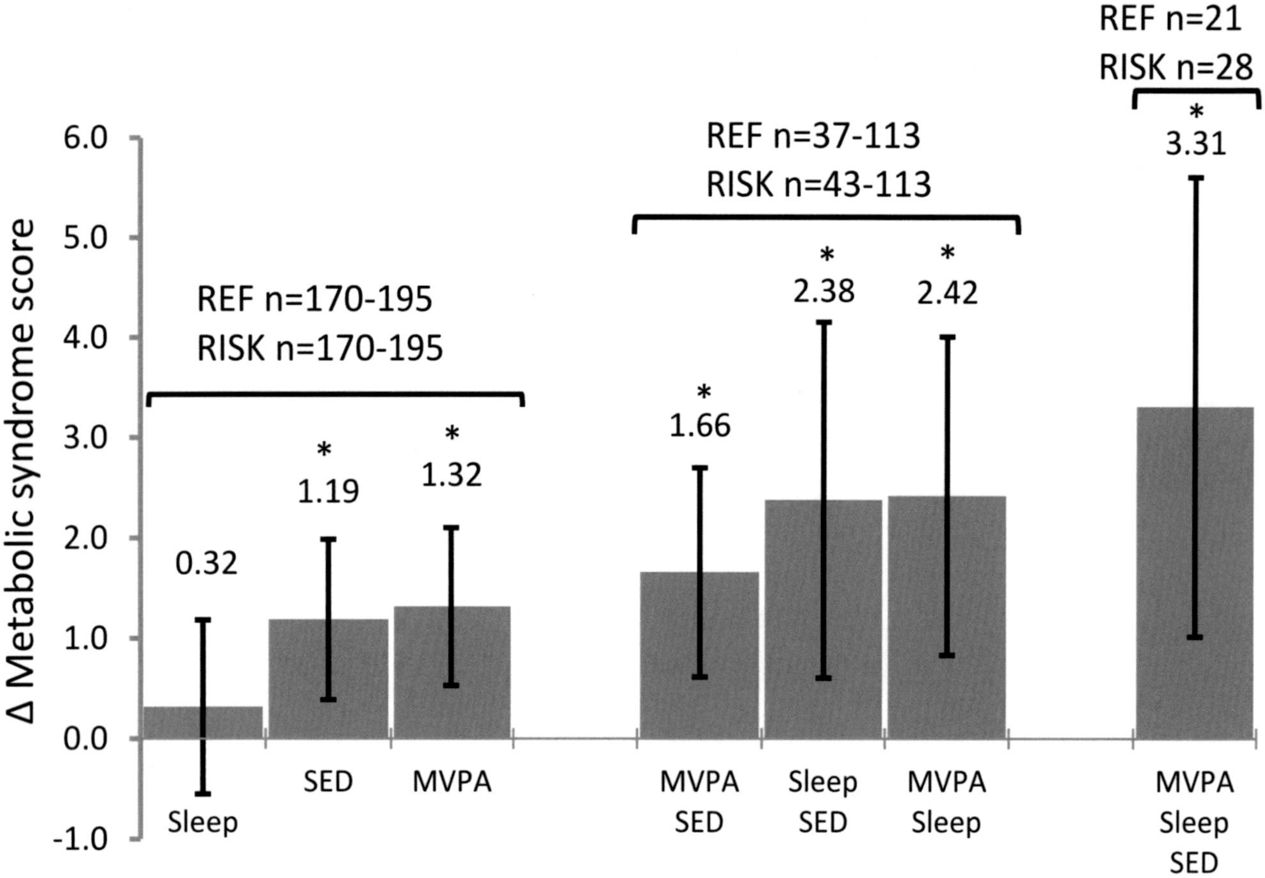

Figure 1. Combined associations between changes in movement behaviors and changes in the metabolic syndrome (MetS) score[1] over a 200-day follow-up period in Danish children. Change in movement behaviors between baseline and day 200 was divided into tertiles using the 1st and 3rd tertile as a reference group (REF) and a risk group (RISK). Data are presented as unstandardized regression coefficients (β) with 95% confidence intervals (CI) between reference group and risk group using a linear mixed model. Sleep, sleep duration (RISK<-24.8 vs. REF>-5.5 min/night); SED, sedentary time (RISK>1.6 vs. REF<-3.4%); MVPA, moderate-to-vigorous physical activity (RISK<0.3 vs. REF>15.2 min/day). Adjusted for days of follow up [1]MetS-score = (age, sex, pubertal status and sex-pubertal status interaction standardised z-scores of) waist circumference+MAP+HOMA$_{IR}$+triglycerides – HDL-C. *P = 0.001 to 0.009.

reported sleep disturbances were associated with several risk markers. However, none of these sleep measures were associated with the MetS-score in our cross-sectional analysis. Another study using accelerometers in obese adolescents found no association between sleep duration and the prevalence of metabolic syndrome [38]. Other studies using accelerometer-determined sleep duration and quality found a negative association with blood pressure [39] or no association [40], whereas evidence for a link between short sleep duration and insulin resistance [41–45] or waist circumference [46] is more evident.

To our knowledge, no study has assessed changes in accelerometer-determined sedentary time or sleep duration with changes in a clustered cardio-metabolic risk score in children, and only a single study has assessed this for PA finding no prospective association between MVPA and the MetS-score, but an inverse association between vigorous PA and the MetS-score [47]. Results from exercise interventions have reported favourable changes in waist circumference, HDL-C, triglycerides and insulin levels in obese children [48] and reduced systolic blood pressure in normotensive adolescents [49]. Although we did not find changes in total PA and MVPA to be associated with all of these cardio-metabolic risk markers, we found that increased total PA and MVPA were associated with decreased MetS-score. The prospective association between sedentary time and MetS-score disappeared after adjusting for MVPA; however, MVPA and sleep duration were independently associated with the MetS-score even after adjusting for sedentary time.

Quality of fat intake has been proposed to be important in the etiology of cardiovascular diseases [29] and intake of saturated fatty acids has been found to be positively associated with insulin levels and systolic blood pressure in children [50]; however, adjusting for intake of dietary fat quality only changed the beta-coefficients slightly. Instead, the prospective associations between movement behaviours and the MetS-score became non-significant after controlling for FMI, indicating that adiposity partly explains the reported associations. In another large cross-sectional study of children and adolescents, the association between PA and clustered cardio-metabolic risk was found to be independent of skinfold thickness [32]. The authors suggest that their precise measurement of activity (accelerometers) explains why they were able to show an association between activity and CVD risk independent of fatness [51]; however, this could also have been caused by the suboptimal adiposity measure. A recent study supports our finding as their cross-sectional association between PA/sedentary time and insulin sensitivity disappeared after controlling for adiposity [52].

In a recent cross-sectional study of 536 children with at least one obese parent, waist circumference and diastolic blood pressure were lower and HDL-C higher among children in the upper tertile of MVPA and lower tertile of sedentary time when compared to the opposite ($P<0.01$) [4]. Likewise, a large cross-sectional study of approximately 20,000 children and adolescents, using the same tertiles of MVPA and sedentary time (combined associations), found the expected differences in waist circumference, systolic blood pressure, insulin, triglycerides and HDL-C ($P<0.05$) [5]. This was despite the fact that some markers (especially insulin) appeared to be better with higher sedentary time across all MVPA tertiles. As these studies did not compare tertiles of MVPA and sedentary time separately, it is difficult to evaluate the potential synergistic effect when combined. We did so in our longitudinal analyses and found a gradual, although not significant, increase in the MetS-score when going from one to three movement behaviors (sleep duration, MVPA and sedentary time). Therefore, despite the fact that sedentary time and MVPA were not independently associated with the MetS-score, combined associations were evident between sedentary time/MVPA/sleep duration and the MetS-score. Our data, therefore, suggest that multiple movement behaviors should be targeted to improve cardio-metabolic risk markers in childhood.

The magnitude of the cross-sectional associations between movement behaviors and cardio-metabolic risk markers were relatively small, which is most likely because movement behaviors are highly variable in children [10] and because our measurements are only proxies of the behaviors we are trying to assess. Moreover, the children are mainly healthy; however, waist circumference, triglycerides and HDL-C had higher beta-values than what was observed in two recent studies [4,5], despite the fact that our children were less obese. The most likely explanation for this is that our use of an average of three seasons removed some of the within-person variability (including season specific differences and longitudinal trends) and thereby got better estimates of habitual behavior. Results from the combined analyses in movement behaviors were more substantial. Children in the tertiles with the most favorable changes in MVPA, sleep duration and sedentary time during the follow-up period compared with those in the least favorable tertiles of changes had remarkably lower $HOMA_{IR}$ and higher HDL-C. These differences are comparable to what has been observed from a successful 12-week aerobic exercise program for obese children [48]. The magnitude of changes observed in cardio-metabolic risk markers due to healthy movement behaviors in our study, therefore, seems to be meaningful from a public health standpoint.

The strength of our study included repeated measures of a large and well-characterized sample of children (demographics, diet, accelerometer-determined movement behaviors and FMI) that allowed us to adjust for a number of variables when looking at changes occurring over time. Another strength is the MetS-score, which mainly stems from the fact that there is no clear definition of the MetS in children or adolescents and that the prevalence rate is relatively low. The approach is more sensitive and statistically less prone to errors compared to the dichotomous approach. However, sample-specific values cannot be compared to other studies and cannot determine the prevalence of MetS. Strengths and limitations of the accelerometer-derived movement behaviours including attachment site, epoch length, cut-points, season variation and the possible influence of cycling, have been discussed previously [10,53,54]. Even though we used a longitudinal approach, we cannot determine cause and effect associations, although it is unlikely that the cardio-metabolic risk markers led to impaired movement behaviors, except from adiposity [5,54].

In summary, low MVPA and short sleep duration were associated with an increased cardio-metabolic risk profile over a 200-day follow-up period in a sample of Danish children. Furthermore, simultaneous unfavorable changes in MVPA, sedentary time and sleep duration synergistically increased the cardio-metabolic risk profile of children. The present findings indicate that multiple movement behaviors should be targeted to improve cardio-metabolic risk markers in childhood and that this is possibly mediated by adiposity.

Acknowledgments

The authors are very grateful to the participants and would also like to acknowledge the school staff as well as other researchers and staff in the OPUS project for their participation and contribution to the study.

Author Contributions

Conceived and designed the experiments: AA KFM IT SMD CTD AS MFH. Performed the experiments: MFH CTD SMD RA. Analyzed the data: MFH. Wrote the paper: MFH. Discussed the analysis and interpretation of the data: MFH AS CR JPC. Reviewed the manuscript critically and approved the final manuscript: MFH JPC CTD SMD RA AA KFM IT CR AS.

References

1. Spruyt K, Molfese DL, Gozal D. (2011) Sleep duration, sleep regularity, body weight, and metabolic homeostasis in school-aged children. Pediatrics 127: 345–352.
2. Andersen LB, Harro M, Sardinha LB, Froberg K, Ekelund U, et al. (2006) Physical activity and clustered cardiovascular risk in children: A cross-sectional study (the european youth heart study). Lancet 368: 299–304.
3. Sardinha LB, Andersen LB, Anderssen SA, Quitério AL, Ornelas R, et al. (2008) Objectively measured time spent sedentary is associated with insulin resistance independent of overall and central body fat in 9-to 10-year-old portuguese children. Diabetes Care 31: 569–575.
4. Chaput J, Saunders TJ, Mathieu M, Henderson M, Tremblay MS, et al. (2013) Combined associations between moderate to vigorous physical activity and sedentary behavior with cardiometabolic risk factors in children. Appl. Physiol. Nutr. Metab. 38: 477–483.
5. Ekelund U, Luan J, Sherar LB, Esliger DW, Griew P, et al. (2012) Moderate to vigorous physical activity and sedentary time and cardiometabolic risk factors in children and adolescents. JAMA 307: 704–712.
6. Eisenmann JC. (2008) On the use of a continuous metabolic syndrome score in pediatric research. Cardiovascular diabetology 7: 17–22.
7. Morrison JA, Friedman LA, Wang P, Glueck CJ. (2008) Metabolic syndrome in childhood predicts adult metabolic syndrome and type 2 diabetes mellitus 25 to 30 years later. J Pediatr 152: 201–206.
8. Kristensen PL, Møller N, Korsholm L, Wedderkopp N, Andersen LB, et al. (2008) Tracking of objectively measured physical activity from childhood to adolescence: The european youth heart study. Scand J Med Sci Sports 18: 171–178.
9. Damsgaard CT, Dalskov SM, Petersen RA, Sørensen LB, Mølgaard C, et al. (2012) Design of the OPUS school meal study: A randomised controlled trial assessing the impact of serving school meals based on the new nordic diet. Scand J Public Health 40: 693–703.
10. Hjorth MF, Chaput J, Michaelsen K, Astrup A, Tetens I, et al. (2013) Seasonal variation in objectively measured physical activity, sedentary time, cardio-respiratory fitness and sleep duration among 8–11 year-old danish children: A repeated-measures study. BMC Public Health 13: 808–817.
11. Trost SG, Loprinzi PD, Moore R, Pfeiffer KA. (2011) Comparison of accelerometer cut points for predicting activity intensity in youth. Med Sci Sports Exerc 43: 1360–1368.
12. World Health Organization (2010) Global recommendations on physical activity for health. Available: http://apps.who.int/iris/bitstream/10665/44399/1/9789241599979_eng.pdf.
13. National Sleep Foundation (2013) Children and sleep. Available: http://www.sleepfoundation.org/article/sleep-topics/children-and-sleep.
14. Sadeh A, Sharkey KM, Carskadon MA. (1994) Fundamental research activity-based sleep-wake identification: An empirical test of methodological issues. Sleep 17: 201–207.

15. Damsgaard CT, Stark KD, Hjorth MF, Biltoft-Jensen A, Astrup A, et al. (2013) n-3 PUFA status in school children is associated with beneficial lipid profile, reduced physical activity and increased blood pressure in boys. Br J Nutr 110: 1304–1312.
16. Cutfield WS, Jefferies CA, Jackson WE, Robinson EM, Hofman PL. (2003) Evaluation of HOMA and QUICKI as measures of insulin sensitivity in prepubertal children. Pediatric diabetes 4: 119–125.
17. Dulloo A, Jacquet J, Solinas G, Montani J, Schutz Y. (2010) Body composition phenotypes in pathways to obesity and the metabolic syndrome. Int J Obes 34: 4–17.
18. Onis M, Onyango AW, Borghi E, Siyam A, Nishida C, et al. (2007) Development of a WHO growth reference for school-aged children and adolescents. Bull World Health Organ 85: 660–667.
19. Cole TJ, Bellizzi MC, Flegal KM, Dietz WH. (2000) Establishing a standard definition for child overweight and obesity worldwide: International survey. BMJ 320: 1240–1245.
20. Cole TJ, Flegal KM, Nicholls D, Jackson AA. (2007) Body mass index cut offs to define thinness in children and adolescents: International survey. BMJ 335: 194–201.
21. Lambert M, Delvin EE, Levy E, O'Loughlin J, Paradis G, et al. (2008) Prevalence of cardiometabolic risk factors by weight status in a population-based sample of quebec children and adolescents. Can J Cardiol 24: 575–583.
22. Tresaco B, Bueno G, Pineda I, Moreno L, Garagorri J, et al. (2005) Homeostatic model assessment (HOMA) index cut-off values to identify the metabolic syndrome in children. J Physiol Biochem 61: 381–388.
23. National High Blood Pressure Education Program Working Group on High Blood Pressure in Children and Adolescents. (2004) The fourth report on the diagnosis, evaluation, and treatment of high blood pressure in children and adolescents. Pediatrics 114: 555–576.
24. Tremblay MSTMS, LeBlanc AGLBAG, Janssen IJI, Kho MEKME, Hicks AHA, et al. (2011) Canadian sedentary behaviour guidelines for children and youth. Applied Physiology, Nutrition, and Metabolism 36: 59–64.
25. Morris NM, Udry JR. (1980) Validation of a self-administered instrument to assess stage of adolescent development. Journal of youth and adolescence 9: 271–280.
26. Owens JA, Spirito A, McGuinn M. (2000) The children's sleep habits questionnaire (CSHQ): Psychometric properties of a survey instrument for school-aged children. Sleep 23: 1043–1052.
27. Biltoft-Jensen A, Bysted A, Trolle E, Christensen T, Knuthsen P, et al. (2012) Evaluation of web-based dietary assessment software for children: Comparing reported fruit, juice and vegetable intakes with plasma carotenoid concentration and school lunch observations. Br J Nutr 110: 186–195.
28. Biltoft-Jensen A, Trolle E, Christensen T, Islam N, Andersen L, et al. (2012) WebDASC: A web-based dietary assessment software for 8–11-year-old danish children. J Hum Nutr Diet doi: 10.1111/j.1365-277X.2012.01257.x
29. Mensink RP, Zock PL, Kester AD, Katan MB. (2003) Effects of dietary fatty acids and carbohydrates on the ratio of serum total to HDL cholesterol and on serum lipids and apolipoproteins: A meta-analysis of 60 controlled trials. Am J Clin Nutr 77: 1146–1155.
30. Black A. (2000) The sensitivity and specificity of the goldberg cut-off for EI: BMR for identifying diet reports of poor validity. Eur J Clin Nutr 54: 395–404.
31. Steele RM, Brage S, Corder K, Wareham NJ, Ekelund U. (2008) Physical activity, cardiorespiratory fitness, and the metabolic syndrome in youth. J Appl Physiol 105: 342–351.
32. Ekelund U, Brage S, Froberg K, Harro M, Anderssen SA, et al. (2006) TV viewing and physical activity are independently associated with metabolic risk in children: The european youth heart study. PLoS medicine 3: 2449–2457.
33. Steele RM, van Sluijs EM, Cassidy A, Griffin SJ, Ekelund U. (2009) Targeting sedentary time or moderate-and vigorous-intensity activity: Independent relations with adiposity in a population-based sample of 10-y-old british children. Am J Clin Nutr 90: 1185–1192.
34. Cliff DP, Okely AD, Burrows TL, Jones RA, Morgan PJ, et al. (2013) Objectively measured sedentary behavior, physical activity, and plasma lipids in overweight and obese children. Obesity 21: 382–385.
35. Colley RC, Garriguet D, Janssen I, Wong SL, Saunders TJ, et al. (2013) The association between accelerometer-measured patterns of sedentary time and health risk in children and youth: Results from the canadian health measures survey. BMC Public Health 13: 200–208.
36. Atkin AJ, Ekelund U, Møller NC, Froberg K, Sardinha LB, et al. (2012) Sedentary time in children: Influence of accelerometer processing on health relations. Med Sci Sports Exerc 45: 1097–1104.
37. Chaput J, Klingenberg L, Astrup A, Sjödin A. (2011) Modern sedentary activities promote overconsumption of food in our current obesogenic environment. Obesity Reviews 12: e12–e20.
38. Sung V, Beebe DW, VanDyke R, Fenchel MC, Crimmins NA, et al. (2011) Does sleep duration predict metabolic risk in obese adolescents attending tertiary services? A cross-sectional study. Sleep 34: 891–898.
39. Javaheri S, Storfer-Isser A, Rosen CL, Redline S. (2008) Sleep quality and elevated blood pressure in adolescents. Circulation 118: 1034–1040.
40. Martikainen S, Pesonen A, Feldt K, Jones A, Lahti J, et al. (2011) Poor sleep and cardiovascular function in children. Hypertension 58: 16–21.
41. Javaheri S, Storfer-Isser A, Rosen CL, Redline S. (2011) Association of short and long sleep durations with insulin sensitivity in adolescents. J Pediatr 158: 617–623.
42. Klingenberg L, Chaput J, Holmbäck U, Visby T, Jennum P, et al. (2012) Acute sleep restriction reduces insulin sensitivity in adolescent boys. Sleep 36: 1085–1090.
43. Flint J, Kothare SV, Zihlif M, Suarez E, Adams R, et al. (2007) Association between inadequate sleep and insulin resistance in obese children. J Pediatr 150: 364–369.
44. Koren D, Katz LEL, Brar PC, Gallagher PR, Berkowitz RI, et al. (2011) Sleep architecture and glucose and insulin homeostasis in obese adolescents. Diabetes Care 34: 2442–2447.
45. Matthews KA, Dahl RE, Owens JF, Lee L, Hall M. (2012) Sleep duration and insulin resistance in healthy black and white adolescents. Sleep 35: 1353–1358.
46. Chaput JP, Lambert M, Gray-Donald K, McGrath JJ, Tremblay MS, et al. (2011) Short sleep duration is independently associated with overweight and obesity in quebec children. Canadian journal of public health 102: 369–374.
47. Ried-Larsen M, Grøntved A, Møller NC, Larsen KT, Froberg K, et al. (2013) Associations between objectively measured physical activity intensity in childhood and measures of subclinical cardiovascular disease in adolescence: Prospective observations from the european youth heart study. Br J Sports Med. doi:10.1136/bjsports-2012-091958.
48. Zorba E, Cengiz T, Karacabey K. (2011) Exercise training improves body composition, blood lipid profile and serum insulin levels in obese children. J Sports Med Phys Fitness 51: 664–669.
49. Buchan D, Ollis S, Thomas N, Buchanan N, Cooper S, et al. (2011) Physical activity interventions: Effects of duration and intensity. Scand J Med Sci Sports 21: e341–e350.
50. Aeberli I, Spinas GA, Lehmann R, Molinari L, Zimmermann M. (2009) Diet determines features of the metabolic syndrome in 6-to 14-year-old children. International Journal for Vitamin and Nutrition Research 79: 14–23.
51. Andersen LB, Froberg K, Brage S, Ekelund U, Anderssen S. (2006) Physical activity and cardiovascular risk in children – authors' reply. The Lancet 368: 1326–1327.
52. Henderson M, Gray-Donald K, Mathieu M, Barnett TA, Hanley JA, et al. (2012) How are physical activity, fitness, and sedentary behavior associated with insulin sensitivity in children? Diabetes Care 35: 1272–1278.
53. Hjorth MF, Chaput JP, Damsgaard CT, Dalskov SM, Michaelsen KF, et al. (2012) Measure of sleep and physical activity by a single accelerometer: Can a waist-worn actigraph adequately measure sleep in children? Sleep Biol Rhythms 10: 328–335.
54. Hjorth MF, Chaput J-P, Ritz C, Dalskov S-M, Andersen R, et al. (2014) Fatness predicts decreased physical activity and increased sedentary time, but not vice versa: support from a longitudinal study in 8–11 year old children. Int J Obes. doi: 10.1038/ijo.2013.229.

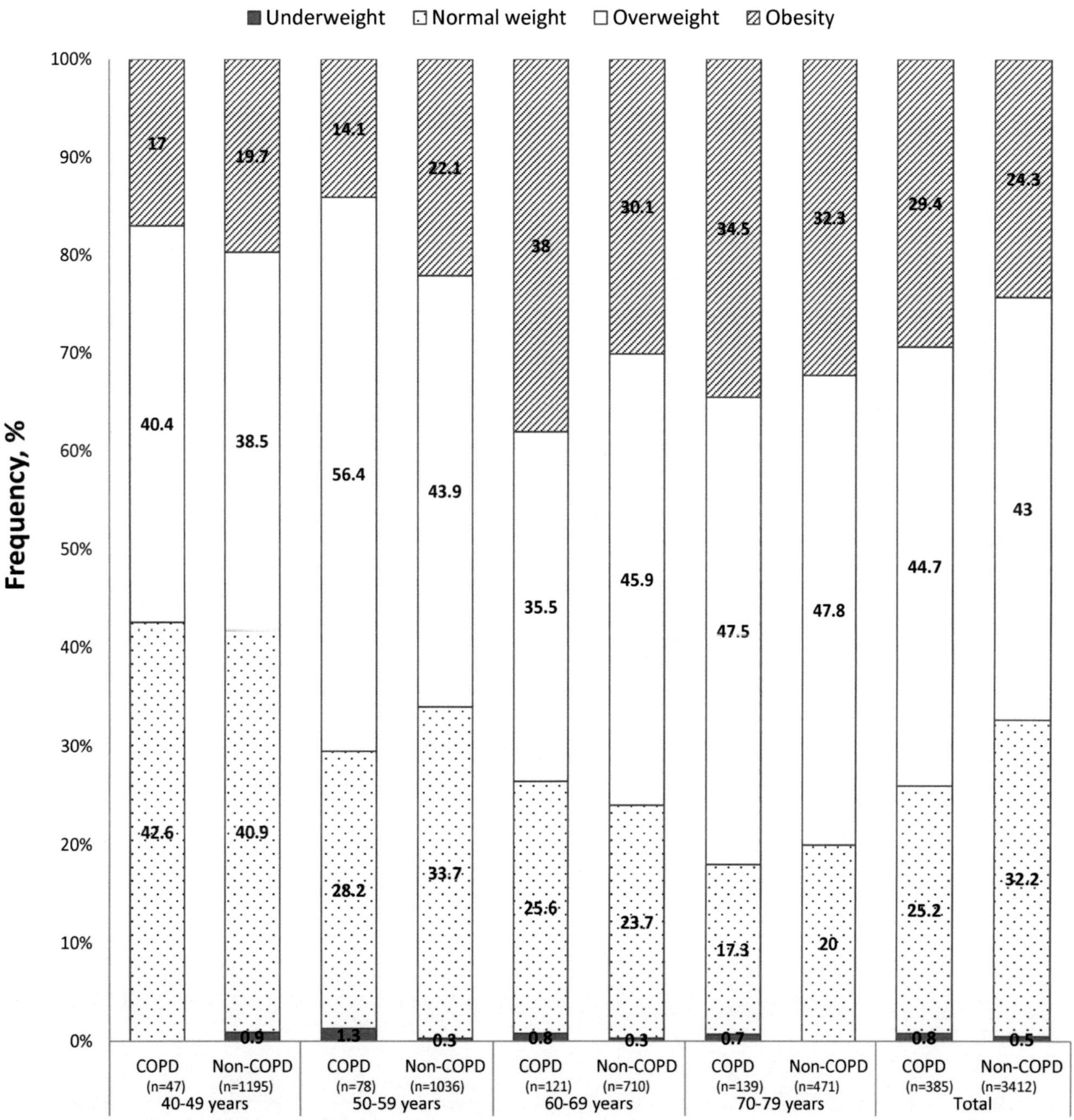

Figure 1. Distribution of BMI classifications according to age group in COPD and non-COPD subjects.

Although low BMI and muscle wasting have traditionally been the focus of nutritional assessment in COPD [7], recent data indicate that obesity is becoming frequent in this disease [8] and some evidence suggests that obesity might contribute to respiratory symptoms and exercise limitation, regardless of airflow obstruction [9]. However, the current evidence of a possible association between obesity and poorer COPD disease state is still limited.

Most studies concerning the prevalence of nutritional alterations in COPD have been performed in selected populations [10–12] and the impact of BMI on health status and prognosis seems to differ with COPD stage. In fact, in some studies, obese patients with more severe COPD appear to have better outcomes ("obesity paradox") [6]. Little information is available regarding the BMI distribution in COPD patients from population-based studies [13,14], which is necessary to more accurately represent the total spectrum of patients with the disease, and to provide more unbiased inferences.

We have analyzed the EPI-SCAN study [15,16] aiming to characterize the BMI distribution in a population-based sample of COPD patients and to evaluate the impact of obesity on health status, exercise tolerance, daily physical activity, systemic inflammation and comorbidity.

18

Impact of Obesity on the Clinical Profile of a Population-Based Sample with Chronic Obstructive Pulmonary Disease

Francisco García-Rio[1]*, Joan B. Soriano[2], Marc Miravitlles[3], Luis Muñoz[4], Enric Duran-Tauleria[5], Guadalupe Sánchez[6], Victor Sobradillo[7], Julio Ancochea[8]

1 Servicio de Neumología, Hospital Universitario La Paz, IdiPAZ, Madrid, Spain, and CIBER de Enfermedades Respiratorias, Madrid, Spain, **2** Fundación Caubet-CIMERA Illes Balears, Bunyola, Illes Balears, Spain, and CIBER de Enfermedades Respiratorias, Illes Balears, Spain, **3** Pneumology Department, Hospital Universitario Vall d'Hebron, Barcelona, Spain, **4** Pneumology Department, Hospital Reina Sofía, Córdoba, Spain, **5** Centro de Investigación en Epidemiología Ambiental – CREAL, Barcelona, Spain, **6** Medical Department, GlaxoSmithkline S.A., Madrid, Spain, **7** Pneumology Department, Hospital de Cruces, Bilbao, Spain, **8** Servicio de Neumología, Hospital Universitario de La Princesa, Instituto de Investigación Sanitaria Princesa, Madrid, Spain

Abstract

Aims: To characterize the distribution of BMI in a population-based sample of COPD patients and to evaluate the impact of obesity on their health status, exercise tolerance, systemic inflammation and comorbidity.

Methods: A population-based sample of 3,797 subjects aged 40–80 years from the EPI-SCAN study was selected. Subjects were categorized according their body mass index (BMI) as underweight (<18.5 kg/m^2), normal weight (18.5–24.9 kg/m^2), overweight (25.0–29.9 kg/m^2) or obese (BMI≥30.0 kg/m^2). Subjects were evaluated with post-bronchodilator spirometry and 6-minute walk tests. Smoking habits, respiratory symptoms, generic and specific quality of life, daily physical activities, comorbidities and systemic inflammatory biomarkers were recorded.

Results: The prevalence of obesity or being overweight was higher in the 382 COPD patients than in the subjects without airflow limitation (29.4%, 95%CI 24.8–33.9% vs. 24.3, 95%CI 22.9–25.8; and 44.7%, 95%CI 39.7–49.6% vs. 43.0%, 95%CI 41.3–44.6, respectively; p = 0.020). In the COPD subgroup, obese subjects presented more dyspnea and less chronic cough, chronic bronchitis or chronic phlegm than normal-weight patients, as well as a worse health status. Moreover, reduced exercise tolerance and higher plasmatic C-reactive protein levels were found in the obese patients, who also presented a greater prevalence of cardiovascular disease (adjusted odds ratio 4.796, 95%CI 1.806–12.736, p = 0.002).

Conclusions: In a population-based sample, obesity is more prevalent in COPD patients than in subjects without airflow limitation. Furthermore, obesity affects the clinical manifestations, quality of life and exercise tolerance of COPD patients, and it may contribute to a phenotype characterized by increased systemic inflammation and greater frequency of cardiovascular comorbidity.

Editor: Juan P. de Torres, Clinica Universidad de Navarra, Spain

Funding: Funding for the EPI-SCAN study was provided by GlaxoSmithKline. The funder provided support in the form of salaries for authors (GS), but did not have any additional role in the study design, data collection and analysis, decision to publish, or preparation of the manuscript. The specific roles of these authors are articulated in the "author contributions" section.

Competing Interests: One of coauthors (GS) is a full-time employee of GlaxoSmithKline, drug manufacturer and sponsor of the study. However, the subject of the study is epidemiological with no drugs involved. This does not alter the authors' adherence to PLOS ONE policies on sharing data and materials. The rest of authors do not have any conflict of interest with relation to the contents of the manuscript.

* Email: fgr01m@gmail.com

Introduction

Chronic obstructive pulmonary disease (COPD) is characterized by a range of pathophysiologic changes that contribute to a highly variable clinical presentation as well as heterogeneity among patients. In addition to airflow limitation, the integral evaluation of COPD needs to consider at least several aspects, such as symptoms, exacerbations and comorbidities [1,2].

Comorbidities occur frequently in COPD patients but show great variability in reported prevalence [3]. COPD is often associated with significant nutritional abnormalities in particular. Extra-pulmonary manifestations such as low body weight, low body mass index (BMI) and depletion of fat-free mass have been extensively reported [4,5], and they are recognized as independent prognostic factors in COPD patients [6,7], often considered in the more advanced, late COPD stages and an indication of an emphysematous phenotype.

Table 1. General characteristics, functional status and severity of the COPD groups.

	Normal weight (18.5–24.9 Kg/m²)	Overweight (25–29.9 Kg/m²)	Obesity (>30 Kg/m²)	Total	p
Patients, n	97	172	113	382	
Males, %	63.9%	75.6%	68.1%	70.4%	0.108
Age, yr.	61±10	64±11[‡]	66±9[†]	64±10	0.001
BMI, Kg/m²	22.9±1.7	27.4±1.5	33.7±3.7	28.1±4.7	<0.001
Smoking status					<0.001
Current smoker, %	50.5	33.7	19.5	33.8	
Former smoker, %	33.0	39.0	48.7	40.3	
Never smoker, %	16.5	27.3	31.9	25.9	
Smoking exposure, pack-years	34.1±21.6	43.3±29.1[‡]	46.1±24.9[‡]	41.4±26.3	0.009
Self-reported exposure to vapors, gases, dusts or fumes, %	38.1	34.9	43.4	38.2	0.354
Occupational exposure					
Biological dusts, %	25.8	19.8	30.1	24.3	0.130
Mineral dusts, %	28.9	24.4	25.7	25.9	0.725
Gases or fumes, %	25.8	15.7	24.8	20.9	0.073
Retired or disabled, %	67.0	72.7	87.5	75.6	0.001
Education level					0.096
Less than primary school, %	14.6	14.0	20.4	16.0	
Primary school, %	34.4	37.2	47.8	39.6	
Secondary school, %	25.0	27.3	21.2	24.9	
University degree, %	24.0	19.8	10.6	18.1	
Pulmonary function					
Post-bronchodilator FVC, % pred.	110±20	107±21	100±21[†§]	106±21	0.002
Post-bronchodilator FEV_1, % pred.	85±20	85±19	79±19	83±20	0.037
Post-bronchodilator FEV_1/FVC, %	62±9	62±7	62±7	62±8	0.976
Post-bronchodilator IC, % pred.	103±28	109±26	106±27	106±27	0.239
Reversibility (positive bronchodilator test) (%)	20.2	31.0	25.9	26.8	0.161
6-min walk test					
Distance, m	468±122	460±114	405±131[†¶]	447±123	0.001
Walk work (m. Kg)	30723±8645	36152±10280[†]	39329±12504[†¶]	35251±10912	<0.001
Δ SpO_2, %	−1.13±2.09	−0.69±2.02	−1.01±3.35	−0.90±2.49	0.377
Δ Borg	0.87±1.22	0.78±1.12	0.98±1.24	0.86±1.17	0.451
Δ Borg/distance walked, %/100 m	0.23±43	0.19±0.32	0.36±0.93	0.25±0.59	0.085
Comorbidity					
Cardiovascular diseases, %	9.3	15.7	31.9	18.8	<0.001
Diabetes mellitus, %	7.2	9.3	19.5	11.8	0.009
Peptic ulcer disease, %	10.3	7.6	5.3	7.6	0.395
Neoplasm, %	7.2	6.4	5.3	6.3	0.848
Charlson index	0.90±1.01	0.84±0.96	1.29±1.15[‡¶]	0.99±1.04	0.001
GOLD risk stage					<0.001
A, %	66.0	59.3	33.6	53.4	
B, %	20.6	32.0	47.8	33.8	
C, %	2.1	1.2	4.4	2.4	
D, %	11.3	7.6	14.2	10.5	
BODE index	1.10±1.55	0.86±1.23	1.61±1.78[§]	1.13±1.53	0.001
ADO index	2.28±1.69	2.58±1.64	3.31±1.52[†¶]	2.72±1.66	<0.001
COPD previous diagnosis, %	29.9	20.9	33.6	27.0	0.046
Current treatment					

Table 1. Cont.

	Normal weight (18.5–24.9 Kg/m²)	Overweight (25–29.9 Kg/m²)	Obesity (>30 Kg/m²)	Total	p
Short-acting beta-agonists, %	13.4	11.6	27.4	16.9	0.001
Long-acting beta-agonists, %	17.5	17.4	30.1	21.2	0.023
Anticholinergics, %	14.4	11.0	20.4	14.7	0.094
Methylxanthines, %	2.1	0	4.4	1.8	0.024
Inhaled corticosteroids, %	18.6	19.8	31.9	23.0	0.029

Values are mean ±SD or frequency. Abbreviations: BMI = body mass index; FVC = forced vital capacity; FEV_1 = forced expiratory volume in 1 second; IC = inspiratory capacity; SpO_2 = oxyhemoglobin saturation.
Comparisons between groups by ANOVA with Bonferroni post-hoc comparisons: †p<0.01 vs. normal weight group; ‡p<0.05 vs. normal weight group; ¶p<0.01 vs. overweight group; §p<0.05 vs. overweight group.

Materials and Methods

The study was approved by the corresponding ethics committees (Hospital Clinic, Barcelona, Spain). All participants gave written informed consent to participate in the study.

Study population

We used data from the EPI-SCAN study, a multicenter, cross-sectional, population-based study conducted at 11 locations throughout Spain. Out of a total of 4,274 subjects who had been randomly contacted by telephone at the 11 sites, 3,885 agreed to participate in the study and a final group of 3,797 (88.8%) were available for analysis (complete minimum data set on gender, age and lung function). The 389 (9.1%) who refused to take part in the survey were slightly older and there were more women as well as never and former smokers. Complete details of the methodology, detailed descriptions of participation rates, and sample characteristics of the EPI-SCAN study have been published elsewhere [16]. For the present study, our source population included 3,797 non-institutionalized participants aged 40–80 who completed acceptable spirometry [17].

Procedures

Body weight was assessed with a beam scale (measured to the nearest 0.1 kg) with subjects standing barefoot and in light clothing. Height was measured by a clinical stadiometer in bare or stocking feet. BMI, defined as weight (kg) divided by the square of height (meters), was calculated. Patients were categorized by World Health Organization (WHO) criteria as [18]: underweight (BMI<18.5 kg/m^2), normal weight (BMI 18.5–24.9 kg/m^2), overweight (BMI 25.0–29.9 kg/m^2) and obese (BMI≥30.0 kg/m^2).

Patient-reported data for smoking history, educational level, domestic and occupational exposures, respiratory history and symptoms, previous medication and use of health services during the preceding year were collected. Any respiratory exacerbation that required a change in regular medication was considered mild, while a respiratory exacerbation treated with a course of oral corticosteroids or antibiotics was considered moderate. Self-reported comorbidity was documented using the Charlson index. The presence of heart failure, ischemic heart disease, peripheral vascular disease or cerebrovascular disease was coded as cardiovascular disease.

Baseline dyspnea was assessed by the Modified Medical Research Council (mMRC) scale, and subjects completed the ECSC respiratory symptoms questionnaire, the Spanish versions of the London Chest Activity of Daily Living (LCADL) scale, the EQ-5D questionnaire and the St. George's Respiratory Questionnaire.

Blood samples were collected using standardized procedures and stored at −80°C for biomarker analysis, as previously described [19]. The biomarkers analyzed were: C-reactive protein (CRP), TNF-α, interleukin (IL)-6, IL-8, fibrinogen and nitrites/nitrates (NOx).

Pre- and post-bronchodilator spirometries were performed at each center using the same equipment and in accordance with current recommendations, as described in previous publications [15,16]. A bronchodilator test was considered positive when there was an increase in FEV_1 or FVC≥12% and ≥200 ml. Six-minute walk tests were performed following current guidelines [20]. To control for a learning effect, 2 walks were performed with a 30-minute rest in between. Walk-work was defined as 6-min walk distance × weight (in kg).

COPD was defined by a post-bronchodilator FEV_1/FVC ratio <0.70 [1] and, in accordance with the new GOLD 2011 stage grades [1], COPD patients were classified in groups A (low risk, fewer symptoms), B (low risk, more symptoms), C (high risk, fewer symptoms) or D (high risk, more symptoms), using predicted FEV_1, mMRC and exacerbation history. COPD severity was determined by the BODE [7] and ADO [21] indices. Subjects with a post-bronchodilator FEV_1/FVC ratio ≥0.70 were considered not to have COPD.

Statistical analysis

Values are expressed as mean ± standard deviation or count and percentage. Differences between study groups were analyzed using the Chi-squared test or ANOVA with post-hoc analysis by the Bonferroni test. In this analysis, a logarithmic transformation was used in those variables not normally distributed, to reduce their skewness. The effect of possible confounding factors was assessed using a generalized linear model analysis adjusted for age, gender, pack-years and post-bronchodilator FEV_1 (% pred.).

In order to examine associations between variables, odds ratios were calculated by logistic regression. We developed multiple logistic regression models with adjustment for age, gender, pack-years and post-bronchodilator FEV_1 (% pred.).

Analyses were performed with SPSS 14.0 for Windows (SPSS, Inc., Chicago, IL). A two-sided p value <0.05 was considered statistically significant.

Table 2. Comparison of symptoms, previous exacerbations, health status and systemic biomarker levels between the study groups.

	Normal weight (18.5–24.9 Kg/m²)	Overweight (25–29.9 Kg/m²)	Obesity (>30 Kg/m²)	Total	p
Symptoms					
Chronic cough, %	39.6	32.0	25.0	31.8	0.079
Chronic bronchitis, %	29.9	18.6	12.6	19.7	0.007
Chronic phlegm, %	39.2	31.4	21.4	30.4	0.020
Dyspnea, %	20.6	23.4	44.2	28.9	<0.001
mMRC	1.49±0.86	1.52±0.75	1.92±0.91[†¶]	1.63±0.84	<0.001
Wheezing, %	64.9	58.1	72.6	64.1	0.045
Mild respiratory exacerbations in the previous year, n per patient	0.10±0.47	0.30±1.77	0.31±0.80	0.25±1.29	0.411
Moderate respiratory exacerbations in the previous year, n per patient	0.45±1.07	0.33±1.05	0.48±0.81	0.40±0.99	0.380
Hospitalizations in the previous year, n per patient	0.02±0.20	0.06±0.41	0.06±0.41	0.05±0.37	0.613
Health-related quality of life					
SGRQ symptoms	29.1±22.8	23.8±21.1	29.2±22.5	26.8±22.1	0.088
SGRQ activity	26.1±27.0	25.6±23.1	38.7±24.9[†¶]	29.5±25.3	<0.001
SGRQ impact	14.6±18.7	12.0±15.1	16.6±17.2	14.0±16.8	0.109
Total SGRQ	20.7±20.2	18.4±16.5	25.7±18.1[¶]	21.1±18.2	0.008
EQ-5D VAS score	71.6±16.7	73.1±15.6	66.7±18.6[§]	70.8±17.0	0.013
EQ-5D utility score	0.83±0.24	0.90±0.19	0.83±0.21	0.86±0.21	0.022
LCADL total	17.1±8.1	15.6±4.1	17.7±7.2[§]	16.6±6.4	0.030
Systemic biomarkers					
CRP, log (mg/l)	0.37±0.31	0.51±0.45	0.60±0.40[†]	0.50±0.41	0.003
TNF-alpha, log (pg/ml)	0.97±0.27	1.06±0.28[‡]	1.06±0.52	1.04±0.27	0.036
IL-6, log (pg/ml)	0.48±0.34	0.46±0.34	0.54±0.35	0.49±0.34	0.216
IL-8, log (pg/ml)	0.51±0.64	0.43±0.60	0.41±0.55	0.44±0.60	0.482
Fibrinogen, g/l	3.24±0.91	3.57±1.13	3.77±1.08[†]	3.54±1.08	0.005
NOx, log (nmol/l)	1.43±0.18	1.42±0.25	1.40±0.22	1.42±0.23	0.625

Values are mean ± SD or frequency. Abbreviations: BMI = body mass index; mMRC = modified Medical Research Council dyspnea scale; SGRQ = St. George's Respiratory Questionnaire; EQ-5D = EuroQol 5 Dimensions questionnaire; VAS = Visual analogue scale; LCADL = London Chest Activities of Daily Living; CRP = C-reactive protein; TNF = tumor necrosis factor; IL = interleukin; NOx = nitrites/nitrates.
Comparisons between groups by ANOVA with Bonferroni post-hoc comparisons: [†]p<0.01 vs. normal weight group; [‡]p<0.05 vs. normal weight group; [¶]p<0.01 vs. overweight group; [§]p<0.05 vs. overweight group.

Results

From the population-based sample of 3,797 subjects, 385 (10.1%) had post-bronchodilator $FEV_1/FVC<0.7$. In comparison with the non-COPD subjects, COPD patients showed a higher prevalence of obesity (29.4%, 95%CI 24.8–33.9% vs. 24.3, 95%CI 22.9–25.8) and of being overweight (44.7%, 95%CI 39.7–49.6% vs. 43.0%, 95% CI 41.3–44.6%) (p = 0.020). In the global sample, being underweight was very uncommon, both in COPD patients (0.8%, 95% CI 0.0–1.7%) as well as in non-COPD subjects (0.5%, 95%CI 0.2–0.7%). Figure 1 shows the BMI distribution in the COPD and non-COPD subjects according to age strata.

Table 1 demonstrates the main characteristics of the normal-weight, overweight and obese COPD groups. In comparison with the normal-weight COPD patients, overweight and obese patients were older and had greater smoking intensity, whereas no differences in gender, occupational exposure or education level were found. FVC and FEV_1 were slightly lower in obese COPD patients than in the other groups, without significant differences in inspiratory capacity or reversibility. Moreover, obese COPD patients walked less distance during six minutes, with a higher walk work than COPD patients with normal weight or overweight. Similarly, comorbidities were more frequent in obese COPD patients than in the other two groups, often associated with the presence of cardiovascular disease or diabetes mellitus. GOLD 2011 grade distribution was also different among the COPD patient groups. Obese COPD patients also showed higher multidimensional severity indices than the other groups and they more frequently used respiratory medication, specifically beta-agonists, methylxanthines and inhaled corticosteroids.

The comparison of symptoms, exacerbation history, health status and systemic inflammatory biomarkers of the three study groups are presented in table 2. Dyspnea and wheezing were more frequent in obese COPD patients, while chronic bronchitis and phlegm resulted more frequent in COPD patients with normal

Table 3. Adjusted comparisons of health status, exercise tolerance and systemic inflammatory biomarkers between the study groups.

	Normal weight (18.5–24.9 Kg/m²)	Overweight (25–29.9 Kg/m²)	Obesity (>30 Kg/m²)	p
mMRC	1.58±0.09	1.48±0.07	1.81±0.09§	0.017
Health-related quality of life				
SGRQ symptoms	29.3±2.6	24.5±2.0	26.5±2.6	0.332
SGRQ activity	28.4±2.8	24.9±2.2	35.9±2.8¶	0.008
SGRQ impact	15.2±1.9	11.6±1.5	14.6±2.0	0.250
Total SGRQ	21.8±2.1	18.0±1.6	23.3±2.1	0.098
EQ-5D VAS score	71.3±1.9	74.0±1.5	67.9±2.0§	0.048
EQ-5D utility score	0.82±0.02	0.91±0.02	0.86±0.03‡	0.017
LCADL total	17.3±0.7	15.4±0.6	16.8±0.7	0.097
Distance 6-min walking test, m	450±14	471±11	422±15§	0.043
Walk work, m. Kg	28144±1246	36815±981†	40232±1302†	<0.001
Systemic biomarkers				
CRP, log (mg/l)	0.40±0.05	0.54±0.04‡	0.57±0.05‡	0.033
TNF-alpha, log (pg/ml)	0.97±0.03	1.05±0.03	1.03±0.04	0.218
IL-6, log (pg/ml)	0.48±0.04	0.48±0.03	0.57±0.04	0.231
IL-8, log (pg/ml)	0.53±0.07	0.42±0.06	0.42±0.07	0.416
Fibrinogen, g/l	3.4±0.1	3.5±0.1	3.6±0.1	0.431
Albumin, g/l	45.2±0.3	45.4±0.3	46.0±0.4	0.188
NOx, log (nmol/l)	1.44±0.03	1.44±0.02	1.41±0.03	0.589

Values are mean ± SEM. Comparisons adjusted by gender, age, pack-year and FEV_1 (% pred). Abbreviations: mMRC = modified Medical Research Council dyspnea scale; SGRQ = St. George's Respiratory Questionnaire; EQ-5D = EuroQol 5 Dimensions questionnaire; VAS = Visual analogue scale; LCADL = London Chest Activities of Daily Living; CRP = C-reactive protein; TNF = tumor necrosis factor; IL = interleukin; NOx = nitrites/nitrates.
Post-hoc comparisons between groups by Bonferroni test: †p<0.001 vs. normal weight group; ‡p<0.05 vs. normal weight group; ¶p<0.01 vs. overweight group; §p<0.05 vs. overweight group.

weight. Significant differences in health-related quality of life, daily physical activity and inflammatory biomarker levels were noted among the three groups. In the adjusted comparison, both dyspnea and health status were worse in obese COPD patients than in overweight COPD patients (Table 3). Reduced exercise tolerance and higher walk work were found in obese patients, although daily physical activity did not reach significant differences between the study groups. Finally, systemic pro-inflammatory state was increased in obese or overweight COPD patients compared with COPD patients with normal weight, showing higher plasmatic CRP levels. Mild and moderate exacerbations and hospitalizations were not significantly different among the three groups.

After multivariate adjustment, differences in multidimensional COPD assessment and in the Charlson index remained among the three study groups (Figure 2). Consistently, BODE and ADO indices were higher in obese COPD patients than in overweight COPD subjects. In turn, comorbidities were more frequent in the obese patients than in the other two COPD groups.

Adjusted odds ratios for comorbidity and respiratory symptoms by COPD group are shown in Figure 3. In comparison with normal-weight COPD patients, the obese patients presented a greater prevalence of cardiovascular diseases (adjusted odds ratio [OR] 4.796, 95%CI 1.806–12.736, p = 0.002) and a different symptomatic profile. The obese COPD patients had lower risk for presenting chronic cough (adjusted OR 0.364, 95% CI 0.178–0.743, p = 0.005), chronic bronchitis (adjusted OR 0.321, 95%CI 0.142–0.724, p = 0.006) or chronic phlegm (adjusted OR 0.398, 95%CI 0.197–0.804, p = 0.010) than COPD patients with normal weight, whereas they had more dyspnea (adjusted OR 2.679, 95%CI 1.307–5.489, p = 0.007).

Discussion

Our study shows that being underweight is uncommon in a population-based series of COPD patients, while obesity affects more than 29% of patients and is more frequent than in subjects without airflow limitation. Also, the presence of obesity determines the clinical behavior of COPD, with more prevalence and severity of dyspnea and less frequency of cough and expectoration, worse quality of life, reduced exercise tolerance, more systemic inflammation and major cardiovascular comorbidity.

Although a previous population study [13] reported a slightly higher incidence (6.7%) of underweight patients, it used a different cut-point than that established by the WHO (BMI<20 Kg/m^2). Our results concur with a series from the US Department of Veterans Affairs Puget Sound Health Care System, which reported only 1.1% of patients with a BMI<18.5 Kg/m^2 [22]. In another study, a prevalence of self-reported underweight lower than 4% has been reported [14]. With regards to obesity, the prevalence observed in our COPD patients (29%) concurs with a large Canadian pulmonary function laboratory database (29%) [23], the PLATINO study (23%) [13] and Canadian National Health Survey (24.6%) studies [14]. Moreover, our data confirm that obesity is more prevalent in patients with COPD than in the general population, which probably depends on the severity of

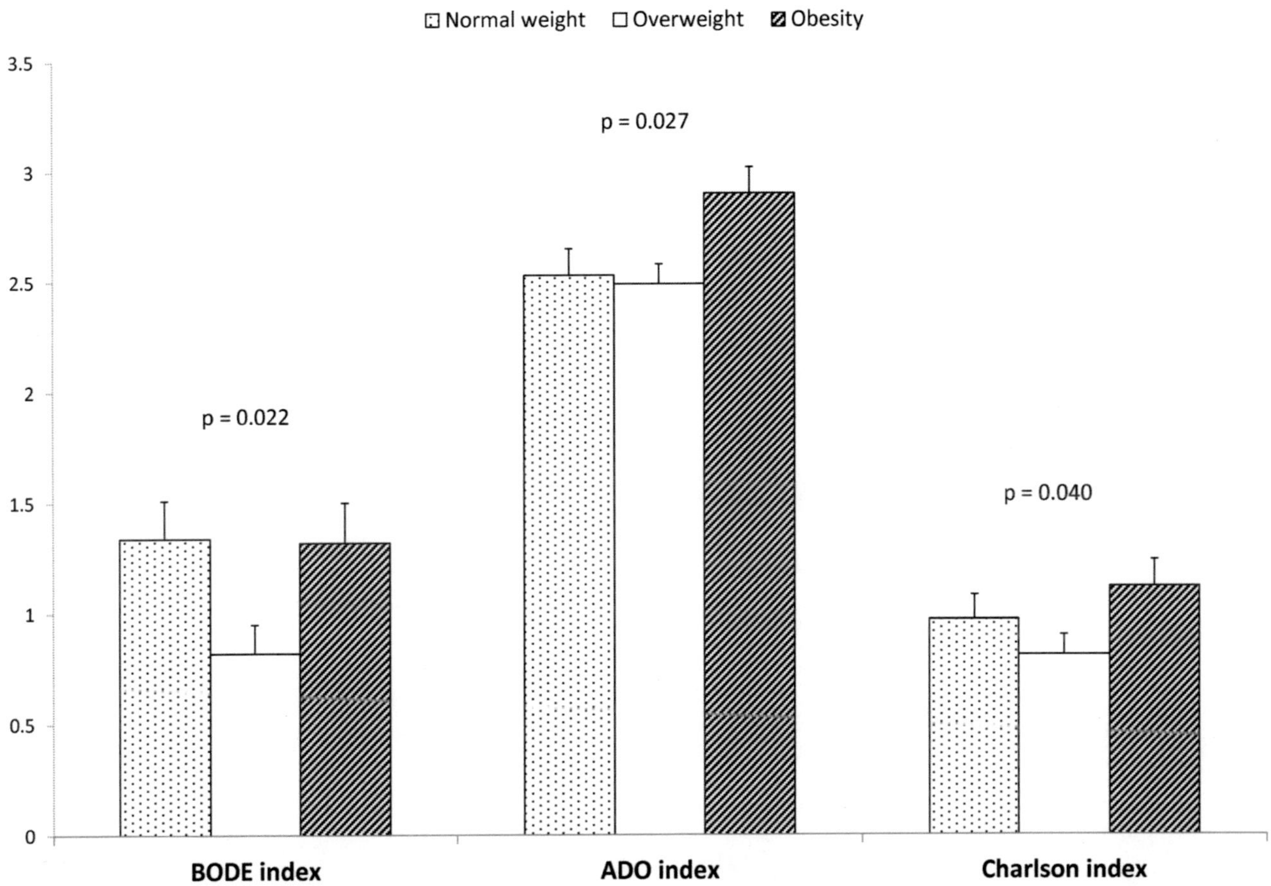

Figure 2. Adjusted comparisons of multidimensional indices and comorbidity between the three groups of COPD patients. Mean values are adjusted for gender, age, packs-year and FEV_1 (% pred.). Error bars represent SEM.

chronic airflow limitation. In fact, there is evidence for higher prevalence of obesity in patients with early stage COPD [9] and it has been reported that obesity is more prevalent in COPD patients with mild obstruction than in severe patients [24]. It is likely that the correlation with severity justifies both the high prevalence of obesity as well as the very low incidence of underweight patients in population studies in which the patient group is mainly comprised of subjects with mild-moderate disease.

The three COPD groups (normal weight, overweight and obese) compared in our study were not homogenous in age or smoking history. Obese patients were older, probably reflecting the physiological weight increase that happens with age and sedentarism associated with exercise- and effort-induced dyspnea [25]. Moreover, and in agreement with Cecere et al. [22], obese patient groups had a lower frequency of current smokers, although the cumulative smoking exposure was higher, probably due to an age effect.

As for lung function, the FVC and FEV_1 of our obese patients were lower than those of normal-weight patients. These findings, which have also been identified in other studies [22,26], coincide with common physiological abnormalities classically associated with simple obesity, such as decreased chest wall and lung compliance, small airway dysfunction and expiratory flow limitation [27]. Contrarily, the lack of differences in inspiratory capacity among our patient groups contradicts with previous information from O'Donnell et al. [23], who reported a directly proportional relationship between BMI and resting IC, suggesting that obesity might reduce lung hyperinflation. This discordance could be attributed to the differing severity and age of the patients included in the two studies, and particularly to the fact that in the O'Donnell study the obese patients were younger than the patients with normal weight, while in our study the opposite was true.

Possibly one of the most prominent findings of our study lies in the impact of obesity on the symptoms profile of COPD patients, where patients with obesity had more dyspnea and less cough and expectoration than patients with normal weight. An analysis of the PLATINO study [13] also reported a higher frequency of dyspnea and wheezing in obese patients, although there were no variations in cough or phlegm. In addition to being more frequent, dyspnea is also more intense in obese patients compared with normal-weight patients, even after adjusting for airflow limitation and other variables. Compared with a small clinical series of COPD patients [28] that identified lower baseline dyspnea in obese patients, which was attributed to lower resting hyperinflation, other more extensive clinical series confirm that obese patients with COPD more frequently experience moderate or severe dyspnea than normal-weight patients [22,26]. A greater perception of the dyspnea associated with obesity may contribute to this finding [29]. Moreover, obesity might differ between various clinical phenotypes of COPD, as suggested in the Tucson prospective cohort study [8].

The crude comparison between the patient groups shows that obese COPD patients presented a greater use of respiratory medication and a poorer health-related quality of life. In the

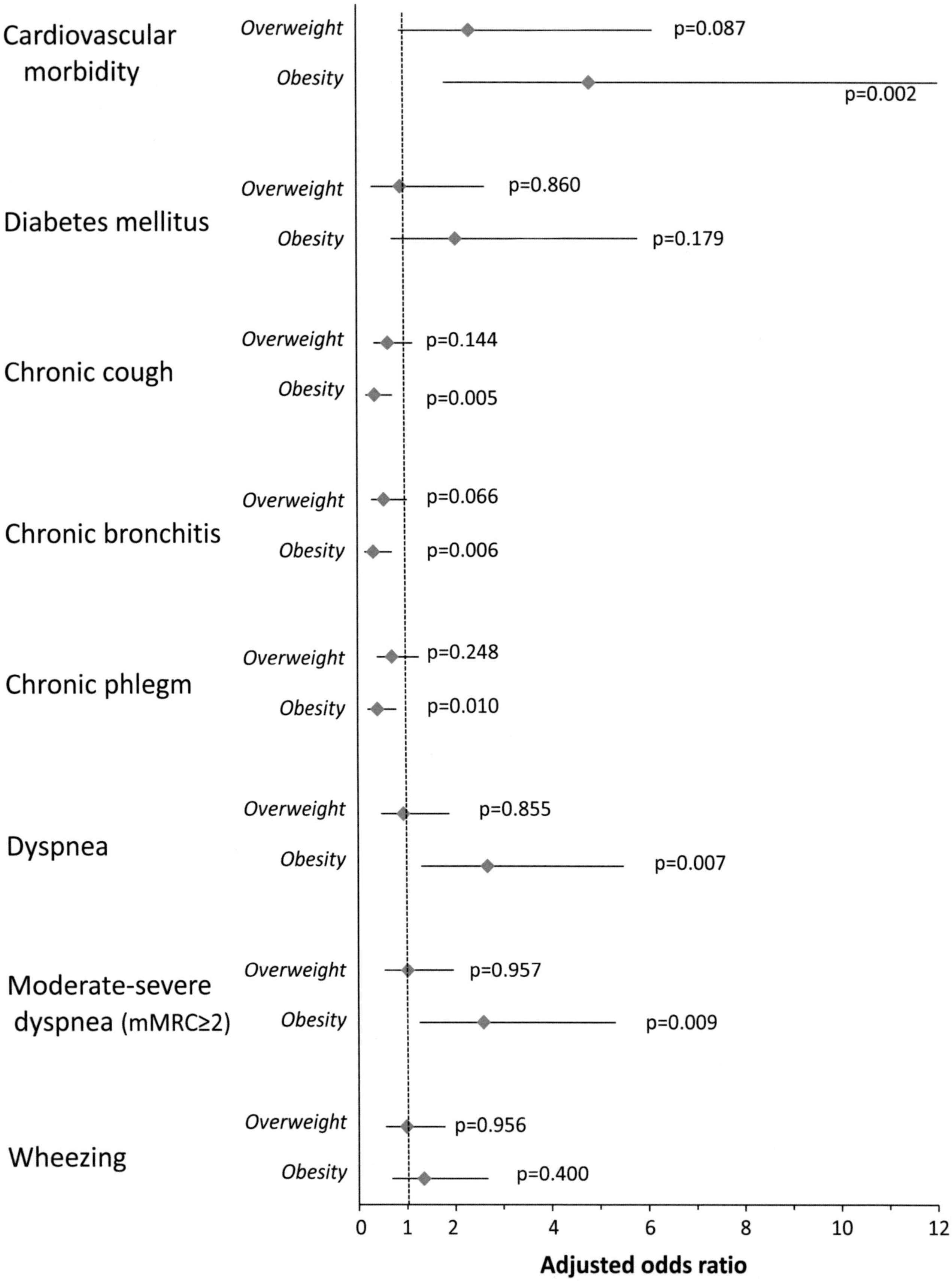

Figure 3. Adjusted risk of comorbidity and respiratory symptoms in overweight and obese COPD patients compared with normal-weight COPD patients. Values are adjusted for gender, age, packs-year and FEV_1 (% pred.).

adjusted analysis, however, only the EuroQoL showed significant differences between groups, while the SGRQ did not reach statistical significance, possibly reflecting the contribution of other determinants (that are not exclusively respiratory in nature) to the poorer quality of life of obese patients.

An aspect that is particularly important is the potential effect of obesity on the perception of symptoms of patients with asthma-COPD overlap syndrome. Taking into account the fact that obesity notably contributes to the breathlessness of asthma patients [30,31] and that some 17% of patients with COPD in our study were categorized as asthma-COPD phenotype [32], one could speculate that the clinical impact of obesity was provided exclusively by this patient subgroup. To assess this possibility, Tables S1-S4 in File S1 present the comparisons between groups while excluding patients with asthma-COPD overlap syndrome, which demonstrates that the effects of obesity on clinical manifestations, quality of life, exercise tolerance and systemic inflammation persist in the remaining COPD patients.

There is a certain discrepancy around the effect of obesity on exercise tolerance in COPD. While reduced tolerance to exercise has been reported [23], other authors do not identify such effect [28,33]. Our results confirm that adjusted exercise tolerance is lower in obese patients who reach a shorter distance walked during the 6-minute walk test. Although the mechanisms of exercise intolerance in obese patients with COPD may be complex due to disease heterogeneity and the existence of serious comorbidities, the neuromechanical uncoupling of the respiratory system seems to play some type of role. Compared to normal-weight COPD patients, obese patients have a higher metabolic demand at any given power output as a result of the high oxygen cost of lifting heavy limbs [23]. Moreover, obese patients with COPD have increased ventilatory demand and more frequently abnormal ventilatory mechanics. In fact, ventilatory requirements are higher in obese COPD patients compared with those of normal weight as a result of combined increased metabolic loading, high fixed physiological dead space and possibly earlier metabolic acidosis [28]. Given the increase in ventilatory demand and the mechanical limitation of ventilation, the muscular effort required to sustain ventilation during exercise is also higher [23]. The net effect of these abnormalities is the increased work and oxygen cost of breathing at any given power output compared with normal-weight individuals, which would be expected to contribute to exercise limitation. This hypothesis coincides with our results that obese patients develop greater walk-work, defined as 6 min walk distance × weight (in kg), and the results of others who demonstrated that obese COPD patients had higher peak symptom-limited oxygen uptake than non-obese patients [28,34].

In the general population, obesity is a strong risk factor for the development and progression of hypertension, dyslipidemia, metabolic syndrome, and type-2 diabetes mellitus [35]. Our results confirm this effect in COPD patients and that the presence of obesity almost multiplies five-fold the risk for presenting cardiovascular comorbidity. In this sense, it has been reported that the application of cluster analysis to segregate COPD patients into different phenotypes has been able to identify a group characterized by obesity and cardiovascular disease [36]. This association is particularly relevant because several studies have shown that cardiovascular diseases, along with lung cancer, are among the main causes of death in COPD patients not selected by severity criteria [37,38]. In spite of this, there continues to be controversy about the potential protective effect of obesity in COPD. Although it has been shown that, in patients with COPD, being overweight or obese had a protective effect against mortality [39], an analysis of the NHANES III cohort has reported that obesity is associated with increased mortality among participants with obstructive lung disease [40]. Furthermore, the increase in dyspnea induced by obesity could worsen the prognosis of these patients. In fact, it has been reported that persistent dyspnea and dyspnea development are risk factors for all-cause, cardiovascular and respiratory mortality in COPD patients, and that dyspnea effects on mortality are more pronounced in obese and older subjects [41].

Our results give supporting data to link obesity with the systemic inflammatory COPD phenotype. In COPD patients, the association between circulating CRP levels and BMI has previously been demonstrated [42]. Is has also been shown that the presence of elevated plasma CRP concentrations is associated with increased risk for the development of cardiovascular comorbidity [43]. From the PAC-COPD study, one of the three COPD subtypes included patients with milder airflow limitation and a high proportion of obesity, cardiovascular disorders, diabetes and systemic inflammation [36]. Most of the features of the so-called metabolic syndrome, including obesity, higher levels of triglycerides, diabetes, ischemic heart disease, arterial hypertension and elevated serum levels of C-reactive protein and fibrinogen, were clustered in this COPD subtype. So, obesity might be a marker for the proposed "chronic systemic inflammatory syndrome", which contributes to the comorbidities that frequently co-exist in patients with COPD [44].

Our study, however, presents several limitations. The evaluation of the nutritional state of the patients was based on BMI and we did not have any information regarding body composition. We do not have a longitudinal follow-up of the patients; therefore, it was not possible to evaluate the relationship between obesity throughout the progression of the disease. Furthermore, our sample presents a very small number of patients with severe or very severe disease because it provides a representative sample of the population distribution seen in COPD, with a predominance of milder patients.

To conclude, our study provides evidence of the higher prevalence of obesity in a population-based sample of patients with COPD. Moreover, our results show that obesity affects the clinical manifestations, quality of life and exercise tolerance of COPD patients, and that obesity might help define a phenotype characterized by increased systemic inflammation and greater frequency of cardiovascular comorbidity.

Supporting Information

File S1 Comparisons between COPD subgroups excluding patients with asthma-COPD overlap syndrome. Combined file includes Table S1-S4. **Table S1**. General characteristics, functional status and severity of the COPD groups excluding the patients with mixed COPD-asthma phenotype. **Table S2**. Comparison of symptoms, previous exacerbations, health status and systemic biomarker levels between the study groups excluding the patients with mixed COPD-asthma phenotype. **Table S3**. Adjusted comparisons of health status, exercise tolerance and systemic inflammatory biomarkers between the study groups excluding the patients with mixed COPD-asthma phenotype. **Table S4**. Adjusted risk of comorbidity and respiratory symptoms in overweight and obese COPD patients compared with normal-weight COPD patients excluding the subjects with mixed phenotype COPD-asthma. Values are adjusted for gender, age, packs-year and FEV1 (% pred.).

Author Contributions

Conceived and designed the experiments: FGR JBS MM LM EDT GS VS JA. Performed the experiments: FGR JBS MM LM EDT GS VS JA. Analyzed the data: FGR JBS MM LM EDT GS VS JA. Contributed reagents/materials/analysis tools: FGR JBS MM LM EDT GS VS JA. Contributed to the writing of the manuscript: FGR JBS MM LM EDT GS VS JA. Obtained permissions for the study: GS FGR JA MM. Vouched for the veracity and completeness of the data and the data analyses: FGR JBS MM LM EDT VS JA.

References

1. Global initiative for chronic obstructive lung disease. Global strategy for the diagnosis, management, and prevention of chronic obstructive pulmonary disease (Revised 2011). Available: http://www.goldcopd.org. Accessed: 2014 Apr 2.
2. Task Force for GesEPOC (2012) Clinical practice guideline for the diagnosis and treatment of patients with chronic obstructive pulmonary disease (COPD) – Spanish guideline for COPD (GesEPOC). Arch Bronconeumol 48 (Suppl 1): 2–58.
3. Chatila WM, Thomashow BM, Minai OA, Criner GJ, Make BJ (2008) Comorbidities in chronic obstructive pulmonary disease. Proc Am Thorac Soc 5: 549–555.
4. Schols AM, Slangen J, Volovics L, Wouters EF (1998) Weight loss is a reversible factor in the prognosis of chronic obstructive pulmonary disease. Am J Respir Crit Care Med 157: 1791–1797.
5. Bernard S, Leblanc P, Whittom F, Carrier G, Jobin J, et al. (1998) Peripheral muscle weakness in patients with chronic obstructive pulmonary disease. Am J Respir Crit Care Med 158: 629–634.
6. Landbo Ch, Prescott E, Lange P, Vestbo J, Almdal TP (1999) Prognostic value of nutritional status in chronic obstructive pulmonary disease. Am J Respir Crit Care Med 160: 1856–1861.
7. Celli BR, Cote CG, Marin JM, Casanova C, Montes de Oca M, et al. (2004) The body-mass index, airflow obstruction, dyspnoea, and exercise capacity index in chronic obstructive pulmonary disease. N Engl J Med 350: 1005–1012.
8. Guerra S, Sherrill DL, Bobadilla A, Martinez FD, Barbee RA (2002) The relation of body mass index to asthma, chronic bronchitis, and emphysema. Chest 122: 1256–1263.
9. García Rodríguez LA, Wallander MA, Tolosa LB, Johansson S (2009) Chronic obstructive pulmonary disease in UK primary care: incidence and risk factors. COPD 6: 369–379.
10. Schols AM, Soeters PB, Dingemans AM, Mostert R, Frantzen PJ, et al. (1993) Prevalence and characteristics of nutricional depletion in patients with stable COPD eligible for pulmonary rehabilitation. Am Rev Respir Dis 147: 1151–1156.
11. Gray-Donald K, Gibbons L, Shapiro SH, Macklem PT, Martin JG (1996) Nutritional status and mortality in chronic obstructive pulmonary disease. Am J Respir Crit Care Med 153: 961–966.
12. Chailleux E, Laaban JP, Veale D (2003) Prognostic value of nutritional depletion in patients with COPD treated by long-term oxygen therapy: data from the ANTADIR observatory. Chest 123: 1460–1466.
13. Montes de Oca M, Tálamo C, Perez-Padilla R, Jardim JRB, Muiño A, et al. (2008) Chronic obstructive pulmonary disease and body mass index in five Latin America cities: The PLATINO study. Respir Med 102: 642–650.
14. Vozoris NT, O'Donnell DE (2012) Prevalence, risk factors, activity limitation and health care utilization of an obese population-based sample with chronic obstructive pulmonary disease. Can Respir J 19: e18–e24.
15. Ancochea J, Badiola C, Duran E, García Río F, Miravitlles M, et al. (2009) Estudio EPI-SCAN: resumen del protocolo de un estudio para estimar la prevalencia de EPOC en personas de 40 a 80 años de edad en España. Arch Bronconeumol 45: 41–47.
16. Miravitlles M, Soriano JB, García-Río F, Muñoz L, Duran-Tauleria E, et al. (2009) Prevalence of COPD in Spain: Impact of undiagnosed COPD on quality of life and daily life activities. Thorax 64: 863–868.
17. Miller MR, Hankinson J, Brusasco V, Burgos F, Casaburi R, et al. (2005) Standardisation of spirometry. Eur Respir J 26: 319–338.
18. World Health Organization (1995) Physical status: the use and interpretation of anthropometry. Report of a WHO Expert Committee. World Health Organ Tech Rep Ser 854: 1–452.
19. García-Río F, Miravitlles M, Soriano JB, Muñoz L, Duran-Tauleria E, et al. (2010) Systemic inflammation in chronic obstructive pulmonary disease: a population-based study. Respir Res 11: 63.
20. ATS Statement: Guidelines for the six-minute walk test (2002) Am J Respir Crit Care Med 166: 111–116.
21. Puham MA, Garcia-Aymerich J, Frey M, Riet G, Antó JM, et al. (2009) Expansion of the prognostic assessment of patients with chronic obstructive pulmonary disease: the updated BODE index and the ADO index. Lancet 374: 704–711.
22. Cecere LM, Littman AJ, Slatore CG, Udris EM, Bruson CL, et al. (2011) Obesity and COPD: associated symptoms, health-related quality of life, and medication use. COPD 8: 275–284.
23. O'Donnel DE, Deesomchok A, Lam YM, Guenette JA, Amornputtisathaporn N, et al. (2011) Effects of BMI on static lung volumes in patients with airway obstruction. Chest 140: 461–468.
24. Čekerevac I, Lazić Z (2011) Obesity and chronic obstructive pulmonary disease. Srp Arh Celok Lek 139: 322–327.
25. Rennard SI, Calverley P (2003) Rescue! Therapy and the paradox of the Barcalounger. Eur Respir J 21: 916–917.
26. Van den Bemt L, van Wayenburg CAM, Smeele IJM, Schermer TRJ (2009) Obesity in patients with COPD, an undervalued problem?. Thorax 64: 640.
27. Franssen FME, O'Donnell DE, Goossens GH, Blaak EE, Schols AMWJ (2008) Obesity and the lung: 5-Obesity and COPD. Thorax 63: 1110–1117.
28. Ora J, Laveneziana P, Ofir D, Deesomchok A, Webb KA, et al. (2009) Combined effects of obesity and chronic obstructive pulmonary disease and exercise tolerance. Am J Respir Crit Care Med 180: 964–971.
29. Salome CM, Munoz PA, Berend N, Thorpe CW, Schachter LM, et al. (2008) Effect of obesity on breathlessness and airway responsiveness to methacholine in non-asthmatic subjects. Int J Obes (Lond) 32: 502–509.
30. Deesomchok A, Fisher T, Webb KA, Ora J, Lam YM, et al. (2010) Effects of obesity on perceptual and mechanical responses to bronchoconstriction in asthma. Am J Respir Crit Care Med 181: 125–133.
31. Shim YM, Burnette A, Lucas S, Herring RC, Weltman J, et al. (2013) Physical deconditioning as a cause of breathlessness among obese adolescents with a diagnosis of asthma. PLoS ONE 8: e61022.
32. Miravitlles M, Soriano JB, Ancochea J, Muñoz L, Duran-Tauleria E, et al. (2013) Characterisation of the overlap COPD-asthma phenotype. Focus on physical activity and health status. Respir Med 107: 1053–1060.
33. Ischaki E, Papatheodorou G, Gaki E, Papa I, Koulouris N, et al. (2007) Body mass and fat-free mass indices in COPD. Relation with variables expressing disease severity. Chest 132: 164–169.
34. Laviolette L, Sava F, O'Donnell DE, Webb KA, Hamilton AL, et al. (2010) Effect of obesity on constant work rate exercise in hyper inflated men with COPD. BMC Pulm Med 10: 33.
35. Lavie CJ, Milani RV (2003) Obesity and cardiovascular disease: the Hippocrates paradox? J Am Coll Cardiol 42: 677–679.
36. Garcia-Aymerich J, Gomez FP, Benet M, Farrero E, Basagaña X, et al. (2011) Identification and prospective validation of clinically relevant chronic obstructive pulmonary disease (COPD) subtypes. Thorax 66: 430–437.
37. Mannino DM, Doherty DE, Buist S (2006) Global Initiative on Obstructive Lung Disease (GOLD) classification of lung disease and mortality: findings from the atherosclerosis risk in communities (ARIC) study. Respir Med 100: 115–122.
38. Nicholas R, Anthonisen MD, Melissa A, Skeans MS, Wise MD, et al. (2005) The effects of a smoking cessation intervention on 14.5-year mortality. Ann Intern Med 142: 233–239.
39. Cao C, Wang R, Wan J, Bunjhoo H, Xu Y, et al. (2012) Body mass index and mortality in chronic obstructive pulmonary disease: a meta-analysis. PLoS ONE 7: e43892.
40. Jordan JG Jr, Mann JR (2010) Obesity and mortality in persons with obstructive lung disease using data from the NHANES III. South Med J 103: 323–330.
41. Figarska SM, Boezen HM, Vonk JM (2012) Dyspnea severity, changes in dyspnea status and mortality in the general population: the Vlagtwedde/Vlaardingen study. Eur J Epidemiol 27: 867–876.
42. Broekhuizen R, Wouters EF, Creutzberg EC, Schols AM (2006) Raised CRP levels mark metabolic and functional impairment in advanced COPD. Thorax 61: 17–22.
43. Sin DD, Man SF (2003) Why are patients with chronic obstructive pulmonary disease at increased risk of cardiovascular diseases? the potential role of systemic inflammation in chronic obstructive pulmonary disease. Circulation 107: 1514–1519.
44. Fabbri LM, Rabe KF (2007) From COPD to chronic systemic inflammatory syndrome? Lancet 370: 797–799.

Table 1. Self-reported intake of banned substances in the Doped group.

Subject	Substances and dosage in recent 5 years	Substances and dosage >5 years ago
D1	Testosterone (1250 mg w^{-1}) Dianabol (8 mg d^{-1}) Insulin (10–12 IU d^{-1}) IGF I (50 µg d^{-1})	Testosterone (1250 mg w^{-1})Dianabol (8 mg day^{-1}) Trenbolone (262.5 mg w^{-1})
D2	Testosterone (2000 mg w^{-1}) Deca-durabolin (600–800 mg w^{-1}) Dianabol (50 mg d^{-1}) Insulin (12 IU d^{-1}) Ephedrine (60 mg d^{-1})	Testosterone (2500 mg w^{-1}) Insulin (18 IU day^{-1})
D3	Testosterone (1500 mg w^{-1}) Deca-durabolin (800–1600 mg w^{-1}) Boldone (500 mg w^{-1}) Ephedrine (4–6 IU d^{-1}, 6 days w^{-1})	Testosterone (1500 mg w^{-1}) Deca-durabolin (600 mg w^{-1})
D4	Testosterone 500 mg w^{-1} GH (Somatropin) (4–6 IU d^{-1}, 6 days w^{-1}) Deca-durabolin (600 mg w^{-1})	Testosterone (500 mg w^{-1}) Deca-durabolin (600 mg w^{-1})
D5	Testosterone (500 mg w^{-1}) Deca-durabolin (250 mg w^{-1}) Dianabol (175–350 mg w^{-1}) Ephedrine (10000 IU total)	Testosterone (500 mg w^{-1}) Deca-durabolin (250 mg w^{-1}) Trenbolone (75 mg w^{-1})
D6	Testosterone (500 mg w^{-1}) Deca-durabolin (200 mg w^{-1}) Dianabol (200 mg w^{-1})	Testosterone (500 mg w^{-1}) Deca-durabolin (200 mg w^{-1})
D7	Testosterone (250 mg w^{-1}) Dianabol (175 mg w^{-1})	Testosterone (250 mg w^{-1})
D8	Testosterone (250 mg w^{-1}) Deca-durabolin (200 mg w^{-1}) Dianabol (200 mg w^{-1}) Oxar (175 mg w^{-1})	Testosterone (250 mg w^{-1}) Deca-durabolin (200 mg w^{-1}) Oxar (175 mg w^{-1})
D9	Testosterone (1000 mg w^{-1}) Boldone (1000 mg w^{-1}) Dianabol (105 mg w^{-1})	Testosterone (1000 mg w^{-1}) Boldone (250 mg w^{-1})
D10	Testosterone (500 mg w^{-1}) Deca-durabolin (400 mg w^{-1}) Trenbolone (150 mg w^{-1}) Dianabol (150–200 mg w^{-1})	Testosterone (500 mg w^{-1}) Deca-durabolin (400 mg w^{-1})

steroid users compared to the non-steroid users. In addition, in the steroid users, significant increase in frequency of fibers expressing developmental myosin heavy chain (MyHC) isoforms was also observed compared to the non-steroid users [14,15]. On basis of the results, we concluded that intake of anabolic steroids in combination with strength training induced both fiber hypertrophy and fiber hyperplasia (formation of new muscle fibres), in which the activation of satellite cells is a key process. However, the studies did not reveal whether the changes in muscle morphology were accompanied by improvement in muscle strength as well as body composition.

In anti-doping campaign, blood and urine samples are the major materials to be tested [5]. However, due to the fast metabolic character of most AAS, remnants of AAS or its metabolites are traceable only for a short time in blood or urine after AAS intake, while the effects of AAS on skeletal muscles will remain for a long period, perhaps lifetime [16]. So far, no study has compared muscle morphology and strength between long-term AAS abusing, and clean athletes.

It has been proposed that the effects of AAS on muscle are dose-dependent [2,5,8,17]. Twenty weeks of testosterone administration increases skeletal muscle mass, leg strength and power in a dose-dependent fashion, but did not improve muscle fatigability or physical function [17]. However, the effects of AAS dosage on skeletal muscles have never been studied over a period of several years.

The present study will investigate the effects of long term supplementation of AAS on muscle strength and morphology, and explore the relationships between AAS dosage, muscle strength and morphology in elite athletes. We proposed that strength training athletes using AAS will have a higher enhancement in muscle strength through morphological adaptations compared with strength training athletes without using AAS. In addition, the effects of long term AAS supplementation on skeletal muscles will be dose-dependent. Thus, the muscular responses to long term AAS supplementation can be detected and used to separate Doped from Clean athletes.

Materials and Methods

Ethics Statement

All participants were informed about the design of the study and written informed consent was obtained from all participants. The study protocol was approved by the Ethics Committee for northern Sweden at Umeå University. This was not an intervention study and no actions were taken to influence the participants' exercise training regime, diet, AAS administration or other activities. Manuscript data is confidential and protected by the Swedish personal integrity law (Personuppgiftslagen 1998:204) and the permission from the ethical board for northern Sweden (www.epn.se) at Umeå University (EPN Nr 08–145M).

Subjects

To investigate the long term effects of AAS supplementation on athletes, we recruited 17 strength training elite athletes through personal contact. All subjects were individually interviewed regarding doping substances, physical activity, smoking habits, known illnesses and medication intake. Ten were current users of AAS or AAS derivatives (Doped; age 41.1±8.0 years) and seven reported that they had never used AAS (Clean; age 29.1±6.2 years). Clean subjects had signed a contract with their local clubs and the Swedish Power Lifting Federation, committing them to never use any drugs, under sever monetary punishment. The subjects have been continuously doping-tested with negative results.

The ten Doped subjects were asked to report all banned-substances including doses and intervals taken for the past years. Detailed information of the banned substances and dosage is shown in Table 1. The AAS administration regimen includes both "stacking" (simultaneous use of several types of AAS) and "cycling" (a drug-free period followed by times when doses and types of drugs taken were initiated or increased). Intake usually follows a pyramid schedule with increased intake over time to avoid equation of AAS levels.

All the subjects reported that they had trained regularly between 4–6 times per week for at least five years. The physical training

Effects of Long Term Supplementation of Anabolic Androgen Steroids on Human Skeletal Muscle

Ji-Guo Yu[1], Patrik Bonnerud[2], Anders Eriksson[2], Per S. Stål[4], Yelverton Tegner[2], Christer Malm[1,3]*

1 Department of Surgical and Perioperative Sciences, Sports Medicine Unit, and School of Sport Sciences, Umeå University, Umeå, Sweden, **2** Department of Health Sciences, Luleå University of Technology, Luleå, Sweden, **3** Winternet, Boden, Sweden, **4** Department of Integrative Medical Biology, Section for Anatomy, Umeå University, Umeå, Swenden

Abstract

The effects of long-term (over several years) anabolic androgen steroids (AAS) administration on human skeletal muscle are still unclear. In this study, seventeen strength training athletes were recruited and individually interviewed regarding self-administration of banned substances. Ten subjects admitted having taken AAS or AAS derivatives for the past 5 to 15 years (Doped) and the dosage and type of banned substances were recorded. The remaining seven subjects testified to having never used any banned substances (Clean). For all subjects, maximal muscle strength and body composition were tested, and biopsies from the vastus lateralis muscle were obtained. Using histochemistry and immunohistochemistry (IHC), muscle biopsies were evaluated for morphology including fiber type composition, fiber size, capillary variables and myonuclei. Compared with the Clean athletes, the Doped athletes had significantly higher lean leg mass, capillary per fibre and myonuclei per fiber. In contrast, the Doped athletes had significantly lower absolute value in maximal squat force and relative values in maximal squat force (relative to lean body mass, to lean leg mass and to muscle fiber area). Using multivariate statistics, an orthogonal projection of latent structure discriminant analysis (OPLS-DA) model was established, in which the maximal squat force relative to muscle mass and the maximal squat force relative to fiber area, together with capillary density and nuclei density were the most important variables for separating Doped from the Clean athletes (regression = 0.93 and prediction = 0.92, $p<0.0001$). In Doped athletes, AAS dose-dependent increases were observed in lean body mass, muscle fiber area, capillary density and myonuclei density. In conclusion, long term AAS supplementation led to increases in lean leg mass, muscle fiber size and a parallel improvement in muscle strength, and all were dose-dependent. Administration of AAS may induce sustained morphological changes in human skeletal muscle, leading to physical performance enhancement.

Editor: Stephen E. Alway, West Virginia University School of Medicine, United States of America

Funding: This work was supported by grants from the Swedish National Centre for Research in Sports and WADA (Grant 08C15CM). The funders had no role in study design, data collection and analysis, decision to publish, or preparation of the manuscript.

Competing Interests: Christer Malm has part-time employment at the non-profit organization (an economical union) Winternet, Boden, Sweden since 2001. Some of the work for the manuscript was executed using equipment at Winternet. All data, ethical permission, potential patents etc. are filed under Sports Medicine Unit, Umeå University (EPN nr 08–145M). Thus, all past and present data belong to Umeå University. This does not alter the authors' adherence to PLOS ONE policies on sharing data and materials.

* Email: Christer.malm@idrott.umu.se

Introduction

Testosterone and other anabolic androgen steroids (AAS) are used by increasing population of professional and recreational athletes with the intention to increase muscle size and improve muscle strength [1–3]. Even though athletes using AAS claim significant gain in performance, a large number of academic studies investigating the performance-enhancing effects of AAS have described discordant and often contradictory outcomes [4,5]. Some studies revealed significant gains in strength and muscle mass/girth [6–8] whereas others reported no effects of AAS on muscle mass/girth and/or muscle strength [9,10]. Such conflicting results have been attributed to poor study design including non-blinded condition, no placebo control, small sample size and AAS dose variation. Above all, in most studies, out of ethic consideration, AAS administration was usually no longer than 6 months. Such a short period of AAS administration obviously could not reflect the reality of AAS abuse in athletes and sport enthusiasts. In reality, AAS usage was estimated to sustain for several years or the whole competition period in athletes [11]. Thus, the difference in AAS administration period between AAS abusers and subjects in most academic studies might be one of the major reasons leading to the different conclusions.

Short term AAS administration has been shown to induce muscle strength enhancement. The increased muscle strength has been attributed to increased muscle mass which was associated with muscle fiber hypertrophy of both type I and type II fibers [12,13]. Effects of long term AAS administration on muscle morphology in relation with muscle strength as well as with body composition are, however, still unclear. In our early studies on strength training subjects with long period AAS self-administration (9±3.3 years), analysis of muscle biopsies revealed significant increases in mean fiber area for both type I and type II fibers, number of myonuclei and proportion of central nuclei in the

Table 2. Anthropometry, muscle strength and morphology in Clean and Doped athletes [mean ± SD or median (min-max)].

Variable	Doped	Clean	p
Anthropometry	N = 10	N = 7	
Body weight (kg)	108±17	110±13	0.85
Lean body mass (kg)	89.8±8.2	74.6±6.8	0.06
Lean leg mass (kg)	28.6±2.5	25.5±1.4	0.01
Performance	**N = 9**	**N = 7**	
Personal Bench record (kg)#	205 (155–320)	190 (145–230)	0.79
Personal Squat record	254±11	265±35	0.53
Personal Deadlift record (kg)#	257 (150–300)	269 (245–300)	0.86
Maximal Squat force (N)	2416±633	3302±274	0.004
Maximal Squat force/Lean body mass (N kg^{-1})	29.5±4.0	49.8±5.8	0.001
Maximal Squat force/Lean leg mass (N kg^{-1})	88±17	130±14	<0.001
Maximal Squat force/Mean fiber area (N μm^{-2})	0.33±0.09	0.50±0.05	0.001
Maximal Squat force/Type I fiber area (N μm^{-2})	0.38±0.12	0.64±0.06	<0.001
Maximal Squat force/Type IIa fiber Area (N μm^{-2})	0.28±0.08	0.40±0.06	0.009
Muscle morphology	**N = 10**	**N = 6**	
Fiber area (μm^2)#	7744 (4731–16330)	6733 (5668–8567)	0.70
Type I fiber area (μm^2)#	6511 (3734–15208)	5189 (4408–6139)	0.30
Type IIa fiber area (μm^2)#	9066 (4820–17446)	8489 (7144–11448)	0.78
Capillary density (n μm^{-2}); CD	218±43	182±41	0.12
Capillaries/Fiber (n); CAF	3.93±0.70	3.05±0.42	0.02
Capillaries/Type I fiber (n); CAFI	4.24±0.60	3.16±0.49	0.003
Capillaries/Type IIa fiber (n); CAFIIa	4.08±0.66	2.94±0.37	0.002
Capillaries/Mean fiber area (n μm^{-2}); CAFA	0.55±0.12	0.46±0.11	0.20
Capillaries/Type I fiber area (n μm^{-2}); CAFAI	0.69±0.16	0.62±0.11	0.33
Capillaries/Type IIa fiber area (n μm^{-2}); CAFAIIa	0.45±0.10	0.36±0.09	0.09
Nuclei/Type I fiber (n); NIFI	2.20±0.11	1.83±0.13	0.04
Nuclei/Type IIa fiber (n)#; NIFIIa	3.84 (2.5–6.0)	3.34 (2.6–4.1)	0.25
Nuclei/Type I fiber area (n μm^{-2}) × 1000; NIFAI	0.37±0.10	0.36±0.08	0.83
Nuclei/Type IIa fiber area (n μm^{-2}) × 1000; NIFAIIa	0.46±0.10	0.40±0.06	0.21
Internal nuclei/Fiber (n)#; INIF	0.07 (0.01–0.25)	0.07 (0.01–0.36)	0.98

#Wilcoxon signed rank test [median (min-max)].

was defined as self-reported mean hours of exercise training each week during the past five years, and consisted mainly of high intensity resistance training. The Doped group consists of a mixture of bodybuilders, strongmen competitors and weightlifters whereas the Clean group consists of weightlifters only. The mode of resistance training differs slightly between the two groups; the Doped group used both 1–4 repetitions/set and 8–12 repetitions/set, while the Clean group used mainly 1–4 repetitions/set. We have to emphasize that this is the only ethically feasible approach to study long term effects of AAS abuse on athletes.

Muscle strength and body composition

Subjects performed static squats at a 105° knee angle in a custom-made Smith squat machine and ground reaction forces were recorded by AMTI force plates (464 × 508 mm, Advanced Mechanical Technology Incorporated, Massachusetts, USA). Forces were recorded in x, y and z directions at 100 Hz using the Qualisys Track Manager (QTM) software (Qualisys AB, Gothenburg, Sweden). Maximal force (one single recording), Mean of the highest 50 recordings and Mean of 0.1 sec highest recordings according to rank (highest to lowest) were used for statistical analysis. Personal records (PR) from competition (without tight suits) or equivalent (not all participants had competed in all disciplines) for Bench press, Squat lift and Deadlift were also used for comparisons.

Blood samples

Blood sample of 10 ml was collected from all subjects the same time in the morning after overnight fasting by venipuncture from the cubital vein. Because we could not perform regular doping tests on the subjects and the Doped subjects were not on a "cycle", indirect indicator of blood hormone level was used to prove/disprove the use of AAS.

Muscle samples

Skeletal muscle biopsies were obtained from the vastus lateralis muscle using standard needle or forceps biopsy technique [18,19]. The biopsies were taken from the middle part of the muscle, mounted in OCT compound (Tissue Tek, Miles laboratories, Naperville, IL, USA) and then frozen in liquid propane chilled

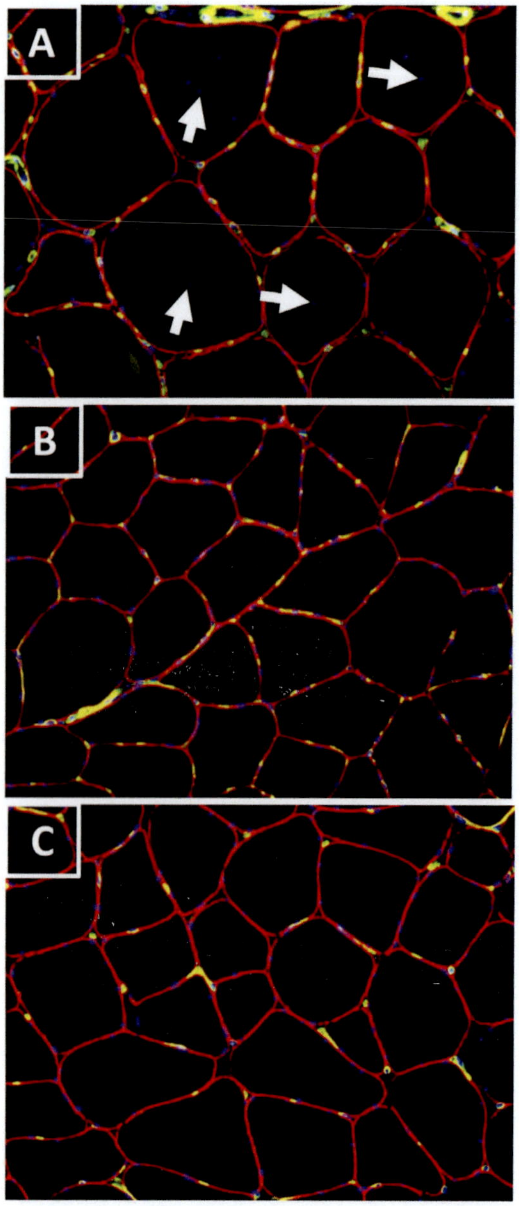

Figure 1. Multiple labeled muscle cross-sections with DAPI (Blue) for nuclei, mAb 4C7 (green) for capillary and mAb 5H2 (red) for fiber membrane. Sections from one Doped athlete using higher (A; >2500 mg·week^{-1}) and one using lower doses AAS (B;< 500 mg·week^{-1}), and from one Clean athlete (C). Doped athletes with higher doses AAS showed larger fiber areas (A) than Doped athletes with lower AAS doses (B) and Clean athletes (C). More capillaries and nuclei around each type I fiber were observed in the Doped athletes (A and B) compared to Clean (C). Internal nuclei are marked with arrows in A.

with liquid nitrogen and stored at −80°C until further processing. Due to technical problems, one biopsy from the Clean group was discarded, leaving 6 biopsies in the Clean group for analysis.

Biopsy processing

Serial muscle cross-sections were cut at −20°C by using a Reichert Jung cryostat (Leica, Nussloch, Germany). Eight µm thick sections were stained with haematoxylin-eosin and a modified Gomori trichrome staining for basic histopathology including detection of degenerative processes and inflammation [20].

Five µm thick transverse sections were processed for IHC with different and previously characterized antibodies. For fiber phenotype type classification, serial sections were stained with monoclonal antibodies (mAbs) against different MyHC isoforms: A4.840 (strong affinity for MyHCI; [20]), A4.74 (strong affinity for MyHCIIa; [20]), N2.261 (strong affinity to MyHCIIa, weak affinity for MyHCI, no affinity for MyHCIIx; [20]), BF-35 (strong affinity for all MyHC isoforms except IIx; [20]). All antibodies were obtained from the Developmental Studies Hybridoma Bank, developed under the auspices of the National Institute of Child Health and maintained by the University of Biological Sciences, Iowa City, Iowa, USA.

For fiber size measurement and capillary visualization, mAb 5H2 against laminin α2 chain in muscle fiber basement membrane (Nova Castra Lab, Newcastle, UK) and mAb 4C7 against laminin α5 in capillary basement membrane (Chemicon, Temecula, Calif., USA) were used [21].

The IHC staining process is the same as described earlier [22]. Visualization of bound primary antibody was performed using indirect unconjugated immunoperoxidase technique and/or indirect immunofluorescence technique with affinity-purified Abs specifically prepared for multiple labelling and conjugated with flurochromes with different emission spectra, fluorescein (FITC), Rhodamine red-X (RRX) and Cyanine 5 (Cy5). Nuclei were identified with 4′, 6-diamidino-2 phenylindole (DAPI) provided in the mounting media (Vectashield, Vector laboratories Inc, Burlingame CA 94010 USA). All antibodies were diluted in 0.01 M PBS containing 0.1% bovine serum albumin (Dako, Glostrup, Denmark) and used at their optimal dilution. Control sections were treated similarly except that the primary antibodies were exchanged with non-immune serum.

Morphometric analysis

Randomly chosen areas from each section were scanned using a light microscope (Leica DM6000B, Leica Microsystems CMS GmbH, Wetzlar, Germany) equipped with a high-speed fluorescence digital CCD camera (Leica DFC360 FX) connected to an image analysis system (Leica, QWin plus). For each muscle sample, more than 50 fibres (mean 227) were individually analysed in order to obtain a robust morphometric analysis [23].

Based on the staining pattern for the different MyHC mAbs, the fibers were classified as fibers containing solely MyHCI, MyHCIIa or MyHCIIx, or as hybrid fibers co-expressing two MyHC isoforms: MyHCI+IIa or MyHCIIa+IIx. Detailed description of fiber type classification has been described in our earlier study [24].

Estimation of fiber area and number of capillary has been described in detail in a publication from our laboratory [21]. An average of 855 capillaries (range 298–1616) per muscle sample cross section was counted. Capillary density (CD) was calculated as the total number of capillaries per µm^2 muscle cross sectional area (capillary · µm^{-2}). The number of capillaries around each fiber (CAF) included all capillaries within a distance of 6 µm from each individual muscle fiber, as outlined by staining for laminin α5. The number of capillaries around each fiber relative to fiber cross sectional area (CAFA) was calculated according to the formula: CAF/(fiber cross sectional area) × 10^3, representing the cell volume supplied by each capillary.

Nuclei in each fiber (NIF) were calculated as all nuclei within each muscle fiber. The number of nuclei in each fiber relative to fiber area (NIFA) was calculated as: NIF/(cross sectional area for each fiber) × 10^3. This variable measures the nuclear domain in

Table 3. Blood hormone levels [median (min-max)].

Variable	*Biomarker for*	*Clinical range**	*Control*	*Doped*	*p*
Lutenizing hormone (LH; E • L^{-1})	Pituitary gland	1.2–9.6	2.5 (1.2–4.8)	0 (0–1.2)	<0.001
Folicular stimulating hormone (FSH; E • L^{-1})	Pituitary gland	1.0–12.5	3.0 (1.0–4.2)	0 (0–2.3)	<0.001
17-alfa-Hydroxiprogesteron (17-OH-prog; nmol • L^{-1})	Adrenal glands	< 10	1.85 (0.70–7.00)	0.30 (0.30–0.70)	0.001
Alanine aminotransferas ALAT (μkat • L^{-1})	Liver	< 1.2	0.55 (0.48–0.70)	0.77 (0.59–2.08)	0.005
Aspartate aminotransferas ASAT (μkat • L^{-1})	Liver	< 0.76	0.47 (0.33–0.65)	0.68 (0.39–1.92)	0.01
Prolactin (Prol; μg • L^{-1})	Pituitary gland	3–13	6 (4–13)	10 (6–16)	0.01
Urea (mmol L^{-1})	Muscle/Kidney	3.2–8.1	7.4 (4.5–9.6)	4.8 (2.3–5.7)	0.02
Creatin Kinase (CK; μkat • L^{-1})	Muscle	0.8–6.7	4.8 (3.9–11.8)	11.8 (4.2–85.2)	0.03
Testosterone (Testo; nmol • L^{-1})	Androgen	6.3–16	11 (7.1–18)	35 (3.8–130)	0.08
Pro-brain natriuretic peptide (ProBNP; ng • L^{-1})	Heart	< 84	14 (9–31)	10 (0–32)	0.09
Androstendione (nmol • L^{-1})	Adrenal glands	3.2–9.9	2.0 (1.2–2.8)	3.1 (0.6–14)	0.09
Creatinin (Crea; μmol • L^{-1})	Muscle/Kidney	< 100	94 (84–133)	88 (77–112)	0.12
Apolipoprotein B (ApoB, g • L^{-1})	Liver/Intestine	0.50–1.50	0.87 (0.76–1.44)	1.24 (0.83–1.61)	0.16
Sexual hormone binding globuline (SHBG; nmol • L^{-1})	Liver	15–56	29 (18–46)	23 (3.9–54)	0.19
Apolipoprotein A (ApoA; g • L^{-1})	Liver/Intestine	1.10–1,80	1.19 (1.02–1.60)	1.09 (0–1.36)	0.20
Troponin I (Trop I; μg • L^{-1})	Heart	< 0.03	0 (0–0.11)	0 (0–0)	0.20
Estradiol (E2K; pmol • L^{-1})	Estrogen	50–150	81 (55–102)	182 (25–425)	0.25
Growth hormone (GH; μg • L^{-1})	Hypophysis	none	0.10 (0.01–4.80)	0.05 (0–3.1)	0.33
Insulin like growth factor IGF-I (μg • L^{-1})	Anabolism	120–420	194 (95–384)	158 (114–259)	0.35
Dehydroepiandrosterone sulfate (DHEAS; μmol • L^{-1})	Adrenal glands	2.4–13	8.4 (6.0–11)	7.8 (1.3–12)	0.36
Cystatin C (CystC; mg • L^{-1})	Kidney	< 0.99	0.89 (0.70–0.96)	0.84 (0.75–1.00)	0.59
High sensitive C –reactive protein (HCRP; mg • L^{-1})	Heart/Inflammation	< 3	0.4 (0.3–5–4)	1.37 (0–25.6)	0.73
Lipoprotein (a) (Lp(a); mg • L^{-1})	Heart	< 700	356 (84–1463)	372 (222–782)	0.81
Thyroid stimulating hormone (TSH; mE • L^{-1})	Metabolism	0.4–4.7	1.5 (0.6–2.0)	1.7 (0.8–2.8)	0.85
Cortisol (Cortis; nmol • L^{-1})	Adrenal glands	100–800	415 (281–550)	402 (146–498)	0.87
Alkaline phosphatase (ALP; μkat • L^{-1})	Liver	< 1.20	1.0 (0.7–1.6)	1.15 (0.70–1.70)	0.88

Wilcoxon signed rank test [median (min-max)]. * From the Karolinska University Laboratory (www.karolinska.se/Karolinska-Universitetslaboratoriet/)

each fiber. Analysis of internal nuclei in each fiber (INIF) was calculated as all the nuclei within each fiber, but without contact to the cell membrane outline by staining for laminin α5.

Statistical analysis

Normal distribution of data was tested using the Shapiro-Wilk's test and visually inspected through normal quantile plot. Student's unpaired t-test was used to compare measurements between the two groups, but when data was significantly skewed ($p<0.05$), then the Wilcoxon signed-rank two-sample test with normal approximation was applied. Accordingly, mean and standard deviation (SD) or median and range were used for descriptive statistics. Correlation analysis between AAS dosage and other variables was performed using Pearson correlation and linear regression, and skew data was log-transformed. Orthogonal projections of latent structures discriminant analysis (OPLS-DA) models were used to separate groups (Clean from Doped). One predictive component was calculated (Y), where R2Y display the cumulative percent of the modelled variation in Y, using the X model. Q2Y values display the cumulative percent of the variation in Y that can be predicted by the model according to cross validation (leave one out methods and seven groups), using the X model. The variation modelled of X, using all predictive components and orthogonal components in X, R2X (cum) is a measure of fit, i.e. how well the model fits the X data. JMP 11 (SAS Institute Inc., USA) and SIMCA 13.0 (Umetrics AB, Sweden) were used for all statistical calculations.

Results

Maximal muscle strength and anthropometry

Group values of maximal muscle strength and anthropometry were presented in Table 2. The two groups had similar personal records, but compared to the Clean group, the Doped athletes presented significantly higher lean leg mass ($P<0.01$) and lower maximal squat force in both absolute and relative terms. For subject G, data of both AAS intake and Type IIa fiber area were outside normal distribution ($p<0.05$), even after log-transformation. Therefore, results were presented separately with or without the data of the subject.

Muscle morphology

Group values of measurements were presented in Table 2. The vastus lateralis muscle was predominated by fibers expressing slow MyHCI and fast MyHCIIa fibers in both groups, and there was no difference in fiber type proportion in the muscle between the two groups. Hybrid fibers co-expressing MyHCIIa+IIx or MyHCI+IIa isoforms were rare (< 3%) in some athletes from both groups.

No significant difference in mean fiber area of either type I or type IIa was observed between the Doped and the lean athletes.

Table 4. Correlations between AAS dosage and measured variables.

Variable	All subjects (N = 10)		Excluding subject G (N = 9)	
	r	p	r	p
Anthropometry				
Body Weight (kg)	0.33	0.35	0.21	0.59
Lean body mass (kg)	0.62	0.05	0.43	0.25
Lean leg mass (kg)	0.53	0.12	0.27	0.48
Performance				
Maximal Squat force (N)	0.65	0.06	0.75	0.03
Maximal Squat force/Lean body mass ($N \cdot g^{-1}$)	0.51	0.17	0.83	0.01
Maximal Squat force/Lean leg mass ($N \cdot g^{-1}$)	0.55	0.13	0.88	0.004
Maximal Squat force/Mean fiber area ($N \cdot \mu m^{-2}$)	−0.01	0.98	0.76	0.01
Maximal Squat force/Type I fiber area ($N \cdot \mu m^{-2}$)	−0.01	0.98	0.80	0.02
Maximal Squat force/Type IIa fiber Area ($N \cdot \mu m^{-2}$)	−0.08	0.85	0.60	0.12
Morphology				
Mean fiber area $(\mu m^2)^{Log10}$	0.69	0.02	0.24	0.53
Type I fiber area $(\mu m^2)^{Log10}$	0.70	0.06	0.25	0.51
Type IIa fiber area $(\mu m^2)^{Log10}$	0.62	0.06	0.24	0.53
Capillary density (μm^2); CD	−0.33	0.35	0.52	0.15
Capillaries/Fiber (n); CAF	0.47	0.17	0.59	0.10
Capillaries/Type I fiber (n); CAFI	0.64	0.05	0.61	0.08
Capillaries/Type IIa fiber (n); CAFIIa	0.29	0.41	0.49	0.18
Capillaries/Mean fiber area ($n \cdot \mu m^{-2}$); CAFA	−0.39	0.27	0.57	0.11
Capillaries/Type I fiber area ($n \cdot \mu m^{-2}$); CAFAI	−0.43	0.22	0.47	0.20
Capillaries/Type IIa fiber area ($n \cdot \mu m^{-2}$); CAFAIIa	−0.45	0.2	0.45	0.23
Nuclei/Fiber (n); NIF	0.30	0.40	0.21	0.59
Nuclei/Type I fiber (n); NIFI	0.26	0.47	0.14	0.73
Nuclei/Type IIa fiber $(n)^{LOG}$; NIFIIa	0.33	0.36	0.28	0.46
Nuclei/Fiber area ($n \cdot \mu m^{-2}$); NIFA	−0.63	0.05	−0.11	0.78
Nuclei/Type I fiber area ($n\ \mu m^{-2}$); NIFAI	−0.64	0.05	−0.16	0.69
Nuclei/Type IIa fiber area ($n \cdot \mu m^{-2}$); NIFAIIa	−0.61	0.06	−0.09	0.81
Inner Nuclei/Fiber (n); INIF	0.55	0.10	0.12	0.76

Log_{10}; transformed for normal distribution before calculations.

However, the doped athletes presented 15% larger in mean fibre area and large variation in fibre area compared to the clean athletes (Fig. 1). In the Doped group, one individual had extremely large fibers (> 15000 μm^2; Fig. 1).

When capillary measurements were expressed as CD, no difference between the Doped and the Clean groups was observed; however, when expressed as CAF, the Doped group had significantly higher values in both type I and type IIa fibers. When CAF was compensated for fiber area (CAFA), the significant difference between the two groups disappeared for both fiber types (Table 2).

More nuclei per fiber (NIF) were observed in type I fiber of the Doped group compared to the clean group (Table 2). When NIF was compensated for fiber area (NIFA), no difference was observed in any fiber type between the two groups.

The average number of INIF (internal nuclei/fiber) was very low and did not show statistical difference between the two groups.

Hormone level

Because most blood hormone concentration were not normally distributed, data was analysed by non-parametric statistics (Wilcoxon signed rank, Chi^2 approximation), and presented as median and minimum - maximum (Table 3). Several blood hormone concentrations linked to hypophysis and liver function differed significantly ($p<0.05$) between Clean and Doped groups, and were outside clinical ranges. Most notably were LH, where all, and FSH where all but one, Doped subjects had below the clinical range indicating disturbed pituitary gland function. For ASAT and ALAT two, and for CK four, Doped subject were above the clinical range, possibly indicating liver and muscle damage. Seven Doped subjects had testosterone levels above clinical range, but as a group not significantly different from Clean.

Correlation analysis

Table 4 was the results of correlation analysis between AAS dosage and all the other measurements. Among the morphological parameters, AAS dose was significantly correlated to fiber area of both type I and type IIa fiber, to CAF of type I, and NIFA of type I

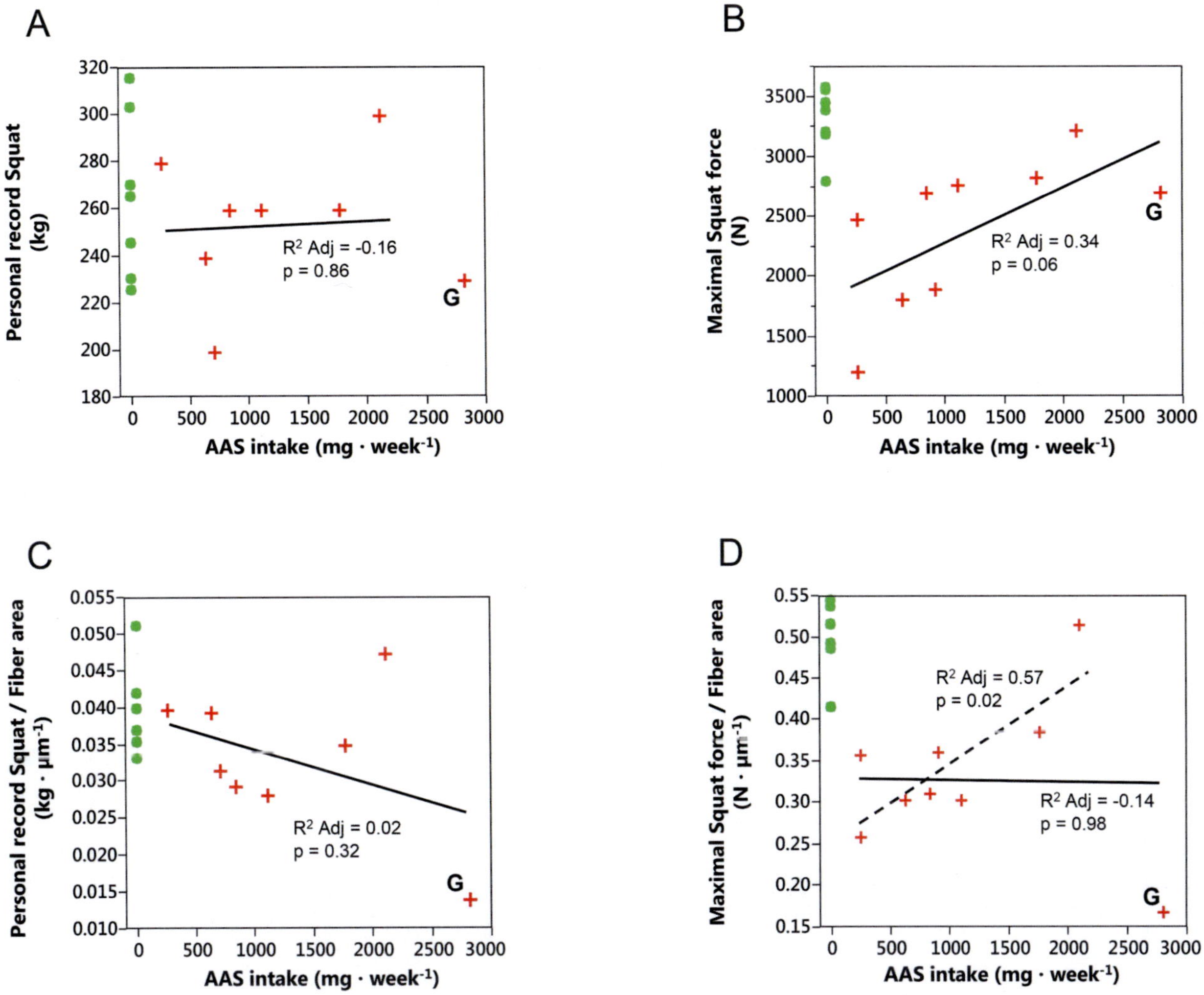

Figure 2. Regression models for the effects of AAS intake on muscle performance. Correlations between AAS weekly intake and muscle performance: A) personal record (kg; $R^2 = -0.16$, $p = 0.86$) and B) maximal squat force (N; $R^2 = 0.34$, $p = 0.06$), and models for the effects of AAS intake on relative muscle performance: C) maximal squat force per lean leg mass ($N \cdot g^{-1}$; $R^2 = 0.02$, $p = 0.32$) and D) maximal squat force per fiber area ($N \cdot \mu m^{-1}$; $R^2 = -0.14$, $p = 0.98$). The residual of subject G is outlier ($p = 0.003$, Shapiro-Wilk W test) and when removed, the regression is significant between force per fiber area and AAS intake ($N \cdot \mu m^{-1}$; $R^2 = 0.57$, $p = 0.02$).

fibers. Some linear regression models were presented in Figure 2. A significant regression was found for mean muscle fiber area (R^2 Adj = 0.40, p = 0.003, not shown), but not for personal record (Fig. 2*A*), nor for personal record relative to fibre area (Fig. 2*C*). A trend (R^2 Adj = 0.34, p = 0.06) towards significant correlation was observed between AAS intake and maximal squat force (Fig. 2*B*). Subject G had extremely high dose of AAS and skewed regression residuals (p = 0.003). When subject G, the outlier was excluded, a significant linear correlation (R^2 Adj = 0.57, p = 0.02) between AAS dose and maximal squat force relative to muscle fiber area was observed (Fig. 2*D*). When subject G was excluded, a second-degree fitting reveals a decreasing trend (R^2 Adj = −0.14, p = 0.98) for maximal squat force relative to fiber area.

OPLS-DA model

In OPLS-DA analysis, a score scatter plot (Fig. 3) out of eight morphological and performance measurements separated clearly the Doped from the Clean athletes (Fig. 4). Of the eight variables, four morphological measurements were higher and the other four of relative maximal squat force were lower in the Doped than in the Clean athletes.

Discussion

The main findings of the study were that the doped athletes had higher lean mass, capillary density and myonuclei density, but lower maximal squat force relative to muscle mass and to fiber area, compared to the clean athletes. The Doped group also had a tendency towards larger fibers, although not significant, most likely due to large variations in fibre area. Low levels of LH and FSH, and high levels of prolactin in some individuals indicate a disturbed pituitary gland function with possible negative effects on reproductive function. High levels of ALAT, ASAT and CK in some individuals suggest that long term use of AAS could damage both liver and muscle tissue. However, no correlations between AAS intake and hormone levels was observed. Thus, testosterone levels at time of sampling cannot explain alternations in these variables, rather concentrations outside clinical limits must stem from long-term supplementation of AAS. Multivariate statistics

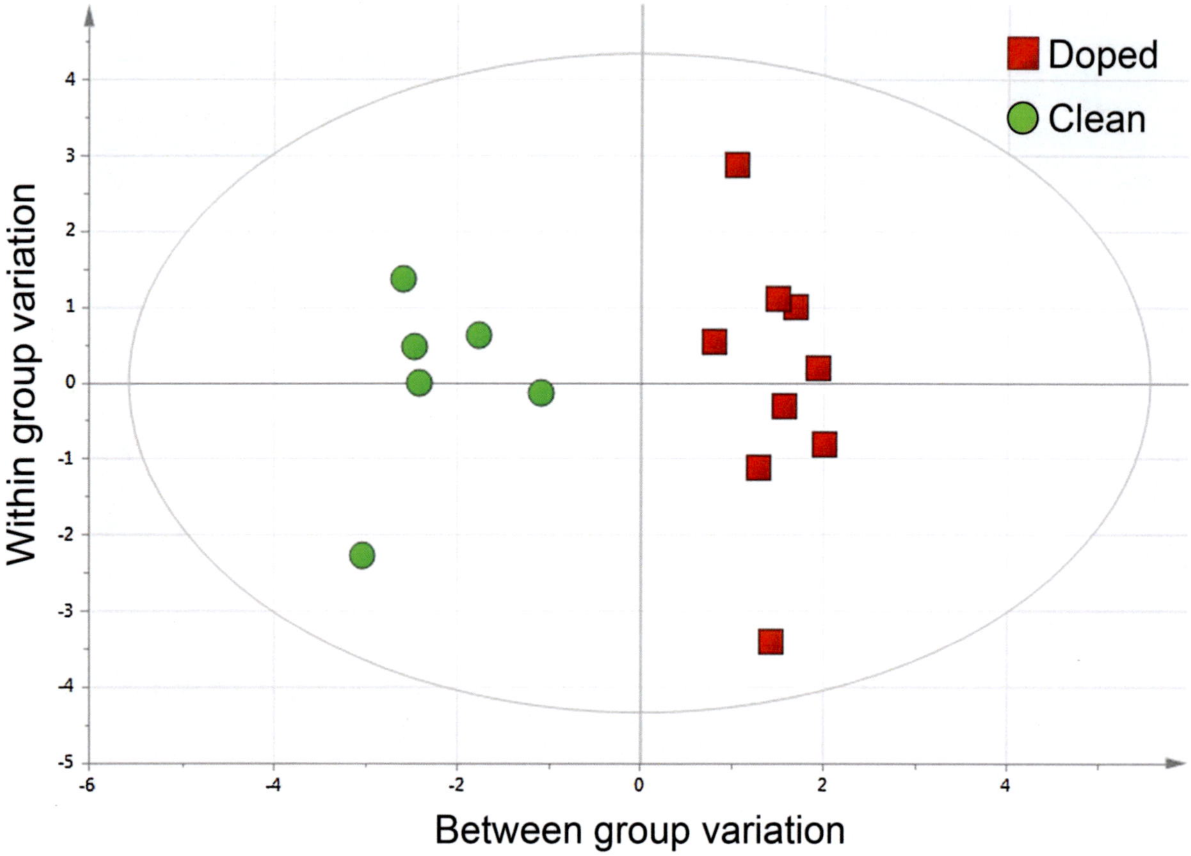

Figure 3. The OPLS-DA model scores scatter plot of combined performance and morphological separates Doped from Clean athletes. Morphological and performance variables (N = 8) are used in an OPLS-DA model to separate Doped (N = 9) from Clean (N = 6) subjects. Regression = 0.93, and prediction by cross-validation = 0.92, $p<0.0001$, Fisher's exact probability test. All nine Doped subjects and six of seven Clean are correctly classified, leaving one Clean un-classified. Variables of importance are displayed in Figure 4.

showed that a combination of eight morphological parameters could clearly separate the doped from the clean athletes. Correlation analysis revealed significant positive correlations between AAS dosage and relative muscle force. The results support previous findings that AAS administration could induce enhancement in both muscle mass and muscle strength, and that the improvements are AAS dose-dependent [5,8,12,25,26]. This is the first study to confirm previous laboratory findings in active doping athletes.

AAS and Muscle Mass, Muscle Morphology and Muscle Strength

Despite abundant studies on the effects of AAS on skeletal muscle, many results are contradictory [5]. Some studies have shown gains in body weight, girth, fat-free mass or lean body mass, but not in muscle strength [27–29], whereas others have shown gains in both muscle mass/girth and muscle strength [5,8,17,30,31], or in neither muscle mass/girth nor muscle strength after short term (from 17 days to 16 weeks) [32–35] or long term (2 years) [36] AAS administration. The present study showed that athletes with long term AAS supplementation had significantly higher leg lean mass compared to Clean athletes. The higher lean leg mass in the Doped subjects has been revealed to be mainly due to increased muscle mass, as shown in our previous study on the same group of doped athletes [37].

Increased muscle mass in subjects using AAS has been proposed to result from muscle hypertrophy alone [12] or from both muscle hypertrophy and hyperplasia [38]. Muscle hypertrophy is often evident by increased muscle fiber size and increased number of myonuclei. The latter is associated with satellite cell activation and myoblast infusion with the existing muscle fibers, leading to greater numbers of myonuclei in larger myofibers [39]. In previous studies on subjects with long term AAS supplementation (9 ± 3.3 years), we observed significant higher frequency of newly formed myofibers in AAS users than in the non-AAS users, indicating that steroid can induce both muscle hypertrophy and hyperplasia [14,15]. In the present study, long term AAS supplementation was only associated with higher lean leg mass, but not with larger fiber size, indicating that muscle fiber hyperplasia may play a role in the muscle mass enhancement. Coincidently, the number of myonuclei in type I fibers in the doped athletes was significantly higher than in the clean athletes, which may indicate satellite cell activation for muscle fiber hyperplasia.

Not many studies have examined the effects of AAS on muscle capillaries. In a previous study of 20 weeks of graded testosterone enanthate injection (25, 50, 125, 300, or 600 mg), Sinha-Hikim et al. [12] did not observe significant difference in capillary density among the five treatment groups. The authors suggested that it is not unlikely that a significant increase in capillaries takes longer than 20 weeks. In the present study, we observed more capillaries around both type I and type IIa fibers in the Doped athletes

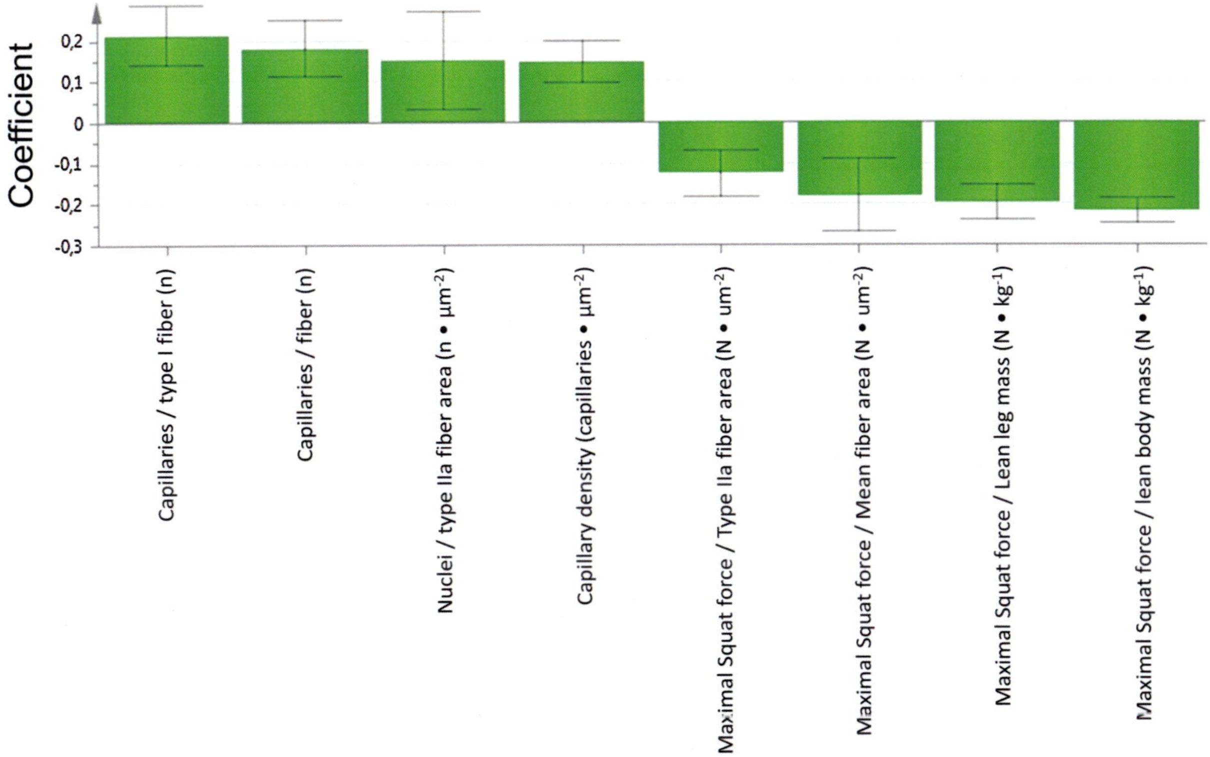

Figure 4. The coefficient plot of variables of importance in the OPLS-DA model. From the OPLS-DA model in Figure 3, the significant important muscle morphological and performance variables separating Doped from Clean subjects are displayed with 95% confidence interval using jack-knifing test. Bars indicate scaled ratios between the Doped and the Clean groups, with higher ratios of the Doped group to the left, and lower ratios to the right.

compared to the Clean group. Importantly, when the parameter of capillaries per fiber (CAF) was calculated by fiber area (CAFA), the significant difference in CAF between the two groups disappeared, indicating proportional and simultaneous increases in number of capillary around each fiber and in muscle fiber size in the Doped group. These are the first results demonstrating an association between long term AAS supplementation and muscle capillarization. Consequently, AAS will enhance not only muscle strength, but also muscle endurance.

It has been shown that combined administration of androgens and resistance training is associated with greater gains in lean body mass, muscle size, and maximal voluntary strength than either intervention alone [31]. The greater increase in maximal voluntary strength is often attributed to greater increase in lean body mass and/or muscle size [5]. However, some studies using lower AAS doses and shorter supplementation times have shown no gains in muscle strength [31], regardless if lean body mass and muscle size were increased or not [5]. Similarly, in the present study, the Doped group had higher lean leg mass, but lower leg strength. Thus, for long-term AAS abusers, increase in muscle mass/lean body mass may be not directly associated with muscle strength improvement.

It is worth to notice that compared to the Clean group, the Doped group presented larger variations in many of the measurements like leg lean mass (Doped, 24.6–32.6 kg vs. Clean, 22.8–26.9 kg), leg maximal strength (Doped, 1823–3242 N vs. Clean, 2799–3570 N) and muscle fibre size (Doped, 6055–16330 μm^2 vs. Clean, 5668–8567 μm^2). Giorgi et al. [40] have reported that much of the gains in body weight and maximum bench press obtained during, and immediately after, 12 weeks of steroid administration and resistance training was lost during a subsequent 12 week period when androgens were not administered. In the present study, not all Doped athletes were in the same "AAS cycle", indicating that during the study, some of the Doped subjects were taking AAS whereas the others were in a "clean" period, i.e. AAS effects on muscles were stacking in some subjects but diminishing in the others. This may explain, among other factors, the large variations in some of the measurements, and resulted in the non-significant differences between the two groups [2]. Of course, the large variations in AAS dosage may also explain some of the variations.

AAS dose-dependent muscular adaptations

Previous studies have shown that testosterone administration was associated with a dose-dependent increase in skeletal muscle mass, leg strength and power [2,17,41]. However, similar correlation between AAS dosage and leg lean mass (or fat free body mass) was not observed in the present study. One previous study has shown that 180 days of transdermal testosterone treatment resulted in increase in leg press by 90 days but did not induce further improvement by 180 days [42]. Another study by [43] has shown that major effects of AAS on muscle strength and lean body mass occurred over the first 12 months of testosterone administration to older men. In the present study, because the Doped athletes were not in the same AAS intake "cycle", the time-dependent effects of AAS on muscles may explain some of the variations in data [2].

In line with laboratory intervention studies [12,26], we observed that AAS dosage was significantly correlated with fiber area and nuclei number (NIFA; Table 4). Some studies have shown more fiber size enhancement in type I fibers than in type IIa fibers both after short term [44] and long term [14,45] AAS self-administration. However, our results of fibre size changes in the doped athletes did not show similar fiber type specificity. Finally, if subject G, with extremely high AAS dose, was taken into calculation of correlation between AAS intake and maximal squat force relative to muscle fiber area, there seem to be an upper limit for AAS intake, beyond which further increase in AAS intake will suppress muscular adaptation and performance.

Study Limitations

While all the Doped athletes have used AAS, the mix and quality of the substance are unknown. This may confound the estimation of AAS dosage as well as the effects on muscle morphology and performance. Additionally, post-study subjects de-coding revealed that Doped group was older and composed of athletes involved in bodybuilding and strongmen events, while Clean athletes were all power-lifters. Consequently, training regiments were slightly different, even though all aiming at increasing muscle strength. Consequences for interpretation of data are several: 1) Doping controls implemented for power-lifters in Sweden has reduced the number of doped athletes, while the same anti-doping efforts have not been taken in other power events. 2) Because the higher age in the Doped group, it can be speculated that athletes in their later career are more prone to AAS. 3) The dose-response effects of AAS on muscle morphology and performance were in agreement with previous intervention studies.

To further explore the effects of long term AAS supplementation on skeletal muscles, more advanced techniques, such as proteomics and metabolomics should be applied in tissue analysing. Again, we have to emphasize that the current study design is hard to be replicated in laboratory due to the extreme doses and duration of AAS supplementation.

Acknowledgments

We thank M Enerstedt, A-K Olofsson and P Boman for excellent technical assistance. Associate Professor, MD Stefan Arver is acknowledged for consultation when selecting blood variables for analysis.

Author Contributions

Conceived and designed the experiments: CM AE YT PB. Performed the experiments: CM PS AE YT PB. Analyzed the data: JGY CM PS AE YT PB. Contributed reagents/materials/analysis tools: CM PS. Contributed to the writing of the manuscript: JGY CM PS AE YT PB.

References

1. Weitzel LR, Sandoval PA, Mayles WJ, Wischmeyer PE (2009) Performance-enhancing sports supplements: role in critical care. Crit Care Med 37: S400–409.
2. Saad F, Aversa A, Isidori AM, Zafalon L, Zitzmann M, et al. (2011) Onset of effects of testosterone treatment and time span until maximum effects are achieved. Eur J Endocrinol 165: 675–685.
3. Thiblin I, Petersson A (2005) Pharmacoepidemiology of anabolic androgenic steroids: a review. Fundamental & clinical pharmacology 19: 27–44.
4. Kuhn CM (2002) Anabolic steroids. Recent Prog Horm Res 57: 411–434.
5. Hoffman JR, Kraemer WJ, Bhasin S, Storer T, Ratamess NA, et al. (2009) Position stand on androgen and human growth hormone use. J Strength Cond Res 23: S1–S59.
6. Boone JB, Jr., Lambert CP, Flynn MG, Michaud TJ, Rodriguez-Zayas JA, et al. (1990) Resistance exercise effects on plasma cortisol, testosterone and creatine kinase activity in anabolic-androgenic steroid users. Int J Sports Med 11: 293–297.
7. Friedl KE, Dettori JR, Hannan CJ, Jr., Patience TH, Plymate SR (1991) Comparison of the effects of high dose testosterone and 19-nortestosterone to a replacement dose of testosterone on strength and body composition in normal men. J Steroid Biochem Mol Biol 40: 607–612.
8. Storer TW, Magliano L, Woodhouse L, Lee ML, Dzekov C, et al. (2003) Testosterone dose-dependently increases maximal voluntary strength and leg power, but does not affect fatigability or specific tension. J Clin Endocrinol Metab 88: 1478–1485.
9. Elashoff JD, Jacknow AD, Shain SG, Braunstein GD (1991) Effects of anabolic-androgenic steroids on muscular strength. Ann Intern Med 115: 387–393.
10. Friedl K (2000) Effect of anabolic steroid use on body composition and physical performance. In: CE Y, editor. Anabolic Steroids in Sport and Exercise. Champaign, IL: Human Kinetics. pp. 139–174.
11. Berning JM, Adams KJ, Stamford BA (2004) Anabolic steroid usage in athletics: facts, fiction, and public relations. J Strength Cond Res 18: 908–917.
12. Sinha-Hikim I, Artaza J, Woodhouse L, Gonzalez-Cadavid N, Singh AB, et al. (2002) Testosterone-induced increase in muscle size in healthy young men is associated with muscle fiber hypertrophy. Am J Physiol Endocrinol Metab 283: E154–164.
13. Sinha-Hikim I, Roth SM, Lee MI, Bhasin S (2003) Testosterone-induced muscle hypertrophy is associated with an increase in satellite cell number in healthy, young men. Am J Physiol Endocrinol Metab 285: E197–205.
14. Kadi F, Eriksson A, Holmner S, Thornell LE (1999) Effects of anabolic steroids on the muscle cells of strength-trained athletes. Medicine and Science in Sports and Exercise 31: 1528–1534.
15. Eriksson A, Kadi F, Malm C, Thornell LE (2005) Skeletal muscle morphology in power-lifters with and without anabolic steroids. Histochemistry and cell biology 124: 167–175.
16. Eriksson A (2006) Strength training and anabolic steroids: a comparative study of the vastus lateralis, a thigh muscle and the trapezius, a shoulder muscle, of strength-trained athletes. Umeå: Umeå University.
17. Storer TW, Woodhouse L, Magliano L, Singh AB, Dzekov C, et al. (2008) Changes in muscle mass, muscle strength, and power but not physical function are related to testosterone dose in healthy older men. J Am Geriatr Soc 56: 1991–1999.
18. Malm C, Nyberg P, Engstrom M, Sjodin B, Lenkei R, et al. (2000) Immunological changes in human skeletal muscle and blood after eccentric exercise and multiple biopsies. J Physiol 529 Pt 1: 243–262.
19. Malm C, Sjodin B, Sjoberg B, Lenkei R, Renstrom P, et al. (2004) Leukocytes, cytokines, growth factors and hormones in human skeletal muscle and blood after uphill or downhill running. J Physiol 556: 983–1000.
20. Dubowitz V, Sewry CA, Lane RJM (2007) Muscle Biopsy: A Practical Approach: Saunders.
21. Stal PS, Lindman R (2000) Characterisation of human soft palate muscles with respect to fibre types, myosins and capillary supply. J Anat 197 (Pt 2): 275–290.
22. Yu JG, Thornell LE (2002) Desmin and actin alterations in human muscles affected by delayed onset muscle soreness: a high resolution immunocytochemical study. Histochemistry and cell biology 118: 171–179.
23. McCall GE, Byrnes WC, Dickinson AL, Fleck SJ (1998) Sample size required for the accurate determination of fiber area and capillarity of human skeletal muscle. Can J Appl Physiol 23: 594–599.
24. Yu JG, Liu JX, Carlsson L, Thornell LE, Stal PS (2013) Re-evaluation of sarcolemma injury and muscle swelling in human skeletal muscles after eccentric exercise. PLoS One 8: e62056.
25. Bhasin S, Calof OM, Storer TW, Lee ML, Mazer NA, et al. (2006) Drug insight: Testosterone and selective androgen receptor modulators as anabolic therapies for chronic illness and aging. Nat Clin Pract Endocrinol Metab 2: 146–159.
26. Sinha-Hikim I, Cornford M, Gaytan H, Lee ML, Bhasin S (2006) Effects of testosterone supplementation on skeletal muscle fiber hypertrophy and satellite cells in community-dwelling older men. The Journal of clinical endocrinology and metabolism 91: 3024–3033.
27. Isidori AM, Giannetta E, Greco EA, Gianfrilli D, Bonifacio V, et al. (2005) Effects of testosterone on body composition, bone metabolism and serum lipid profile in middle-aged men: a meta-analysis. Clin Endocrinol (Oxf) 63: 280–293.
28. Snyder EM, Snyder SA, Giesy JP, Blonde SA, Hurlburt GK, et al. (2000) SCRAM: A scoring and ranking system for persistent, bioaccumulative, and toxic substances for the North American Great Lakes. Part II: Bioaccumulation potential and persistence. Environmental science and pollution research international 7: 116–121.
29. Emmelot-Vonk MH, Verhaar HJ, Nakhai Pour HR, Aleman A, Lock TM, et al. (2008) Effect of testosterone supplementation on functional mobility, cognition, and other parameters in older men: a randomized controlled trial. JAMA 299: 39–52.
30. Rogerson S, Weatherby RP, Deakin GB, Meir RA, Coutts RA, et al. (2007) The effect of short-term use of testosterone enanthate on muscular strength and power in healthy young men. J Strength Cond Res 21: 354–361.
31. Bhasin S, Storer TW, Berman N, Callegari C, Clevenger B, et al. (1996) The effects of supraphysiologic doses of testosterone on muscle size and strength in normal men. The New England journal of medicine 335: 1–7.
32. Fowler WM, Jr., Gardner GW, Egstrom GH (1965) Effect of an anabolic steroid on physical performance of young men. J Appl Physiol 20: 1038–1040.

33. Weiss U, Muller H (1968) [On the problem of influencing strength training with anabolic hormones]. Schweiz Z Sportmed 16: 79–89.
34. Fahey TD, Brown CH (1973) The effects of an anabolic steroid on the strength, body composition, and endurance of college males when accompanied by a weight training program. Med Sci Sports 5: 272–276.
35. Crist DM, Stackpole PJ, Peake GT (1983) Effects of androgenic-anabolic steroids on neuromuscular power and body composition. J Appl Physiol 54: 366–370.
36. Zahner L, Puder JJ, Roth R, Schmid M, Guldimann R, et al. (2006) A school-based physical activity program to improve health and fitness in children aged 6–13 years ("Kinder-Sportstudie KISS"): study design of a randomized controlled trial [ISRCTN15360785]. BMC Public Health 6: 147.
37. Nordstrom A, Hogstrom G, Eriksson A, Bonnerud P, Tegner Y, et al. (2012) Higher muscle mass but lower gynoid fat mass in athletes using anabolic androgenic steroids. J Strength Cond Res 26: 246–250.
38. Hartgens F, Kuipers H (2004) Effects of androgenic-anabolic steroids in athletes. Sports Med 34: 513–554.
39. Herbst KL, Bhasin S (2004) Testosterone action on skeletal muscle. Curr Opin Clin Nutr Metab Care 7: 271–277.
40. Giorgi A, Weatherby RP, Murphy PW (1999) Muscular strength, body composition and health responses to the use of testosterone enanthate: a double blind study. J Sci Med Sport 2: 341–355.
41. Bhasin S, Woodhouse L, Casaburi R, Singh AB, Bhasin D, et al. (2001) Testosterone dose-response relationships in healthy young men. Am J Physiol Endocrinol Metab 281: E1172–1181.
42. Wang C, Swerdloff RS, Iranmanesh A, Dobs A, Snyder PJ, et al. (2000) Transdermal testosterone gel improves sexual function, mood, muscle strength, and body composition parameters in hypogonadal men. J Clin Endocrinol Metab 85: 2839–2853.
43. Page S, Matsumoto AM (2008) Effects of testosterone therapy in older men. JAMA 299: 1900, ; author reply 1900–1901.
44. Kuipers H, Peeze Binkhorst FM, Hartgens F, Wijnen JA, Keizer HA (1993) Muscle ultrastructure after strength training with placebo or anabolic steroid. Can J Appl Physiol 18: 189–196.
45. Hartgens F, Kuipers H, Wijnen JA, Keizer HA (1996) Body composition, cardiovascular risk factors and liver function in long-term androgenic-anabolic steroids using bodybuilders three months after drug withdrawal. Int J Sports Med 17: 429–433.

20

Differential and Conditional Activation of PKC-Isoforms Dictates Cardiac Adaptation during Physiological to Pathological Hypertrophy

Shaon Naskar, Kaberi Datta, Arkadeep Mitra, Kanchan Pathak, Ritwik Datta, Trisha Bansal, Sagartirtha Sarkar*

Genetics and Molecular Cardiology Laboratory, Department of Zoology, University of Calcutta, Kolkata, West Bengal, India

Abstract

A cardiac hypertrophy is defined as an increase in heart mass which may either be beneficial (physiological hypertrophy) or detrimental (pathological hypertrophy). This study was undertaken to establish the role of different protein kinase-C (PKC) isoforms in the regulation of cardiac adaptation during two types of cardiac hypertrophy. Phosphorylation of specific PKC-isoforms and expression of their downstream proteins were studied during physiological and pathological hypertrophy in 24 week male Balb/c mice (*Mus musculus*) models, by reverse transcriptase-PCR, western blot analysis and M-mode echocardiography for cardiac function analysis. PKC-δ was significantly induced during pathological hypertrophy while PKC-α was exclusively activated during physiological hypertrophy in our study. PKC-δ activation during pathological hypertrophy resulted in cardiomyocyte apoptosis leading to compromised cardiac function and on the other hand, activation of PKC-α during physiological hypertrophy promoted cardiomyocyte growth but down regulated cellular apoptotic load resulting in improved cardiac function. Reversal in PKC-isoform with induced activation of PKC-δ and simultaneous inhibition of phospho-PKC-α resulted in an efficient myocardium to deteriorate considerably resulting in compromised cardiac function during physiological hypertrophy via augmentation of apoptotic and fibrotic load. This is the first report where PKC-α and -δ have been shown to play crucial role in cardiac adaptation during physiological and pathological hypertrophy respectively thereby rendering compromised cardiac function to an otherwise efficient heart by conditional reversal of their activation.

Editor: Sudhiranjan Gupta, Texas A & M, Division of Cardiology, United States of America

Funding: This work was funded by grants from Council of Scientific and Industrial Research [Grant#37(1393)/10/EMR-II]; Department of Science and Technology, Govt. of India [Grant#F.No.SR/SO/HS-100/2009] to S. Sarkar. S. Naskar was supported by Research Fellowship from University Grants Commission. The funders had no role in study design, data collection and analysis, decision to publish, or preparation of the manuscript.

Competing Interests: The authors have declared that no competing interests exist.

* Email: sagartirtha.sarkar@gmail.com

Introduction

Cardiac hypertrophy is defined as an increase in cardiac mass and two forms of cardiac hypertrophy viz. physiological and pathological are currently recognized. Physiological increase in cardiac mass is considered to be an adaptive beneficial response which occurs normally during development, pregnancy and in response to sustained exercise [1] that enhances normal cardiac structure and normal or improved cardiac function with no evidence of myocyte apoptosis [2,3]. In contrast, pathological cardiac hypertrophy occurring in response to diverse stimuli including hypertension, valve disease, genetic mutations etc. [4] is detrimental resulting in loss of cardiac function, accumulation of collagen, loss of cardiomyocytes and ultimately heart failure [5].

Among various signaling pathways involved in promoting cardiac hypertrophy protein kinase-C (PKC) has been identified as an important component used by myocytes in response to a variety of extracellular stimuli [6]. PKC, a class of phospholipid dependent serine/threonine kinase, is activated by second messenger molecules formed via receptor-dependent activation of phospholipase-C. Cardiomyocytes express multiple PKC-isoforms with distinct biological functions in different cardiac diseases [7,8]. PKC-α is involved in the development of cardiac hypertrophy though extracellular-signal-regulated kinase-1/2 (ERK-1/2) [9] whereas, activation of PKC-ε has positive effect on cell growth during ventricular hypertrophy [10]. PKC-ε has also been shown to protect post-conditioned cardiomyocytes from programmed cell death [11]. Several reports have shown involvement of PKC-α, -β, and -δ in development of cardiac hypertrophy [7, 8 &12]. Increased PKC-δ expression and decreased expression of PKC-α, -β, -ε, and -ζ was observed in aortic banding model of cardiac hypertrophy [13]. PKC-isoforms have been shown to have either pro (PKC-δ) or anti (PKC-λ, -ζ and -α) apoptotic function in different cell types [14].

Several researchers have shown cardio-protective role of regular exercise in individuals suffering from cardiovascular diseases [15] and endurance training could convert pathological cardiac hypertrophy into physiological form with improved cardiac performances [16]. Although a recent study has reported cardiac damage after bouts of exercise in apparently healthy individuals [15] it is debated whether effect of exercise during physiological hypertrophy is truly a physiological incident that does not lead to pathological LV remodeling and cardiac dysfunction or long term chronic exercise training is maladaptive leading to compensated cardiac function and sudden death [5]. Researchers have pointed out increased cardiac risks in young athletes during or immediately after prolonged exercise training [5,15]. However, the precise mechanism for such cardiac adaptation is not yet fully understood. Our study for the first time has identified specific isoforms of PKC associated to either physiological or pathological hypertrophy and also addressed the mechanism of such diverse cardiac adaptation by PKC-isoform switch.

Materials and Methods

Animal used

Balb/c mice (*Mus musculus*) used in this study were procured from National Institute of Nutrition, Hyderabad, AP, India. All experimental animals were maintained on standard mice chow and water ad libitum in a climate-controlled, light-regulated space with 12-hour light and dark cycles in the departmental animal facility of the University of Calcutta.

Ethics statement

The investigation conforms to the Guidelines for the Care and Use of Laboratory Animals published by the US National Institute of Health (NIH Publication No. 85-23, revised 1996) and was also approved by the Institutional Animal Ethics Committee, University of Calcutta (Registration #885/ac/05/CPCSEA), registered under "Committee for the Purpose of Control and Supervision of Experiments on Laboratory Animals" (CPCSEA), Ministry of Environment and Forests, Government of India.

In vivo generation of cardiac hypertrophy models

24 weeks old male Balb/c mice (n = 20) were used to generate various models for this study. Pathological cardiac hypertrophy was generated in a group of mice designated as H, by ligating right renal artery for 3 weeks described previously with some modifications [17]. Another group of mice designated as H^X, were subjected to exercise training for the last 2 weeks of the 3 weeks tenure of renal artery ligation. Sham operated mice were used as controls.

Physiological cardiac hypertrophy was induced via swim exercise training for 3 weeks as described previously [18,19] with some modifications (mice designated as E) whereas, another group designated as E^R, was first subjected to exercise training for 3 weeks and maintained for 2 more weeks after exercise withdrawal. For time point specific studies, animals were rested for different time frames (viz., 3, 7, 15, 20, 30 and 45 days) after exercise withdrawal (n = 5). 24 week old male sedentary mice for similar period were used as control for this set. Each group of mice was sacrificed after the treatment period and the cardiac tissue was processed accordingly for various experimental purposes as described below.

Isolation of cardiomyocytes from hearts of all experimental groups

Adult myocytes were isolated from hearts of all experimental mice groups following the procedure described previously [20]. ~90% pure isolated cardiomyocytes were confirmed by staining with sarcomeric alpha-actinin antibody (Abcam, MA).

Cardiac fibroblast culture and treatment

Fibroblast cells were isolated from 24 week old male mice hearts by the collagenase dispersion method [21]. 75–80% confluent and 24 h serum-starved cells were treated for 24 h with 10^{-8} mol/liter (Sar1)-Angiotensin-II (Bachem, CA). Ang-II-treated cells were used as positive controls for all subsequent experiments. Untreated cells were used as controls.

In vivo treatment with chemical inhibitors and siRNA against PKC-δ and PKC-α

PKC-δ specific chemical inhibitor Rottlerin (Cat# R5648, Sigma-Aldrich, MO) and PKC-α specific chemical inhibitor Gö6976 (Cat# G1171, Sigma-Aldrich) [22] were dissolved in DMSO. Then along with 1X PBS, inhibitors were injected intraperitoneally in all three groups of experimental mice (C, H and E) at a dose of 600 μg/day/kg body weight during the last seven days of the experimental period as described earlier [23].

siRNAs against PKC-δ (siRNA ID: 151130; Catalogue no. # AM16708, Ambion, Life Technologies, NY) and PKC-α (siRNA ID: 151124; Catalogue no. # AM16708, Ambion, Life Technologies) as well as a nonspecific siRNA (Catalogue no. #4457289, Ambion, Life Technologies) at a concentration of 10 nmoles in 1X PBS was injected in ventricles in all three groups of experimental mice (C, H and E) following manufacturer's protocol during the last seven days of the experimental period as described previously [24] with slight modification.

Treatment of cardiac fibroblasts with PKC-δ Inhibitor and siRNA

Rottlerin at a concentration of 3 μM and PKC-δ siRNA at a concentration of 10 nmoles were used in this study. Inhibitors were added 45 min before Ang-II treatment. Cells treated with equivalent concentration of DMSO and nonspecific siRNA (Catalogue no. #4457289, Ambion, Life Technologies, NY) were used as controls.

Histology

All heart tissues were fixed in Karnovsky's fixative, paraffin-embedded, and cut into 4 μm sections as described earlier [25]. Sections (taken from same areas of the heart of all the experimental animals) were stained with hematoxylin/eosin and all the stained sections were observed and captured under the microscope (BX-51, Olympus, PA) and myocyte dimensions were quantitated by a computer morphometric program (ImageJ, NIH). The cross-sectional areas were quantified in (>100) myocytes from each experimental group.

Reverse transcriptase-PCR (RT-PCR)

Total RNA was isolated from all cardiac ventricular tissues using TRIzol reagent (Invitrogen, CA). Reverse transcription was done using Cloned AMV First-Strand cDNA Synthesis Kit (Invitrogen, CA) to check the expression of pathological hypertrophy marker genes, *Atrial natriuretic factor* (*ANF*) and *β Myosin heavy chain* (*β-MHC*) [17,25] and *Insulin-like growth factor-1* (*IGF-1*) marker for physiological hypertrophy [15] using forward (F) and reverse (R) primers (IDT, San Diego, CA). *Glyceraldehyde-3-phosphate dehydrogenase* (*GAPDH*) was used as internal loading control.

[*ANF*-F5'-TGCCGGTAGAAGATGAGGTC-3′& R5'-AAG-CTGTTGCAGCCTAGTCC-3′

β-MHC-F5'-CGGATGCCATACAGAGGAC-3′& R5'-CCT-CATAGGCGTTCTTGAGC-3′

IGF-1-F5'-TGAGCTGGTGGATGCTCTCAGTT-3′& R5'-TCTGAGTCTGGGCATGTCATGT-3′

GAPDH-F5'-ACTCCACTCACGGCAAATTC-3′& R5'-TGTTGCTGTAGCCGTAT-3′]

Protein extraction

After the experimental period, hearts were dissected out and perfused with chilled 1X phosphate buffered saline (PBS). Then the heart tissues were homogenized in protein extraction buffer [50 mM Tris, 250 mM NaCl 0.5% NP-40, 10% Glycerol, 5 mM EDTA, 0.1 M EGTA, 0.1 M PMSF, 1 M DTT, protease inhibitor (aprotinin, leupeptin and pepstatin) and phosphatase inhibitor cocktail (Sigma-Aldrich, MO)] and the supernatants were collected from each sample and concentrations of protein were estimated by Bradford assay at 595 nm using UV-vis Spectrophotometer (UV1700, Shimadzu Corporation, Kyoto, Japan) as described earlier [26].

Protein from adult cardiomyocytes was isolated using M-PER Mammalian protein extraction reagent (Thermo Scientific, IL). Mitochondrial and nuclear fraction from both cell and tissue samples were isolated by differential centrifugation method as described earlier [27,28].

Western blotting

30 μg of total protein and 200 μg of phospho protein samples were separated by SDS-PAGE and transferred to PVDF^{+} membrane (Millipore, MA), followed by incubation with primary antibodies against PKC-δ, phospho-PKC-δ (Thr 505), phospho-PKC-α (Ser 657 and Tyr 658), phospho-PKC-α/βII (Thr 638/641), PKC-α, PKC-βII, phospho-PKC-ε (Ser 729), PKC-ε, phospho-PKC-μ (Ser 744/748 and Ser 916), PKC-μ, phospho-PKC-δ/θ (Ser 643/676), phospho-PKC-θ (Thr 538), PKC-θ, phospho-PKC-ζ/λ (Thr 410/403), PKC-ζ, cytochrome-c, caspase-3, poly ADP ribose polymerase (PARP), phospho-P53 (Ser 46 and Ser 15), protein kinase-B (Akt), phospho-Akt, extracellular-signal-regulated kinase-1/2 (ERK-1/2), phospho-ERK1/2, STAT3, p38 MAPK, phospho-STAT3-Tyr-705, phospho-STAT3-Ser-727 and phospho-p38 MAPK (Cell Signaling, MA), bcl-2-associated X-protein (Bax) (BD Pharmingen, MD), P53, bH3-interacting domain death agonist (Bid), phospholipid scramblase-3 (PLS3) (Abcam, MA). 60S ribosomal protein L-32 (RPL32) (Abcam), Lamin-B and cytochrome-c Oxidase Subunit IV (COX IV) (Cell Signaling) were used as loading control for cytosolic proteins, nuclear proteins and mitochondrial proteins respectively. Immunoreactive bands were visualized using Immobilon Western chemiluminescence HRP substrate (Millipore, MA). The blots were scanned and quantitated using Gel Doc XR system and Quantity One software version 4.6.3 (Bio-Rad, CA).

Total collagen estimation by hydroxyproline assay

Hydroxyproline assay was performed to measure ventricular collagen concentration both for *in vivo* experimental tissues as well as fibroblast culture supernatant (24 h treatment) [29]. Briefly, the tissue samples and fibroblast culture supernatants were subjected to acid digestion followed by vacuum drying. After resuspension in citrate acetate buffer, the samples were incubated with isopropyl alcohol, chloramine T, and Ehrlich's reagent at 25°C for 18 h, and intensity of the red color was measured at 558 nm using Varioskan Multimode Reader (Thermo Fisher, IL). With the help of a standard curve, hydroxyproline content in the unknown samples was calculated. The amount of collagen was calculated by multiplying hydroxyproline content by a factor of 8.2.

Caspase activity assay

Caspase activity was measured from all experimental cardiac tissues using ApoAlert caspase-3 and –9 Fluorescent Assay Kit (Clontech Laboratories, CA) following manufacturer's protocol [17]. Briefly, tissue samples were homogenized in chilled protein extraction buffer. Then, 50 μl of 2X Reaction Buffer/DTT mix and 1 μl of Caspase-3 Inhibitor DEVD-CHO (for negative control) or 1 μl of DMSO (for other samples) was added to 50 μl of supernatant obtained from each sample. After incubation on ice for 30 min 5 μl of 1 mM Caspase-3 Substrate (DEVD-AFC; 50 μM final conc.) was added to each tube and incubated at 37°C for 1 hr. Fluorescence was measured at 400 nm excitation and 505 nm emission wavelengths (Varioskan Multimode Reader, Thermo Fisher, IL). For Caspase-9 activity, 5 μl of Caspase-9 Substrate (LEHD-AMC; 50 μM final conc.) was added to each tube and after incubation for 1 hr, fluorescence was measured at 380 nm excitation and 460 nm emission wavelength.

Immunohistochemistry

Frozen ventricular tissue sections (4 μm) were prepared using cryostat CM1850 (Leica, CA) from all experimental groups. Tissue sections were fixed and stained with antibodies against phospho-PKC-δ and phospho-PKC-α (Cell signaling) and sarcomeric α-actinin (Abcam), followed by incubation with labeled secondary antibodies Alexafluor 488, and Alexa fluor 633 (Molecular Probes, OR) as described earlier [17]. After mounting with Vectashield [with DAPI] (Vector Laboratories, CA), tissue sections were visualized under confocal FV1200 microscope (Olympus, PA).

Determination of cardiac function

Two-dimensional echocardiography was performed to determine cardiac function *in vivo* using ultrasound system (Vivid S5 system, GE Healthcare, WI) as described earlier [17]. M-mode views were used to assess the left ventricular chamber dimensions and functional parameters using digitized images captured during examination of each mouse.

Statistical analysis

Results were expressed as mean ± S.E. of >3 independent experiments. Data was analyzed by independent samples t-test and ANOVA using SPSS (v13.0; IBM, NY). Values of $P<0.05$ were considered as significant.

Results

Assessment of cardiac hypertrophy in all the experimental groups

Significant increase in the heart weight to body weight ratio (HW/BW) was observed in pathological as well as physiological hypertrophy (group H: 5.97±0.11 and group E: 5.12±0.12) compared to control group (4.34±0.06). Interestingly, the HW/BW ratio significantly increased in mice after exercise withdrawal (group E^R: 5.65±0.09) compared to E and decreased in pathological hypertrophy group undergoing exercise training (group H^X: 5.07±0.16; Figure 1A). Significant increase in expression of *ANF* and *β-MHC* in group E^R (1.97±0.12-fold for *ANF* and 2.02±0.12-fold for *β-MHC*) compared to E, whereas, exercise training in pathological hypertrophy group showed significant down regulation in expression of both these hypertrophy marker genes (*ANF*: 2.44±0.03-fold and *β-MHC*: 2.14±0.02-fold in H^X compared to H; Figure 1C, Figure S3). On the other hand, expression of *IGF-1*, the marker for physiological hypertrophy, that was increased significantly in group E (2.5±0.12-fold) compared to H or C, was drastically down regulated in group E^R (1.78±0.02-fold) compared to E (Figure 1C, Figure S3). The cross-sectional area of cardiomyocytes was significantly increased in group H (288.62±7.75 μm^2) and E (227.9±8.53 μm^2) compared to C (157.45±4.99 μm^2). However, the myocyte cross-

sectional area was significantly increased in group E^R (260.1±9.38 μm^2) compared to E (Figure 1B). Similarly, ventricular collagen concentration was significantly increased in group H (0.613±0.02 μg/mg) compared to E and C. Interestingly, ventricular collagen concentration was significantly increased in mice after exercise withdrawal (group E^R: 0.693±0.01 μg/mg) compared to E and was significantly decreased in pathological hypertrophy group undergoing exercise training (group H^X) (0.517±0.04 μg/mg) compared to H (Figure 1D). Left ventricular chamber dimensions assessed by M-Mode echocardiography revealed significantly increased inter ventricular septum thickness (IVST) and posterior wall thickness (PWT) in group H (0.62±0.02 mm for IVST and 0.51±0.08 mm for PWT) and E (0.51±0.05 mm for IVST and 0.41±0.10 mm for PWT) compared to C (IVST 0.42±0.01 mm and PWT 0.26±0.06 mm) (Figure S1). Both IVST (0.47±0.01 mm) and PWT (0.31±0.04 mm) were significantly reduced in H^X animals compared to group H indicating exercise after pathological hypertrophy ameliorates ventricular chamber thickness. Withdrawal from exercise in group E^R revealed markedly increased IVST (0.59±0.02 mm), PWT (0.46±0.04 mm) (Figure S1) along with increased LVDD (3.07±0.05 mm) and decreased %FS (39±0.02%) compared to group E (LVDD 2.24±0.12 mm and 62.5±0.04%FS) manifesting severely compromised cardiac function in group E^R, while cardiac function was markedly improved in group H^X (LVDD 2.44±0.03 mm and %FS 55±0.33%) compared to group H (2.94±.05 mm for LVDD and 33±0.02% for %FS; Figure S2).

Activation of PKC-isoforms during pathological and physiological hypertrophy

Phosphorylation status of different PKC-isoformswas estimated in C, H and E mice groups. Western blot analysis revealed no significant difference in phosphorylation levels of PKC-ε (Ser 729), PKC-α/βII (Thr 638/641), PKC-δ/θ (Ser 643/676), PKC-θ (Thr 538), PKC-ζ/λ (Thr 410/403), PKC-μ (Ser 744/748) and PKC-μ (Ser 916) in any of these groups (Figure S4 A). However, expression levels of total PKC-ε, PKC-ζ and PKC-θ increased significantly in group E and H compared to control, with no change in expression levels of total PKC-βII and PKD (Figure S4 A).

However, phosphorylation level of PKC-δ (Thr 505) was found to be significantly high exclusively in group H (4.00±0.08-fold) compared to either C or E; whereas, significant increase in PKC-α phosphorylation level (Ser 657 and Tyr 658) was recorded in group E (6.13±0.02-fold) compared to either C or H (Figure 2A, 2B and S4 B). Interestingly, withdrawal from exercise in group E^R showed significant down regulation in phospho-PKC-α level (4.73±0.07-fold) and induced phospho-PKC-δ level (2.75±0.11-fold) compared to group E, akin to what was observed in group H. On the contrary, significant increase in the levels of phospho-PKC-α (5.10±0.10-fold) and decrease in phospho-PKC-δ level (3.61±0.14-fold) was observed in group H^X compared to H (Figure 2A, 2B and S4 B), similar to what is seen in group E. Total PKC-α expression increased in groups H (1.58±0.04-fold), E (1.30±0.04-fold) and H^X compared to groups C and E^R (Figure 2A). On the other hand, expression of total PKC-δ was increased in group H (4.97±0.07-fold) and E^R (4.17±0.07-fold) compared to either C or E (Figure 2A). The western blot results were corroborated further by immunofluorescence studies that showed pronounced phosphorylation of PKC-δ in groups H and E^R compared with either group C or E. On the other hand, phosphorylation of PKC-α was increased in groups E and H^X compared to E, H or E^R (Figure 2D).

Expression of PKC-δ and-α was studied in exercised withdrawn animals with increasing period of rest (3, 7, 15, 20, 30 and 45 days post exercise). Phosphorylation of PKC-δ was observed in exercise withdrawn animals from the 15thday of rest and was maximally induced on the 45th day of rest period. Phosphorylation of PKC-δ was increased by 2.73±0.3-fold on the15th day, 2.79±0.06-fold on the 20th day, 2.88±0.15-fold on the 30th day and 3.24±0.08-fold on the 45th day of rest compared to exercised animals (E). However, phosphorylation of PKC-α was observed till the 3rd day after exercise withdrawal but could not be detected with increasing time of rest (Figure 2C). Cardiac function was also found to deteriorate from 15th day of rest and was almost equally compromised till 45th day rest period as evidenced by significantly increased LVDD and reduced %FS, compared to 0 or 3 days of post exercise rest (Table 1).

PKC-δ induces apoptotic signals in myocytes after exercise withdrawal during physiological hypertrophy

Subcellular fractionation followed by western blot analysis in different experimental groups revealed cleavage of PKC-δ and translocation of its active subunit (41 kD) to mitochondria and nucleus in group H and to a lesser extent in group H^X (Figure 3A). No translocation of PKC-δ active subunit was observed in groups C or E. However, when exercise was withdrawn in physiological hypertrophy (group E^R), nuclear translocation was observed (Figure 3A and 3B). Similar translocation pattern of active PKC-δ fragment was observed in isolated adult cardiomyocytes from animals of all experimental groups (Figure 3D).

Expression level of total and phosphorylated p53 (ser-46, ser-15) was observed in group H compared to groups C and E. However, phosphorylated p53 band reappeared in group E^R (4.43±0.12-fold for total p53, 4.66±0.20-fold at ser-46 and 3.56±0.2-fold at ser-15 compared to E; Figure 3A) and phosphorylation level in group H^X was significantly reduced compared to H (Figure 3A).

The expression of proapoptotic proteins downstream to PKC-δ, such as phospholipid scramblase-3 (PLS3), bcl-2 associated X-protein (Bax), cleavage of bH3-interacting domain death agonist (Bid) to truncated-Bid (t-Bid) and cytosolic/mitochondrial ratio of cytochrome-c were significantly increased in group E^R (1.91±0.02-foldfor PLS3, 2.83±0.08-fold for Bax and 11.09±0.13-fold for cytochrome-c) as was induced in group H compared to either C or E (Figure 3B).

Western blot analysis with whole heart and isolated cardiomyocytes from different experimental groups revealed active catalytic fragments (19 kD and 17 kD) of cleaved caspase-3 during exercise withdrawal group E^R that were absent in group E (Figure 3C and 3D). Caspase-3 activity assay showed similar trend with significantly induced activity in group H and E^R (3.28±0.69-fold) compared to E (Figure 3C). Appearance of cleaved 89 kD active fragment of Poly ADP ribose polymerase (PARP) which is a hallmark of pathological hypertrophy (H) was also detected in group E^R (Figure 3D). In tune with this, significant increase in phosphorylation of STAT3 (at Tyr-705 and Ser-727) and P38 MAPK was observed in group E^R compared to groups E or C (Figure 3E).

Both phosphorylated and total PKC-δ expression was significantly reduced in PKC-δ siRNA treated pathological hypertrophy group (H) along with significant down regulation of Bax (2.91±0.06-fold), cytosolic/mitochondrial ratio of cytochrome-c (6.29±0.08-fold) and cleavage of PARP compared to nonspecific siRNA treated group H (Figure 4A and S5). The PKC-δ siRNA treatment also resulted in significant reduction in activities of caspase-3 and -9in group H (7.83±0.53 and 3.56±0.28-fold respectively) compared to nonspecific siRNA treated group H

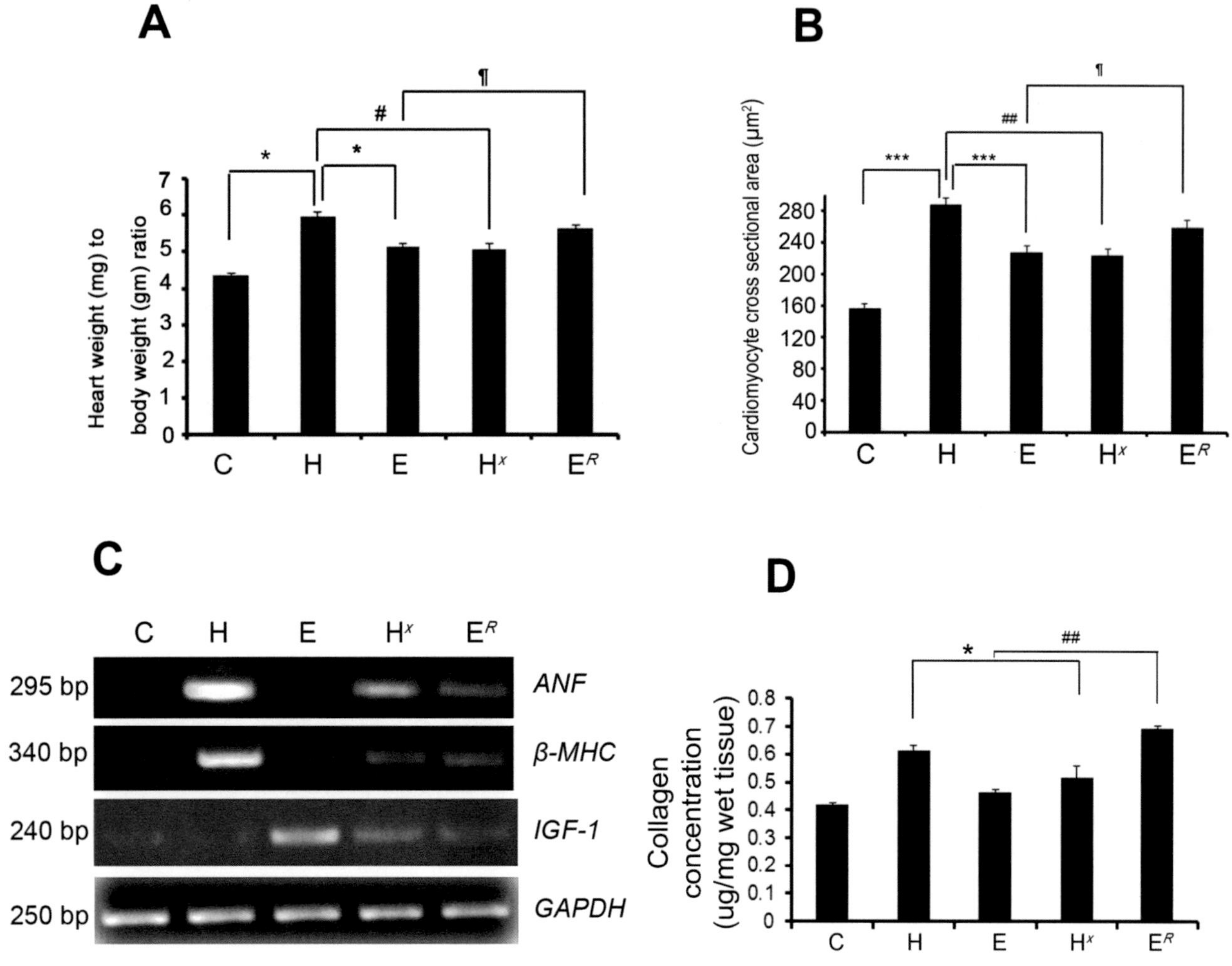

Figure 1. Assessment of hypertrophy and estimation of collagen in all the experimental groups. (**A**) Graph showing HW/BW ratio in all five experimental models: pathological hypertrophy (H), physiological hypertrophy (E), exercise-trained pathological hypertrophy (H^X), mice kept at rest after 4 weeks of exercise training (E^R) and representative control (C) (*$p<0.05$ for H versus E or C; #$p<0.05$ for H versus H^X; ¶$p<0.05$ for E versus E^R). (**B**) Graph showing cardiomyocyte cross-sectional area (in μm^2) in groups C, H, E, H^X, and E^R (***$p<0.001$ for H versus E or C; ##$p<0.01$ for H versus H^X; ¶$p<0.05$ for E versus E^R). (**C**) Expression profile of pathological hypertrophy markers (*ANF* and *β-MHC*) and physiological hypertrophy marker (*IGF-1*) estimated by RT-PCR. *GAPDH* was used as loading control. (**D**) Graph showing ventricular collagen concentration in groups C, H, E, H^X, and E^R estimated by hydroxyproline assay.

mice (Figure 4B). Similar results were observed when group H mice were treated with chemical inhibitor Rottlerin compared to vehicle treated ones (data not shown). PKC-δ siRNA or Rottlerin treatment did not alter the expression of these proteins during physiological hypertrophy (data not shown).

Down regulation of PKC-α promotes deactivation of Akt and ERK-1/2 mediated cell survival pathway during exercise withdrawal

The phosphorylation status of Akt and ERK-1/2, downstream pro-survival targets of PKC-α, was studied in all the experimental groups. Western blot analyses revealed phosphorylation of Akt (serine 473) only in group E and phospho-Akt to Akt ratio was decreased by 1.52±0.02-fold during exercise withdrawal in group E^R (Figure 5A and S6) whereas, exercise regimen during pathological hypertrophy (H^X) resulted in Akt phosphorylation that was absent in group H (data not shown). Similarly, phospho-ERK-1/2 to ERK-1/2 ratio was increased significantly in group E (5.3±0.02-fold) compared to C but decreased in group E^R (1.44±0.15-fold) compared to E (Figure 5A and S6). Activity assay of proapoptotic caspase-9 protein revealed significant down regulation in group E compared to H (5.95±0.67-fold). Interestingly, caspase-9 activity was found to increase significantly in group E^R (5.17±0.50-fold) compared to E (Figure 5B). Cardiomyocytes isolated from experimental groups showed similar trend in phosphorylation level of PKC-α and Akt (Figure 5D).

Pro-survival role of PKC-α during physiological hypertrophy was further confirmed by treating exercised mice group (E) with PKC-α siRNA. Significant down regulation in the levels of phospho and total PKC-α along with phospho-Akt and phospho-ERK-1/2 levels was observed in group E mice treated with PKC-α siRNA compared to nonspecific siRNA treatment (Figure 5C and S7). G6976 (chemical inhibitor of PKC-α) treatment showed similar results for phosphorylation of Akt and ERK levels (data not shown). Inhibition of PKC-α activity did not alter phosphorylation status of either Akt or ERK-1/2 during pathological hypertrophy (H) (data not shown).

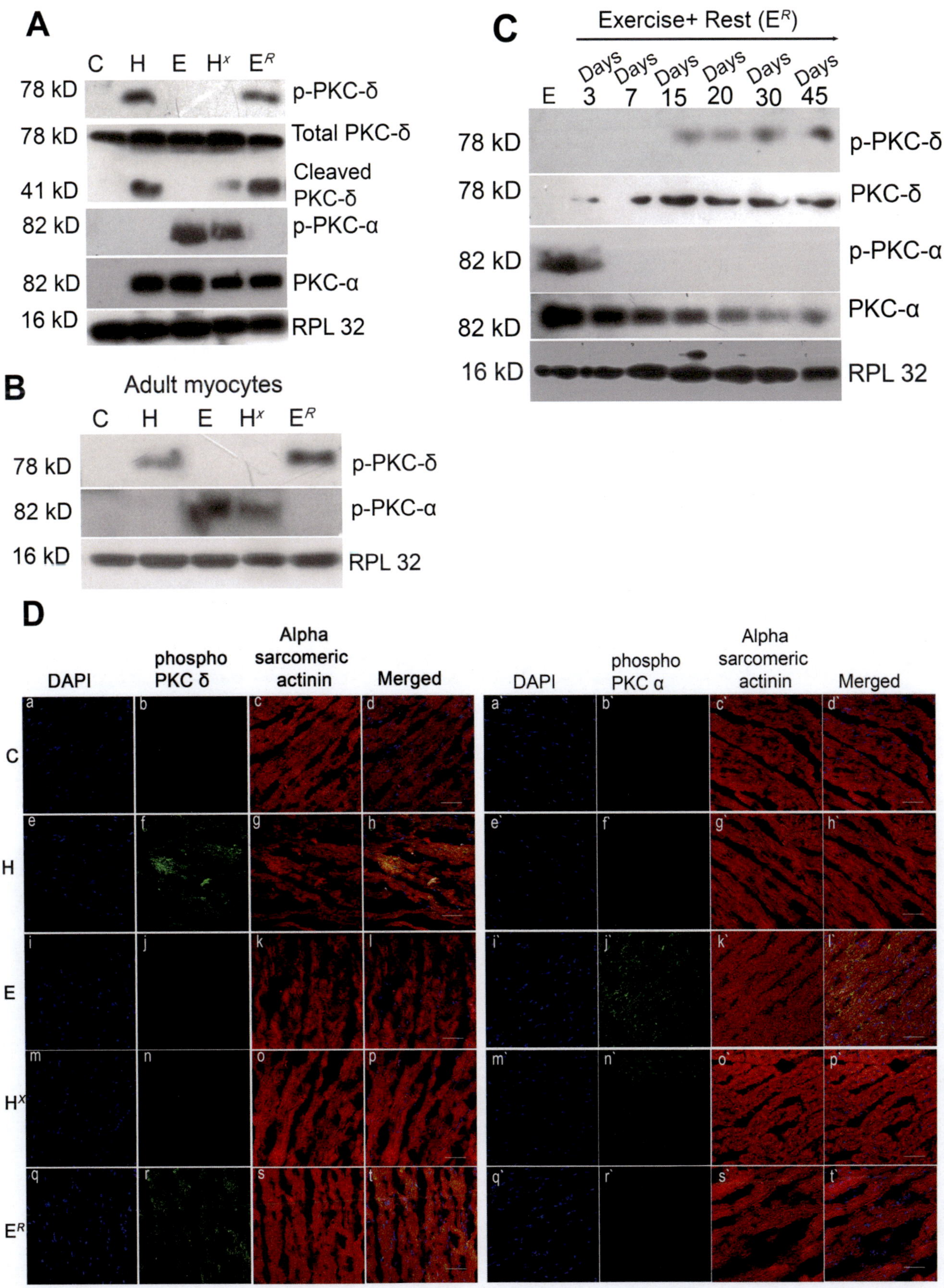
A
C H E Hˣ Eᴿ
78 kD p-PKC-δ
78 kD Total PKC-δ
41 kD Cleaved PKC-δ
82 kD p-PKC-α
82 kD PKC-α
16 kD RPL 32
B
Adult myocytes
C H E Hˣ Eᴿ
78 kD p-PKC-δ
82 kD p-PKC-α
16 kD RPL 32
C
Exercise+ Rest (Eᴿ)
E Days 3 Days 7 Days 15 Days 20 Days 30 Days 45
78 kD p-PKC-δ
78 kD PKC-δ
82 kD p-PKC-α
82 kD PKC-α
16 kD RPL 32
D
DAPI
phospho PKC δ
Alpha sarcomeric actinin
Merged
DAPI
phospho PKC α
Alpha sarcomeric actinin
Merged
C
H
E
Hˣ
Eᴿ

Figure 2. Differential expression profile of Protein Kinase-C isoforms. (**A**) Western blot analyses showing change in expression of PKC α and PKC-δ (phospho and total) in groups C, H, E, H^X and E^R. PKC-δ cleavage product (41 kD) is exclusive in group H, H^X and E^R. RPL32 was used as loading control. (**B**) Western blot analyses showing phosphorylation of PKC-δ and PKC-α in adult cardiomyocytes isolated from different experimental groups. RPL32 was used as loading control. (**C**) Western blot analyses showing changes in expression of phosphorylated and total PKC-δ and PKC-α in exercise withdrawn animals (E^R) rested for different time periods. RPL32 was used as loading control. (**D**) Immunofluorescence study showing expression of phospho-PKC-δ and -α in different experimental group. Tissue sections showing phospho-PKC-δ expression in panels b, f, j, n and r and phospho-PKC-α in panels b′, f′, j′, n′ and r′ (green fluorescence). Sections were counter stained with alpha sarcomeric actinin antibody (panels c, g, k, o and s for PKC-δ and panels c′, g′, k′, o′ and s′ for PKC -α; red fluorescence). Nuclei were stained with DAPI (panels a, e, i, m and q for PKC-δ and panels a′, e′, i′, m′ and q′ for PKC-α; blue fluorescence) and merged images are shown in panels d, h, l, p and t for PKC-δ and panels d′, h′, l′, p′ and t′ for PKC-α. Increased expression of phospho-PKC-δ was observed in groups H and E^R whereas, phospho-PKC-α expression was induced in group E and H^X (Scale bar = 50 μm, Magnification = 40X).

Inhibition of PKC isoforms reverses cardiac adaptation during pathological and physiological hypertrophy

PKC-α inhibition activates PKC-δ during physiological hypertrophy. PKC-α siRNA treatment during physiological hypertrophy led to significant increase in the phospho-PKC-δ level in group E mice along with increase in ratio of cytosolic/mitochondrial cytochrome-c (8.74±0.2-fold, $p<0.01$) and cleavage of caspase-3 compared to nonspecific siRNA treated group E mice (Figure 6A). Significantly induced caspase-3 (10.54±0.06-fold, $p<0.05$) and caspase-9 (14.42±2.16-fold, $p<0.05$) activities were also recorded in PKC-α siRNA treated group E samples (Figure 6B). However, inhibition of PKC-α during pathological hypertrophy did not show alteration of phospho-PKC-δ expression and apoptotic markers in group H (data not shown). Apart from induced apoptotic signaling, altered activation from PKC-α to PKC-δ resulted in compromised cardiac function with significantly increased LVDD and decrease in %FS in PKC-α siRNA treated group E mice, compared to nonspecific siRNA treated mice of the same group (LVDD: 2.87±0.02 mm vs 2.24±0.12 mm; %FS: 49.8±0.02% vs 62.5±0.04%; $p<0.05$) (Figure S8).

Inhibition of PKC-δ activates PKC-α isoform and subsequent Akt-ERK 1/2 activation during pathological hypertrophy. PKC-δ siRNA treated group H mice on the other hand, showed significant increase in the level of both phospho-PKC-α (5.73±0.33-fold, $p<0.01$) and total PKC-α (1.54±0.04-fold, $p<0.01$) level compared to nonspecific siRNA treated pathological hypertrophy group (Figure 6C). Inhibition of PKC-δ also significantly increased the expression of phospho-Akt (2.57±0.04-fold, $p<0.01$) and phospho-ERK-1/2 (2.61±0.02-fold, $p<0.01$) in this mice group (Figure 6C). However, PKC-δ inhibition did not alter expression of phospho-Akt, phospho-ERK-1/2 in group E (data not shown). Inhibition of PKC-δ and subsequent activation of phopho-PKC-α level in group H resulted in notably improved cardiac function with significant decrease in LVDD (1.75±0.05 mm, $p<0.05$) and increase in %FS (72.6±0.03%, $p<0.05$) compared to otherwise severely compromised functional parameters in nonspecific siRNA treated mice with pathlogical hypertrophy (Figure S9).

Inhibition of PKC-δ modulates collagen concentration via STAT3 and P38 MAPK

Inhibition of PKC-δ resulted in significant regression of ventricular collagen concentration in siRNA treated pathological hypertrophy (H) (0.377±0.02 μg/mg) samples as well as in Ang-II treated cardiac fibroblast (2.90±0.01 ng/ml) compared to nonspecific siRNA treated group H (0.597±0.01 μg/mg) and cardiac fibroblast (4.06±0.21 ng/ml) respectively (Figure 7A).

PKC-δ siRNA treated pathological hypertrophy mice group (H) and Ang-II treated cardiac fibroblast showed significantly reduced phosphorylation status of PKC-δ along with P38 MAPK. The inhibitor treatment also resulted in reduction of phosphorylation of STAT3 (Tyr-705 and Ser-727) in group H mice as well as in Ang-II treated cardiac fibroblast compared to nonspecific siRNA treated group H and cardiac fibroblast (Figure 7B). *In vivo* and *in vitro* treatment with PKC-δ siRNA had no significant effect on total P38 and STAT3 (data not shown). Similar reduction in expression of these proteins was observed following Rottlerin treatment in group H mice and Ang-II treated cardiac fibroblast (data not shown).

Discussion

PKC has been identified as an important player during cardiac hypertrophy [6]. However, isoform specific roles of PKC during pathological and physiological hypertrophy have never been reported. This study for the first time revealed how differential activation and switch of PKC-isoforms dictate cardiomyocyte adaptation via key downstream modulators to regulate cardiac efficiency during physiological and pathological hypertrophy.

Table 1. M-mode echocardiography data.

Experimental Groups	LVDD in mm	%FS	PW thickness in mm	IV septum thickness in mm
C	2.17±0.05	61±0.08%	0.26±0.06	0.42±0.01
H	2.94±0.05	33±0.02%	0.51±0.08	0.62±0.02
H^X	2.44±0.03	55±0.02%	0.31±0.04	0.47±0.03
E	2.24±0.12	62.5±0.04%	0.37±0.01	0.5±0.05
$E^{R\ 3days}$	2.30±0.15	57.5±1.32%	0.35±0.03	0.45±0.05
$E^{R15days}$	3.07±0.05	39±0.03%	0.46±0.04	0.6±0.02
$E^{R45days}$	2.99±0.06	37.5±2.33%	0.49±0.02	0.67±0.03

LVDD, left ventricular diastolic dimensions; FS, fractional shortening; PW thickness, posterior wall thickness; IV thickness, interventricular septum thickness.

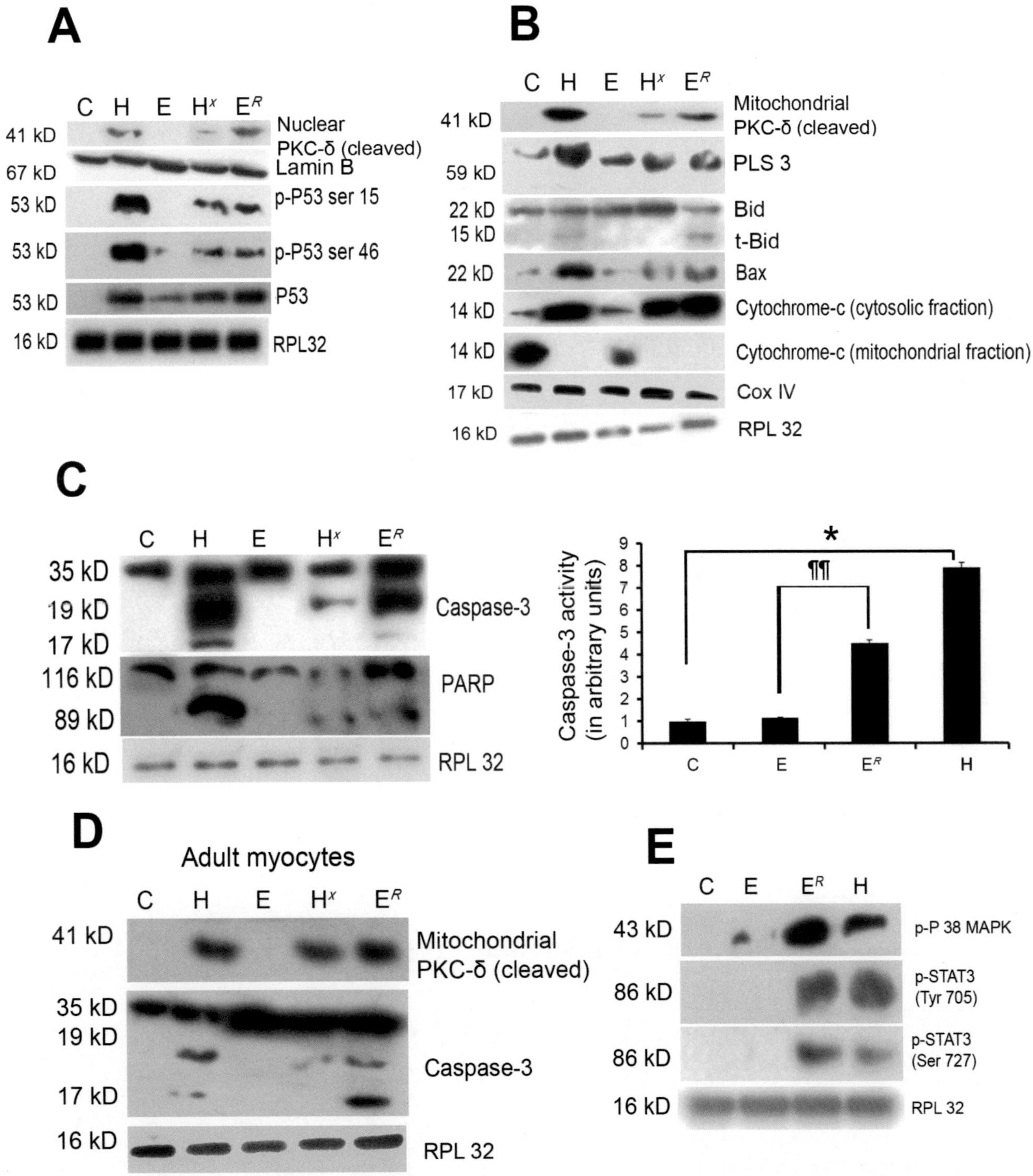

Figure 3. PKC-δ associated downstream target proteins. (**A**) Western blot analysis with the nuclear protein revealed significantly increased translocation of cleaved PKC-δ (41 kD) to nucleus in group H, H^X and E^R compared to either C or E. Significantly increased phospho-p53 (at Ser 46 and Ser 15) and total p53 was observed in group H and E^R compared to E or C whereas significantly reduced phospho-p53 (at Ser 46 and Ser 15) and total p53 was observed in groups E and H^X compared to H or E. RPL32 and Lamin B were used as loading control for cytosolic proteins and nuclear proteins respectively. (**B**) Subcellular fractionation followed by western blot analyses with mitochondrial protein showing significantly increased translocation of cleaved PKC-δ (41 kD) to mitochondria in group H, H^X and E^R compared to either C or E along with increased expression of PLS3, t-Bid, Bax, cytochrome-c proteins. RPL32 and COX IV were used as loading control for cytosolic proteins and mitochondrial proteins respectively. (**C**) Western blot analysis showingcleavage of caspase-3 and PARP in group H and E^R compared to C or E. RPL32 was used as loading control. Caspase-3 activity assay showing similar changes in all the experimental groups. No significant difference in caspase-3 activity was detected between groups E and C (*$p<0.05$ for H versus C; ###$p<0.001$ for H versus H^X; ¶¶$p<0.01$ for E versus E^R). (**D**) Subcellular fractionation followed by western blot analyses showed significantly increased translocation of cleaved PKC-δ (41 kD) to mitochondria along with caspase-3 cleavage in adult cardiomyocytes isolated from group H and E^R compared to either C or E or H^X. RPL32 was used as loading control. (**E**) Western blot analysis showing phosphorylation status of STAT3 and P38 MAPK in groups C, E, E^R and H.

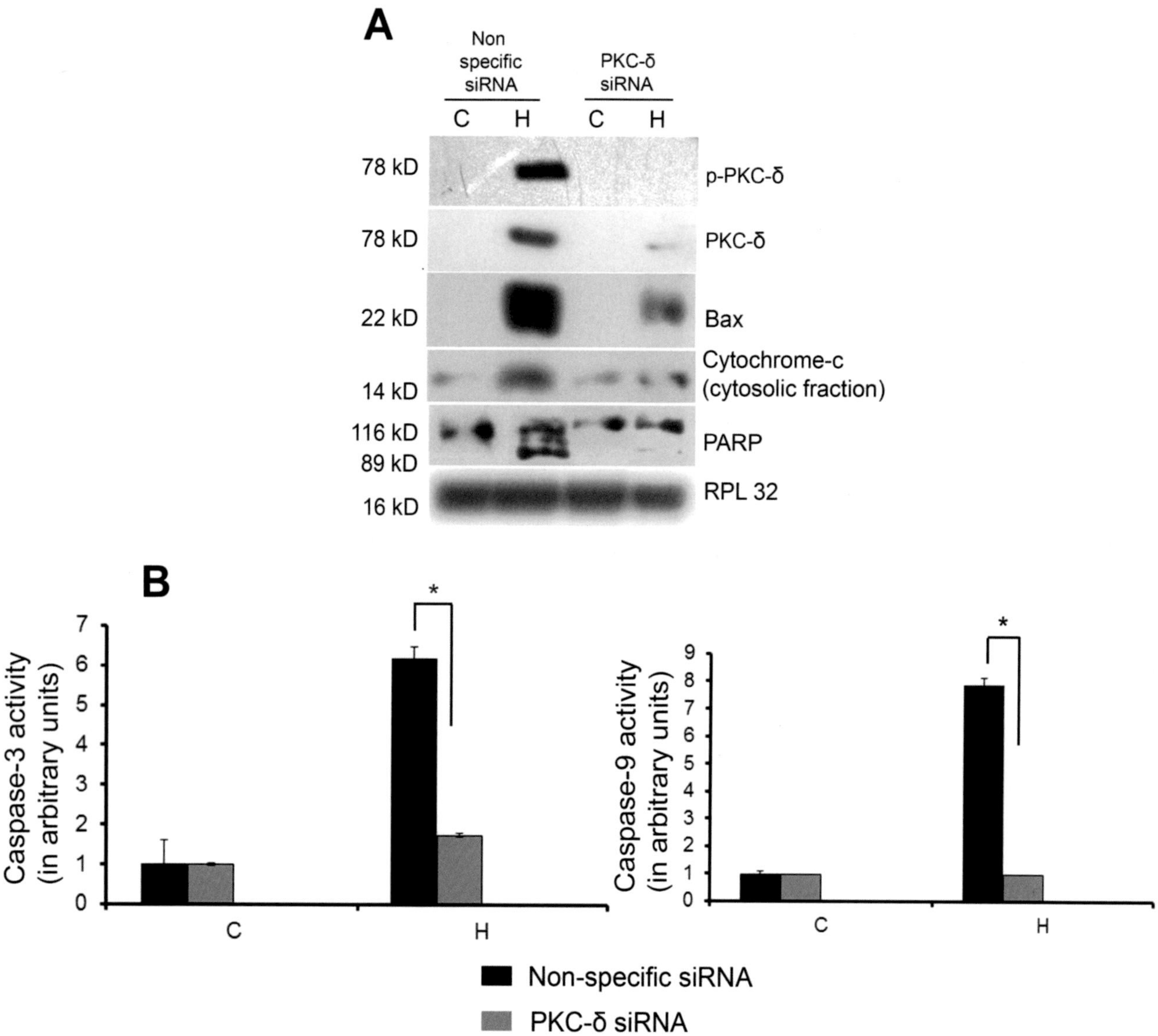

Figure 4. Inhibition of PKC-δ reduces expression of downstream targets. (**A**) Western blot analysis showing successful down regulation in expression of both phospho and total PKC-δ along with significant decrease in the level of bax, cytosolic cytochrome-c and PARP cleavage in mice treated with PKC-δ siRNA in group H. RPL32 was used as loading control. (**B**) Graph showing caspase-3 and caspase-9 activities in the two experimental groups (C and H) treated with siRNA and nonspecific siRNA. Significant decrease in caspase-3 and caspase-9 activities occurred in mice treated with PKC-δ siRNA compared to mice treated with nonspecific siRNA [*$p<0.05$ for H (nonspecific siRNA) versus H (PKC-δ siRNA)].

Pathological hypertrophy in group H was confirmed by significant increase in HW/BW ratio, induced expression of hypertrophy markers *ANF* and *β-MHC* along with ventricular collagen concentration, a marker of cardiac fibrosis [17,25]. Physiological hypertrophy by exercise training was characterized by increase in HW/BW ratio and *IGF-1* expression in group E [15]. Cardiomyocyte cross-sectional areas were increased significantly in both groups H and E compared to C (Figure 1A, 1C, 1D and S3). Left ventricular chamber dimensions showed significant thickening during pathological hypertrophy (Group H) as evidenced by increased IVST, PWT, LVDD (Figure S1 and S2) and decreased %FS (Figure S2) confirming severely compromised cardiac function. Physiological hypertrophy (Group E) was marked by increased LVDD but no significant change in %FS with that of control animals confirming efficient cardiac contractibility. Interestingly, when group E mice were withdrawn from the exercise regimen for two weeks (group E^R) significant up regulation of *ANF* and *β-MHC* and severely compromised cardiac function was observed indicating development of pathological hypertrophy, akin to group H (Figure 1A, 1C, 1D and S1, S2, S3).

Several studies had already indicated a prominent role of PKC during cardiac hypertrophy [7–12] but the precise role of specific PKC-isoforms encompassing various forms of hypertrophy processes is still not understood. Our study revealed altered expression and differential phosphorylation of PKC-α and -δ in group E and H respectively, while activation of other PKC-isoforms remained more or less unaltered among different mice groups (Figure 2A and S4 A-S4 B). Phosphorylation of PKC-δ at Thr 505 was detected exclusively in group H while phosphorylated PKC-α at Ser 657 and Tyr 658 was observed in group E, suggesting their exclusive activation during pathological and physiological hypertrophy respectively (Figure 2A–2B, 2D and S4 B). On the

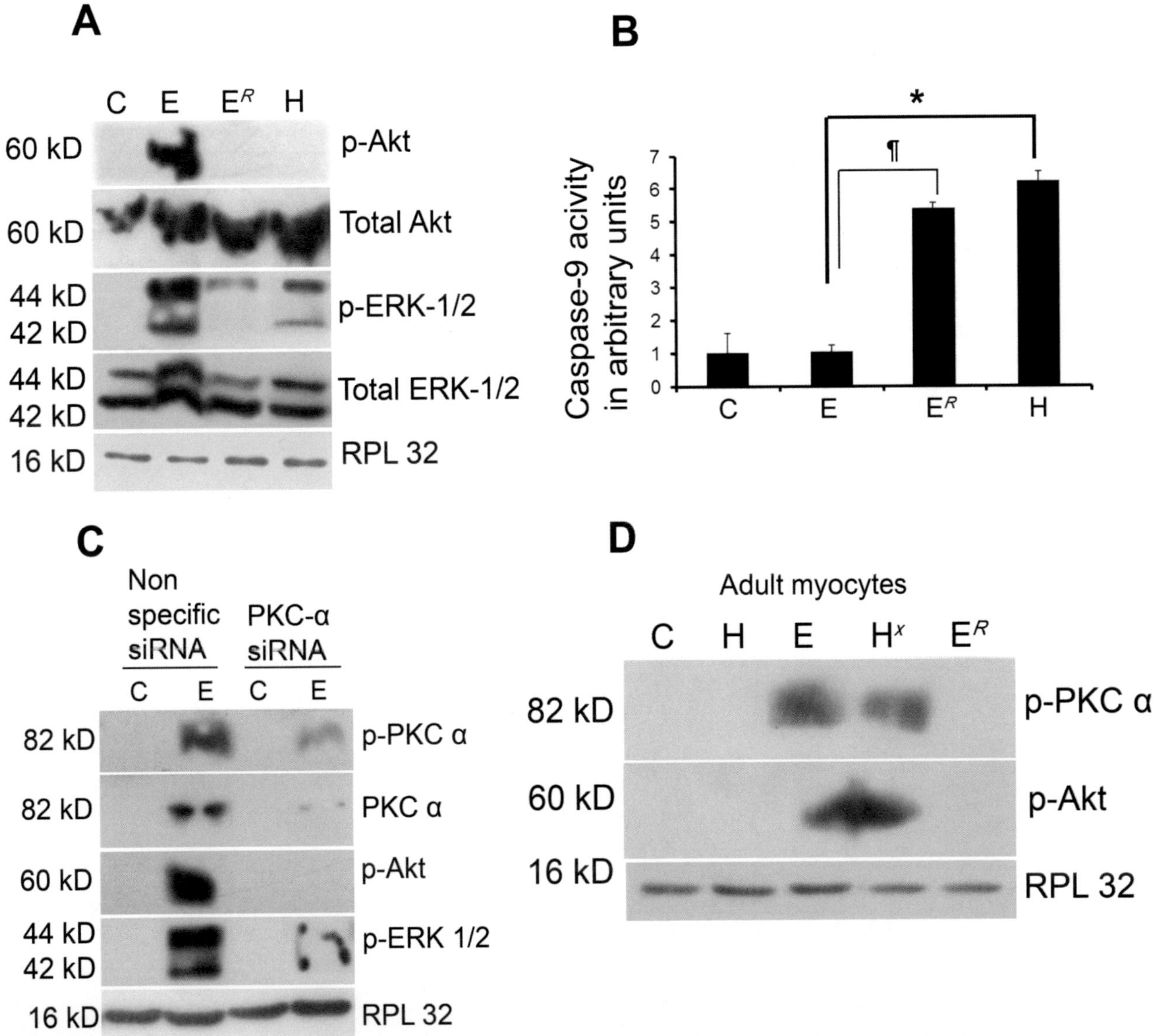

Figure 5. PKC-α and survival kinases. (**A**) Western blot analysis showing phospho-Akt to Akt and phospho-ERK-1/2 to ERK-1/2 ratio to be significantly increased in group E compared to either H or C. phospho-Akt/Akt and phospho-ERK-1/2 to ERK-1/2 ratio was significantly decreased in group E^R compared to E. RPL32 was used as loading control. (**B**) Graph showing caspase-9 activity in groups C, E, E^R and H. (*$p<0.05$ for H versus E; ¶$p<0.05$ for E versus E^R). (**C**) Western blot analyses reveal successful knockdown of phospho and total PKC-α along with significant decrease in the phosphorylation level of Akt and ERK-1/2 in mice treated with PKC-α siRNA. RPL32 was used as loading control. (**D**) Phosphorylation of PKC-α and Akt was observed by western blot analysis in adult cardiomyocytes isolated from group E and H^X compared to C, H and E^R. RPL32 was used as loading control.

contrary, withdrawal from exercise regimen in group E^R resulted in reduction in phospho-PKC-α level compared to E with significant increase in total and phospho-PKC-δ whereas, significant increase in phospho-PKC-α and reduced phospho-PKC-δ level were the hallmarks of group H^X (Figure 2A–2B, 2D and S4 B). This is the first report where involvement of specific PKC-isoforms -δ and -α was recorded in pathological and physiological hypertrophy respectively with strategic reversal of the same during reversed hypertrophic conditions evidenced by PKC-δ activation in E^R and PKC-α in H^X groups suggesting that transition from PKC-α to -δ activation could dictate alteration from adaptive to compromised cardiac hypertrophic condition in animal model. Time point study with E^R group of mice showed increasing trend of phosphorylation of PKC-δ from 15thday of rest which increased progressively till the 45thday (Figure 2C), with progressive deterioration in cardiac performance (Table 1). Phosphorylation of PKC-α, on the other hand, started declining progressively from the 3rdday onwards after exercise withdrawal. This was an interesting observation as our data suggests that post exercise rest period could lead towards negative cardiac remodeling in hearts with efficient performances during physiological hypertrophy.

Study of downstream signaling pathways regulated by the specific PKC-isoforms during pathological and physiological hypertrophy revealed that induced PKC-δ phosphorylation and its increased translocation to mitochondria and nucleus during

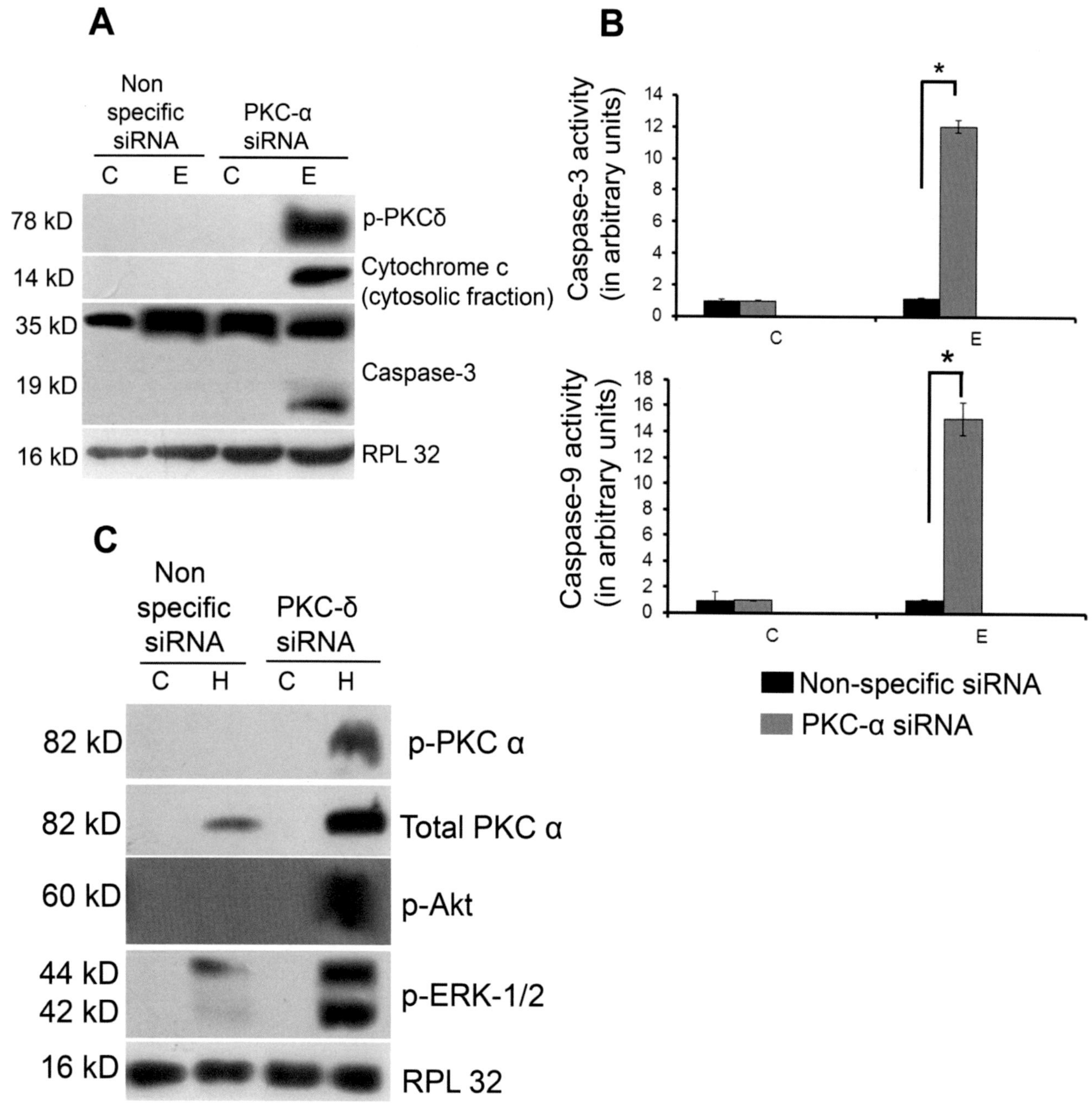

Figure 6. Reversal of PKC isoforms modulates hypertrophy regulators. (**A**) Western blot analysis showing inhibition of PKC-α in physiological hypertrophy mice with PKC-α siRNA resulting in significant phosphorylation of PKC-δ and translocation of active PKC-δ (41 kD), cytosolic cytochrome-c and caspase-3 cleavage compared to nonspecific siRNA treated physiological hypertrophy mice. RPL32 was used as loading control. (**B**) Graph showing PKC-α siRNA treatment during physiological hypertrophy generation showed significant increase in caspase-3 and caspase-9 activities compared to nonspecific siRNA treatment during physiological hypertrophy [* $p<0.05$ for E (nonspecific siRNA) versus E (PKC-α siRNA)]. (**C**) Western blot analyses showing significantly increased phosphorylation of PKC-α, Akt and ERK-1/2 and PKC-α expression in pathological hypertrophy mice treated with PKC-δ siRNA. RPL32 was used as loading control.

pathological hypertrophy (Figure 3A, 3B and 3D) could induce cardiomyocyte apoptosis in group H, as reported earlier where overexpression of PKC-δ catalytic fragment and its translocation to subcellular organelles induced apoptosis in various cell types and overexpression of PKC-δ kinase 'dead mutants' protected cells from apoptosis [30]. Translocated active PKC-δ interacts with PLS3 [31] that increases cardiolipin expression on the outer mitochondrial membrane [32] thereby recruiting.

t-Bid for eventual cytochrome-c release via formation of Bax/Bak pores [33]. Significant increase in activation and translocation of PLS3, cleavage of Bid to t-Bid, Bax, cytosolic cytochrome-c, phospho-P53 level [30] along with induced cleavage of caspase-3, an upstream activator of PKC-δ [34] and PARP, a known substrate of caspase-3 [28] was observed in group H compared to other groups (Figure 3A–3D). Proapoptotic role of PKC-δ during pathological hypertrophy was further confirmed by inhibiting both phosphorylated and total PKC-δ activity in group H mice that

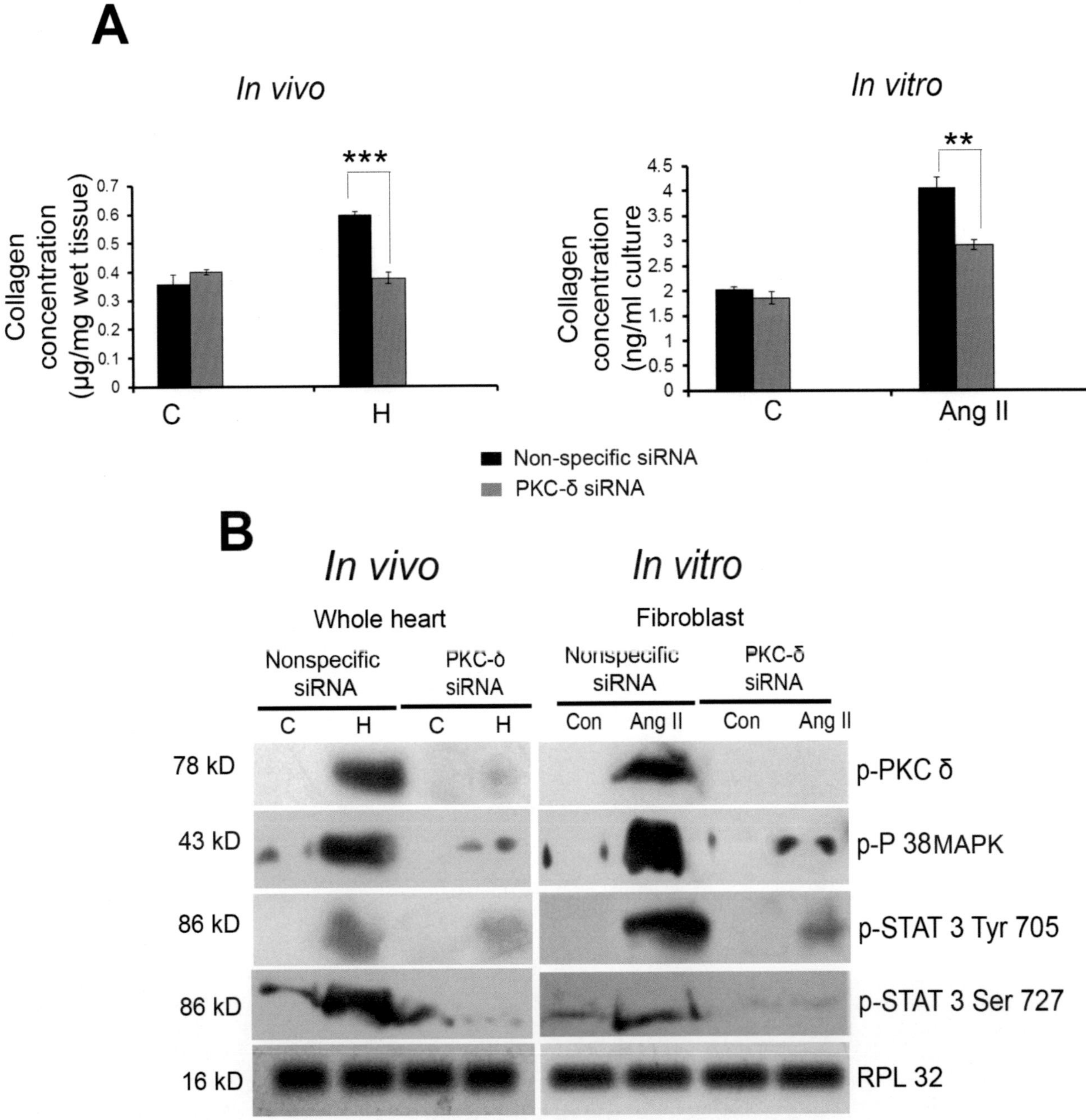

Figure 7. Effect of PKC-δ down regulation on collagen synthesis during pathological hypertrophy. (**A**) Graph showing ventricular collagen concentration in groups C, H and H + PKC-δ siRNA (*in vivo*) and in groups C, Ang-II and Ang-II + PKC-δ siRNA (*in vitro*) estimated by hydroxyproline assay. [***p<0.01 for H (nonspecific siRNA) versus H (PKC-δ siRNA) and **p<0.01 for Ang-II (nonspecific siRNA) versus Ang-II (PKC-δ siRNA)]. (**B**) Western blot analysis showing status of phospho PKC-δ, phospho P38, phospho STAT3 (Tyr 705 and Ser 727), STAT3 following PKC-δ siRNA treatment along with pathological hypertrophy (H) in comparison to hypertrophy alone *in vivo* as well as *in vitro*. RPL32 was used as loading control.

showed significant reduction in the levels of apoptotic regulators (Figure 4A, 4B and S5). In tune with our earlier results all these markers were increased significantly in E^R after exercise withdrawal in physiological hypertrophy group (Figure 3A–3D). Thus, it can be inferred that PKC-δ activation during pathological hypertrophy induces cardiomyocyte apoptotic load resulting in compromised cardiac function [17,28] similar to what was recorded in E^R mice that has been withdrawn from a continuous exercise training regimen during physiological hypertrophy. Our results also suggest that exercise training could play a crucial role in the deactivation of proapoptotic PKC-δ and its downstream modulators resulting in improved cardiac efficiency during pathological hypertrophy in group H^X (Figure 3A–3D).

Activation of caspase-3 via the intrinsic pathway is a critical mediator of the hypertrophic responses [28,35]. In addition to regulation of hypertrophic responses, caspase-3 has been shown to cleave PKC-δ for its activation during apoptosis in vascular smooth muscle cells as well as in a wide range of other cell types [30,34]. Our data has shown translocations of cleaved PKC-δ into mitochondria and nucleus (Figure 3A–3B) which in turn induces caspase-9 mediated caspase-3 cleavage thus forming a feedback loop that further exacerbates the hypertrophic responses [30]. These results cumulatively demonstrate that caspase mediated signaling is a key driver of the pathologic hypertrophy state and establish a clear link between caspase-3 signaling and cleavage activation of various PKC isoforms [36,37].

PKC-α on the other hand, has been reported by many to be a pro-survival isoform that promotes cell survival via direct phosphorylation of Akt at serine 473 [38] and also as a negative regulator of cardiac functional efficiency shown by its increased expression in various models of cardiac injury or failure [12,39]. PKC-α dependent regulation of cardiomyocyte hypertrophy requires ERK-1/2 activation [9] for cardio-protection during ischemia reperfusion injury through activation of the several anti-apoptotic and pro-survival signaling cascades [40]. Our study has revealed significantly increased phosphorylation of Akt and ERK-1/2 along with exclusive activation of PKC-α in group E during physiological hypertrophy (Figure 5A and S6). Their pro-survival role in these animals was also ascertained by significantly decreased caspase-9 activity (Figure 5B), corroborating earlier reports that claimed responsibility of these kinases for the inactivation of proapoptotic caspase-9 [41]. Inhibition of both phosphorylated and total PKC-α during physiological hypertrophy resulting in significant deactivation of phospho-ERK-1/2 and -Akt level further confirms the pro-survival role of PKC-α (Figure 5C and S7) and indicates that exercise training could play a crucial role in the activation of PKC-α and its downstream pro-survival proteins. In contrast, deactivation of PKC-α along with decreased phosphorylation of Akt and ERK-1/2 leading to the activation of pro-apoptotic caspase-9 recorded in group E^R (Figure 5A–5B and 5D) again confirms that withdrawal from exercise training during physiological hypertrophy leads to onset of pathological hypertrophic characters marked by induction of myocyte apoptosis and compromised cardiac function in group E^R. Moreover PKC-δ inhibition in group H interestingly, led to the reactivation of PKC-α along with induced downstream pro-survival markers viz. phospho-Akt and phospho-ERK-1/2 with significant improvement of cardiac function during pathological hypertrophy (Figure 6C and S9) similar to the condition achieved through exercise training during pathological hypertrophy in group H^X. This result was corroborated by an earlier report where PKC-δ inhibition led to activation of PKC-α isoform in prostate cancer cells [42]. Simultaneously, PKC-δ inhibition also resulted in significant decrease in ventricular collagen concentration in both *in vivo* and *in vitro* models of pathological hypertrophy along with significant reduction of phospho-STAT3 (at Tyr-705 and Ser-727; Figure 7A and 7B), an important regulator of ventricular collagen synthesis as described earlier by our group [25].

On the other hand, PKC-α inhibition during physiological hypertrophy resulted in activation of PKC-δ in group E along with induction of apoptotic regulator proteins and severely compromised cardiac function (Figure 6A–6B and S8) similar to the phenotypes observed in group E^R. This result corroborates with an earlier report that showed induced PKC-δ dependent apoptotic program upon inhibition of PKC-α in salivary epithelial cells [14].

Thus, our study clearly demonstrated that PKC-α and -δ isoforms are the prime modulators of cardiac adaptation during physiological and pathological hypertrophy respectively. Further, this study also established that cardiac adaptive processes during transition of an efficiently functioning heart to a functionally compromised heart could be modulated by reversal of activation of PKC-α to-δ isoform.

Supporting Information

Figure S1 M-mode echocardiography parameters. Graph showing IVST and PWT in all experimental groups (*$p<0.05$ for H versus E or C; #$p<0.05$ for H versus H^X; ¶$p<0.05$ for E versus E^R).

Figure S2 M-mode echocardiography parameters. Graph showing LVDD and %FS in all experimental groups (*$p<0.05$ for H versus E or C; #$p<0.05$ for H versus H^X; ¶$p<0.05$ for E versus E^R).

Figure S3 Band intensities of hypertrophy markers. Graph showing pathological hypertrophy markers (*ANF* and *β-MHC*) and physiological hypertrophy marker (*IGF-1*) estimated by RT-PCR. *GAPDH* was used as loading control. (For *ANF* ***$p<0.001$ for E versus E^R; ###$p<0.001$ for H versus H^X; For *β-MHC* ****$p<0.001$ for E versus E^R; ###$p<0.001$ for H versus H^X; For *IGF-1* ***$p<0.001$ for E versus H; ###$p<0.001$ for E versus E^R).

Figure S4 Expression level of different PKC-isoforms. **(A)** Western blot analyses showing status of phospho-PKC-isoforms [PKC-ε (Ser 729), PKC-α/βII (Thr 638/641), PKC-δ/θ (Ser 643/676), PKC-θ (Thr 538), PKC-ζ/λ (Thr 410/403), PKC-μ (Ser 744/748) and PKC-μ (Ser 916)] and total PKC-isoforms (PKC-ε, PKC-ζ, PKC-βII and PKD) in group C, H and E. RPL32 was used as loading control. **(B)** Graph showing relative band intensity of phospho-PKC-δ and phospho-PKC-α in C, H, E, H^X and E^R as revealed by western blot analysis (For phospho-PKC-δ: ***$p<0.001$ for H versus C or E; ###$p<0.001$ for H versus H^X; ¶¶$p<0.01$ for E versus E^R. For phospho-PKC-α: **$p<0.01$ for E versus H or C; ###$p<0.001$ for H versus H^X; ¶¶$p<0.01$ for E versus E^R).

Figure S5 Silencing of PKC-δ results in down regulation of apoptotic markers. Graph showing significantly decreased phospho-PKC-δ, Bax and cytochrome-c (cytosolic/mitochondrial ratio) in mice treated with PKC-δ siRNA compared to nonspecific siRNA treated mice [*$p<0.05$ for H (nonspecific siRNA) versus H (PKC-δ siRNA)].

Figure S6 Relative expression of Akt and ERK-1/2. Graph showing phospho-Akt/Akt and phospho-ERK-1/2/ERK-1/2 ratio in group C, E, E^R and H (For phospho-Akt/Akt ratio: ***$p<0.001$ for E versus C; ¶¶$p<0.01$ for E versus E^R. For phospho-ERK-1/2/ERK-1/2 ratio: ***$p<0.001$ for E versus C; ¶¶$p<0.01$ for E versus E^R.

Figure S7 Silencing of PKC-α results in down regulation of prosurvival markers. Graph showing significantly decreased phospho-PKC-α along with significant decrease in the phosphorylation level of Akt and ERK-1/2 in mice treated with PKC-α siRNA compared with nonspecific siRNA treated mice [*$p<0.05$ for E (nonspecific siRNA) versus E (PKC-α siRNA)].

Figure S8 Cardiac functional parameters after PKC-α silencing. Graph showing significant increase in LVDD and decrease in %FS in mice treated with PKC-α siRNA compared to nonspecific siRNA treated mice [*p<0.05 for E (nonspecific siRNA) versus E (PKC-α siRNA)].

Figure S9 Cardiac functional parameters after PKC-δ silencing. Graph showing significant decrease in LVDD and increase in %FS in mice treated with PKC-δ siRNA compared to nonspecific siRNA treated mice [*p<0.05 for H (nonspecific siRNA) versus H (PKC-δ siRNA)].

Acknowledgments

We gratefully acknowledge Dr. Mamta Chawla Sarkar, National Institute of Cholera and Enteric Diseases, Kolkata, for her valuable input during manuscript preparation.

Author Contributions

Conceived and designed the experiments: SS SN. Performed the experiments: SN KD AM KP RD TB. Analyzed the data: SS SN AM KD. Wrote the paper: SS SN AM KD. Handled animals: SN RD KD. Statistical analysis: KP.

References

1. Catalucci D, Latronico MV, Ellingsen O, Condorelli G (2008) Physiological myocardial hypertrophy: how and why? Front Biosci 1: 312–324.
2. Fagard RH (1997) Impact of different sports and training on cardiac structure and function. Cardiol Clin 15: 397–412.
3. Jin H, Yang R, Li W, Lu H, Ryan AM, et al. (2000) Effects of exercise training on cardiac function, gene expression, and apoptosis in rats. Am J Physiol Heart Circ Physiol 279: 2994–3002.
4. Seidman JG, Seidman C (2001) The genetic basis for cardiomyopathy: from mutation identification to mechanistic paradigms. Cell 104: 557–567.
5. Weeks KL, McMullen JR (2011) The athlete's heart vs. the failing heart: can signaling explain the two distinct outcomes? Physiology 26: 97–105.
6. Takeishi Y, Ping P, Bolli R, Kirkpatrick DL, Hoit BD, et al. (2000) Transgenic overexpression of constitutively active Protein Kinase C epsilon causes concentric cardiac hypertrophy. Circ Res 86: 1218–1223.
7. Koide Y, Tamura K, Suzuki A, Kitamura K, Yokoyama K, et al. (2003) Differential induction of protein kinase C isoforms at the cardiac hypertrophy stage and congestive heart failure stage in Dahl salt-sensitive rats. Hypertens Res 26: 421–426.
8. Sil P, Kandaswamy V, Sen S (1998) Increased protein Kinase C activity in myotrophin-induced myocyte growth. Circ Res 82: 1173–1188.
9. Braz JC, Bueno OF, De Windt LJ, Molkentin JD (2002) PKC-α regulates the hypertrophic growth of cardiomyocytes through extracellular signal–regulated kinase1/2 (ERK-1/2). J cell Biol 156: 905–919.
10. Duquesnes N, Lezoualc'h F, Crozatier B (2011) PKC-delta and PKC-epsilon: foes of the same family or strangers? J Mol Cell Cardiol 51: 665–673.
11. Dong Y, Morris-Natschke SL, Lee KH (2011) Biosynthesis, total syntheses, and antitumor activity of tanshinones and their analogs as potential therapeutic agents. Nat Prod Rep 28: 529–542.
12. Liu Q, Molkentin JD (2011) Protein kinase C-α as a heart failure therapeutic target. J Mol Cell Cardiol 51: 474–478.
13. Churchill E, Budas G, Vallentin A, Koyanagi T, Mochly-Rosen D, et al. (2008) PKC isozymes in chronic cardiac disease: possible therapeutic targets? Annu Rev Pharmacol Toxicol 48: 569–599.
14. Matassa AA, Kalkofen RL, Carpenter L, Biden TJ, Reyland ME (2003) Inhibition of PKC-α induces a PKC-δ-dependent apoptotic program in salivary epithelial cells. Cell Death Differ 10: 269–277.
15. Ellison GM, Waring CD, Vicinanza C, Torella D (2012) Physiological cardiac remodeling in response to endurance exercise training: cellular and molecular mechanisms. Heart 98: 5–10.
16. Garciarena CD, Pinilla OA, Nolly MB, Laguens RP, Escudero EM, et al. (2009) Endurance training in the spontaneously hypertensive rat: conversion of pathological into physiological cardiac hypertrophy. Hypertension 53: 708–714.
17. Mitra A, Basak T, Datta K, Naskar S, Sengupta S, et al. (2013) Role of α-crystallin B as a regulatory switch in modulating cardiomyocyte apoptosis by mitochondria or endoplasmic reticulum during cardiac hypertrophy and myocardial infarction. Cell Death Dis 4: e582.
18. Evangelista FS, Brum PC, Krieger JE (2003) Duration-controlled swimming exercise training induces cardiac hypertrophy in mice. Braz J Med Biol Res 36: 1751–1759.
19. Galindo CL, Skinner MA, Errami M, Olson LD, Watson DA, et al. (2009) Transcriptional profile of isoproterenol-induced cardiomyopathy and comparison to exercise-induced cardiac hypertrophy and human cardiac failure. BMC Physiol 9: 9–23.
20. Pathak M, Sarkar S, Vellaichamy E, Sen S (2001) Role of myocytes in myocardial collagen production. Hypertension 37: 833–840.
21. Sil P, Sen S (1997) Angiotensin II and myocyte growth: role of fibroblasts. Hypertension 30: 209–216.
22. Pabla N, Dong G, Jiang M, Huang S, Kumar MV, et al. (2011) Inhibition of PKCδ reduces cisplatin-induced nephrotoxicity without blocking chemotherapeutic efficacy in mouse models of cancer. J Clin Invest 121: 2709–2722.
23. Chintalgattu V, Katwa LC (2009) Role of protein kinase C-delta in angiotensin II induced cardiac fibrosis. Biochem Biophys Res Commun 386: 612–616.
24. Mut M, Amos S, Hussaini IM (2010) PKC alpha phosphorylates cytosolic NF-kappaB/p65 and PKC delta delays nuclear translocation of NF-kappaB/p65 in U1242 glioblastoma cells. Turk Neurosurg 20: 277–285.
25. Mir SA, Chatterjee A, Mitra A, Pathak K, Mahata SK, et al. (2012) Inhibition of signal transducer and activator of transcription 3 (STAT3) attenuates interleukin-6 (IL-6)-induced collagen synthesis and resultant hypertrophy in rat heart. J Biol Chem 287: 2666–2677.
26. Sarkar S, Vellaichamy E, Young D, Sen S (2004a) Influence of cytokines and growth factors in Ang II-mediated collagen up regulation by fibroblasts in rats: role of myocytes. Am J Physiol Heart Circ Physiol 287: 107–117.
27. Bhowmick R, Halder UC, Chattopadhyay S, Chanda S, Nandi S, et al. (2012) Rotaviral enterotoxin nonstructural protein 4 targets mitochondria for activation of apoptosis during infection. J Biol Chem 287: 35004–35020.
28. Chatterjee A, Mir SA, Dutta D, Mitra A, Pathak K, et al. (2010) Analysis of p53 and NF-kB signaling in modulating the cardiomyocyte fate during hypertrophy. J Cell Physiol 226: 2543–2554.
29. Stegemann H, Stalder K (1967) Determination of hydroxyproline. Clin Chim Acta 18: 267–273.
30. Zhao M, Xia L, Chen GQ (2012) Protein Kinase C-δ in apoptosis: a brief overview. Arch Immunol Ther Exp 60: 361–372.
31. He Y, Liu J, Grossman D, Durrant D, Sweatman T, et al. (2007) Phosphorylation of mitochondrial phospholipid scramblase-3 by protein kinase C-delta induces its activation and facilitates mitochondrial targeting of t-Bid. J Cell Biochem 101: 1210–1221.
32. Liu J, Dai Q, Chen J (2003b) Phospholipid scramblase-3 controls mitochondrial structure, function, and apoptotic response. Mol Cancer Res 1: 892–902.
33. Dave KR, Bhattacharya SK, Saul I, DeFazio RA, Dezfulian C, et al. (2011) Activation of protein kinase C delta following cerebral ischemia leads to release of cytochrome-c from the mitochondria via bad pathway. PLoS One 6: e22057.
34. Kato K, Yamanouchi D, Esbona K, Kamiya K, Zhang F, et al. (2009) Caspase-mediated protein kinase C-delta cleavage is necessary for apoptosis of vascular smooth muscle cells. Am J Physiol Heart Circ Physiol 297: 2253–2261.
35. Putinski C, Abdul-Ghani M, Stiles R, Brunette S, Dick SA, et al. (2013) Intrinsic-mediated caspase activation is essential for cardiomyocyte hypertrophy. Proc Natl Acad Sci U S A 110: E4079–4087.
36. Datta R, Kojima H, Yoshida K, Kufe D (1997) Caspase-3-mediated cleavage of protein kinase C theta in induction of apoptosis. J Biol Chem 272: 20317–20320.
37. Endo K1, Oki E, Biedermann V, Kojima H, Yoshida K, et al. (2000) Proteolytic cleavage and activation of protein kinase C μ by caspase-3 in the apoptotic response of cells to 1-beta-D-arabinofuranosylcytosine and other genotoxic agents. J Biol Chem 275: 18476–18481.
38. Partovian C, Simons M (2004) Regulation of protein kinase B/Akt activity and Ser473 phosphorylation by protein kinase C alpha in endothelial cells. Cell Signal 16: 951–957.
39. Steinberg SF (2012) Cardiac actions of protein kinase C isoforms. Physiology (Bethesda) 27: 130–139.
40. Cuadrado I, Fernández-Velasco M, Boscá L, de Las Heras B (2011) Labdanediterpenes protect against anoxia/reperfusion injury in cardiomyocytes: involvement of Akt activation. Cell Death Dis 2: e229.
41. Lee SW, Won JY, Lee HY, Lee HJ, Youn SW, et al. (2011) Angiopoietin-1 protects heart against ischemia/reperfusion injury through VE-cadherin dephosphorylation and myocardiac integrin-β1/ERK/caspase-9 phosphorylation cascade. Mol Med 17: 1095–1106.
42. Tanaka Y, Gavrielides MV, Mitsuuchi Y, Fujii T, Kazanietz MG (2003) Protein kinase C promotes apoptosis in LNCaP prostate cancer cells through the activation of p38 MAPK and inhibition of the Akt survival pathway. J Biol Chem 278: 33753–33762.

A Behavioral Mechanism of How Increases in Leg Strength Improve Old Adults' Gait Speed

Azusa Uematsu[1]*, Kazushi Tsuchiya[2], Norio Kadono[3], Hirofumi Kobayashi[4], Takamasa Kaetsu[5], Tibor Hortobágyi[6,7], Shuji Suzuki[1]

1 Faculty of Human Sciences, Waseda University, Tokorozawa, Japan, **2** Graduate School of Human Sciences, Waseda University, Tokorozawa, Japan, **3** Advanced Research Center for Human Sciences, Waseda University, Tokorozawa, Japan, **4** Graduate School of Arts and Sciences, The University of Tokyo, Meguro-ku, Japan, **5** School of Human Sciences, Waseda University, Tokorozawa, Japan, **6** University Medical Center Groningen, University of Groningen, Groningen, The Netherlands, **7** Department of Sport, Exercise and Rehabilitation, Northumbria University, Newcastle-upon-Tyne, United Kingdom

Abstract

We examined a behavioral mechanism of how increases in leg strength improve healthy old adults' gait speed. Leg press strength training improved maximal leg press load 40% ($p = 0.001$) and isometric strength in 5 group of leg muscles 32% ($p = 0.001$) in a randomly allocated intervention group of healthy old adults (age 74, $n = 15$) but not in no-exercise control group (age 74, $n = 8$). Gait speed increased similarly in the training (9.9%) and control (8.6%) groups (time main effect, $p = 0.001$). However, in the training group only, in line with the concept of biomechanical plasticity of aging gait, hip extensors and ankle plantarflexors became the only significant predictors of self-selected and maximal gait speed. The study provides the first behavioral evidence regarding a mechanism of how increases in leg strength improve healthy old adults' gait speed.

Editor: Stephen E. Alway, West Virginia University School of Medicine, United States of America

Funding: This study was supported in part by Waseda University Grant for Special Research Projects (2013A-943 and 2013B-224) (http://www.waseda.jp/rps/en/index.html). The funders had no role in study design, data collection and analysis, decision to publish, or preparation of the manuscript.

Competing Interests: The authors have declared that no competing interests exist.

* Email: uematsu@aoni.waseda.jp

Introduction

The decline in self-selected habitual gait speed can reach 16% per decade starting at age 60 [1–5]. A decline in gait speed is normally associated with deteriorating health. Consequently, self-selected habitual gait speed measured on a level surface in middle ages predicts many clinical conditions later in life, including daily function, late-life mobility, independence, falls, fear of falls, fractures, mental health, cognitive function, adverse clinical events, hospitalization, institutionalization, and survival [2,6–15]. A gait speed of ~0.6 m/s has been identified as a threshold for frailty and represents an additional risk factor for functional decline in old adults [2]. Therefore, maintaining gait speed over this threshold or even over 0.8 m/s, as suggested in some studies, is clinically important because slow gait can potentially lead to motor passivity: as the time needed to cross the street or reach a destination becomes longer, old adults become less motivated to ambulate [16].

Leg strength and power can help maintain gait speed in old age. Some studies reported a significant association between gait speed and old adults' ability to produce force during a maximal voluntary contraction (MVC). For example, plantarflexor [4] and knee extensor MVC forces [17,18], and leg power [3,19–21] are associated with gait speed. In other studies, however, hip and knee extensor strengths did not correlate with gait speed [22]. Novel compared with a simple type of exercise interventions tend to increase gait speed somewhat more reliably [8]. However, a careful analysis in recent review revealed a statistically significant but weak association between the training-induced increases in leg muscle strength and gait speed ($r^2 = 0.21$, $p = 0.018$) [23]. Furthermore, the coefficient of determinations between increases in plantarflexor MVC and gait speed in 6 studies and between the increases in leg power and gait speed in 8 studies, respectively, was $r^2 = 0.16$ ($p = 0.421$), and $r^2 = 0.00$ ($p = 0.996$) [23]. Therefore, the mechanism of how strength and power training increases gait speed remains unclear.

A critical element that these studies have not yet addressed is how, if at all, does a strength intervention affect the relationship between leg strength and gait speed. More specifically, it is unknown as to how the increase of an individual leg muscle group's strength contributes to gait speed after the intervention and if muscles that improve the most also predict the increases in gait speed most accurately. Because the ankle plantarflexors contribute over 70% to the total leg mechanical output in the propulsion phase of gait [23], even small increases in ankle strength could play a significant role in increasing gait speed. Yet, old compared with young adults use their hip extensors more and ankle planter flexors less during gait [24]. This is the concept of biomechanical plasticity of the aging gait [23,24] that suggests a shift in function to the proximal hip from distal ankle extensors, implying that any increase in hip function could hypothetically be also a factor in improving gait speed. Taken together, the purposes of the present study were: 1) to determine the effects of lower extremity strength training on maximal strength of 5 leg muscle groups including hip abductor, hip adductors, hip extensors, knee extensors, and ankle plantarflexors; 2) to examine the relationship between leg strength of each muscle group and gait speed before and after the intervention; and 3) to test the hypothesis that, according to the concept of biomechanical plasticity of gait, hip and ankle functions become significant predictors of gait speed in healthy old adults. If these expectations were correct, the results would provide the first behavioral evidence regarding the mechanism of how increase in leg strength actually improves gait speed in old adults.

Methods

Ethics statement

The Human Ethics Committee at Waseda University approved the study protocol. Before the start of the study, each participant read and signed a written informed consent. All procedures were conducted according to the Declaration of Helsinki.

Subjects and design

Twenty-five 70–81-year-old healthy community-dwelling volunteers (12 males, 13 females) participated in this study. All participants were healthy enough to visit the laboratory on their own by car, bicycle, or on foot.

The study had a 2-group pre-test and post-test design. We assigned participants randomly to control (3 males and 5 females; age = 74.3±3.9 years; height = 156.3±10.6 cm; weight = 54.3±10.7 kg) and exercise-training groups (9 males and 8 females). One female participant withdrew from the study due to knee joint pain caused by an accident. Another female participant dropped out of the study after the 1st training session due to time conflicts. Thus, 9 males and 6 females (age = 74.3±3.4 years; height = 158.8±6.8 cm; weight = 57.7±7.3 kg) completed all the training and testing sessions. We tested all participants for walking ability, physical performance, and isometric strengths of 5 muscle groups at baseline and after 8 weeks of leg press training or no training.

Testing protocol

Participants completed the short physical performance battery (SPPB) and maximal isometric strength testing of five muscle groups against a hand-held dynamometer on the initial day of the study. The 1-repetition maximum (1RM) leg strength was tested 2 or 3 days later on a second testing day in the training group.

Short physical performance battery (SPPB). The SPPB is valid and reliable functional tests of old adults' balance, walking speed, and leg strength [25]. Briefly, SPPB quantifies standing balance, gait speed over 4 m level surface, and leg strength through 5, timed chair rises. Subjects were allowed to practice as needed so that they could become familiar with these tests. Experimenter recorded the time required to perform each test using a stopwatch (S123-4000, SEIKO).

Walking speed. We measured participants' self-selected walking speed on flat surface over 4 m and maximal walking speed on flat surface over 7 m. The 4-m self-selected walking speed was determined as a part of the SPPB test. The instruction was as follows: "Walk at your usual speed, just as if you were walking down the street to go to the store." For the maximal walking speed, participants stood behind a line and walked past a target line set at 7 m. The instruction was: "Walk as fast as you safely can as if you tried to catch a bus but do not run". Subjects practiced the maximal walking speed test 1–2 times before the data collection. Walking speed was recorded to the 10th of a second accuracy with the stopwatch.

Leg strength. We measured maximal voluntary isometric strength of the right leg during hip extension, abduction, and adduction and during knee extension and ankle plantarflexion using a hand-held dynamometer (MT-100, SAKAI Medical Company, Japan). We adopted a highly standardized testing protocol validated previously (Intraclass correlation coefficients > 0.90) [26,27]. We performed all of the measurements with a calibrated load-cell sensitive to pull forces up to 980 N (MT-110, SAKAI Medical Company, Japan), placed in series within a 2.5-cm wide non-stretch plastic strap. For hip extension, subjects lay prone across an examination table with the left leg straight and the right knee flexed 90° and positioned 10–15 cm past the table edge. The top end of the strap loop was just superior to the popliteal fossa and the other end was anchored tautly to the floor. Subjects performed maximal hip extension by pressing upwards into the strap. For hip abduction, subjects lay supine with both legs straight on the examination table 30° apart and the strap looping around both knees. Subject performed maximal hip abduction by pressing the straight right leg outward into the strap. Subjects assumed the same position on the table for hip adduction, but the strap was looped around the subject's right knee and around the left thigh of the experimenter, standing next to the examination table on the right side of the subject. For knee extension, subjects sat in an armless chair and flexed the knee 90°. One end of the strap loop was placed on the shank just above the right lateral malleolus and the other end around the right rear leg of the chair. The foot sole was about 1 cm above the floor. For ankle plantarflexion, subjects assumed the same body position as for hip extension. One end of the strap loop was around the distal end of the metatarsals and the other end around the table leg. The ankle was in anatomical position. For all tests, subjects were allowed to grasp the table or chair edge. Participants first practiced each test at 40–50% of maximal effort then performed 1–2 trials at 70–80% of maximal effort. Subjects performed 2 maximal effort trials for 5 seconds each with strong verbal encouragement. There was 30 s of rest between each strength test. One researcher administered all of the strength tests in a randomized order between subjects. The higher of the 2 scores was used in the analysis.

1RM leg strength. On a separate day, we measured leg strength during a bilateral 1RM seated leg press on a weight-stacked leg press machine (maximum load: 218 kg, Nautilus), used also in the exercise training intervention. Subjects started the leg press movement with the hip and knee joints flexed 90° and completed the movement with the hip and knees extended and plantarflexed. Subjects were instructed to complete the press movement in 1 continuous, smooth, and brisk motion and then return to the starting position slowly and smoothly. After a thorough familiarization with the test, subjects performed several trials at 30–40% and then 2–3 trials at 70–80% of their anticipated maximal load. The load, based on preliminary work, was then increased in about 9 kg steps until the 1RM load. Subjects performed no more than 4 steps to reach 1RM and had no difficulty in executing the leg press testing. There was 60 s of rest between each trial. To minimize the potential effects of 1RM testing on mobility, only the training group performed the 1RM testing.

Training protocol

We chose leg press as an exercise stimulus because preliminary work revealed that the electromyographic activation of the hip, knee, and ankle extensors during leg press was ~80% of activation measured during single-joint exercise and because these muscles

Table 1. Changes in the dependent variables.

Parameter	Interaction/main effect	Group	Pre	Post
Gait speed (m/s)				
Self-selected	Time	CG	1.10±0.18	1.19±0.14
		EG	1.05±0.15	1.19±0.16
Maximal	Time	CG	1.43±0.16	1.56±0.13
		EG	1.56±0.21	1.66±0.24
Maximal strength (kg)	Group×Time			
Plantarflexion		CG	8.26±4.37	8.85±5.13
		EG	8.13±5.76	12.87±4.83
Knee extension		CG	22.69±6.65	21.76±7.69
		EG	27.97±13.22	29.13±14.69
Hip extension		CG	11.39±6.70	14.20±8.30
		EG	13.57±11.08	22.69±14.00
Hip abduction		CG	16.26±7.04	17.13±4.57
		EG	18.20±5.41	20.46±6.03
Hip adduction		CG	14.33±5.32	14.11±4.89
		EG	16.13±5.26	18.01±6.48

Values are mean ± SD. CG, control group. EG, exercise group. Group×Time, group by time interaction ($p = 0.002$). Time, time main effect (all $p = 0.001$).

are also involved in the stance phase of gait. For example, compared with a single joint maximal voluntary isometric contraction, during a 1RM leg press the activation of the hip extensor biceps femoris, the knee extensor vastus lateralis, and the ankle plantarflexor gastrconemius medialis was, respectively, 87% (±16), 92% (±22), and 78% (±19) (n = 6 young adults, age 21.2).

The training program consisted of 16 sessions administered over 8 weeks. Each session was about 30 minutes long and started with a standard 5–10 minutes of warm-up that included: rhythmical bouncing and bending exercise, stretching of hip, knee, and ankle muscles, side-to-side torso flexion, and arm rotations. The training load was then set at 30–40% of 1RM and participants performed 3 bouts of 10 repetitions. Subjects remained seated in the leg press machine during the 2-minutes-long inter-bout rest period. Subjects were instructed to perform each repetition rapidly and forcefully. The training load was adjusted throughout the training program. We selected a light load, higher movement velocity to increase the specificity of the training stimulus to gait speed, as suggested previously [28–30]. The same staff person supervised each training session. After the training, there was a 5-minute-long cool down period and subjects performed stretching. Members of the control group continued their habitual activities.

Statistical analyses. The data are reported as mean ± SD. The main analysis was a Group (intervention, control) by Time (pre, post) analysis of variance repeated-measures on Time. In case of a significant interaction, a Bonferroni's post-hoc contrast was used to determine the means that were different. We computed a Pearson's product correlation coefficient between gait speed and expressions of leg strength. We used a step-wise, multiple-regression analysis to directly test the hypothesis as to which muscle group predicted gait speed after the intervention. We also compared the simple linear regression coefficients before and after training using a small sample t-test. Statistical significance was set for all analysis at $p<0.05$.

Results

Training stimulus

In each of the 8 weeks, the mass lifted by the subjects during the leg press averaged 44 kg (or 39% of the pre-test 1RM), 53 kg (47%), 62 kg (55%), 71 kg (63%), 79 kg (70%), 86 kg (76%), 89 kg (79%), and 90 kg (79%), respectively. The average training load was a moderate 59% relative to pre-test 1RM. Because we instructed the participants to move the loads rapidly, the combination of training volume, movement speed, and the number repetitions – as planned - qualified the training stimulus as power training.

Changes in SPPB and 1RM

There was no group by time interaction for the SPPB score ($p = 0.162$) and the groups were also similar at baseline ($p = 0.064$). The time main effect revealed 7.5% or 0.8 units of improvement ($p = 0.002$), caused by the 11.1% in the control compared with the 4.2% change in training group. Leg press training improved leg press 1RM 40.4% (±26.3) to 155.9 (±46.2) from 113.0 kg (±35.6) at baseline ($p<0.001$).

Changes in gait speed and muscle strength

Table 1 shows that there was no group by time interaction for the 4-m self-selected ($p = 0.340$) and 7-m maximal ($p = 0.560$) gait speed, respectively. The time main effect revealed 11.2% or 0.12 m/s improvements in self-selected ($p = 0.001$) and 7.2% or 0.11 m/s increases in maximal gait speed ($p = 0.001$). The 2 groups' gait speeds were similar at baseline (control vs. training group: self-selected: 1.10 vs. 1.05 m/s; maximal: 1.43 vs. 1.56 m/s, both $p>0.05$).

Table 1 also shows the changes in maximal voluntary strength measured by manual muscle testing in 5 muscle groups. There was no group by muscle group by time interaction ($p = 0.394$). The group by time interaction ($p = 0.002$) revealed that the 32.0% or 4.0 kg average improvement in the 5 muscle groups combined was greater than the 6.3% or 0.6 kg gain in the control group ($p = 0.002$). When each muscle group's contribution to the summed strength score was computed in the training group before and after the intervention, there was a muscle group by time interaction ($p = 0.004$). Table 2 shows that the plantarflexors (3.7%) and hip extensors (6.8%) increased and the knee extensors decreased (5.9%) the contribution to the changes in total strength (all $p<0.001$). The hip abductors and adductors decreased ~2% the contributions to the total strength change (both $p = 0.060$).

Correlations analyses

Table 3 shows the correlation coefficients between walking speed and leg strength in the exercise group. Before the intervention, the correlations (range: $r = 0.00$ to 0.55) were low and except for 1 (hip abduction) of 10 correlation coefficients, not significant ($p>0.05$). After the intervention, 8 of 10 correlations were statistically significant, ranging from $r = 0.53$ ($p = 0.040$) to $r = 0.75$ ($p = 0.001$). In 4 of 5 muscles the coefficients were somewhat higher for the maximal ($r = 0.60$) compared with the self-selected gait speed ($r = 0.53$). The increase in the correlation was similar between self-selected gait velocity and leg strength ($r = 0.32$ increase in correlation) and maximal walking speed and leg strength ($r = 0.27$ increase in correlation).

At baseline, a forward step-wise, multiple-regression selected hip abductor strength as significant predictor of maximal gait speed (adjusted $R^2 = 0.25$, $p = 0.034$). After the intervention, hip extensor strength became the predictor of self-selected walking speed (adjusted $R^2 = 0.29$, $p = 0.024$) and plantar flexor strength predicted maximal gait speed (adjusted $R^2 = 0.53$, $p = 0.001$). Finally, the regression coefficient became significant for the relationship between self-selected walking speed and plantarflexor and hip extensor strength, respectively (Figure 1, panel A and B) and between maximal gait speed and plantarflexor strength (Figure 1, panel C) (all $p<0.05$).

Discussion

The main finding of the present study was that 40.4% increase in leg press 1RM training load and 32.0% increase in maximal isometric strength in 5 leg muscles did not improve gait speed more (9.9%) than what the changes were in the control group (8.6%). However, after the exercise intervention there was a modification in how 5 measures of leg strength contributed to gait speed with hip extensors and ankle plantarflexors becoming the only significant predictors of self-selected and maximal gait speed. We discuss these findings within the framework of biomechanical plasticity of the aging gait.

Leg strength interventions normally improve gait speed [8,23]. Based on 20 studies, the 22% increase in leg strength was coupled with an 11.7% increase in self-selected gait speed (1.25 to 1.38 m/s) in 815 healthy old adults age 72 [23]. In several of the 20 studies the changes in gait speed were not significant [31] reaching only 5 to 7% [32–34] with some studies reporting actually up to 7% decrease instead of an increase in gait speed [35–37]. Therefore, our results are not an unusual finding that a strength or power intervention resulted in modest increases in gait speed. Adjusting for height removed the large difference in gait speed between samples consisting of predominantly Caucasian subjects in the review (1.25 m/s) and studies that enrolled Japanese participants only (the present study and [38]) (1.05 m/s) (0.77 vs. 0.76 speed/height ratio), suggesting that the height-adjusted baseline gait speed was similar in our sample and those published previously. Similarly to the 11.7% increase in gait speed in the 20 studies, our subjects increased self-selected gait speed 13.3%. The 8.2% increase in the control group occurred despite rigorously standardized instructions and a measurement environment that was, to smallest details, kept identical throughout the study, suggesting a learning effect due to the repeat testing. The same phenomenon was also observed previously [39,40]. Therefore, we assume that gait speed can also increase in control subjects as a result of learning.

According to exercise prescription guidelines and recent recommendations, our participants performed power training by moving light-medium loads rapidly [21,41]. It has been suggested that power vs. strength training may be more suitable to increase gait speed [19,21,42–44]. While our and other types of power training was successful and improved leg power and strength 34.7% based on data from 8 studies in 150 subjects age 73, a 13.1% increase in self-selected gait speed to 1.38 from 1.25 m/s after those interventions was similar to the 11.7% increase produced by strength training [23]. Thus, the data from the literature suggest that strength and power interventions can improve self-selected gait speed and these changes are often similar after the 2 types of intervention. At least under the current experimental conditions, in healthy but sedentary seniors the exercise adaptations could include a substantial element of learning induced by the testing protocol. This conclusion is further confirmed by the 9.0 and 6.4% increase in maximal gait speed in the control and intervention groups, respectively (time main effect, $p = 0.001$), a variable that is less often reported in intervention studies [29,30,40]. In particular, considering the ~1.0 m/s self-selected gait speed at baseline, which is well above the 0.8 m/s designated as a marker for median life expectancy [10] and the 0.6 m/s as a threshold for frailty [2], it is likely that the subjects' mobility level at baseline in our and these previous studies [29,30,40] was too high and a ceiling effect blunted the gait responses to the training intervention. Another reason could be that the laboratory environment was restrictive and instructions

Table 2. Contribution by each of the 5 muscle groups to the summed strength score in the training group ($n = 15$).

Muscle group	Pre	Post	Significance
Plantarflexors	8.99±3.42	12.73±3.42	**
Knee extensors	33.14±5.41	27.23±3.81	**
Hip extensors	14.54±5.47	21.34±6.48	**
Hip abductors	23.01±5.04	20.84±5.41	
Hip adductors	20.31±4.83	17.87±2.97	

Values are percent of the summed strength score for each muscle (mean ± SD). Time by Muscle group interaction ($p = 0.004$).
**, significant change between pre and post ($p<0.01$).

Table 3. Pearson product moment correlation coefficients between maximal leg strength and gait speed before and after exercise intervention (n = 15).

Maximal strength	Gait speed	Pre		Post	
		r	p	r	p
Plantarflexion	Self-selected	−0.01	0.98	0.50	0.06
	Maximal	0.02	0.54	0.75	0.00
Knee extension	Self-selected	0.34	0.21	0.56	0.04
	Maximal	0.51	0.06	0.56	0.03
Hip extension	Self-selected	0.06	0.84	0.58	0.02
	Maximal	0.16	0.56	0.54	0.04
Hip abduction	Self-selected	0.36	0.19	0.56	0.00
	Maximal	0.55	0.03	0.61	0.02
Hip adduction	Self-selected	0.29	0.29	0.47	0.08
	Maximal	0.42	0.12	0.53	0.04

p, 2-tailed probability values for the correlation coefficient.

were inadequate stimuli for participants to motivate themselves and walk faster [45].

The disproportionality between the large increase in leg strength and the clinically small increase in (maximal) gait speed suggests the possibility that an increase in leg strength in high-mobility old adults does not correlate with an increase in gait speed in a simple manner. Previous studies reported that leg muscle strength declines gradually with age [46] but the usual gait speed

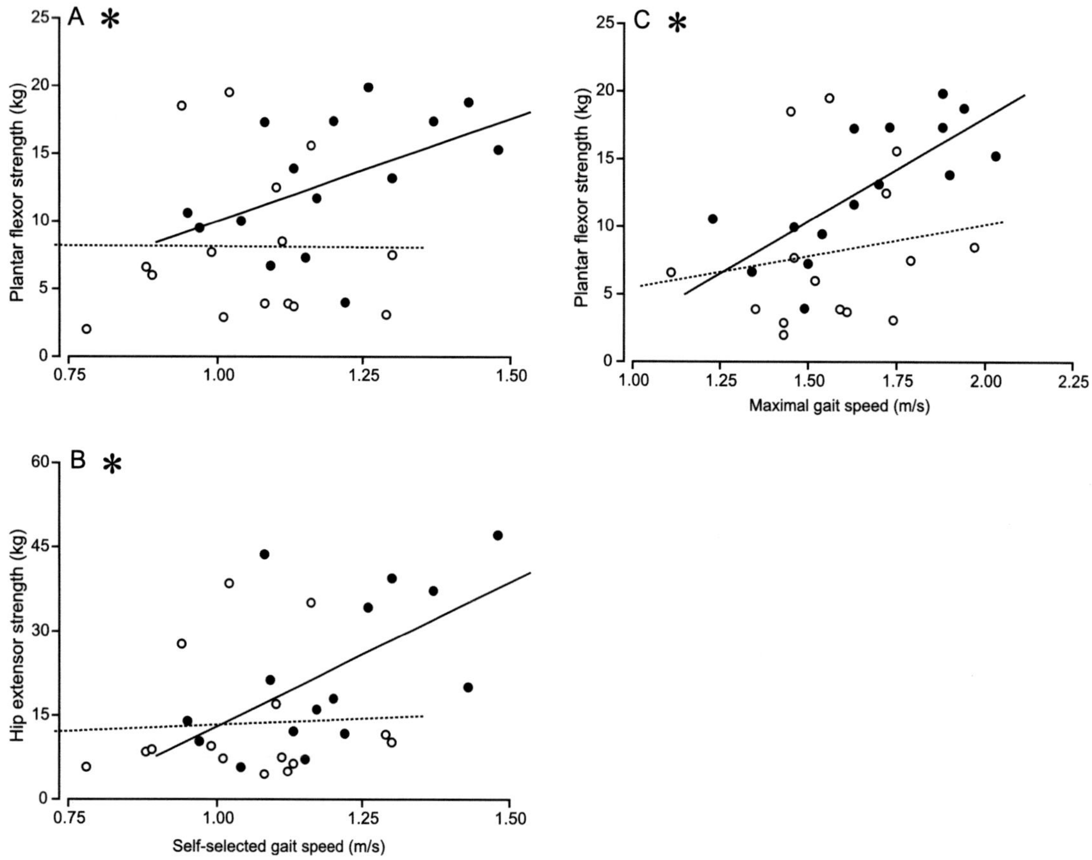

Figure 1. Linear regression of self-selected and maximal gait speed on leg strength before (open symbols, dashed regression lines) and after 16 sessions of leg press training (n = 15). Panel A: before, y = 8.38–0.24x, after, y = 8.84+15.16x; Panel B: before y = 8.89+4.44x, after, y = −35.80+49.91x; Panel C: before, y = 0.84+4.66x, after, y = −12.92+15.50x. The * denotes a significant ($p<0.05$) difference in the slopes of the regression coefficient before and after training determined by small sample t-test.

can decrease rapidly over age 80 [47]. Participants in the present study had such levels of leg muscle strength at baseline that affected functional abilities to only a small extent. Although the intervention was successful in increasing leg strength, the increases in gait speed in the intervention group were much smaller because the functional level in gait was higher compared with the age-related level of relative strength loss. A logical next step for future studies is to examine neuromuscular adaptations to strength and power interventions and determine if such adaptations explain more of the variation in gait speed in functionally less capable old adults than the subjects in the present study.

Leg press has been often a choice of exercise to target the lower extremity extensor mechanism in an effort to improve mobility, including gait speed in old age [28,29,39,40]. A new observation was how the intervention modified the contribution of leg strength to gait speed. Ankle plantarflexor strength increased 58.3% ($p = 0.001$) and its contribution to total leg strength still increased ~4% ($p<0.05$). The intervention also increased hip extension strength 73.6% ($p = 0.001$) and its contribution to the total leg strength still increased ~7% ($p<0.05$). In contrast, the knee extensor and hip abductor strength increased much less, 4 to 12%, and their contribution to the total leg strength did not change or even decreased ~6% (knee extensors).

Our findings are especially insightful in combination with additional analysis of the data revealing that individual leg strength measures showed low or no association with gait speed at baseline ($r = -0.01$ to 0.55, 1 of 10 correlations $p<0.05$, Table 3). However, after the intervention stepwise regression analyses identified the hip extensors and ankle plantar flexors, muscle that increased most their contribution to the total leg strength, the only significant predictors of self-selected and maximal gait speed, respectively only in the training group (Figure 1). These findings agree with the predictions of biomechanical plasticity that assigns a putative role to hip and ankle function in the aging gait [23,24].

Old compared with young adults tend to walk with reduced ankle plantarflexor output and it seems that an increase in hip mechanical output compensates for this reduction in an effort to maintain gait speed [23,24]. Our data further specify this concept by showing a substantial increase in the correlation to $r = 0.75$ ($p = 0.001$) from $r = 0.02$ ($p = 0.540$) between ankle plantarflexor strength and maximal gait speed and to $r = 0.58$ ($p = 0.020$) from $r = 0.06$ ($p = 0.840$) between hip extensor strength and self-selected gait speed (Figure 1). The plantar flexors contribute over 70% to the total support power in the stance phase of gait in young adults which can decrease as much as 20% in old adults with 38% increase in hip power while walking at 1.0 to 1.5 m/s [24,48–54]. The small or no increase after training in the correlation between hip abductor and adductor maximal strength and gait ability, respectively, underscores the specific role of plantarflexors and hip extensors play in gait speed (Table 2). The present data thus show that strength training may not have increased gait speed beyond control subjects' speed but it produced a favorable reconfiguration of the individual joint contributions to gait velocity, providing possibly the first evidence for the incorporation of newly acquired strength into the mechanism that generates gait speed.

Leg press power training improved ankle plantarflexor and hip extensor MVCs but not knee extensor, hip abductor, and hip adductor MVC (all $p>0.05$). The 4% increase in knee extension MVC is unexpectedly low because preliminary testing in young adults revealed 92±22% activation of the vastus lateralis during leg press as a percent of maximal electromyogram measured during maximal isokinetic knee extension. Previous studies that used leg press training reported no knee extension data or used several additional exercises so that our knee extension data are not directly comparable with these studies [28,29,39,40,55]. Perhaps young adults used a different lower extremity alignment in the preliminary study than old adults in the intervention group, resulting in a different muscle activation pattern. Still, it seems that leg press power training at 30–40% of maximal load as a single exercise or embedded in multiple training exercises is safe and effective for the conditioning of multiple muscle groups in old adults who may also prefer these light vs. heavy loads recommended for high-intensity strength training [19,41,42,56,57]. Further, because fast compared with slow muscle contractions are associated with higher motor unit activation at the same load [58], power vs. high-force but low-velocity exercise training is expected to activate a greater number of motor units, resulting in larger neuromuscular and functionally more specific adaptations.

One limitation of the present study was a lack of comprehensive measures of activity of daily living. A second limitation was a lack of biomechanical assessments that could provide more detailed and mechanistic insights into how newly acquired physical abilities became incorporated into the mechanics of gait. Due to the small sample sizes it was not possible to determine if the reported findings differed between men and women.

Conclusion

Light-load leg press power training improved leg press 1RM load 40.4% and 32.0% the maximal force of 5 leg muscles without improving gait speed more in the intervention vs. control groups. However, the intervention modified how 5 measures of leg strength contributed to gait speed: Hip extensors and ankle plantarflexors became the only significant predictors of self-selected and maximal gait speed, respectively. These data provide possibly the first evidence for the incorporation of newly acquired strength into the mechanism that generates gait speed.

Supporting Information

Table S1 Measured variables of physical function test in both groups.

Table S2 1RM and training load progression in training group.

Acknowledgments

We thank Tomoya Ogawa, Madoka Nakamura, and Hanako Okai for their assistance with data collection and for supervising the training program.

Author Contributions

Conceived and designed the experiments: AU HK TH SS. Performed the experiments: AU KT NK HK TK. Analyzed the data: AU KT NK TK. Contributed reagents/materials/analysis tools: AU KT NK TH. Contributed to the writing of the manuscript: AU KT NK HK TK TH SS.

References

1. Abellan van Kan G, Houles M, Vellas B (2012) Identifying sarcopenia. Curr Opin Clin Nutr Metab Care 15: 436–441.

2. Abellan van Kan G, Rolland Y, Andrieu S, Bauer J, Beauchet O, et al. (2009) Gait speed at usual pace as a predictor of adverse outcomes in community-

dwelling older people an International Academy on Nutrition and Aging (IANA) Task Force. J Nutr Health Aging 13: 881–889.
3. Bassey EJ, Fiatarone MA, O'Neill EF, Kelly M, Evans WJ, et al. (1992) Leg extensor power and functional performance in very old men and women. Clin Sci (Lond) 82: 321–327.
4. Bendall MJ, Bassey EJ, Pearson MB (1989) Factors affecting walking speed of elderly people. Age Ageing 18: 327–332.
5. Himann JE, Cunningham DA, Rechnitzer PA, Paterson DH (1988) Age-related changes in speed of walking. Med Sci Sports Exerc 20: 161–166.
6. Atkinson HH, Rosano C, Simonsick EM, Williamson JD, Davis C, et al. (2007) Cognitive function, gait speed decline, and comorbidities: the health, aging and body composition study. J Gerontol A Biol Sci Med Sci 62: 844–850.
7. Dargent-Molina P, Favier F, Grandjean H, Baudoin C, Schott AM, et al. (1996) Fall-related factors and risk of hip fracture: the EPIDOS prospective study. Lancet 348: 145–149.
8. Granacher U, Muehlbauer T, Zahner L, Gollhofer A, Kressig RW (2011) Comparison of traditional and recent approaches in the promotion of balance and strength in older adults. Sports Med 41: 377–400.
9. Guralnik JM, Ferrucci L, Pieper CF, Leveille SG, Markides KS, et al. (2000) Lower extremity function and subsequent disability: consistency across studies, predictive models, and value of gait speed alone compared with the short physical performance battery. J Gerontol A Biol Sci Med Sci 55: M221–231.
10. Studenski S, Perera S, Patel K, Rosano C, Faulkner K, et al. (2011) Gait speed and survival in older adults. JAMA 305: 50–58.
11. Ijmker T, Lamoth CJ (2012) Gait and cognition: the relationship between gait stability and variability with executive function in persons with and without dementia. Gait Posture 35: 126–130.
12. Potter JM, Evans AL, Duncan G (1995) Gait speed and activities of daily living function in geriatric patients. Archives of Physical Medicine and Rehabilitation 76: 997–999.
13. Viccaro LJ, Perera S, Studenski SA (2011) Is timed up and go better than gait speed in predicting health, function, and falls in older adults? J Am Geriatr Soc 59: 887–892.
14. Watson NL, Rosano C, Boudreau RM, Simonsick EM, Ferrucci L, et al. (2010) Executive function, memory, and gait speed decline in well-functioning older adults. J Gerontol A Biol Sci Med Sci 65: 1093–1100.
15. Weuve J, Kang JH, Manson JE, Breteler MM, Ware JH, et al. (2004) Physical activity, including walking, and cognitive function in older women. JAMA 292: 1454–1461.
16. Bollard E, Fleming H (2013) A study to investigate the walking speed of elderly adults with relation to pedestrian crossings. Physiother Theory Pract 29: 142–149.
17. Fiatarone MA, Marks EC, Ryan ND, Meredith CN, Lipsitz LA, et al. (1990) High-intensity strength training in nonagenarians. Effects on skeletal muscle. JAMA 263: 3029–3034.
18. Miyazaki J, Murata S, Horie J, Uematsu A, Hortobagyi T, et al. (2013) Lumbar lordosis angle (LLA) and leg strength predict walking ability in elderly males. Arch Gerontol Geriatr 56: 141–147.
19. Fielding RA, LeBrasseur NK, Cuoco A, Bean J, Mizer K, et al. (2002) High-velocity resistance training increases skeletal muscle peak power in older women. J Am Geriatr Soc 50: 655–662.
20. Fielding RA, Rejeski WJ, Blair S, Church T, Espeland MA, et al. (2011) The Lifestyle Interventions and Independence for Elders Study: design and methods. J Gerontol A Biol Sci Med Sci 66: 1226–1237.
21. Reid KF, Doros G, Clark DJ, Patten C, Carabello RJ, et al. (2012) Muscle power failure in mobility-limited older adults: Preserved single Wber function despite lower whole muscle size, quality and rate of neuromuscular activation. European Journal of Applied Physiology 112: 2289–2301.
22. Brown M, Sinacore DR, Host HH (1995) The relationship of strength to function in the older adult. J Gerontol A Biol Sci Med Sci 50 Spec No: 55–59.
23. Beijersbergen CM, Granacher U, Vandervoort AA, DeVita P, Hortobagyi T (2013) The biomechanical mechanism of how strength and power training improves walking speed in old adults remains unknown. Ageing Res Rev 12: 618–627.
24. DeVita P, Hortobagyi T (2000) Age causes a redistribution of joint torques and powers during gait. J Appl Physiol (1985) 88: 1804–1811.
25. Guralnik JM (05 June 2013) Assessing Physical Performance in the Older Patient. Available: http://www.grc.nia.nih.gov/branches/leps/sppb/. Accessed 01 September 2014.
26. Hirano Y, Yamamoto T (2013) Reliability of soleus muscle measurement with a hand-held dynamometer. Rigakuryoho Kagaku 28: 115–118.
27. Kamiya A, Nagoya H, Takei H (2010) Reliability of measurements of pelvic lateral tilt in the supine and standing positions: Rater's measurement error and reproducibility of subject's posture. Rigakuryoho Kagaku 25: 919–922.
28. Bottaro M, Machado SN, Nogueira W, Scales R, Veloso J (2007) Effect of high versus low-velocity resistance training on muscular fitness and functional performance in older men. Eur J Appl Physiol 99: 257–264.
29. Capodaglio P, Capodaglio Edda M, Facioli M, Saibene F (2007) Long-term strength training for community-dwelling people over 75: impact on muscle function, functional ability and life style. Eur J Appl Physiol 100: 535–542.
30. Kalapotharakos VI, Michalopoulos M, Tokmakidis SP, Godolias G, Gourgoulis V (2005) Effects of a heavy and a moderate resistance training on functional performance in older adults. J Strength Cond Res 19: 652–657.
31. Buchner DM, Cress ME, de Lateur BJ, Esselman PC, Margherita AJ, et al. (1997) The effect of strength and endurance training on gait, balance, fall risk, and health services use in community-living older adults. J Gerontol A Biol Sci Med Sci 52: M218–224.
32. Judge JO, Underwood M, Gennosa T (1993) Exercise to improve gait velocity in older persons. Arch Phys Med Rehabil 74: 400–406.
33. Judge JO, Whipple RH, Wolfson LI (1994) Effects of resistive and balance exercises on isokinetic strength in older persons. J Am Geriatr Soc 42: 937–946.
34. Lord SR, Lloyd DG, Nirui M, Raymond J, Williams P, et al. (1996) The effect of exercise on gait patterns in older women: a randomized controlled trial. J Gerontol A Biol Sci Med Sci 51: M64–70.
35. Buchner DM, Wagner EH (1992) Preventing frail health. Clin Geriatr Med 8: 1–17.
36. Skelton DA, Young A, Greig CA, Malbut KE (1995) Effects of resistance training on strength, power, and selected functional abilities of women aged 75 and older. J Am Geriatr Soc 43: 1081–1087.
37. Symons TB, Vandervoort AA, Rice CL, Overend TJ, Marsh GD (2005) Effects of maximal isometric and isokinetic resistance training on strength and functional mobility in older adults. J Gerontol A Biol Sci Med Sci 60: 777–781.
38. Cao ZB, Maeda A, Shima N, Kurata H, Nishizono H (2007) The effect of a 12-week combined exercise intervention program on physical performance and gait kinematics in community-dwelling elderly women. J Physiol Anthropol 26: 325–332.
39. Liu-Ambrose T, Nagamatsu LS, Graf P, Beattie BL, Ashe MC, et al. (2010) Resistance training and executive functions: a 12-month randomized controlled trial. Arch Intern Med 170: 170–178.
40. Schlicht J, Camaione DN, Owen SV (2001) Effect of intense strength training on standing balance, walking speed, and sit-to-stand performance in older adults. J Gerontol A Biol Sci Med Sci 56: M281–286.
41. American College of Sports Medicine (2009) American College of Sports Medicine position stand. Progression models in resistance training for healthy adults. Med Sci Sports Exerc 41: 687–708.
42. Henwood TR, Riek S, Taaffe DR (2008) Strength versus muscle power-specific resistance training in community-dwelling older adults. J Gerontol A Biol Sci Med Sci 63: 83–91.
43. Marsh AP, Miller ME, Rejeski WJ, Hutton SL, Kritchevsky SB (2009) Lower extremity muscle function after strength or power training in older adults. J Aging Phys Act 17: 416–443.
44. Miszko TA, Cress ME, Slade JM, Covey CJ, Agrawal SK, et al. (2003) Effect of strength and power training on physical function in community-dwelling older adults. J Gerontol A Biol Sci Med Sci 58: 171–175.
45. Fitzsimons CF, Greig CA, Saunders DH, Lewis SH, Shenkin SD, et al. (2005) Responses to walking-speed instructions: implications for health promotion for older adults. J Aging Phys Act 13: 172–183.
46. Hunter SK, Thompson MW, Adams RD (2000) Relationships among age-associated strength changes and physical activity level, limb dominance, and muscle group in women. J Gerontol A Biol Sci Med Sci 55: B264–273.
47. Schrack JA, Simonsick EM, Chaves PH, Ferrucci L (2012) The role of energetic cost in the age-related slowing of gait speed. J Am Geriatr Soc 60: 1811–1816.
48. Cofre LE, Lythgo N, Morgan D, Galea MP (2011) Aging modifies joint power and work when gait speeds are matched. Gait Posture 33: 484–489.
49. Judge JO, Davis RB, 3rd, Ounpuu S (1996) Step length reductions in advanced age: the role of ankle and hip kinetics. J Gerontol A Biol Sci Med Sci 51: M303–312.
50. Kerrigan DC, Todd MK, Della Croce U, Lipsitz LA, Collins JJ (1998) Biomechanical gait alterations independent of speed in the healthy elderly: evidence for specific limiting impairments. Arch Phys Med Rehabil 79: 317–322.
51. McGibbon CA, Krebs DE (2004) Discriminating age and disability effects in locomotion: neuromuscular adaptations in musculoskeletal pathology. J Appl Physiol (1985) 96: 149–160.
52. Monaco V, Rinaldi LA, Macrì G, Micera S (2009) During walking elders increase efforts at proximal joints and keep low kinetics at the ankle. Clinical Biomechanics 24: 493–498.
53. Savelberg HH, Verdijk LB, Willems PJ, Meijer K (2007) The robustness of age-related gait adaptations: can running counterbalance the consequences of ageing? Gait Posture 25: 259–266.
54. Silder A, Heiderscheit B, Thelen DG (2008) Active and passive contributions to joint kinetics during walking in older adults. J Biomech 41: 1520–1527.
55. Wallerstein LF, Tricoli V, Barroso R, Rodacki AL, Russo L, et al. (2012) Effects of strength and power training on neuromuscular variables in older adults. J Aging Phys Act 20: 171–185.
56. Caserotti P, Aagaard P, Larsen JB, Puggaard L (2008) Explosive heavy-resistance training in old and very old adults: changes in rapid muscle force, strength and power. Scand J Med Sci Sports 18: 773–782.
57. Skelton DA, Greig CA, Davies JM, Young A (1994) Strength, power and related functional ability of healthy people aged 65–89 years. Age Ageing 23: 371–377.
58. Masakado Y, Akaboshi K, Nagata M, Kimura A, Chino N (1995) Motor unit firing behavior in slow and fast contractions of the first dorsal interosseous muscle of healthy men. Electroencephalogr Clin Neurophysiol 97: 290–295.

member of the TNF-α receptor superfamily produced by osteoblasts and vascular endothelial and smooth muscle cells [11], which may be involved in the regulation of vascular calcification and mortality [12].

Although nitric oxide (NO) has an important protective role in cardiovascular function, evidence indicates that higher NO levels are present in subjects with MetS [13] and diabetes [14]. Both disorders have been associated with increased atherogenic risk. Furthermore, elevated NO production may lead to insulin resistance [15] being another component to those of MetS, which may be involved in the disease pathophysiology [13].

Furthermore, it has been shown that increased levels of physical activity and functional capacity may reduce MetS incidence and seem to be key components for treatment and prevention [16]. Previous investigations have shown that chronic exercise training reduces the production of pro-inflammatory mediators, enhancing anti-inflammatory mediator activity, including interleukin-10 (IL-10). Such functional properties confer to exercise an important strategy to reduce the low grade inflammatory status of patients with MetS [17].

Studies with resistance training revealed improvements in lean mass, strength gain and reduced levels of inflammatory cytokines, while aerobic training is reported to be effective in improving maximal oxygen consumption (VO_2max), high density lipoprotein (HDL) levels and reducing the level of triglycerides found in the plasma [18-20]. Moreover, the combination of aerobic and resistance training could optimize both cardiovascular and neuromuscular adaptations [21], which are extremely important for women with MetS.

According to Stensvold et al. [33], the optimal training regime to treat MetS and its associated cardiovascular abnormalities remains uncertain. Furthermore, no previous study focused on the effects of combined training on OPG, NO and quality of life in women with MetS.

Thus, this study aims to evaluate the effects of combined aerobic and resistance training (CT) on cardiometabolic risk factors, inflammatory blood markers, quality of life and functional capacity in adult women with MetS. The initial hypothesis is that CT improves cardiometabolic profile, increases functional capacity and reduces inflammatory blood markers in women with MetS.

Materials and Methods

Ethics Statement. The protocol for this trial and supporting CONSORT checklist are available as supporting information; see Checklist S1 and Protocol S1.

All participants provided and signed a written informed consent document prior to participation in the study. All procedures were approved by the Catholic University of Brasilia Research Ethics Committee for Human Use at November, 29, 2012 (protocol CEP/UCB, #279/2010) and the study was conducted according to the principles expressed in the Declaration of Helsinki. The study was conducted at the laboratory of resistance training of the Catholic University of Brasilia.

The trial of this study was registered after patient recruitment began, because only the approval of the Research Ethics Committee was necessary to conduct the study at the Catholic University of Brasilia. The authors confirm that all ongoing and related trial for this intervention is registered.

Participants. Initially, 20 women from the local community (Vila Telebrasilia, Brazil) volunteered to participate and were recruited from posters and lectures about the study from January to April. Each participant received personal explanation after being informed about the study protocol. Although verbal encouragement was given to increase compliance during follow-up (May to July), only 13 completed the study, with two excluded due to caloric restriction and five excluded from the statistical analysis because they missed more than 25% of the training sessions. Individuals completed a thorough physical examination, including a medical history, resting and exercise electrocardiogram [22]. Moreover blood pressure assessments, anthropometric and orthopedic evaluations prior to participation in the experimental protocols were also performed. As inclusion criteria, the only participants included were those aged between 18–40 y, classified with MetS, and those without consistent resistance training for the past six months before the study period. According to ATP III [2], MetS is defined as the presence of 3 or more of the following 5 criteria: increased waist circumference (≥88 cm), hypertriglyceridemia (≥150 mg/dL), low HDL (<50 mg/dL), hypertension (≥ 130/85 mm Hg), and high fasting glucose (≥110 mg/dL). A modified z score was calculated for each variable using individual subject data using the ATP III criteria. The equations used to calculate the MetS z score were as follows: {z score = [(50 - HDL)/11.8] + [(TG −150)/66.2] + [(fasting blood glucose - 110)/10.4] + [(waist circumference - 88)/9.2] + [(mean arterial pressure - 100)/8.7]/100}. Women with physical disabilities, under caloric restriction, diagnosis of diabetes, cardiovascular diseases, uncontrolled hypertension (systolic blood pressure >140 mmHg and diastolic blood pressure >90 mmHg), musculoskeletal disease, recent use of medication and smoking or drug/alcohol abuse were excluded from the trial. A sedentary state was defined by the International physical activity questionnaire (IPAQ).

Study design. We conducted a 10-week prospective quasi-experimental design. Participants and those assessing the outcomes were not blinded to study condition assignment. Subjects were advised to maintain their normal daily eating habits throughout the study. Prior to physical evaluation, participants reported to the laboratory between 08:00–10:00 am following an overnight fast, for blood sampling from the antecubital vein for subsequent analysis of the biochemical variables. Volunteers completed two weeks of familiarization prior to testing (3 sessions/week, with one exercise for each main muscle group which were the same exercises used during resistance training), where they were advised regarding the execution of proper technique. After the familiarization period, one-repetition maximum (1-RM) test and re-test were performed on the chest press on two nonconsecutive days with 48–72 h between tests. The CT protocol began three days after 1-RM testing and was performed on three non-consecutive days of the week, comprising 30 min of moderate to moderate-high intensity on a treadmill at 70–80% reserve heart rate and three sets of 8–12 repetition maximum (RM) of twelve exercises for whole body, and 1-minute rest intervals between sets and exercises.

Exercise Training. Training sessions lasted ~60 min in a facility dedicated to research and under the supervision of exercise physiologists.

Aerobic training. The aerobic component of the program consisted of 30 min of moderate to moderate-high intensity on a treadmill at 70–80% reserve heart rate, with heart rate being continuously monitored throughout each session.

Resistance training. Subjects completed two weeks of familiarization prior to the resistance training program. During the familiarization weeks, individuals were advised regarding proper resistance training technique and completed 3 sessions/week, with one exercise of each main muscle group consisting of 3 sets of 10–12 submaximal repetitions. After the familiarization period subjects initiated the resistance training program consisting of 3 sessions/week during ten weeks. Resistance training machines

22

Enhancing of Women Functional Status with Metabolic Syndrome by Cardioprotective and Anti-Inflammatory Effects of Combined Aerobic and Resistance Training

Ramires Alsamir Tibana[1]*, Dahan da Cunha Nascimento[1], Nuno Manuel Frade de Sousa[2], Vinicius Carolino de Souza[1], João Durigan[3], Amilton Vieira[3], Martim Bottaro[3], Otávio de Toledo Nóbrega[3], Jeeser Alves de Almeida[1,3], James Wilfred Navalta[4], Octavio Luiz Franco[1,5], Jonato Prestes[1]

1 Catholic University of Brasilia, Graduation Program on Physical Education, Brasilia, Brazil, **2** Laboratory of Exercise Physiology, Faculty Estacio of Vitoria, Espirito Santo, Brazil, **3** University of Brasilia, Brasilia, Brazil, **4** Department of Kinesiology and Nutrition Sciences of the University of Nevada, Las Vegas, Nevada, United States of America, **5** Centro de Analises Proteomicas e Bioquimicas. Programa de Pos-Graduaçao em Ciencias Genomicas e Biotecnologia, Universidade Catolica de Brasilia, Brasilia, Brazil

Abstract

These data describe the effects of combined aerobic plus resistance training (CT) with regards to risk factors of metabolic syndrome (MetS), quality of life, functional capacity, and pro- and anti-inflammatory cytokines in women with MetS. In this context, thirteen women (35.4±6.2 yr) completed 10 weeks of CT consisting of three weekly sessions of ~60 min aerobic training (treadmill at 65–70% of reserve heart rate, 30 min) and resistance training (3 sets of 8–12 repetitions maximum for main muscle groups). Dependent variables were maximum chest press strength; isometric hand-grip strength; 30 s chair stand test; six minute walk test; body mass; body mass index; body adiposity index; waist circumference; systolic (SBP), diastolic and mean blood pressure (MBP); blood glucose; HDL-C; triglycerides; interleukins (IL) 6, 10 and 12, osteoprotegerin (OPG) and serum nitric oxide metabolite (NOx); quality of life (SF-36) and Z-Score of MetS. There was an improvement in muscle strength on chest press ($p = 0.009$), isometric hand-grip strength ($p = 0.03$) and 30 s chair stand ($p = 0.007$). There was a decrease in SBP (p = 0.049), MBP ($p = 0.041$), Z-Score of MetS ($p = 0.046$), OPG (0.42±0.26 to 0.38±0.19 ng/mL, $p<0.05$) and NOx (13.3±2.3 µmol/L to 9.1±2.3 µmol/L; $p<0.0005$). IL-10 displayed an increase (13.6±7.5 to 17.2±12.3 pg/mL, $p<0.05$) after 10 weeks of training. Combined training also increased the perception of physical capacity ($p = 0.011$). This study endorses CT as an efficient tool to improve blood pressure, functional capacity, quality of life and reduce blood markers of inflammation, which has a clinical relevance in the prevention and treatment of MetS.

Trial Registration: Brazilian Clinical Trials Registry (ReBec) - RBR-6gdyvz - http://www.ensaiosclinicos.gov.br/rg/?q=RBR-6gdyvz

Editor: Yiqing Song, Indiana University Richard M. Fairbanks School of Public Health, United States of America

Funding: The authors received no specific funding for this study.

Competing Interests: The authors have declared that no competing interests exist.

* Email: ramirestibana@gmail.com

Introduction

Metabolic syndrome (MetS) combines several metabolic and hemodynamic alterations that increase the risks of cardiovascular diseases and premature death [1]. These risk factors include central obesity, dyslipidemia, hypertension and elevated fasting glucose [2]. Moreover, subjects with MetS present with 78% higher risk of cardiovascular events and death compared with healthy individuals [1]. According to the National Health and Nutrition Examination Survey (NHANES) conducted in the United States between 2003–2006, and the NCEP Adult Treatment Panel III (ATP III) guidelines, an estimated 34% of adults aged >20 years met the MetS criteria [3]. It has been shown that men between 20–50 years of age present higher MetS prevalence, while these numbers are higher in women after 50 years, which increases the attention of menopause transition period [4]. Additionally, the residual hypertension risk is increased by 90% in adult life, classifying this population as a target candidate for prevention from MetS risk factors [5].

Furthermore, MetS is also associated with chronic low-grade inflammation, a condition in which inflammatory blood markers are slightly elevated [6]. Interleukin-6 (IL-6), interleukin-1β (IL-1β) and tumor necrosis factor-α (TNF-α) cytokines play a central role on immune responses and inflammatory processes [7]. The activation of inflammation via Th1 lymphocytes through interleukin-12 (IL-12) has also shown to be involved [8]. Additionally, such inflammatory cytokines are known to contribute to the development of atherosclerosis, insulin resistance and hypertension, which are also criteria for MetS diagnosis [9,10]. Another blood marker to be considered is osteoprotegerin (OPG), a soluble

were from JOHNSON (Landmark Drive, Cottage Grove, USA). All training sessions were carefully supervised by three experienced professionals (ratio of supervision 1:2 – 1 professor for 2 participants). Participants were required to complete at least 85% of the exercise sessions. No major complications or cardiac events occurred during the study period. The resistance training was divided into A (leg press, knee extensor, leg curl, hip adduction, hip abduction, standing calf raise and abdominal crunches), B (chest press, lat pull down, shoulder press, machine elbow flexion, triceps extension and abdominal crunches) and C (leg press, knee extensor, leg curl, chest press, lat pull down, shoulder press and abdominal crunches) regiments. For all listed exercises, three sets with 8–12 RM were performed, with a one-minute rest interval between each set and exercise. Training loads were monitored each session according to the increase in muscle capacity of the participants. The mean duration to complete one repetition was 3–4 s (both concentric and eccentric phases of the movement) and training sessions lasted ~30 min. The number of repetitions and the loads used for each exercise session were recorded. The loads were updated when necessary to keep the number of repetitions within the same range of RM and to provide a progressive overload. Additionally, correct breathing patterns were instructed to avoid Valsalva maneuver.

Outcome Measures

Primary Outcomes

Cytokines. Participants reported to the laboratory between 08:00–10:00 am, after an overnight fast, and after blood collection, samples were centrifuged at room temperature at 2,000 rpm for 15 min. All subjects were encouraged to avoid smoking, alcohol and caffeine consumption as well as unusual physical activity to avoid influence on these parameters. The serum was removed and frozen at 80°C for further analysis. Serum was analyzed for amyloid A using a DADE Dimension RXL clinical chemistry analyzer (Dade-Behring, Inc, Newark, DE, USA). The analyzer was calibrated daily using Liquid-Assayed Multiqual (Bio-Rad, Hercules, CA, USA), and two levels of quality control with known concentrations. In addition, serum IL-10, IL-6 and IL-12 were assessed using commercially available enzyme-linked immunosorbent assay (ELISA) kits (BioLegend's ELISA Max Deluxe, San Diego, CA, USA) and OPG (R&D System Inc., Minneapolis, MN, USA). Standard curves were generated using commercially available microplate reader-compatible statistical software (Micro-Win 2000, Microtek Laborsysteme GmbH, Overath, Germany). All samples were determined in duplicate to guarantee the precision of the results. For all measures the mean intra-assay coefficient of variation was 2.9–9.5%, the inter-assay coefficient of variation was 5.9–7.0%, and the sensitivity was 0.0093 pg/mL.

Nitrite Levels. To perform the analysis, the blood was centrifuged previously. The serum concentration of nitrite was determined by the Griess reaction. In brief, serum samples were deproteinized by adding zinc sulfate (15 mg/mL), followed by centrifugation at 10000 g for 10 min; 100 μL of the supernatant was applied to a microplate well, and following addition of 100 μL vanadium (III) chloride (8 mg/mL) to each well, Griess reagents [50 μL sulfanilamide (2%) and 50 μL N- (1-naphthyl) ethylendiamine dihydrochloride (0.1%)] were added. After 30 min incubation at 37°C, absorbance was read at 540 nm using the ELISA reader (Sunrise, Tecan, Austria). Concentration of NO_2 in serum samples was determined from the linear standard curve established by 0–100 μM sodium nitrite.

Secondary Outcomes

Maximal strength testing. After 2 weeks of adaptation to the exercises and 3–5 days after the last training session, 1-RM test was performed on chest press exercise on 2 different days separated by a minimum of 48 h. The protocol consisted of a light warm-up of 5 min of treadmill walking followed by 8 repetitions at 50% of estimated 1-RM (according to the participants' capacity verified in the 2 weeks of adaptation). After a 1-min rest, subjects performed 3 repetitions at 70% of the estimated 1-RM. Following 3 minutes of rest, participants completed 3–5 attempts interspersed with 3-to-5 min rest intervals, with progressively heavier weights (~5%) until the 1-RM was determined.

Isometric handgrip strength. Isometric handgrip strength was determined by a manual mechanical dynamometer (Takei, T.K.K Grip strength dynamometer 0–100 kg, Japan). Volunteers stood still with both arms extended and the forearm positioned in a neutral rotation. The handgrip width of the dynamometer was individually adjusted for each participant, according to hand size allowing the stem next to the body to be positioned on the second phalanges: index, medial and ring fingers. Three attempts were allowed interspersed with 1 min rest intervals. The best measure was used and relative isometric strength was determined as follows: Relative strength = Absolute strength (kg)/Body mass (kg) [23].

The 6-minute walk test. The 6-minute walk test (6MWT) was performed according to the American Thoracic Society protocol [24]. Functional capacity was determined by the distance walked in a covered 30-meter walkway.

Functional fitness tests. Two components of the functional fitness test [25] were selected as a measure of functional performance. The following test items were conducted as follows: (1) a 30-s chair stand test (the maximum number of times within 30 s that an individual can rise to a full stand from a seated position, without pushing off with the arms), and (2) the sit and reach test evaluated flexibility using the modified chair sit-and-reach test.

Anthropometrics. Height and weight were measured for the calculation of the body mass index (BMI). All circumferences were obtained using non elastic tape, and measurements were obtained in triplicate and averaged to obtain the circumference score. Neck circumference was obtained with the subject sitting with the head in the Frankfort horizontal plane position. Briefly, a measuring tape was applied around the neck inferior to the laryngeal prominence and perpendicular to the long axis of the neck, while the minimal circumference was measured and recorded to the nearest 0.1 cm [26]. Waist circumference was measured at the midpoint between the lower rib margin, hip circumference was measured at the widest portion of the buttocks and the body adiposity index (BAI) was determined by the following formula: (BAI = [(hip circumference)/((height)1.5)–18)] [27].

Blood pressure measurement. Systolic (SBP), diastolic (DBP) were measured with a validated oscillometric device (Microlife 3AC1-1, Widnau, Switzerland) according to the recommendations of the International Protocol of the European Society of Hypertension [28]. The cuff size was adapted to the arm circumference of each participant according to the manufacturer's recommendations, and BP was assessed in triplicate (measurements separated by 5 min) with the mean value used for further analysis after 10 min of seated rest. All BP measurements were taken on the left arm. Mean blood pressure (MBP) was calculated as the sum of DBP and one-third of the pulse pressure. All blood pressure measures were assessed in triplicate (measurements separated by 1 min) with the mean value used for analysis.

Biochemical parameters. Participants reported to the laboratory between 08:00–10:00 am, after an overnight fast, for blood withdrawal from the antecubital vein. Plasma triglycerides, HDL-cholesterol and glucose levels were measured by enzymatic CHOP-POD, homogeneous HDL-cholesterol and Hexokinase methods, respectively.

Quality of life. Health-related quality of life was assessed using the Brazilian version of the Short Form 36 Health Survey (SF-36) [29]. Quality of life is a multidimensional construction characterized by four essential components: psychological well-being; physical functioning; social relations; and functional competence. The measure assesses eight dimensions. For each item, patients were required to select the answer closest to their own experience. The types of answer possible varied from item to item, from yes or no answers to answers on a scale of 1–6. Each domain score ranges from 0 to 100, the highest score indicating better health conditions related to quality of life.

Sample size

The power of the sample size was determined using G*Power version 3.1.3, based on the differences between pre and post primary outcomes and the metabolic syndrome z score. Considering the final sample size of this study and an alpha error of 0.05, the sample power ($1-\beta$) was 1.00 for NO, 0.96 for IL-10/NO ratio and 0.71 for metabolic syndrome z score. Unfortunately, IL-6 ($1-\beta = 0,24$), IL-12 ($1-\beta = 0,25$), IL-10 ($1-\beta = 0,60$) and OPG ($1-\beta = 0,57$) did not reach the recommended power and interpretation of the data must be careful, specially the IL-6 and the IL-12. However, the effect sizes of the correlations involving IL-6 and IL-12 with anthropometric or biochemical variables in this study were large ($|p| > 0.5$), corresponding to a strong sample power for the correlations [30].

Statistical analysis

The results are expressed as means ± standard deviation (SD). Shapiro-Wilk tests were applied to check for normality distribution of study variables. In case of nonparametric distribution, a logarithmic transformation was performed. The anthropometric, biochemical, NO and physical fitness variables were parametrically distributed, however, the SF-36 scores, cytokines and osteoprotegerin were nonparametricly distributed. The pre and post-intervention variables were compared using paired-samples t-test (parametric samples) and the Wilcoxon signed-rank test (nonparametric samples). The Spearman's correlation was used to evaluate the correlation between delta (post-pre) cytokines concentration and anthropometric or biochemical variables and between physical fitness and SF-36 scores after training program. The Cohen's convention (1988) [30] was used for assigning strength of association between the variables. The level of significance was p≤0.05 and SPSS version 20.0 (Somers, NY, USA) software was used.

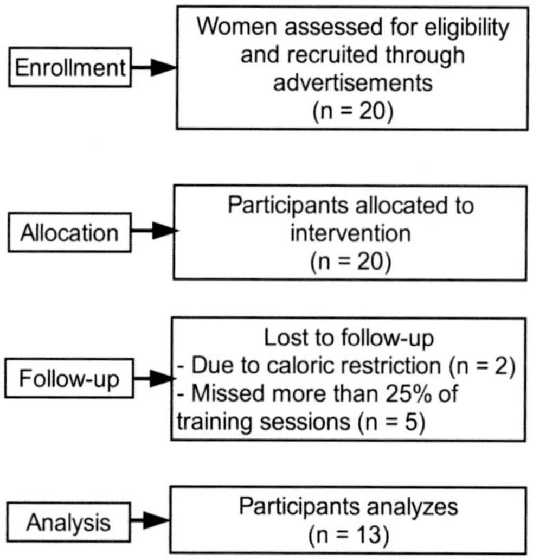

Figure 1. Flow-chart of the participants.

Results

Flow of participants through trial. Initially, 20 women volunteered to participate. Only 13 completed the study, with two excluded due to caloric restriction and five excluded from the

Table 1. Anthropometric and hemodynamic characteristics of the subjects (n = 13) before and after the training program (mean ± SD).

	Pre	Post	*p*-value
Weight, kg	74.8±7.2	74.2±7.5	0.352
Body mass index, kg/m^2	30.0±2.5	29.7±2.0	0.321
Waist circumference, cm	85.8±4.9	84.9±5.6	0.237
Hip circumference, cm	105.9±4.5	105.1±4.3	0.242
Neck circumference, cm	35.2±2.1	35.7±1.6	0.165
Waist to height ratio	0.54±0.04	0.54±0.03	0.468
Waist to hip ratio	0.81±0.04	0.81±0.05	0.514
Body adiposity index, %	26.8±2.6	26.4±1.9	0.238
Systolic blood pressure, mmHg	119.2±14.6	112.7±9.7	0.049*
Diastolic blood pressure, mmHg	79.5±15.6	72.8±10.1	0.051
Mean arterial pressure, mmHg	92.8±14.6	86.1±8.8	0.041*
Metabolic syndrome z score	1.26±0.17	1.19±0.09	0.046*

*Statistically significant (p≤0.05).

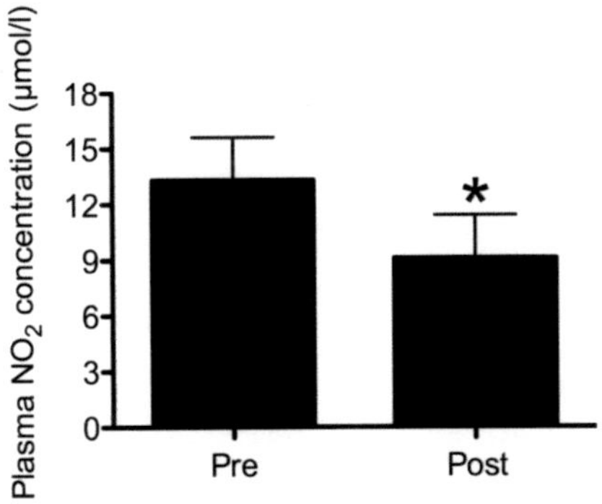

Figure 2. Nitric oxide (NO) concentration before (pre) and after (post) the training program (mean ± SD). *Statistically different compared with pre-values (p≤0.05).

statistical analysis because they missed more than 25% of the training sessions (figure 1).

Subject Characteristics. On average, volunteers attended 20±3 training sessions during the 10-week training program. Table 1 presents the anthropometric and hemodynamic characteristics of the subjects before and after the training program. There were no statistically significant differences after 10-weeks of the training program with respect to anthropometric variables ($p \geq 0.05$).

Metabolic Risk Factors. Analyses of HDL (44.5±9.5 mg/dL pre to 46.4±8.8 mg/dL post training, $p = 0.392$), glucose (88.6±8.4 mg/dL pre to 88.3±4.6 mg/dL post training, $p = 0.882$) and triglyceride (118.0±56.5 mg/dL pre to 118.5±61.8 mg/dL post training, $p = 0.910$) concentrations did not reveal any significant changes. However, there was a significant decrease in systolic (p = 0.049), mean arterial pressure (p = 0.041) and metabolic syndrome z score (p = 0.046).

Inflammation blood markers. After the 10-week training program, the NO plasma concentration had a significant decrease (13.3±2.3 µmol/L to 9.1±2.3 µmol/L; p<0.0005; figure 2). Interestingly, NO was reduced after the training program for all volunteers. The minimum decrease was approximately 15% and the maximum was 60% (31.8±12.1%). There was a significant increase in IL-10 concentration ($p = 0.043$) and a significant decrease in OPG concentration ($p = 0.034$) after the training program. There were no statistically significant differences ($p \geq 0.05$) pertaining to IL-6 or IL-12 concentrations after the training program (table 2). The ratio IL-10/NO also displayed a significant increase ($p = 0.008$) as a result of the training program. The Spearman's correlations between cytokine concentration and anthropometric or biochemical variables are presented in table 3. According to Cohen (1988), the strength of association for all significant correlations (p≤0.05) presented in this study were large correlations.

Functional fitness tests. Table 4 presents the physical fitness tests performed before and after the training program. There was a significant increase for the sitting-rising test ($p = 0.007$), and chest and handgrip strength ($p \leq 0.05$) after completion of the training program. There were no statistically significant increases in flexibility ($p = 0.402$) or the 6-min walking tests ($p = 0.606$).

Quality of life. The SF-36 scores were shown in table 5. Among the eight domains of the SF-36, physical function scale was the only one that had a significant increase ($p = 0.011$) after the training program. There were positive correlations of post 6-min walking test score with post SF-36 scores of physical function ($r = 0.586$, $p = 0.035$), role physical ($r = 0.582$, $p = 0.037$), general health ($r = 0.631$, $p = 0.021$) and role emotional ($r = 0.676$, $p = 0.011$). The post flexibility score after the training program also had a positive correlation with the post SF-36 score of general health ($r = 0.645$, $p = 0.017$).

Discussion

Interpretation

The main findings of the present study provide evidence that 10 weeks of CT decrease chronic inflammation, blood pressure, Z-Score of MetS, and improve muscle strength, quality of life and functional capacity in adult women with MetS, confirming the initial hypothesis. Moreover, although there was no weight loss, women with MetS decreased blood markers of low-grade inflammation associated with overweight and obesity.

CT is widely used due to the unique advantages of aerobic and resistance training. Aerobic training has been shown to improve cardiorespiratory fitness, promoting energy expenditure and fat utilization, while resistance training induces gains in muscle size, strength, endurance, and power. Furthermore, CT has been reported not only to reduce health risks and symptoms associated with physical inactivity, but improves performance of daily living activities [21,31].

MetS is associated with chronic low-grade inflammation, a condition in which inflammatory markers in the circulation are slightly elevated [32]. In our study, there was a significant decrease in blood markers of inflammation (OPG and NO) and an increase of anti-inflammatory cytokines (IL-10) following ten weeks of CT. The change in IL-6 and IL-12 could not be shown, however, because the lack of sample power for these variables, the result warrants confirmation. Meanwhile, it was shown a large correlation between the change in body adiposity index and IL-6 or IL-12

Table 2. Evaluation of Interleukin-10 (IL-10), osteoprotegerin (OPG), interleukin-6 (IL-6) and interleukin-12 (IL-12) concentrations before and after the training program (mean ± SD).

	Pre	Post	*p*-value
IL-10, pg/mL	14.96±7.48	19.38±12.30	0.043*
OPG, pg/mL	0.49±0.26	0.43±0.19	0.034*
IL-6, pg/mL	0.63±1.95	0.13±0.33	0.276
IL-12, mg/dL	1.04±1.49	0.66±0.89	0.237
IL-10/NO	1.21±0.53	2.35±1.36	0.008*

*Statistically significant (p≤0.05).

Table 3. Spearman's correlations between cytokines concentration and anthropometric or biochemical variables.

	IL-10	OPG	IL-6	IL-12
Delta (post-pre) correlations				
Neck circumference	NS	NS	0.616*	NS
Body adiposity index	NS	NS	0.637*	0.572*
HDL	NS	NS	0.649*	0.723*
NO	NS	NS	NS	NS

IL-10, interleukin-10; OPG, osteoprotegerin; IL-6, interleukin-6; IL-12, interleukin-12; HDL, high-density lipoprotein; NO, nitric oxide; NS, non-significant; *Statistically significant ($p \leq 0.05$).

concentrations after CT. Recently, Stensvold et al (2012) [33] reported that after 12 weeks of aerobic interval training the levels of TNF-α were lower as compared to resistance trained and control groups in subjects with MetS. However, different from the present study, total body fat was reduced with aerobic interval training (from 33.9±7.3% to 32.2±7.9%) and resistance training (from 31.2±3.9% to 29.7±3.4%). Similarly, Ho et al (2013) [34] found that 12 weeks of moderate-intensity aerobic (60% heart rate reserve), resistance training (four sets of 8–12 repetitions at 10-RM level of 5 whole body exercises), and CT (15 min of aerobic exercise and 2 sets of 8–12 repetitions of 5 whole body exercises) decreased TNF-α in overweight and obese individuals compared to a control group.

Growing evidence suggests that NO plays an important role in the development of MetS [35,13]. Previous studies reported that increased plasma NO concentration in hypertensive coronary artery disease patients might represent a compensatory response to increased superoxide anion concentration [36]. Moreover, increased shear stress with hypertension might stimulate NO production. Zahedi et al (2008) [13] also have found similar results and suggested that nonspecific tissue damage in MetS and diabetes might increase the activity of inducible nitric oxide synthase (iNOS), and therefore results in the accumulation of NO. In our study, there was a significant decrease in NO levels following 10 weeks of CT. The decrease in NO and OPG in response to CT reveal important protective effects against the deleterious effects of low-grade inflammation in women with MetS.

The increase in the anti-inflammatory response following CT, represented by the increased levels of IL-10 may have contributed to the decrease of blood markers of inflammation (OPG and NO), as shown in previous studies [37,38].

Nevertheless, data reveal that despite improvements in the cardiovascular risk factors of MetS (blood pressure and inflammation) and the increase in functional capacity, no modifications with respect to blood glucose, HDL-C and triglycerides were observed. Similarly, meta-analytic data revealed that isolated exercise programs without caloric restriction induced limited improvements in such parameters. Shaw et al (2006) [39] evaluated 43 studies including 3476 participants and found that exercise without caloric restriction control is associated with a lower decrease of body mass, blood pressure and blood glucose as compared with exercise associated with dietary restriction. Orozco et al (2008) [40] compared the effects of isolated diet and diet plus CT. Results revealed that diabetes risk was lower in the combined group. Additionally, individuals submitted to combined exercise training and diet presented a decrease in blood pressure and obesity anthropometric indexes, which was not observed for the group participating in exercise alone.

Regarding the quality of life, it has been reported that subjects with MetS have reduced perception of quality of life [40]. Recently, Okosun et al (2013) [41] found that MetS is associated with poor physical health (1.65; 95% CI = 1.09−2.50), mental health (1.67; 95% CI = 1.09−2.83) and overall health (1.44; 95% CI = 0.80−2.59) in Mexican-Americans. In the present study, it was observed that CT improved the perception of physical function in adult women with MetS. Our findings were similar to

Table 4. Physical fitness tests performed before and after the training program (mean ± SD).

	Pre	Post	*p*-value
Sitting-rising, rep	20.3±4.0	24.5±4.6	0.007*
Flexibility, cm	28.6±9.3	29.3±8.7	0.402
6-min walking, m	587.4±42.9	581.3±48.2	0.606
Chest press 1RM, kg	55.8±6.8	59.8±9.4	0.009*
Chest press relative strength	0.75±0.09	0.81±0.10	0.002*
Right handgrip, kg	33.7±7.7	35.0±7.7	0.030*
Right handgrip relative strength	0.45±0.09	0.47±0.08	0.008*
Left handgrip, kg	31.1±7.2	32.5±6.1	0.024*
Left handgrip relative strength	0.41±0.09	0.44±0.07	0.016*

1RM, 1-repetition maximum.
*Statistically significant ($p \leq 0.05$).

Table 5. SF-36 scores before and after the training program (mean ± SD).

	Pre	Post	*p*-value
Physical function	76.9±21.0	82.7±19.5	0.011*
Role Physical	75.0±28.9	76.9±37.4	0.666
Bodily pain	60.3±28.1	65.9±23.0	0.498
General health	56.1±17.6	59.0±14.8	0.674
Vitality	57.7±10.3	57.7±12.0	0.300
Social function	78.9±21.9	81.7±23.7	0.944
Role emotional	74.3±30.9	69.2±39.6	0.683
Mental health	58.8±7.7	58.4±11.2	0.860

*Statistically significant ($p \leq 0.05$).

previous trials in subjects with type 2 diabetes [42] and obesity [43]. Imayama et al (2011) [44] examined the individual and combined effects of dietary weight loss and/or exercise interventions (moderate to vigorous aerobic exercise/225 min per week) on health-related quality of life (HRQOL) in overweight/obese postmenopausal women. This same report showed that a combined diet and exercise intervention had positive effects on HRQOL and psychological health, which may be greater than that of exercise or diet alone. Thus, it is likely that the CT program utilized in the present study would provide additional improvements in quality of life parameters if combined with a dietary restriction intervention.

The present study has some limitations that should be considered, such as the limited time of the intervention (only ten weeks), the reduced sample power for cytokines, and the lack of more accurate measures to evaluate body composition (body fat and lean body mass), which may have influenced the results. Another limitation was the lack of a control group, although it has been speculated that a control group is not always necessary, particularly considering that the health of the subjects could be compromised as a result of not participating in CT. Additionally, results from a control group would probably reveal no positive effect on anthropometric, biochemical and cardiovascular risk factors of MetS, as has been reported in a previous study [44]. Finally, the non-significant variation with the biochemical data, such as glucose, triglycerides and HDL-C can be, at least in part attributed to the lack of dietetic control, as well as the limited sample size. It is possible that an interdisciplinary approach would induce more positive results in biochemical and anthropometric variables, as previously found in other studies. However, "significant" results based upon this exploratory research should clearly be labeled as exploratory results. To confirm these results the corresponding hypotheses have to be tested in further confirmatory studies.

In summary, ten weeks of CT reduced blood markers of inflammation such as NO, IL-10 and OPG, blood pressure and metabolic syndrome Z scores in women with MetS. Moreover, the improvement of the quality of life (physical function domain) and functional capacity (leg, chest and handgrip strength) reinforce the clinical relevance of CT for women with MetS. Thus, the results of this study provide further evidence for the recommendation of regular CT to decrease cardiovascular risk factors of MetS.

Author Contributions

Conceived and designed the experiments: RAT DCN JP. Performed the experiments: RAT DCN JP. Analyzed the data: RAT NMFS. Contributed reagents/materials/analysis tools: VCS MB OTN OLF. Wrote the paper: RAT NMFS JD AV MB OTN JAA JN OLF DCN JP.

References

1. Gami AS, Witt BJ, Howard DE, Erwin PJ, Gami LA, et al. (2007) Metabolic syndrome and risk of incident cardiovascular events and death: A systematic review and meta-analysis of longitudinal studies. J Am Coll Cardio 49(4): 403–414.
2. Expert Panel on Detection, Evaluation, and Treatment of High Blood Cholesterol in Adults: Executive Summary of The Third Report of The National Cholesterol Education Program (NCEP) Expert Panel on Detection, Evaluation, And Treatment of High Blood Cholesterol In Adults (Adult Treatment Panel III) (2001) JAMA 285(19): 2486–2497.
3. Ervin RB (2009) Prevalence of metabolic syndrome among adults 20 years of age and over, by sex, age, race and ethnicity, and body mass index: United States, 2003–2006. Natl Health Stat Report 5(13): 1–7.
4. Kim HM, Park J, Ryu SY, Kim J (2001) The effect of menopause on the metabolic syndrome among Korean women: the Korean National Health and Nutrition Examination Survey. Diabetes Care 30(3): 701–6.
5. Vasan RS, Beiser A, Seshadri S, Larson MG, Kannel WB, et al. (2002) Residual lifetime risk for developing hypertension in middle-aged women and men: The Framingham Heart Study. JAMA 287(8): 1003–10.
6. Esposito K, Giugliano D (2004) The metabolic syndrome and inflammation: Association or causation? Nutr Metab Cardiovasc Dis 14(5): 228–232.
7. Dinarello CA (1996) Biologic basis for interleukin-1 in disease. Blood 87(6): 2095–2147.
8. Trinchieri G (1995) Interleukin-12: a proinflammatory cytokine with immuno-regulatory functions that bridge innate resistance and antigen-specific adaptive immunity. Annu Rev Immunol. 13: 251–76.
9. Festa A, D'Agostino R Jr, Howard G, Mykkanen L, Tracy RP, et al. (2000) Chronic subclinical inflammation as part of the insulin resistance syndrome: the Insulin Resistance Atherosclerosis Study (IRAS). Circulation 102(1): 42–47.
10. Robbie L, Libby P (2001) Inflammation and atherothrombosis. Ann N Y Acad Sci 947: 167–179.
11. Aoki A, Murata M, Asano T, Ikoma A, Sasaki M, et al. (2013) Association of serum osteoprotegerin with vascular calcification in patients with type 2 diabetes. Cardiovas Diabetol 9: 12–11.
12. Morena M, Terrier N, Jaussent I, Leray-Moragues H, Chalabi L, et al. (2006) Plasma osteoprotegerin is associated with mortality in hemodialysis patients. J Am Soc Nephrol 17: 262–270.
13. Zahedi Asl S, Ghasemi A, Azizi F (2008) Serum nitric oxide metabolites in subjects with metabolic syndrome. Clin Biochem 41(16–17): 1342–7.
14. Maejima K, Nakano S, Himeno M, Tsuda S, Makiishi H, et al. (2001) Increased basal levels of plasma nitric oxide in Type 2 diabetic subjects. Relationship to microvascular complications. J Diabetes Complications 15(3): 135–43.

15. Dallaire P, Marette A (2004) Obesity-linked insulin resistance: is nitric oxide the missing link? Can J Diabetes 28(1): 59–66.
16. Cornier MA, Dabelea D, Hernandez TL, Lindstrom RC, Steig AJ, et al. (2008) The metabolic syndrome. Endocr Rev 29(7): 777–822.
17. Mathur N, Pedersen BK (2008) Exercise as a mean to control low-grade systemic inflammation. Mediators Inflamm in press.
18. Prestes J, Shiguemoto G, Botero JP, Frollini A, Dias R, et al. (2009) Effects of resistance training on resistin, leptin, cytokines, and muscle force in elderly postmenopausal women. J Sports Sci 27(14): 1607–1615.
19. Tibana RA, Navalta J, Bottaro M, Vieira D, Tajra V, et al. (2013) Effects of eight weeks of resistance training on the risk factors of metabolic syndrome in overweight/obese women - "A Pilot Study". Diabetol Metab Syndr 28; 5(1): 11.
20. Schwingshackl L, Dias S, Strasser B, Hoffmann G (2013) Impact of different training modalities on anthropometric and metabolic characteristics in overweight/obese subjects: a systematic review and network meta-analysis. PLoS One 8(12): e82853.
21. Kang J, Ratamess N (2014) Which comes first? Resistance before aerobic exercise or vice versa? ACSM'S Health & Fitness Journal 18(1): 9–14.
22. Tavel ME (2001) Stress testing in cardiac evaluation: current concepts with emphasis on the ECG. Chest 119(3): 907–925.
23. Prestes J, Tibana RA (2013) Muscular static strength test performance and health: Absolute or relative values? Rev Assoc Med Bras 59(4): 308–309.
24. ATS Committee on Proficiency Standards for Clinical Pulmonary Function Laboratories (2002) ATS statement: guidelines for the six-minute walk test. Am J Respir Crit Care Med 166(1): 111–7.
25. Rikli RE, Jones CJ (1999) Development and validation of a functional fitness test for community-residing older adults. J Aging Phys Act 7: 129–161.
26. Tibana RA, Teixeira TG, Farias DL, Silva Ade O, Madrid B, et al. (2012) Relation of neck circumference and relative muscle strength and cardiovascular risk factors in sedentary women. Einstein (Sao Paulo) 10(3): 329–334.
27. Bergman RN, Stefanovski D, Buchanan TA, Sumner AE, Reynolds JC, et al. (2011) A better index of body adiposity. Obesity 19(5): 1083–1089.
28. Topouchian JA, El Assaad MA, Orobinskaia LV, El Feghali RN, Asmar RG (2005) Validation of two devices for self-measurement of brachial blood pressure according to the International Protocol of the European Society of Hypertension: the SEINEX SE-9400 and the Microlife BP 3AC1-1. Blood Pressure Monitoring 10(6): 325–31.
29. Ciconelli RM, Ferraz MB, Santos W, Meinão I, Quaresma MR (1999) Brazilian Portuguese version of the SF-36. A reliable and valid quality of life outcome measure. Revista Brasileira de Reumatologia 39(3): 143–150.
30. Cohen J (1988) Statistical Power Analysis for the Behavioral Sciences. Psychology Press: Taylor & Francis Groups. 115 p.
31. Fyfe JJ, Bishop DJ, Stepto NK (2014) Interference between Concurrent Resistance and Endurance Exercise: Molecular Bases and the Role of Individual Training Variables. Sports Med in press.
32. Pereira GB, Tibana RA, Navalta J, Sousa NM, Córdova C, et al. (2013) Acute effects of resistance training on cytokines and osteoprotegerin in women with metabolic syndrome. Clin Physiol Funct Imaging 33(2): 122–30.
33. Stensvold D, Slørdahl SA, Wisløff U (2012) Effect of exercise training on inflammation status among people with metabolic syndrome. Metab Syndr Relat Disord 10(4): 267–72.
34. Ho SS, Dhaliwal SS, Hills AP, Pal S (2013) Effects of chronic exercise training on inflammatory markers in Australian overweight and obese individuals in a randomized controlled trial. Inflammation 36(3): 625–32.
35. Kanbak G, Akalin A, Dokumacioglu A, Ozcelik E, Bal C (2011) Cardiovascular risk assessment in patients with type 2 diabetes mellitus and metabolic syndrome: role of biomarkers. Diabetes Metab Syndr 5(1): 7–11.
36. Yoon Y, Song J, Hong SH, Kim JQ (2000) Plasma nitric oxide concentrations and nitric oxide synthase gene polymorphisms in coronary artery disease. Clin Chem 46(10): 1626–30.
37. Pedersen BK, Bruunsgaard H, Klokker M, Kappel N, MacLean DA, et al. (1997) Exercise-induced immunomodulation possible roles of neuroendocrine and metabolic factors. International Journal of Sports Medicine (Suppl 1): S2–7.
38. Bruunsgaard H (2005) Physical activity and modulation of systemic low-level inflammation. Journal of Leukocyte Biology 78(4): 819–835.
39. Shaw K, Gennat H, O'Rourke P, Del Mar C (2006) Exercise for overweight or obesity. Cochrane Database Syst Rev 8(4): CD003817.
40. Orozco LJ, Buchleitner AM, Gimenez-Perez G, Roqué I, Figuls M, et al. (2008) Exercise or exercise and diet for preventing type 2 diabetes mellitus. Cochrane Database Syst Rev 16(3): CD003054.
41. Okosun IS, Annor F, Esuneh F, Okoegwale EE (2013) Metabolic syndrome and impaired health-related quality of life and in non-Hispanic White, non-Hispanic Blacks and Mexican-American Adults. Diabetes Metab Syndr 7(3): 154–60.
42. Williamson DA, Rejeski J, Lang W, Van Dorsten B, Fabricatore AN, et al. (2009) Impact of a weight management program on health-related quality of life in overweight adults with type 2 diabetes. Arch Intern Med 169(2): 163–171.
43. Imayama I, Ulrich CM, Alfano CM, Wang C, Xiao L, et al. (2012) Effects of a caloric restriction weight loss diet and exercise on inflammatory biomarkers in overweight/obese postmenopausal women: a randomized controlled trial. Cancer Res 72(9): 2314–26.
44. Imayama I, Alfano CM, Kong A, Foster-Schubert KE, Bain CE, et al. (2011) Dietary weight loss and exercise interventions effects on quality of life in overweight/obese postmenopausal women: a randomized controlled trial. Int J Behav Nutr Phys Act. 25: 8–118.

amounts of MVPA, participation in OYS does not guarantee MVPA. Studies have found that children and adolescents spend large proportions of time during OYS inactive or in light PA [12,21,22]. Furthermore, coaches spent a considerable proportion of training time in management and knowledge delivery contexts [12], where it is likely that children and adolescents would be relatively inactive [23].

Coaches, therefore, have the opportunity to influence their athletes' PA levels, particularly during training where coaches are better able to dictate the intensity of PA, compared to a game. However, the way coaches perceive themselves with regards to influencing girls' PA is not clear and further exploration is warranted due to the high proportion of children who participate in OYS and the myriad of health and developmental benefits children and adolescents stand to gain through the setting. OYS presents a good opportunity to participate in PA and has the potential to be a powerful health-promoting environment for children and adolescents, where coaches are at the helm.

To our knowledge, no study has explored whether coaches perceive themselves as influential on PA for girls participating in OYS. Further, only a few cross-sectional studies have examined children and adolescents' PA levels in OYS [12,21,22], finding that children and adolescents spent large proportions of time during OYS inactive or in light PA. Coaches' views on their athletes' current PA levels and their opinions on improving their athletes' PA levels, however, have not been investigated. Lastly, coaches' perceived challenges in OYS have also not previously been considered, and as such, this information could provide valuable insight on aspects of the coaching experience that could inform future studies aiming to increase PA in OYS. Accordingly, this study aimed to explore OYS coaches': (1) perceived role as a coach; (2) perception of themselves as role models for PA; (3) views on their athletes' current PA levels; (4) opinions on improving their athletes' PA levels; and (5) their perceived challenges as coaches in OYS.

Methods

Study design and procedures

This study conforms to the consolidated criteria for reporting qualitative research (COREQ) developed by Tong, Sainsbury, and Craig [24]. Between July and August 2012, each of the 30 coaches recruited took part in one in-depth semi-structured interview with the primary author (JMG). Interviewing is one of the most commonly used methods in qualitative research [25] and is a method capable of providing rich and comprehensive data [26]. Semi-structured interviews also provide the interviewer with the flexibility to further explore participants' responses [27].

The interview questions, prompts, and probes used in this study are outlined in Table 1. The development of the interview questions was guided by the aforementioned study aims. Most interview questions were open-ended to elicit a wide range of responses and prompts and probes were used to encourage further discussion, when required. To ensure content validity, the interview guide was iteratively developed by all members of the research team; reviewing content, structure, and wording of the questions. The research team also assessed the ordering of the interview questions and length of the interview. The questions were pilot tested on three adults who had coaching experience in a range of sports to ensure appropriate face validity.

Each participant was informed that the current study would be disseminated as part of JMG's doctoral thesis and associated publications, and all participants provided verbal and written informed consent prior to participating in their interview. All interviews were conducted face-to-face, and the majority of the interviews took place at a training ground prior to one of the participants' regular scheduled training sessions (23/30 interviews). Interviews were also conducted at participants' homes (5/30) or at a local café (2/30 interviews), as these locations were most convenient for the coaches. Each interview was conducted in a private or semi-private location and only the participant and the primary author were present during the interviews. The interviews lasted approximately 30 minutes, ranging from 28–40 minutes. At the conclusion of each interview, the participant received a $50 gift card as compensation for their time. Following each interview, field notes were made by JMG reflecting any key moments or quotes that occurred.

All interviews were conducted by JMG, who has conducted prior research on the chosen organised sports [12]. He has four years of personal experience coaching childrens' organised sport teams, and has played soccer for over 20 years. JMG is also working towards a doctoral degree in the area of PA promotion in children and youth, and currently holds an honours bachelor's degree in community health sciences. This knowledge and experience of sports and coaching was useful, because it helped build rapport with participants, and ensured jargon used by the coaches was understood. Most participants did not have any prior relationship with the research team; however, five coaches were involved in a previous study [12].

Participants

A convenience sample of OYS coaches who coached club and representative level teams of girls aged 9 to 17 years participated in this study. In this study, a club-level coach coaches athletes that have registered with an OYS club and have been assigned to a team. Representative athletes are also registered with an OYS club; however, these athletes were selected members of a team. Representative athletes represent their district and compete in a higher level of competition than club athletes. The representative-level is not the highest level of competition in OYS; however, higher levels of competition were not discussed in this study.

Participants were recruited from OYS clubs playing netball, basketball, and outdoor soccer (football) in the Greater Sydney Metropolitan Area, Australia. These organised sports were chosen because of their popularity amongst girls (in terms of participation rates) in Australia [28]. Initially, a member of each of the organised sport club's executive committee was contacted by the primary author (JMG), to provide information about the study. Clubs then provided contact details (a phone number and/or an email address) of interested participants who were coaching girls' teams in the appropriate age range. Detailed study information was then sent via email to each potential participant and coaches were included based on their willingness to participate in the study. The Human Research Ethics Committee of the University of Western Sydney approved this study.

Participant characteristics are detailed in Table 2. In total, 30 coaches (10 coaches from each of the three organised sports) participated. Coaches were aged 18–69 years (mean age $=42.2\pm13.2$ years) and had an average of 13.3 ± 11.8 years of coaching experience. The majority of the coaches were male (63%), married (57%), educated at a tertiary level (57%), held a form of coaching credential related to their sport (90%), and were overweight (43% with ≥ 25 BMI<30) or obese (30% with BMI≥ 30), based on participants' self-reported height and weight.

Data analysis

Interviews were audio-recorded and transcribed verbatim by JMG. During transcription, further notes were added to the

23

Do Coaches Perceive Themselves as Influential on Physical Activity for Girls in Organised Youth Sport?

Justin M. Guagliano[1]*, Chris Lonsdale[2], Richard R. Rosenkranz[1,3], Gregory S. Kolt[1], Emma S. George[1]

1 School of Science and Health, University of Western Sydney, Sydney, Australia, **2** Institute for Positive Psychology and Education, Australian Catholic University, Sydney, Australia, **3** Department of Human Nutrition, Kansas State University, Manhattan, Kansas, United States of America

Abstract

Participation in organised youth sports (OYS) has been recommended as an opportunity to increase young peoples' physical activity (PA) levels. While coaches can potentially influence athletes' PA levels, what has not been explored is the question; do coaches perceive themselves as influential on PA for girls in OYS? Participants were 30 coaches of girls OYS teams aged 9–17 years in the Greater Sydney Metropolitan Area, Australia. Participants took part in a semi-structured interview that lasted approximately 30 minutes. They responded to questions regarding their perceived role as coaches, their perceptions of themselves as role models for PA, their views on their athletes' current PA levels, their opinions on improving their athletes' PA levels, and their perceived challenges as coaches in OYS. Many coaches considered themselves role models for PA due to their own involvement in organised sports. Coaches felt that they were conscious of girls' PA levels during training and could accurately gauge how active girls were. Coaches perceived their training sessions to provide sufficient PA and thus, did not feel the need to try to increase PA during training. Many coaches were cautious about conducting training sessions where the PA intensity was high for prolonged periods because they believed that it could potentially result in dropout from OYS. Coaches' perceived time commitment to OYS, variability of skill/experience amongst girls, and poor parental support as major challenges they experienced in OYS. This study provided a unique insight from the perspective of coaches in OYS. Most coaches felt that they had the potential to influence PA for girls in OYS; however, coaches may underestimate or not fully realise the impact they can have on the girls they coach. Future research should focus on educating coaches to capitalise on the opportunity they have to promote PA through OYS.

Editor: Naoyuki Hayashi, Tokyo Institute of Technology, Japan

Funding: This study was funded by the School of Science and Health at the University of Western Sydney. The funders had no role in study design, data collection and analysis, decision to publish, or preparation of the manuscript.

Competing Interests: The authors have declared that no competing interests exist.

* Email: j.guagliano@uws.edu.au

Introduction

Organised youth sports (OYS) is a structured physical activity (PA) setting for children and adolescents that is governed by the rules of the sport being played [1]. In OYS, athletes attend training sessions and games under supervision of one or more adults, who most often assume the role of team coach [1,2]. Coaches in OYS are in an ideal position to impact the health and well-being of children and adolescents. Due to their role in OYS, coaches can carry considerable influence, as they are viewed as experts by their athletes [3]. Similarly, Smith and Smoll [4] have suggested that coaches can have a strong impact on children and adolescents within an OYS context due to the amount of direct involvement they have with their athletes on a weekly basis. Coaches also have considerable reach, as high proportions of children and adolescents participate in OYS around the world [5]. The most recent prevalence data indicate that, approximately 66% of all Australian children (67% of all boys and 65% of all girls) participate in at least one OYS (including dance) outside of school hours [6,7]. Through their participation in OYS, children and adolescents have the potential to be exposed to an array of physical and psychosocial health and developmental benefits [8–11].

Arguably, one of the most pertinent attributes of OYS is its potential to contribute significantly to moderate-to-vigorous physical activity (MVPA) levels of participating children [12,13]. Children and adolescents should engage in at least 60 minutes of MVPA daily and vigorous PA, including activity that strengthens muscle and bone, should be incorporated at least three times per week [14–16]. However, since a sizeable proportion of children and adolescents around the world do not meet the recommended levels of daily MVPA [5]. In Australia, a recent report found that less than one-fifth of Australian children and adolescents, aged 5–17, met recommended physical activity guidelines every day of the week [6]. This issue is even more concerning when examining youth PA levels separately, by gender. Girls are less physically active than boys throughout childhood [17,18] and their participation in PA declines more sharply than in boys as they transition into adolescence [17,19]. As such, girls have been identified as a high priority group for PA promotion [20], therefore participating in OYS can have major public health implications. Although participation in OYS provides an ideal opportunity for children and adolescents to accumulate substantial

Table 1. Interview questions, prompts, and probes.

• How do you describe your role as a coach?
• In terms of physical active, do you see yourself as a role model for your athletes?
○ In relation to having a healthy/active lifestyle?
• In what ways do you think you can influence the health behaviours of your athletes?
• How active do you think the athletes are during training?
• Can you tell me about the major demands or challenges you face as a coach?
○ Personal (e.g., lack of time, work or family commitments)
○ Athletes (e.g., lack of motivation, interest, or discipline)
○ Parents
○ Facilities/equipment
• If you were asked to make changes to your team with regard to promotion of greater physical activity levels during training time, what factors would influence your ability to do that?
• How important is it to you that your athletes are physically active during training?
• Can you identify ways you could increase children's physical activity levels during organised sport training?
• How do you plan what you're going to do for a training session? Take me through your process.
• How important is it to you that your athletes are physically active outside of organised sport?
• To what degree do you think you are responsible for influencing the physical activity behaviours of your athletes outside of organised sport?

original field notes made during post-interview reflection. After transcription, 20% of transcripts were returned to corresponding participants for verification. To ensure equal representation, two participants (a male and a female) were selected from each sport for verification. Participants made no changes to their transcripts.

Using a long table approach, content analysis was conducted using guidelines established by Côté, Salmela, Baria, and Russell [29]. Due to the exploratory nature of this study, an interpretational approach to analysis was used [30]. Côté et al. [29], described two separate phases for interpretational qualitative analysis: (1) data organisation (or creating tags) and (2) data interpretation (or creating categories). The process used to analyse the data is illustrated in Figure 1. A decision-making heuristic for the analysis of unstructured qualitative data by Côté and Salmela [31] was also used.

During the data organisation phase, text from each transcript (and corresponding field notes) were divided into segments called meaning units to produce a set of concepts that reflected meaningful pieces of information [29]. Text was divided into meaning units directly on each transcript, where tags were assigned to each meaning unit. Tagging was performed by JMG. A separate document was kept as an inventory of all the accumulated tags for the second phase of the analysis. For the data interpretation phase, the inventory of tags from all transcripts was examined by JMG and ESG. For our purposes, a deductive process was used to underpin the coding framework and help organise tags; where tags fell within five overarching categories (the aims of this study). An inductive process, however, was used to group tags with similar meaning together, which led to the emergence of themes and sub-themes within each overarching category. Disagreements while categorising were discussed with two members of the research team (CL and GSK) until a consensus was reached.

Sample size was determined *a priori* to ensure equal representation of the three organised sports. Transcripts were analysed after all interviews were conducted, in the order in which the interviews were conducted to determine theoretical saturation. Côté et al. [29] stated that theoretical saturation is reached when new data fits adequately into the existing framework. Theoretical saturation was determined to have occurred following the 23rd interview.

In order to assess classification consistency, a random sample of 25% of tags was selected for independent classification under mutually exclusive categories and themes by a member of the research team familiar with the study aims but removed from data analysis until this point (RRR). Agreement was determined by comparing RRR's independent classification of a random sample of tags with the classification of tags conducted by the rest of the research team. Seventy percent agreement was set as the minimum acceptable level of agreement. Agreement was also assessed using Cohen's kappa coefficient. RRR's independent classification of a random sample of tags showed a high level agreement with the rest of the research team (88.6% agreement, kappa coefficient = 0.88).

Results

A summary of the main themes, sub-themes, and example quotes that emerged from the 30 in-depth semi-structured interviews with OYS coaches are presented by category in Tables 3 to 7. The five categories are presented in the following order: (1) participants' perceived role as coaches (five themes, three sub-themes); (2) their perception of themselves as role models for PA (two themes, no sub-themes); (3) their views on their athletes' current PA levels (five themes, no sub-themes); (4) their opinions on improving their athletes' PA levels (five themes, two sub-themes); and (5) their perceived challenges as coaches in OYS (four themes, nine sub-themes).

Perceived role as coaches

Coaches described roles in which they could be influential to their athletes, such as being a mentor or role model. The most common influential perceived role that coaches cited, though, was as a teacher:

Table 2. Characteristics of Participating Coaches.

Variable	Netball (n = 10)	Basketball (n = 10)	Soccer (n = 10)
Mean age (±SD)	41.8(18.8)	38.8(12.3)	45.8(5.4)
Sex, n			
Male	2	8	9
Female	8	2	1
Mean height (cm) (±SD)	165.7(9.4)	179.3(11.4)	176.2(10.8)
Mean weight (kg) (±SD)	74.6(13.1)	83.3(20.2)	94.4(15.2)
Mean body mass index (±SD)	27.2(4.2)	25.6(4.3)	30.3(5.3)
Marital Status, n			
Married	4	5	8
Divorced	1	1	0
Not married	5	4	2
Level of education, n			
University or higher	2	3	1
Certificate/diploma	3	3	5
Trade/apprenticeship	1	0	1
Secondary school	3	2	2
Less than secondary school	1	2	1
Annual income, n			
$100,000+	3	2	7
$80,000–$99,999	1	5	1
$60,000– $79,999	1	0	1
$40,000–$59,999	2	0	1
$20,000–$39,999	0	2	0
<$20,000	3	1	0
Mean years coaching (±SD)	18.5(16.3)	12.8(8.7)	8.5(7.2)
Mean number of sports coaching (±SD)	1(0)	1.1(0.3)	1.5(0.9)
Mean number of age groups coaching (±SD)	1.8(0.6)	2.8(0.8)	1.7(1.0)
Coaches with coaching credentials, n	10	10	7

Note: n = number of coaches.

"Mainly I'm like a teacher and that's what I want to be seen as because that's what I'm doing - teaching the girls about netball… skills, strategy and so on." [Netball coach 13].

Within this theme, coaches described the need to foster sports-related development, promote the development of life skills, and to create a positive environment for their athletes. Sport-specific development was the focal point for many coaches, with a particular focus on teaching athletes skills, tactical/strategic awareness, and preparedness relevant to their sport. Another predominant topic discussed by coaches was their efforts to try to teach life skills through sport. The most frequently discussed life skills were accountability, confidence, respect, and social skills. Many considered generating a positive team environment to be an important aspect of their role as a coach. In particular, coaches identified the need to create an environment that was fun, friendly, and supportive.

Other coaches perceived their role to be that of a facilitator, which was described by coaches as someone who organises aspects of OYS (e.g., plan training sessions, set line ups, ensure equal playing time), or as a disciplinarian, which was described as someone who is strict and resolves conflicts amongst athletes. Perceived roles as a facilitator or disciplinarian, however, were not as common as the previously mentioned perceived roles.

Coaches' perceptions of themselves as role models for PA

When asked, most coaches thought of themselves as a role model for PA, but many had not considered it before.

"I suppose I haven't thought about it before now…. But, I think it's [being a role model] a given, you know, it's just an understanding you have, that if you're coaching and you're still playing they'll look up to you." [Soccer coach 5].

Other coaches cited their participation at training, their current involvement in the sport (as an athlete in a team), a physically active lifestyle, and their age and longevity in the sport as reasons for perceiving themselves as role models for PA for their athletes.

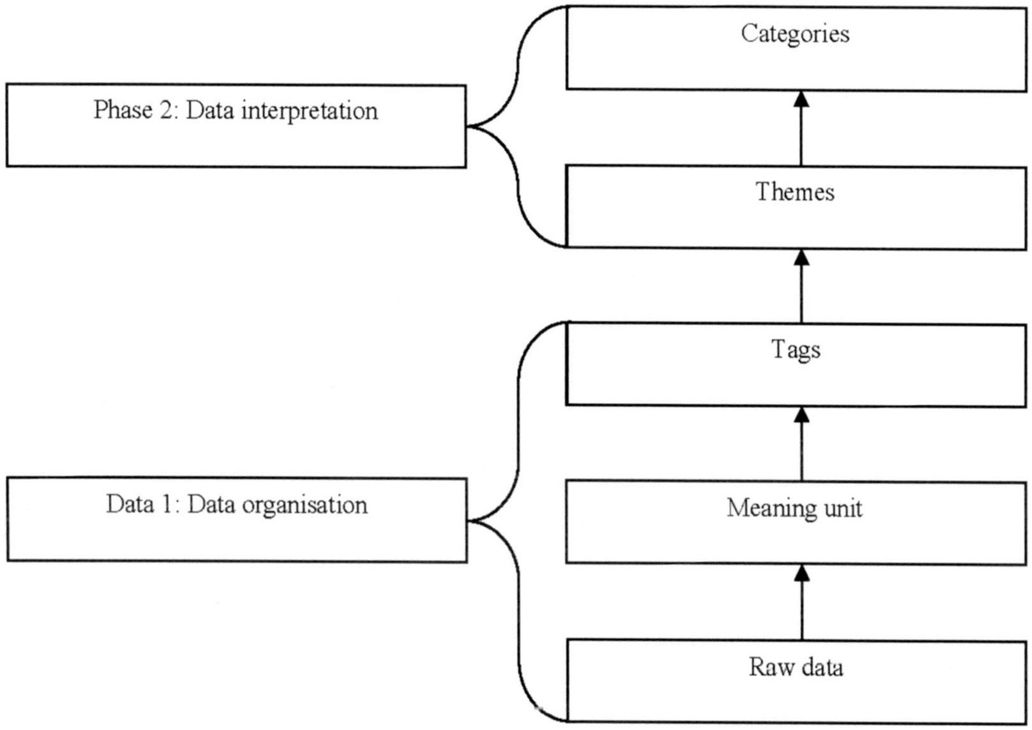

Figure 1. Data analysis process.

While most coaches considered themselves role models for PA, the view was not shared by all coaches. Poor fitness levels, old age, injury or health problems, and retirement from organised sports were the most common reasons for coaches not perceiving themselves as role models. Although some coaches did not perceive themselves as particularly good role models for the

Table 3. Perceived role as coaches: summary of categories, themes, sub-themes, and example quotes.

Category	Themes	Sub-themes	Example quotes
Perceived role as a coach	Teacher	To foster sports-related development	"My main role is to teach them how to be better soccer players. I focus on developing their soccer skills, preparing them for games and keeping them focused" [SC 6].
		To foster the development of other life skills	"For the girls, I would hope I'm seen as kind of like a life coach. I try focus on teaching them things they can learn through sport that can be used later in life like I tell them if you lose a ball, you have to make sure you get back and try to win it back because you are not helping the team if you don't – that's being accountable" [SC 3].
		To create positive environment	"…I'm a bit of a joker at times and I try to keep the atmosphere as light, fun, and friendly as possible and I think I have a pretty good rapport with the kids" [NC 15].
	Role Model		"I see myself as a role model for the girls… I'm only a little bit older than the girls on my team and I want them to know that I don't care if other people judge me because I play sport and if they say things like 'oh it's not girly to be running around playing sport getting sweaty'. I want to show them that it's just sports, I do it, and everyone should be doing it, really. [NC 17].
	Mentor		"I'm more of a mentor, someone who's guiding them to achieve the goals that they want and helping them develop the skills that they need to achieve those goals" [SC 10].
	Facilitator		"I organise their training sessions once a week, prepare them for the game… make sure they are ready to go, that they know what we're doing, adjusting positions, making sure everyone has equal court time… and I take care of all the paperwork."[NC 16].
	Disciplinarian		"A lot of people will tell you I'm a meanie (laughs). So, I suppose I'm a disciplinarian because I'm strict." [BC 20].

SC = soccer coach; NC = netball coach; BC = basketball coach.

Table 4. Coaches' perceptions of themselves as role models for physical activity: summary of categories, themes, sub-themes, and example quotes.

Category	Themes	Sub-themes	Example quotes
Coaches' self-perceptions as role models for athletes	Positive self-perception as a role model for physical activity		"They see me play on Monday nights in the men's comp and I train with them all the time, running around; so hopefully they see me as a role model both for basketball skills as well as the fitness aspect of it." [BC 25].
			"I've never really thought about it, but yeah, I haven't not played sport (laughs)... and most of the kids that I coach know that I've played at a pretty high level too. So I'd consider myself a pretty good role model." [BC 20].
			"I do because this is my lifestyle. I find it odd that people aren't physically active, you know (laughs). I'm a PE teacher, I coach, play, umpire, I'm in an old ladies representative team as well, so you know, it's just what I am about and hopefully some of that rubs off." [NC 13].
			"...not only in the teams that I'm coaching but also in my general life with people around the netball courts. I'm definitely a role model to people around the netball courts in terms of longevity, how long can you do this sport? And people just sort of respect that I think." [NC 8].
	Negative self-perception as a role model for physical activity		"...probably not in the physical activity sense – I'm a bit passed that... I'm not the fittest 50-year old I know." [NC 15].
			"Probably not, you're talking to an old bugger here." [SC 6].
			"Not since my knees have gone on me." [BC 11].
			"Oh look, probably not. I don't actually play netball anymore, I did for 15 years previously, but my physical activity has sort of taken a dip." [NC 16].

SC = soccer coach; NC = netball coach; BC = basketball coach.

reasons listed above, some recognised the importance and the opportunity they had to be role models.

> *"I see the importance of people like me being a role model for our players... the truth is you don't have to be a physically fit person to inspire others to be fit. But, role modelling is always important and there is an opportunity as coaches to be a fantastic role model." [Basketball coach 29].*

Perceived levels and importance of PA

Coaches' perceived importance related to athletes' PA during training. Coaches' perceptions relating to the importance of athlete PA during training were not universal. The majority of coaches, however, perceived PA to be important during training, with some stating that being physically active is more important to them than winning.

> *"...keeping the girls active at training is very important, it's one things I really try to do. I love seeing the girls improve their fitness, their skills... and hey, if we get some wins along the way, that's great too (laughs)." [Basketball coach 11].*

Some coaches mentioned that a physically active training session was needed to keep girls motivated and engaged. Other coaches stated that the athletes would benefit by being physically active during training because their fitness levels will allow them to outperform their opposition late in games.

Also, a few coaches discussed how they front-loaded their training sessions to include higher intensity PA at the beginning of the season and purposefully dropped the PA intensity at training as the season went on. The reason that coaches did this was because they felt girls' fitness levels were not maintained over the off-season, so the focus of training sessions at the beginning of the season was to regain girls' fitness. Once coaches felt the girls' fitness was regained, the focus of their training sessions shifted to skill development, where coaches perceived PA intensity to drop.

> *"Early in the year, fitness training was huge because the girls were pretty low in fitness, you know, they had the summer holidays and they hadn't done much. But, as we move on during the season, ball skills and controlling the ball become paramount... then it's lots of drills and getting their positions right. So the intensity at training drops a bit because we do more drills and focus less on the fitness aspect." [Soccer coach 9].*

Coaches who felt that their athletes' PA level during training was not important tended to believe that it was more important to focus on teaching sport-related skills and skill development. These coaches were willing to sacrifice PA intensity to achieve this.

Perceived levels of PA. Most coaches felt that they were conscious of their athletes' PA levels and that they were able to gauge how active the girls were at training. Furthermore, the majority of coaches considered high intensity PA to be inherent in OYS.

> *"I'm always on them about different things, trying to keep the intensity up... and as a coach you can gauge how the team is training ... so, if the group is down then I can quickly gauge that the intensity is down and I'll try to pick it up." [Basketball coach 20].*
> *"...I try to keep the girls moving and high intensity activity is natural in soccer." [Soccer coach 1].*

Training session preparation. Coaches' training preparation responses were highly variable, ranging from developing a meticulously written training plan to no planning at all. In this sample of coaches, very few coaches actually wrote down their

Table 5. Coaches' perceived levels and importance of physical activity: summary of categories, themes, sub-themes, and example quotes.

Category	Themes	Sub-themes	Example quotes
Coaches' perceived levels and importance of physical activity	Athlete physical activity during training is important		"Yeah because if they get too many drink breaks they shut off, they're not motivated, they're not active, and they talk. Then the training session just drags out and doesn't become a good training session." [SC 24].
			"The more you keep them active at training the easier it'll be coping in game situations when they're under pressure in the final quarter because they'll have that fitness. So, you know, it's really really important for them, far more than the club player who may only play a quarter or two." [NC 23].
			"...at the beginning of the season they're a lot more active and we do a lot more running than they would later in the season later." [SC 6].
	Athlete physical activity during training is not important		"I'd rather they be focused and lazy than running around not listening at all. I think that's more important... I've got to get across what we're trying to do – the skills and how we'll implement that in a game." [NC 16].
	Training planning		"I wing it. I've been coaching for so many years I just make it up as I go." [NC 14].
			"I write down what I want at the beginning of the year, but no, I don't write a formalised plan for each session it's more of a general idea." [BC 11].
			"....the less committed the team is the less time I put into making a training session." [BC 27].
	Athlete physical activity outside of orgnanised youth sport is important		"...anything they can do outside netball is only going to improve performance and make things easier during netball. So, that is important to me but I can't demand it and I don't initiate conversations about be active outside netball." [NC 23].
			"Nowadays what we do as coaches is not enough because the kids aren't doing anything outside of the sports they play." [BC 21].
			"For rep players it's important." [BC 22].
			"If you want to play at an elite level, one 2-hour training session a week is not going to get you there." [BC 19].
	Athlete physical activity outside of orgnanised youth sport is not important		"I believe that people should be active, especially kids, during and outside of sports. But, with the team that I'm coaching now, if I could get them all to training and get them to come to the game, that's two activity sessions a week and I'd be satisfied with that. If I was coaching a rep team, I'd expect them to do more than that." [NC 8].

SC = soccer coach; NC = netball coach; BC = basketball coach.

plan for training, with many claiming that they just mentally prepare for their training sessions.

> *"I usually just plan in my head on my way to training, so it's mentally written down... so, there is the warm up that I want to do, there are certain drills I want to do and there is a cool down...." [Netball coach 12].*

Some coaches discussed having general or thematic (e.g., shooting drills, passing drills) training session plans in mind rather

Table 6. Coaches' perceptions on improving athlete physical activity: summary of categories, themes, sub-themes, and example quotes.

Category	Themes	Sub-themes	Example quotes
Coaches' perceptions on improving athlete physical activity	Perceives a need to increase athlete physical activity during training		"...there probably is a need to increase activity, but it might be hard to convince the girls." [NC 17]
	Does not perceive a need to increase athlete physical activity during training		"No there's no need, I'm fairly happy with where we're at. I've been doing this for a while." [BC 19].
	Methods to increase physical activity during training	Coach-specific methods	"Make sure that you're prepared and organised and that you set out a specific training schedule so that there isn't any down time." [BC 21].
			"focus more on constant running or movement and less standing time, less watching, less waiting, and less listening to instructions from myself...." [BC 30].
		Drill modification	"...using modified drills. So, smaller groups and lots of equipment so they're really just keep chugging through." [NC 13].
	Perceived responsibility to influence physical activity outside of organised youth sports		"No, I don't think I'm responsible for the girls outside of the sport... I don't have that much of an influence outside of soccer." [SC 4].
			"With the rep players we encourage them to do things outside of netball but not with the club players." [NC 23].
			"I don't feel a responsibility, but I'll use the word opportunity again, I think there's a huge opportunity as a coach." [BC 29].
	Coach has the ability to impact health behaviours		"...I think I can because coaches I've had have had an impact on me and my sisters as well, I think I can...." [NC 7].
	Coach does not have the ability to impact health behaviours		"We [as coaches] only see the kids twice a week, once at training and once at the game, so I think parental influence is far outweighing anything I can do as a coach." [NC 15].
			"...because I only see them for probably 2 hours a week I think other influences like parents, schools, and even friends would play a much larger role in influencing their physical activity." [NC 16].

SC = soccer coach; NC = netball coach; BC = basketball coach.

than including specific drills, claiming that they are experienced enough to come up with specific drills on-the-spot. Some even claimed that they would just "wing it" during their training sessions, relying on their coaching experience to develop a session as-they-go. Some coaches with multiple teams admitted that they spent less time preparing training sessions for their less competitive teams. The majority of coaches said that their focus at training was based on observed weaknesses from the previous game.

Coaches' perceived importance related to athletes' PA outside of OYS. Athletes' PA outside of OYS was perceived as being important by most coaches. This was due to the perceived positive effect it would have on performance in OYS. Also, being physically active outside of OYS was perceived as being more important for representative athletes compared to club athletes by coaches; especially if there was a desire to play at an elite level. It appeared that coaches were content if club athletes attended their weekly training session and game, but for representative athletes the expectation to be physically active went beyond weekly training and games; these athletes were expected to be physically active in some way outside of OYS.

Some coaches reflected on changes in norms from their childhood where playing outside was regarded as a norm, compared to now where coaches perceive children to be doing very little outside of OYS.

> *"I remember when I was a kid, you get home from school, you go down to your mate's place and play basketball, footy, soccer, whatever, or you're on your push bike... now you don't see any push bikes or anything like that. It's a completely different lifestyle than when I was a kid. [Basketball coach 21].*

> *"It's not like it used to be back when I was a kid, we used to play outside until it got dark every night after school. Things have changed and I think that the kids have got to do something outside of your training session to get better, I think a lot of kids today come to training and that's it for the week." [Basketball coach 29].*

Coaches' perceptions on improving athlete PA

Perceived need to increase athlete PA during training. Few coaches perceived the need to increase PA because they were content with the level of PA during their training

Table 7. Coaches' perceived challenges: summary of categories, themes, sub-themes, and example quotes.

Category	Themes	Sub-themes	Example quotes
Coaches' perceived challenges	Coaches' perceived personal challenges	Time commitment to coaching	"There's a high level of commitment required in coaching you have the campaign, training, match day, phone calls and emails to organise everyone, etcetera, etcetera. It can be pretty time consuming." [SC 4].
			"After having a whole shift at work all day and then having to organise the drills and getting them down-pat that's one barrier for me because this is my first year coaching." [SC 9].
		Weak in some coaching aspect	"I'm good at the coaching and the motivating and leadership skills; but the technical skills is not my expertise, you know, I haven't really played a lot of soccer." [SC 5].
			" One of my weaknesses is getting kids focused when they need to be focused. When I was a younger coach, kids were having fun but they weren't actually getting better because there would be no focus at training." [BC 27].
			"I'm coaching the kids based on my own experiences, you know, I haven't had any formal training so, that's a big barrier for me." [SC 28].
		Work commitments	"I'm really really busy with work and I really try hard just to find the time to put the effort into being with the girls but often I have to get someone else to run training because I can't make it." [SC 10].
	Coaches' perceived challenges relating to their athletes	Athletes' variability in skill/experience	"I suppose one of the big barriers I have with the 11's is that there is such a wide array of skill and experience. So, I have some girls that are really, really advanced and you have some that aren't, like I've got two girls playing their first year of netball. So, it's hard trying to catch them up as well as making the ones who want to advance not bored." [NC 12].
		Athletes' lack of interest/focus	"...they do chatter a lot and that can be a problem sometimes, to keep them interested and keep them focused on what they're meant to doing." [SC 10].
		Athletes' lack of motivation/commitment	"...lack of motivation is a barrier sometimes. Sometimes the girls probably don't take it as seriously as they should and some girls just see training as a social thing; which it definitely can be. But, it's important that they make an effort to train hard otherwise why bother coming?" [BC 30].
		Athlete management	"Sometimes the girls don't listen to what I tell them to do, like if I tell them to do warm up laps they'll complain and it becomes a negotiation, which wastes time." [NC 17].
			"There's always one or two in most teams where you'll find a personality where you've got to work really hard to work out where they're coming from or what their problem is without having them blow up or getting upset or whatever. It's definitely an obstacle – one that you don't need." [NC 23].
			"I've got one girl who hasn't spoken all year and one who is deaf so, she can't get instructions from me. With those girls in particular, it's been very difficult for me." [SC 5].
	Coaches' perceived challenges relating to their athletes' parents	Managing parental expectations/perceptions	"...dealing with the parents is a big one... playing time; expectations on the teams' performance; their opinions on where I should be playing their daughter; parents who are yelling at refs, opposing parents, players... you name it." [SC 3].
		Parental commitment	"The main barrier is getting the children to training. That's the main barrier. All the children like to play and as a general rule you'll get the children there on a Saturday to play, but the lack of commitment by the parents to get their kids to training is huge" [NC 8].
	Coaches' perceived challenges relating to promoting physical activity.		"There's just not enough time to do anything besides basketball. We only have two sessions a week for two hours." [BC 21].

SC = soccer coach; NC = netball coach; BC = basketball coach.

sessions. Some coaches, however, reported having to reduce the intensity of their training sessions because of the girls' disinclination to train at a high intensity.

> *"...the girls were just not keen to put the effort into the training sessions that I was running.... I've had to re-adjust my focus and my expectations for the girls and I'm happy where we sit now with the level of activity" [Soccer coach 2].*

A major concern raised by coaches was a fear of athlete dropout if the PA intensity during training in OYS was too high.

> *"You can't push some of these girls too much, because they'll quit. You can try to be motivational to get them to be more active, but you can't force them, you know." [Basketball coach 22].*

> *"...there's a lack of fitness in probably two-thirds of the side and there's a reluctance to put the effort in.... So, if I were to step up the intensity, there would be more of a dropout rate. A lot of the girls fake injury to sit out as it is." [Soccer coach 4].*

> *"...they would revolt [if the coach tried to increase PA]. They would just go 'no, I'm not doing it' or they wouldn't come to training. So, you've really got to gauge how far you can push them. [Netball coach 15].*

One coach, however, emphasised the need to take advantage of the time spent in OYS because she has noticed that the girls who she coaches are less active and has noticed changes in body shape and their physical ability.

> *"...compared to 10 years ago, the girls I coach are generally less active, and I've noticed that they don't have the same gross motor skills as they would've had 10 years ago. I definitely see a change in body shape and physical ability. So, I think we need to take advantage of the time kids are at basketball because for some, this is all the activity they get in a week." [Basketball coach 21].*

Methods to increase PA during training. Although most coaches did not feel the need to increase PA during their training sessions, they were, however, able to identify ways to increase training session PA if they needed to. Coaches suggested improving their organisation, increasing preparation for training, developing more specific training plans, and reducing waiting (i.e., in lines during drills or during drill tranisition) and instruction time. They also suggested modifying drills to include smaller groups and having more equipment available.

Perceived responsibility to influence PA outside of OYS. Although most coaches felt that their athletes should be physically active outside of OYS, very few felt it was their responsibility to influence PA outside of OYS. Coaches felt that they had very little influence over their athletes' PA behaviours outside of OYS, most commonly citing parents as more influential in this respect. Peers were also considered by coaches to have a greater influence on PA levels outside of OYS than they did.

The comparison between representative athletes and club athletes emerged once again while discussing coaches' perceived responsibility to influence PA outside of OYS. Some coaches thought it was more likely that they could encourage representative athletes to train in their free time outside of OYS as opposed to club athletes; however, this was seldomly discussed.

Although not feeling a responsibility to influence PA outside of OYS, some acknowledged that coaches in OYS have a substantial opportunity to do so. See Table 6 for supporting quotes.

Coaches' perceived ability to impact health behaviours. When coaches were asked if they felt they had the ability to impact girls' health behaviours, coaches took a very pragmatic approach. Some coaches stated they have had coaches that have had a lasting impact on them, so it was plausible that they could have a lasting impact on their athletes. There were no identifible charateristics that were apparent among coaches with differing opinions of their perceived ability to impact girls' health behaviours (i.e., sport coached, coach's gender, coaching experience).

Interestingly, PA was rarely discussed as a health behaviour when identifying whether coaches thought they could impact their athletes' health behaviours or not. Often the conversation shifted from the designed focus on PA to coaches discussing their attempts to inform their athletes about healthy eating.

> *"I try to encourage healthier eating, like I had one girl that used to eat a meat pie before a game, so I tried to get her in the habit of eating the correct foods before games. That's one area where I think I can leave an impression.... what they eat and how they prepare is important and I think I can help with that." [Netball coach 18].*

Most coaches, though, perceived their ability to impact girls' health behaviours was limited. Insufficient exposure and influence were the main reasons that coaches could not impact girls' health behaviours. Again, parents, teachers, and peers were considered to have a greater influence on girls' health behaviours.

Coaches' challenges in OYS

Coaches' perceived personal challenges relating to OYS. Few coaches felt they had any personal challenges while coaching in OYS. The perceived time needed to commit to OYS was, however, the main issue identified by coaches who did report having personal challenges. The time needed for administrative tasks as well as preparing for training were the two biggest time consumers, with the latter particularly affecting less experienced coaches. Some coaches discussed an over-commitment to their sport; this included coaching and refereeing multiple teams and games, respectively.

> *"Maybe an over-commitment to basketball... I can only be in one place at one time and sometimes it clashes with training. It takes a toll on you, some nights I'm coaching non-stop." [Basketball coach 20].*

> *"...Friday nights I'm here coaching three teams and reffing two, so it's just bang-bang-bang five games in a row." [Basketball coach 25].*

Some coaches felt that they were weak in some aspects of coaching, which they perceived as a limitation in their coaching ability. Perceived coaching weaknesses included poor sport-specific technical skills, difficulty keeping athletes focused on the task at hand, and lack of formal training. Work commitments also emerged as an issue faced by coaches occasionally, but were not commonly discussed.

Coaches' perceived challenges relating to their athletes. A predominant challenge coaches discussed was the wide variation in athletes' skill levels and experience within a team.

Some coaches described the dilemma of trying to find the right balance at training, where the skilled/experienced athletes feel engaged without leaving the less skilled/experienced athletes to fall further behind.

Girls' focus and interest levels posed problems for coaches as well, with the main reported obstacle being that girls talk too much during training. Some coaches described training as a "social gathering" and felt that girls' motivation and commitment was lacking. As a negotiation with the girls, some coaches have implemented "talk time" where they are allowed to talk at certain points of the training session, in an effort to minimise conversations that are not sports-related.

> *"I've had to implement, what I call, 'talk time' to keep the conversations to a minimum during training... see a lot of them went to primary school together and they're at different high schools. So, it's like a reunion every Wednesday night." [Soccer coach 9].*

Athlete management was another theme that emerged as an athlete-related challenge, which related to non-compliance with coach instructions, difficult athletes, and athletes with disabilities. See Table 7. for supporting quotes.

Coaches' perceived challenges relating to their athletes' parents. All coaches, at one point or another, experienced some sort of issue relating to their athletes' parents during their years coaching OYS. Athletes' playing time was one of the most common complaints from parents. Parental commitment to OYS was cited as a major issue for coaches as well, with the main perceived issue being parents' unreliability when it came to getting their daughters to training.

Also, one coach was frustrated with some parents' lack of interest in the sport that their daughter was playing and felt that the lack of parental support could impact on further participation in OYS.

> *"It annoys me when the parents aren't quite on the same wavelength as you because I love this stuff [netball], okay, and I think most of the girls do too. So, it bothers me when parents don't take any interest in it and I'd bet there are probably kids who stop playing netball because they don't have any support from their mum or dad." [Netball coach 13].*

Another coach noticed that, as the girls on his team got older, fewer parents were attending their daughters' training and game sessions.

> *"When I started coaching them at 12... all the parents were there and now, no parents are there." [Soccer coach 1].*

Coaches' perceived challenges relating to promoting PA. Frequency and duration of training sessions were the most commonly cited challenges with regard to promoting PA. Coaches felt they had too little time at training to discuss anything outside of the sport they were coaching.

Discussion

To our knowledge, this is the first study to explore whether coaches perceive themselves as influential on PA for girls participating in OYS. More specifically, we explored coaches' perceived role as coaches, their perception of themselves as role models for PA, their views on their athletes' current PA levels, their opinions on improving their athletes' PA levels, and their perceived challenges during OYS. Our analysis of 30 in-depth semi-structured interviews suggests that most coaches feel that they have the potential to influence PA for girls in OYS. It is possible, though, that coaches may underestimate or not fully realise the impact they can have on the girls they coach in OYS.

When asked about their perceived role as a coach, a range of influential roles were discussed. The perception of being a teacher, role model, or mentor resonated with many of the coaches in this study. The fact that several influential roles resonated with coaches is a positive finding from a PA promotion standpoint, as Smith and Smoll [4] have suggested that coaches can have a strong impact on children and adolescents due to consistent direct involvement with them. Not surprisingly, coaches primarily reported that it was their responsibility to provide sport-specific development (e.g., technical skills, tactical awareness, preparedness). Coaches also reported, however, that it was part of their role to create a positive environment (e.g., fun, friendly, supportive) and to foster the development of life skills, which was also found in recent study by Vella et al. [32]. Those authors also noted that the responsibility coaches felt to develop athletes' life skills was an important extension to existing literature and our study lends support to that finding.

While some coaches had never considered it before the interview, the majority perceived themselves to be role models for PA, particularly if they were still currently involved in organised sports in some capacity (i.e., active participants during training or currently playing in a team). Although no direct comparisons are available, Drummond et al. examined student and health educators' perceptions in relation to role modelling exercise [29]. The authors found that 90% (18 out of 20) of health educators perceived themselves as role models for exercise for their students, citing their participation level as the main reason for this perception [33]. In contrast to our findings, however, nonparticipation in sports was not cited as a reason for health educators not perceiving themselves as role models for exercise in the study by Drummond et al. [33].

Most coaches stated that being physically active during OYS was important. Coaches reported that they were conscious of their athletes' PA levels and had the ability to gauge their athletes' PA levels. The presumption by many, however, was that high-intensity PA was inherent to OYS. So, it is not surprising that most coaches felt it was unnecessary for them to try to increase girls' PA levels and reduce their inactivity during training. Smith and Smoll's [4] research, however, indicates that coaches have limited awareness of their actions during OYS and state that increasing awareness is essential for change to occur. Therefore, low-cost methods, such as pedometers or direct observation systems (e.g., the System for Observing Fitness Instruction Time [34]), could be used to provide coaches with objectively measured feedback on girls' PA levels, and self-monitoring could be introduced to coaches in an effort to assist in optimising time spent in training during OYS.

An interesting theme that emerged was the concern held by coaches that girls might drop out of OYS if, for a prolonged period training, PA intensity was too high. Coaches' recognition that they could be responsible for prompting athletes' withdrawal is a positive finding. Youth athletes in other studies have ranked their coach as the most influential person in making the decision to withdraw from OYS [35], where one study found that coaches influenced nearly one-third of athletes to withdraw from OYS [36]. Of the extensive literature that exists relating to athlete dropout from OYS [37–39], as far as we are aware, high-intensity

PA is not commonly reported as a reason for withdrawal from OYS among athletes. One study sampled nearly 400 athletes and reported over 30 reasons for athlete withdrawal from OYS and none of the athlete-reported reasons related specifically to PA intensity. This is not to say that high-intensity PA cannot influence girls' decision to withdraw from OYS. Though, as far as we are aware, coaches' perception that girls may withdraw from OYS due to high intensity PA does not appear to be in line with athlete-reported reasons for dropping out of OYS. Further exploration on this topic is warranted and should be taken into consideration in any PA promotion interventions in OYS involving girls.

Generally, coaches in this study reported spending little time preparing for training sessions. The majority of coaches said that they relied on their experience to create impromptu training sessions. Mandic and colleagues have suggested that coaches should ensure that training session drills are structured to maximise PA intensity [40]. Further supporting a structured training session, a recent study conducted in a physical education setting found a negative correlation between time spent in management (i.e., drill transition, instruction) and student MVPA [23]. Without prior preparation, there is a greater likelihood that time at training is not being used as efficiently as it can be, and PA intensity could potentially drop.

Coaches reported that they were capable of altering their training sessions to increase girls' PA, if they felt they needed to. Coaches were able to identify numerous strategies that could be employed in their training sessions to increase opportunities to be active, reduce inactivity, and improve their efficiency and management of training. Many of the strategies that coaches identified have also been recommended within a physical education setting; and included: using smaller groups, providing more equipment, reducing waiting, and reducing instruction time to increase girls' opportunities to be physically active [41,42]. However, coaches' awareness of these strategies may not necessarily mean they will employ them because knowledge can be a poor predictor of behaviour [43]; especially if coaches' perception of girls' PA during training is already considered adequate. Approaches are needed, then, to ensure that coaches are not only aware of strategies to increase opportunities to be active (and reduce inactivity), but also have the belief that as a result of implementing these strategies it can lead to positive outcomes (e.g., health benefits) [43].

Most coaches stated that being physically active during OYS was important, however, rarely discussed the health benefits associated with being physically active. Coaches in this study felt confident discussing the sport they coached, but may lack confidence discussing the more general health benefits associated with PA. Coaches' perceived ability to impact girls' health behaviours was also discussed, and few coaches felt that they could have an impact on the health behaviours of the girls they coached. This belief may represent a missed opportunity for coaches to make a meaningful impact on girls' health behaviours as girls can learn behaviours from their coaches, particularly if the girls admire their coach [44]. Coaches did not feel that they were able to impact their girls' health behaviours, and two of the main reasons for this were a perceived lack of influence and limited exposure to their athletes. However, Smith and Smoll [4] suggest the contrary, coaches can greatly impact their athletes. Interestingly, PA was rarely mentioned as a health behaviour that coaches felt they could impact, rather healthy eating was commonly discussed instead. This may be due to coaches' perception that PA is inherent to OYS.

Outside of OYS, coaches discussed changes in norms from their childhood where unstructured leisure-time PA was regarded as a norm. They also perceived there to be a decline in PA amongst children and adolescents, however, very few coaches felt responsible for influencing girls to be physically active outside of OYS. Even though most coaches perceived their role to be one that could be influential to their athletes in OYS, it appears many of them do not perceive their influence to extend outside of OYS. Coaches suggested that parents and peers had a greater influence on PA outside of OYS than coaches did. There is ample evidence to support coaches' claims that parents and peers are influential in supporting children to be physically active [45–47]; however, one study found that physical education teachers were as influential as parents in supporting adolescents' PA outside of school [48]. While this is not a direct comparison, it is possible that OYS coaches can also greatly influence girls' PA outside of OYS and coaches are underestimating the impact they can have.

The most commonly perceived personal challenge experienced by coaches was the amount of time they felt they needed to commit to OYS. Administrative tasks and preparing for training were considered the two biggest perceived consumers of coaches' time. Many coaches, however, stated that they relied on their experience to plan training sessions somewhat spontaneously. Coaches also identified a number of challenges relating to coaching their athletes. The predominant issue was the amount of variation in skill level and experience within their teams. Some coaches found it difficult to keep the skilled/experienced girls engaged during training without having the less skilled/experienced girls falling further behind, likely increasing the amount of instruction needed. These findings could potentially result in training sessions that do not maximise athletes' opportunities to be physically active. These are important findings as previous literature has shown that for the majority of time during OYS athletes are inactive or in light PA [12,13,21,22]. Furthermore, Dudley et al. [23] found negative correlations between instruction/management and MVPA. This valuable insight could inform future studies aiming to increase PA in OYS.

Coaches also reported girls' focus/interest levels, motivation/commitment, and athlete management as challenges. Although coaches identified these as challenges, they seemed confident in their ability to deal with them, often detailing how they overcome them.

When coaches discussed their perceived challenges in relation to parents, an interesting finding from a PA promotion perspective was that some coaches believed that they were able to identify girls on their teams who had low parental support. Coaches reported being frustrated with some parents' lack of commitment and support for their daughters. A coach commented on how annoyed she was with parents who did not take any interest in the sport their daughter played, and suggested that girls with a lack of parental support are likely to stop playing OYS. This is an encouraging finding as there is strong evidence to suggest that parental support is linked with children's PA behaviours [49–52] and children's participation in OYS [53,54]. Furthermore, Lubans, Sylva, and Morgan [55] found that in older adolescents, parental support was significantly correlated with MVPA; however, one coach commented on his observation that parents' presence during OYS has decreased as the girls he coached got older. Given that girls' PA levels tend to decrease sharply in adolescence [17,19], maintaining parental support may be an important factor to consider in efforts to increase and maintain PA levels in girls as they transition into adolescence and adulthood. As coaches in this study were able to identify athletes lacking this much-needed parental support, coaches may be able to play an important role maintaining parental support and should be examined further.

Some potential limitations should be considered when interpreting these findings. Firstly, it is possible that coaches offered socially desirable viewpoints during their interview. Secondly, a convenience sample was used, possibly introducing an element of selection bias. That said, a wide array of responses from a diverse sample of coaches was collected. Lastly, female-coaching perspectives may be underrepresented as our sample contained more men than women; however, male coaches are more prevalent than female coaches in OYS [56]. Despite these limitations, the present study provides unique insight into coaches' perceptions of themselves as being influential on PA for girls in OYS. Also, rigorous research methodology was employed to ensure the trustworthiness of the data. We used several strategies [57] to strengthen the credibility of our data, for example, investigator triangulation during the interpretation phase, individual classification during data analysis, reflexivity, and member checking. Along with aiding in the credibility of the data, the above-mentioned strategies also protected against individual perceptual biases [58]. According to Lincoln and Guba [59], demonstrating credibility may be considered sufficient to support the notion of dependability. Further, we have established acceptable confirmability by using published guidelines to analyse our data [29,31] and, as mentioned above, employed strategies to reduce individual perceptual biases. Lastly, concerning transferability, Lincoln and Guba [59] suggested that transferability is primarily the responsibility of the researcher interested in transferring the findings to another context or population than that of the original study. Lincoln and Guba [59] also state that so long as the original study presents sufficient descriptive data to allow comparisons the issue of transferability has been adequately addressed. The current study provided a thorough description of the research context and adequate descriptive data allowing other researchers to make judgement on how practical a transfer of the results are to a different context or population.

Considering the high proportion of children that participate in OYS, and the myriad of health and developmental benefits associated with the setting, OYS has the potential to be a powerful health-promoting environment for children and adolescents. Recently a number of studies have examined OYS clubs as a setting to promote health [9,10,60]. These studies illustrate a wide range of health-promoting capabilities OYS can provide and the importance of OYS clubs. However, only one study recognised that OYS clubs can play a role in promoting PA [60]. Our study provides a unique perspective on OYS coaches' perceptions of themselves as being influential on PA for girls in OYS. Further, coaches in this study (whilst not the primary focus) indicated that they were confident discussing healthy eating with the girls on their team. They may, however, underestimate or not fully realise the impact they can have. To further enhance the health-promoting capabilities of OYS, there should also be an emphasis placed on educating coaches to capitalise on the opportunity they have to promote PA to the girls they coach. This information on OYS can be used as a platform on which to inform policies, programs, and interventions to develop strategies to increase girls' PA levels through OYS.

Acknowledgments

We would like to thank the coaches for their participation in this study and Dr. Rebecca Olson for her constructive criticism of our research methodology.

Author Contributions

Conceived and designed the experiments: JMG RRR GSK CL. Performed the experiments: JMG. Analyzed the data: JMG CL RRR GSK ESG. Contributed to the writing of the manuscript: JMG CL RRR GSK ESG.

References

1. Janssen I (2014) Active play: An important physical activity strategy in the fight against childhood obesity. Canadian Journal of Public Health 105: e22–e27.
2. Smoll FL, Smith RE (2002) Children and youth in sport: A biopsychosocial perspective (2nd ed.). Dubuque, IA: Kendall-Hunt.
3. Conroy DE, Coatsworth JD (2006) Coach training as a strategy for promoting youth social development. The Sport Psychologist 20: 128–144.
4. Smith RE, Smoll FL (1997) Coaching the coaches: Youth sports as a scientific and applied behavioral setting. Current Directions in Psychological Science 6: 16–21.
5. Tremblay MS, Gray CE, Akinroye K, Harrington DM, Katzmarzyk PT, et al. (2014) Physical activity of children: A global matrix of grades comparing 15 countries. Journal of Physical Activity and Health 11: S113–S125.
6. Active Healthy Kids Australia (2014) Is sport enough? The 2014 Australian report card on physical activity for children and young people. Adelaide, South Australia: Active Healthy Kids Australia. 1–49 p.
7. Australian Bureau of Statistics (2012) Children's participation in sport and leisure time activities, 2003 to 2012. Catalogue No. 4901.0. Canberra: Australian Bureau of Statistics; 2012.
8. Fraser-Thomas J, Côté J, Deakin J (2005) Youth sport programs: An avenue to foster positive youth development. Physical Education & Sport Pedagogy 10: 19–40.
9. Geidne S, Quennerstedt M, Eriksson C (2013) The youth sports club as a health-promoting setting: An integrative review of research. Scandinavian Journal of Public Health 41: 269–283.
10. Kokko S, Kannas L, Villberg J (2009) Health promotion profile of youth sports clubs in Finland: club officials' and coaches' perceptions. Health Promotion International 24: 26–35.
11. Strong WB, Malina RM, Blimkie CJ, Daniels SR, Dishman RK, et al. (2005) Evidence based physical activity for school-age youth. The Journal of Pediatrics 146: 732–737.
12. Guagliano JM, Rosenkranz RR, Kolt GS (2013) Girls' physical activity levels during organized sports in Australia. Medicine & Science in Sports & Exercise 45: 116–122.
13. Wickel EE, Eisenmann JC (2007) Contribution of youth sport to total daily physical activity among 6-to 12-yr-old boys. Medicine & Science in Sports & Exercise 39: 1493–1500.
14. World Health Organization (2010) Global recommendations on physical activity for health.
15. Department of Health and Aging (2014) Australia's physical activity & sedentary behaviour guidelines for children (18–64 years). Canberra: Commonwealth of Australia.
16. Department of Health and Aging (2014) Australia's physical activity & sedentary behaviour guidelines for young people (13–17 years). Canberra: Commonwealth of Australia.
17. Troiano RP, Berrigan D, Dodd KW, Mâsse LC, Tilert T, et al. (2008) Physical activity in the United States measured by accelerometer. Medicine and Science in Sports and Exercise 40: 181–188.
18. Hardy LL, Okely AD, Dobbins TA, Booth ML (2008) Physical activity among adolescents in New South Wales (Australia): 1997 and 2004. Medicine & Science in Sports & Exercise 40: 835–841.
19. Kimm SY, Glynn NW, Kriska AM, Barton BA, Kronsberg SS, et al. (2002) Decline in physical activity in black girls and white girls during adolescence. New England Journal of Medicine 347: 709–715.
20. Camacho-Miñano MJ, LaVoi NM, Barr-Anderson DJ (2011) Interventions to promote physical activity among young and adolescent girls: A systematic review. Health Education Research 26: 1025–1049.
21. Leek D, Carlson JA, Cain KL, Henrichon S, Rosenberg D, et al. (2011) Physical activity during youth sports practices. Archives of Pediatrics & Adolescent Medicine 165: 294–299.
22. Sacheck JM, Nelson T, Ficker L, Kafka T, Kuder J, et al. (2011) Physical activity during soccer and its contribution to physical activity recommendations in normal weight and overweight children. Pediatric Exercise Science 23: 281–292.
23. Dudley DA, Okely AD, Cotton WG, Pearson P, Caputi P (2012) Physical activity levels and movement skill instruction in secondary school physical education. Journal of Science and Medicine in Sport 15: 231–237.
24. Tong A, Sainsbury P, Craig J (2007) Consolidated criteria for reporting qualitative research (COREQ): A 32-item checklist for interviews and focus groups. International Journal for Quality in Health Care 19: 349–357.
25. Bryman A (2012) Social research methods. New York, NY: OUP Oxford.
26. Creswell JW (2012) Qualitative inquiry and research design: Choosing among five approaches. Thousand Oaks, CA: Sage Publications, Inc.

27. Boeije HR (2009) Analysis in qualitative research. Thousand Oaks, CA: Sage Publications Limited.
28. Australian Bureau of Statistics (2009) Children's participation in organised sport and dancing.
29. Côté J, Salmela JH, Baria A, Russell SJ (1993) Organizing and interpreting unstructured qualitative data. The Sport Psychologist 7: 127–137.
30. Tesch R (1990) Qualitative research: Analysis types and software tools. Philadelphia, PA: RoutledgeFlamer, Taylor & Francis Inc.
31. Côté J, Salmela JH (1994) A decision-making heuristic for the analysis of unstructured qualitative data. Perceptual and Motor Skills 78: 465–466.
32. Vella SA, Oades L, Crowe T (2011) The role of the coach in facilitating positive youth development: Moving from theory to practice. Journal of Applied Sport Psychology 23: 33–48.
33. Drummond JL, McGuire JG, Bennett G (2002) Student perceptions of exercise role modelling by secondary health educators. Health Education Journal 61: 78–86.
34. McKenzie TL, Sallis JF, Nader PR (1991) SOFIT: System for observing fitness instruction time. Journal of Teaching in Physical Education 11: 195–205.
35. Rottensteiner C, Laakso L, Pihlaja T, Konttinen N (2013) Personal Reasons for Withdrawal from Team Sports and the Influence of Significant Others among Youth Athletes. International Journal of Sports Science and Coaching 8: 19–32.
36. Armentrout S, Kamphoff C (2011) Organizational barriers and factors that contribute to youth hockey attrition. Journal of Sport Behavior 34: 121–136.
37. Hedstrom R, Gould D (2004) Research in youth sports: Critical issues status. White Paper Summaries of Existing Literature.
38. Fraser-Thomas J, Côté J, Deakin J (2008) Understanding dropout and prolonged engagement in adolescent competitive sport. Psychology of Sport and Exercise 9: 645–662.
39. Fraser-Thomas J, Côté J (2006) Youth sports: Implementing findings and moving forward with research. Athletic Insight 8: 12–27.
40. Mandic S, Bengoechea EG, Stevens E, de la Barra SL, Skidmore P (2012) Getting kids active by participating in sport and doing It more often: focusing on what matters. International Journal of Behavioral Nutrition and Physical Activity 9: 86.
41. Rink J, Hall TJ, Williams LH (2010) Schoolwide physical activity: A comprehensive guide to designing and conducting programs. Champaign, IL: Human Kinetics.
42. Kelder SH, Mitchell PD, McKenzie TL, Derby C, Strikmiller PK, et al. (2003) Long-term implementation of the CATCH physical education program. Health Education & Behavior 30: 463–475.
43. Ajzen I, Joyce N, Sheikh S, Cote NG (2011) Knowledge and the prediction of behavior: The role of information accuracy in the theory of planned behavior. Basic and Applied Social Psychology 33: 101–117.
44. Blomquist KB (1986) Modeling and health behavior: Strategies for prevention in the schools. Health Education 17: 8–11.
45. Fitzgerald A, Fitzgerald N, Aherne C (2012) Do peers matter? A review of peer and/or friends' influence on physical activity among American adolescents. Journal of Adolescence 35: 941–958.
46. Trost SG, Sallis JF, Pate RR, Freedson PS, Taylor WC, et al. (2003) Evaluating a model of parental influence on youth physical activity. American Journal of Preventive Medicine 25: 277–282.
47. Cox M, Schofield G, Kolt GS (2010) Responsibility for children's physical activity: Parental, child, and teacher perspectives. Journal of Science and Medicine in Sport 13: 46–52.
48. McDavid L, Cox AE, Amorose AJ (2012) The relative roles of physical education teachers and parents in adolescents' leisure-time physical activity motivation and behavior. Psychology of Sport and Exercise 13: 99–107.
49. Bélanger M, Casey M, Cormier M, Filion AL, Martin G, et al. (2011) Maintenance and decline of physical activity during adolescence: Insights from a qualitative study. International Journal of Behavioral Nutrition and Physical Activity 8: 117.
50. Bradley R, McRitchie S, Houts R, Nader P, O'Brien M (2011) Parenting and the decline of physical activity from age 9 to 15. International Journal of Behavioral Nutrition and Physical Activity 8: 33.
51. Sallis JF, Prochaska JJ, Taylor WC (2000) A review of correlates of physical activity of children and adolescents. Medicine and science in sports and exercise 32: 963–975.
52. Bauer KW, Nelson MC, Boutelle KN, Neumark-Sztainer D (2008) Parental influences on adolescents' physical activity and sedentary behavior: longitudinal findings from Project EAT-II. International Journal of Behavioral Nutrition and Physical Activity 5: 12.
53. Eime RM, Harvey JT, Craike MJ, Symons CM, Payne WR (2013) Family support and ease of access link socio-economic status and sports club membership in adolescent girls: a mediation study. International Journal of Behavioral Nutrition & Physical Activity 10: 50.
54. Timperio A, van Stralen M, Brug J, Bere E, Chinapaw M, et al. (2013) Direct and indirect associations between the family physical activity environment and sports participation among 10–12 year-old European children: testing the EnRG framework in the ENERGY project. Int J Behav Nutr Phys Act 10: 15.
55. Lubans DR, Sylva K, Morgan PJ (2007) Factors associated with physical activity in a sample of British secondary school students. Australian Journal of Educational & Developmental Psychology 7: 22–30.
56. Leberman S, LaVoi N (2011) Juggling balls and roles, working mother-coaches in youth sport: Beyond the dualistic worker-mother identity. Journal of Sport Management 25: 474–488.
57. Krefting L (1991) Rigor in qualitative research: The assessment of trustworthiness. The American Journal of Occupational Therapy 45: 214–222.
58. Patton MQ (2001) Qualitative research & evaluation methods. Thousand Oaks, CA: Sage Publications Inc.
59. Lincoln YS, Guba EA (1985) Naturalistic inquiry. Beverly Hills, CA: Sage.
60. Kelly B, King L, Bauman AE, Baur LA, Macniven R, et al. (2014) Identifying important and feasible policies and actions for health at community sports clubs: A consensus-generating approach. Journal of Science and Medicine in Sport 17: 61–68.

24

A Randomized Pilot Trial of Remote Ischemic Preconditioning in Heart Failure with Reduced Ejection Fraction

Michael A. McDonald[1]*, Juarez R. Braga[1], Jing Li[2], Cedric Manlhiot[2], Heather J. Ross[1], Andrew N. Redington[2]

1 Division of Cardiology, Peter Munk Cardiac Centre, University of Toronto, Toronto, Canada, **2** Division of Cardiology, Hospital for Sick Children, University of Toronto, Toronto, Canada

Abstract

Background: Remote ischemic preconditioning (RIPC) induced by transient limb ischemia confers multi-organ protection and improves exercise performance in the setting of tissue hypoxia. We aimed to evaluate the effect of RIPC on exercise capacity in heart failure patients.

Methods: We performed a randomized crossover trial of RIPC (4×5-minutes limb ischemia) compared to sham control in heart failure patients undergoing exercise testing. Patients were randomly allocated to either RIPC or sham prior to exercise, then crossed over and completed the alternate intervention with repeat testing. The primary outcome was peak VO2, RIPC versus sham. A mechanistic substudy was performed using dialysate from study patient blood samples obtained after sham and RIPC. This dialysate was used to test for a protective effect of RIPC in a mouse heart Langendorff model of infarction. Mouse heart infarct size with RIPC or sham dialysate exposure was also compared with historical control data.

Results: Twenty patients completed the study. RIPC was not associated with improvements in peak VO2 (15.6+/−4.2 vs 15.3+/−4.6 mL/kg/min; p = 0.53, sham and RIPC, respectively). In our Langendorff sub-study, infarct size was similar between RIPC and sham dialysate groups from our study patients, but was smaller than expected compared to healthy controls (29.0%, 27.9% [sham, RIPC] vs 51.2% [controls]. We observed less preconditioning among the subgroup of patients with increased exercise performance following RIPC ($p<0.04$).

Conclusion: In this pilot study of RIPC in heart failure patients, RIPC was not associated with improvements in exercise capacity overall. However, the degree of effect of RIPC may be inversely related to the degree of baseline preconditioning. These data provide the basis for a larger randomized trial to test the potential benefits of RIPC in patients with heart failure.

Trial Registration: ClinicalTrials.gov NCT01128790

Editor: Yoshihiro Fukumoto, Kurume University School of Medicine, Japan

Funding: The authors have no funding or support to report.

Competing Interests: Andrew Redington is co-holder of a patent and shareholder in a company developing an automated remote preconditioning device. There was no commercial funding or other involvement for this project and an automated device was not used in this study. This does not alter the authors' adherence to PLOS ONE policies on sharing data and materials.

* Email: Michael.mcdonald@uhn.on.ca

Introduction

Exercise impairment in patients with chronic heart failure (HF) is associated with significant morbidity and mortality [1–4]. Objective measures of exercise capacity continue to be important predictors of clinical outcomes, and are widely used to risk stratify HF patients for advanced therapies, including cardiac transplantation [3–5]. The effects of chronic left ventricular dysfunction and HF on exercise capacity are multifactorial, and relate to diminished cardiac output and to alterations in peripheral and respiratory skeletal muscle structure and function [6–9]. Notably, improvements in skeletal muscle function and exercise capacity are associated with improvements in left ventricular function [10], reduced hospitalization [11], and better transplant-free survival [12]. It follows that interventions to improve exercise capacity may translate into significant clinical benefits in the HF population.

Remote ischemic preconditioning (RIPC) is a well-described protective mechanism in which a transient, sub-lethal reduction in blood flow to tissues in one area of the body renders other remote tissues more resistant to subsequent episodes of prolonged ischemia [13]. Although the precise mechanisms are not fully defined, the remote ischemic preconditioning stimulus appears to trigger release of circulating factors [14–16] that result in downstream effects on mitochondrial function within the target organ(s) [13]. Early clinical application of RIPC in cardiac patients has been encouraging; transient limb ischemia, typically involving 2–4 cycles of 5–10 minutes each, has been shown to limit myocardial injury in the setting of elective cardiac or vascular surgery, as well as percutaneous coronary intervention for angina or acute myocardial infarction [17–21].

To date, the impact of RIPC in HF patients has not been explored. However, 'local' ischemic preconditioning of the legs improved maximal power output and maximal oxygen consumption during subsequent bicycle ergometry in healthy volunteers [22]. Recent work from members of our group has demonstrated that RIPC can improve maximal performance in highly trained swimmers, suggesting a salutary effect on peripheral skeletal, respiratory and cardiac muscle function under conditions of exercise induced hypoxic ischemia [23]. We therefore sought to determine whether RIPC would be associated with improvements in exercise capacity in patients with HF due to left ventricular systolic dysfunction.

Methods

The protocol for this trial and supporting CONSORT checklist are available as supporting information; see Checklist S1 and Protocol S1.

Ethics Statement

All patients provided written informed consent, and the study protocol was approved by the Research Ethics Board of the University Health Network, and registered prior to initiation (Identifier: NCT01128790, registered December 2009 at ClinicalTrials.gov). The CONSORT 2010 Statement for clinical trials was followed for the reporting of our study results herein. There are currently no ongoing clinical trials of RIPC intervention from our group at this time.

Patient Population

We performed a randomized, controlled, crossover pilot trial of patients recruited from the Heart Function Clinic at the Toronto General Hospital, a University of Toronto affiliated teaching hospital. The Heart Function Clinic is a large volume multidisciplinary clinic that manages of a broad spectrum of HF patients, including those with advanced HF referred for consideration of transplantation or mechanical circulatory support.

Ambulatory clinic patients scheduled for routine cardiopulmonary stress testing were approached for study inclusion if they met all of the following criteria: ≥18 years of age, left ventricular ejection fraction (LVEF) <40%, history of New York Heart Association (NYHA) class II–IV symptoms, HF for at least 12 weeks, and clinical stability. Patients were initially excluded for any of the following reasons: ischemic cardiomyopathy, cardiovascular related hospitalization within the preceding four weeks, diabetes, peripheral neuropathy, inability to exercise or other contraindications to stress testing, inability or unwillingness to participate in serial exercise testing. Patients were enrolled and followed from September 2009 to February 2011. Following study initiation, there were comparatively few patients from our clinic population with non-ischemic cardiomyopathy who met all other inclusion criteria, and we therefore modified our protocol to include patients with stable underlying coronary disease that were otherwise eligible. All other exclusion criteria were maintained throughout the study.

Study Protocol

Patients were approached for participation and consent was obtained prior to their scheduled cardiopulmonary exercise test. Immediately prior to testing, patients were randomized by one of the investigators (MM or JB) in a 1:1 ratio by computer generated allocation sequence, to the order in which they received either RIPC intervention or sham intervention. Patients then crossed over to receive the alternate intervention at a dedicated follow-up visit for repeat exercise testing. Where possible, patients were scheduled for a second exercise study within four weeks to minimize the potential impact of disease progression or any interim therapeutic intervention on exercise capacity. Throughout the duration of the trial, patients were unaware of the expected effects of the sham or RIPC treatment and investigators (other than those performing the intervention) remained blinded to treatment assignment.

The RIPC stimulus consisted of four cycles of 5 minutes of upper limb ischemia followed by 5 minutes of reperfusion. A blood pressure cuff was placed over the upper arm, and limb ischemia was achieved by inflating the cuff 20 mmHg above the systolic pressure. The sham intervention consisted of four cycles of 5 minutes of blood pressure cuff inflation to only 10 mmHg, interspersed with 5 minutes of cuff deflation to simulate reperfusion. After completing four cycles of either intervention, 30 mL of blood was drawn, placed on ice and transferred to the investigators' laboratory as part of the pre-specified mechanistic sub-study. Immediately thereafter, patients completed a cardiopulmonary exercise test with respiratory gas analysis according to a routine stationary bicycle ramp protocol (10 Watt per minute incremental workload). Testing was symptom limited after achieving a diagnostic workload, defined as a respiratory exchange ratio >1.05. A dedicated exercise physiologist who was unaware of the treatment assignment supervised all tests, and a blinded investigator (HR) reported the results.

The primary outcome measure was peak oxygen consumption (VO2) measured in milliliters of oxygen consumed per kilogram of body mass per minute (mL/kg/min) during peak exercise following sham intervention compared to peak VO2 following RIPC intervention. Secondary outcomes included a comparison of exercise duration, workload achieved, ventilatory anaerobic threshold, absolute peak VO2, and the slope of the minute ventilation (VE) to carbon dioxide production (VCO2) ratio. As this pilot study was exploratory in nature and undertaken for feasibility, no sample size calculations were performed. We estimated that 20 patients with paired exercise data would represent an adequate sample to inform future trial design and generate appropriate study hypotheses.

Sub-study Protocol

We conducted a pre-specified sub-study to assess whether HF patients elaborate circulating protective factor(s) in response to a RIPC stimulus. The animal protocols used for this study were approved by the Animal care and Use Committee of the Hospital for Sick Children in Toronto and conformed with the Guide for the Care and Use of Laboratory Animals published by the National Institutes of Health (publication # 85-23, revised 1996). The 30 mL of blood drawn immediately following the RIPC or sham intervention was collected in heparinized tubes and placed on ice. It was subsequently centrifuged at 3000 rpm for 20 minutes at room temperature and the plasma fraction was dialyzed against a 20 fold volume of Krebs-Henseleit solution across a 12–14 kDa dialysis membrane. The dialysate was then prepared for use in a mouse heart Langendorff model as previously described [23]. Briefly, the dialysate was made isotonic and adjusted to pH 7.4 with sodium bicarbonate and glucose. Prior to perfusion of the mouse hearts, D-glucose, $NaHCO_3$ and EDTA were added to a final concentration of 15 mM, 25 mM and 0.5 mM in the dialysate, respectively. Mice were anesthetized with pentobarbital in standard fashion and the hearts were excised, cannulated at the aorta, and perfused with modified Krebs-Ringer buffer at 37°C. A water-filled latex balloon was inserted into the left ventricle, connected to a pressure transducer and maintained at 7–10 mmHg to allow beat to beat measurement of left ventricular pressures (PowerLab data acquisition system AD Instruments; Colorado Springs, CO, USA). Dialysate derived from each patient for both sham and RIPC conditions was used to perfuse 2–4 mouse hearts, and data from each preparation was averaged.

Following a 20 minute stabilization period, the hearts were perfused with the study patient dialysate solution and then subjected to 30 minutes of no-flow ischemia followed by 60 minutes of reperfusion. After completing the protocol, the hearts were frozen at −80°C. Each heart was then sectioned into 1 mm thick slices and stained with 1.25% 2,3,5-triphynyltetrazolium chloride to distinguish areas of infarcted tissue (white colour) from non-infarcted tissue (red colour). The slices were formalin fixed and scanned into Photoshop. Using this method, it was possible to trace the area of infarcted tissue and express this as a proportion of the total area of LV myocardium at risk. The primary endpoint of this Langendorff sub-study was infarct area in hearts perfused with sham dialysate versus infarct area in hearts perfused with RIPC dialysate. Secondary endpoints included LV developed pressure, LV end-diastolic pressure, maximum rate of systolic pressure rise (dP/dt max) and fall (dP/dt min). Infarct size observed after sham or RIPC dialysate exposure in heart failure patients described above was also compared with infarct size observed using an identical sham and RIPC procedure to prepare dialysate from 4 healthy subjects serving as historical controls (4 males, age range 25–50 years).

Statistical Analysis

Continuous data are reported as means with standard deviation, and categorical data are reported as frequencies. Normality of the distribution of continuous variables was tested using the Shapiro-Wilks test. Differences in exercise outcomes between sham control and RIPC intervention were assessed using paired t-tests. Logistic regression model was used to identify factors associated with response to RIPC, with relative difference between RIPC and Sham used as a dependent variable and each categorical variable or each tertile of continuous variables as independent predictors. A p-value of <0.05 was considered significant for all comparisons. All analyses were performed using SPSS for Windows v 11.0 (SPSS Inc., Chicago, IL).

Results

Main Study

Figure 1 outlines the patient flow through the study. In total, 22 patients consented to participate from September 2009 to January 2011, and all 22 were randomized and subsequently completed the assigned first intervention prior to undergoing the initial cardiopulmonary exercise stress test. Two patients, both allocated to the initial sham control group, withdrew from the study and declined to undergo follow-up exercise testing. Therefore, the final study population included in the analysis consisted of 20 patients who completed the protocol with both sham and RIPC interventions.

The baseline characteristics of the study patients are shown in Table 1. As outlined, the majority were males with non-ischemic cardiomyopathy. All patients were treated with beta blockers and ACE inhibitors, 70% required loop diuretics, and a large proportion of patients had received a defibrillator and/or cardiac resynchronization therapy. Although all patients had previously been characterized as NYHA class II, III, or IV, most were minimally symptomatic at the time of enrollment.

The majority of patients in this study (16/20) completed sequential cardiopulmonary exercise tests within 30 days as planned. Two patients were unable to return for scheduled follow-up testing for logistical reasons and completed the protocol within 90 days, and an additional two patients completed follow-up by 180 days. There were no adverse effects observed for any of our study patients. The results for the primary outcome, peak VO2 for RIPC compared to sham intervention, are shown in Figure 2 and Table 2. Overall, RIPC prior to cardiopulmonary exercise testing was not associated with improvements in peak VO2 in this population (15.6+/−4.2 mL/kg/min vs 15.3+/−4.6 mL/kg/min; p = 0.53, for sham and RIPC, respectively). With respect to the secondary outcomes, there was no observed benefit of RIPC on exercise duration, workload achieved, anaerobic threshold, or VE/CO2 slope (Table 2). Excluding patients that did not complete the protocol within 30 days had no impact on our results. Moreover, post-hoc exploratory analysis did not identify any baseline clinical characteristics, (including age, gender, duration of heart failure, functional class, BNP level) associated with an improved peak VO2 following RIPC intervention. Finally, the sequence of testing did not appear to have an effect on our results, as there were no significant differences in peak VO2 from the initial exercise study compared to the follow-up study, irrespective of the treatment allocation.

Langendorff Sub Study

In the Langendorff study, there was no significant difference in infarct area between mouse hearts perfused with sham dialysate and those perfused with RIPC dialysate (29.0+/−7.9% versus 27.9+/−6.8%; p = 0.62). Additionally, the secondary endpoint hemodynamic measurements were not significantly different at any stage following perfusion with either sham or RIPC derived dialysate.

Using this Langendorff model, we undertook a further exploratory comparison of infarct size following perfusion with dialysate derived from our heart failure study population versus infarct size following perfusion with dialysate derived from plasma from healthy controls undergoing sham/RIPC intervention. The infarct size observed in hearts perfused with dialysate from our heart failure patients was nearly 45% less than the infarct size observed in hearts perfused with healthy control dialysate following sham intervention. Moreover, the infarct area seen in our study approximates the infarct area seen with exposure to dialysate from healthy control subjects following RIPC intervention (Figure 3).

In order to determine whether the apparent lack of effect of RIPC in our study population could be explained by a high degree of baseline preconditioning, we assessed infarct size in the Langendorff model according to clinical response to RIPC treatment. In this post hoc analysis, mouse infarct size was significantly smaller among the subgroup of patients who had no improvement in exercise capacity following RIPC intervention, suggesting that the overall absence of a clinical response to RIPC in our study population may relate to a higher degree of preconditioning at baseline for the majority of patients (Figure 4).

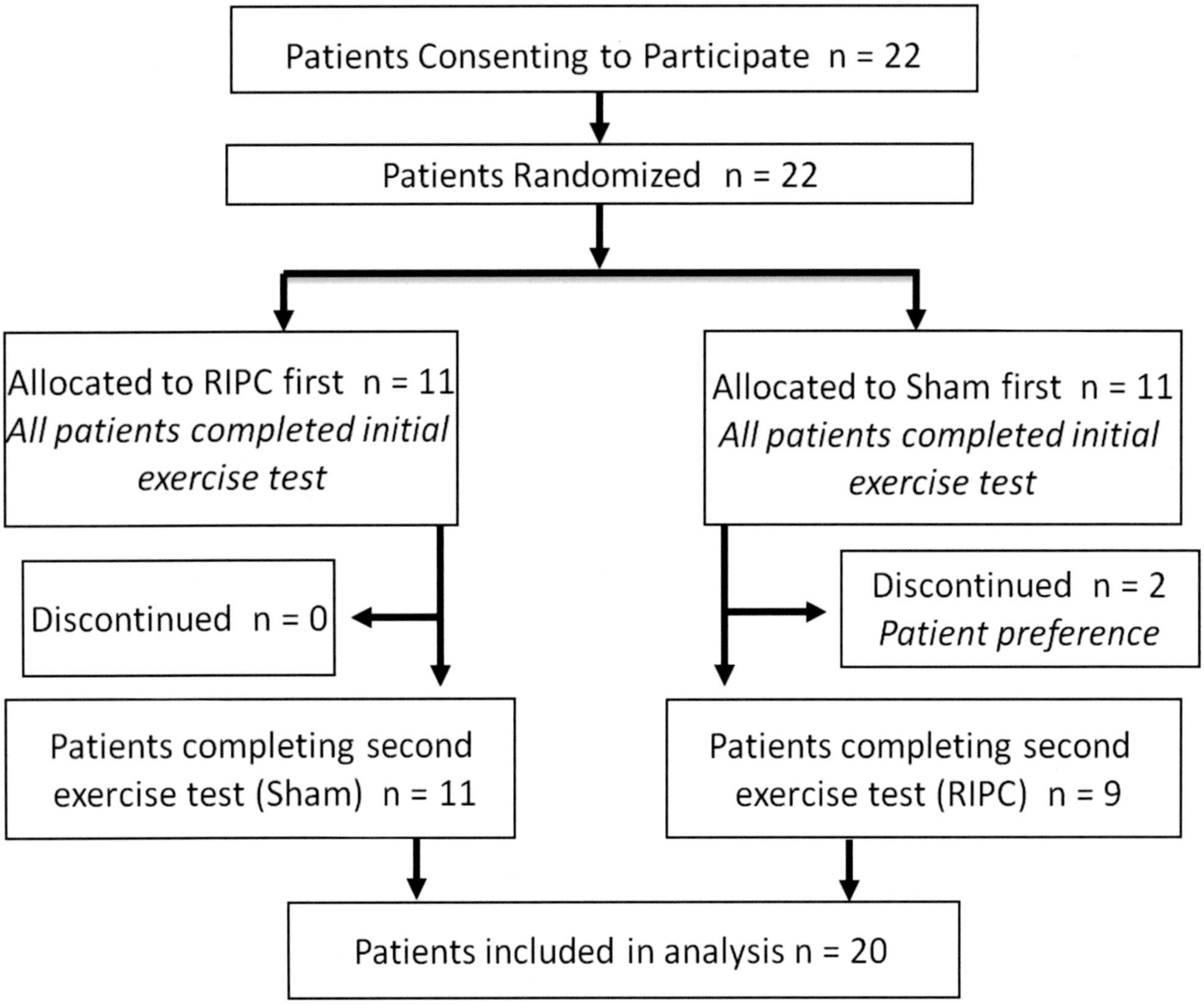

Figure 1. Patient flow through the study. 22 patients consented to participate in the study. Two patients declined repeat testing and were excluded from the analysis; 20 patients complete the study protocol with paired testing.

Discussion

In this randomized crossover pilot study, RIPC was not associated with improvements in objective measures of exercise capacity in ambulatory HF patients with left ventricular dysfunction. Specifically, there was no overall benefit with respect to any of the prognostically important exercise variables, including peak VO2, exercise duration, workload achieved or VE/VCO2 slope during cardiopulmonary stress testing. A principle finding from our Langendorff sub-study was that RIPC in this study population does not appear to confer additional protection against ischemia reperfusion injury through release of circulating preconditioning factor(s). This observation is in contrast with the effects of RIPC in a healthy control population [23]; moreover our results suggest that patients with chronic HF may already be relatively preconditioned.

To our knowledge, this is the first clinical trial to evaluate the effect of RIPC in a heart failure population. There is a growing body of evidence that suggests RIPC induced by transient limb ischemia, similar to the protocol used in our study, is associated with a significant reduction in end organ injury due to a variety of ischemic stressors. One of the earliest clinical studies of RIPC was a randomized controlled trial of 37 pediatric patients undergoing cardiopulmonary bypass for corrective cardiac surgery [17]. In this study, four 5-minute cycles of limb ischemia and reperfusion resulted in less troponin elevation, lower inotrope requirements, and better lung function in the early post-operative setting. RIPC with lower limb ischemia was also shown to attenuate myocardial and renal injury in a randomized controlled trial of 82 patients undergoing elective abdominal aortic aneurysm repair [19]. These early trials have supported the observation that RIPC confers multisystem protection in an ischemic environment.

Maximal exercise performance is limited by 'relative' ischemia of skeletal muscle and is associated with tissue hypoxia and lactic acid accumulation, and thus can be considered a form of ischemic stress. Recently, the potential benefits of ischemic preconditioning have extended into the domain of exercise performance in healthy individuals. de Groot and colleagues showed that ischemic preconditioning of each leg prior to bicycle exercise testing improved both maximal workload and maximal oxygen consumption [22] in healthy volunteers. Members of our group have shown that RIPC induced by transient upper limb ischemia immediately

Table 1. Baseline characteristics of the study population.

Age (years)	56.3+/−11.8
Male	18 (90)
Duration of heart failure (months)	71.3+/−63.4
Etiology:	
Ischemic	4 (20)
Non-ischemic	16 (80)
LVEF (%)	29.3+/−6.8
NYHA functional class:	
I	5 (25)
II	10 (50)
III	5 (25)
IV	-
HTN*	3 (15)
Smoking history:	
Never	11 (55)
Prior	8 (40)
Current	1 (5)
Atrial fibrillation	6 (30)
Medications:	
ACE inhibitor/ARB†	20 (100)
Beta blocker	20 (100)
Spironolactone	10 (50)
Digoxin	7 (35)
Loop diuretic	14 (70)
Nitrate	2 (10)
AICD‡	12 (60)
CRTˡ	5 (25)
Systolic blood pressure (mmHg)	105.7+/−12.8
Diastolic blood pressure (mmHg)	69+/−9.9
Heart rate (beats/min)	64.8+/−7.8
Height (cm)	178.6+/−8.6
Weight (kg)	94.7+/−22.5
Hemoglobin (g/L)	145.4+/−14.8
Serum creatinine (μmol/L)	94+/−22.5
Serum sodium (mmol/L)	138.5+/−2.7
BNP# (pg/mL)	Range 10.0–1616.0

(N = 20).
Values are expressed as means +/− standard deviation, or numbers and percentages.
*HTN: hypertension.
†ARB: angiotensin receptor blocker.
‡AICD: automated implantable cardioverter-defibrillator.
ˡCRT: cardiac resynchronization therapy.
#BNP: B-type natriuretic peptide.

prior to exercise was associated with significant improvements in competitive swim times in elite athletes [23]. Furthermore, dialyzed serum taken from the swimmers following RIPC (but not serum taken before) was shown to carry a circulating "protective factor" that significantly reduced infarct size in a mouse Langendorff model of ischemia-reperfusion [23], confirming the importance of humoral-mediated pathways discussed earlier [14–16]. Prior to performing our study, we hypothesized that RIPC may have a favorable impact on exercise capacity of HF patients who are subject to musculoskeletal and cardiac ischemia as they reach an anaerobic state at peak exercise. These patients have poor exercise tolerance secondary to reduced cardiac output, abnormalities in myocyte fibre composition, and reduced mitochondrial density [7–9]. Any intervention to improve exercise performance in a HF population with various physiologic limitations could potentially translate into important clinical benefits.

Why then was there no overall impact of RIPC on exercise capacity in this study, despite using a conventional preconditioning protocol? The answer to this question may be multifactorial, but

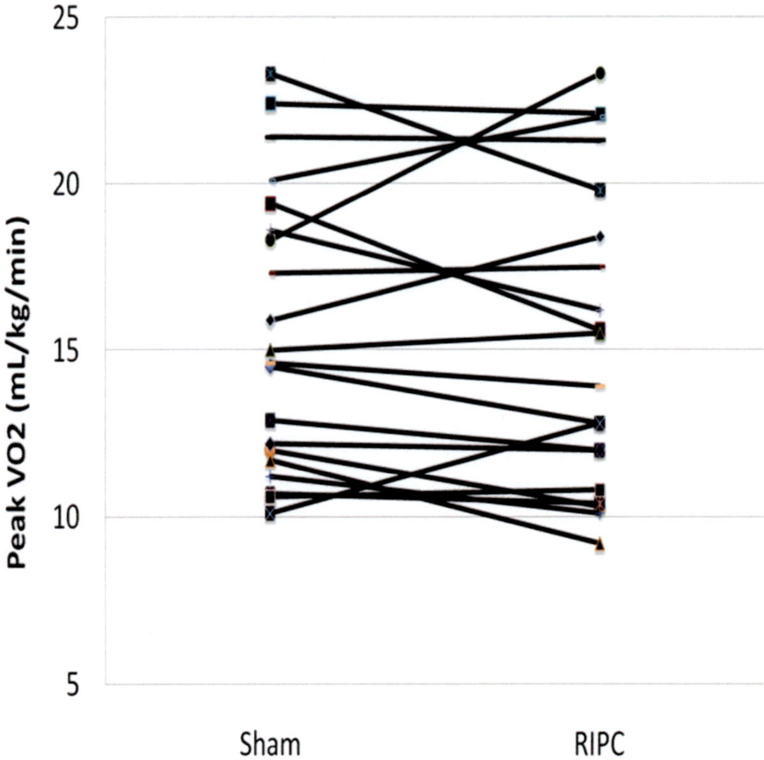

Figure 2. Individual exercise test results for sham versus RIPC intervention. Peak VO2 is shown for all study subjects undergoing exercise stress testing immediately following sham and RIPC interventions.

our Langendorff study provides important new evidence to suggest that these patients may already be in a 'preconditioned state'. Indeed, our results show that plasma obtained after sham intervention already contained dialyzable circulating cardioprotective factors characteristic of those liberated by remote preconditioning stimuli [14–16]. Consequently, overall the level of cardioprotection observed in control dialysate from the heart failure patients was similar to that seen after RIPC in normal volunteers, and was unaffected by additional RIPC. The reason for this is less clear however. There is emerging evidence that vigorous exercise in healthy subjects itself is a stimulus for release of cardioprotective factors [24]. We speculate that daily activities in HF patients may act as a similar stimulus to the release of cardioprotective factors as a result of skeletal muscle ischemia. It is also possible that the heart may act as a paracrine organ for the release of cardioprotective factors. For example, Dickson and colleagues have shown that coronary effluent from hearts subjected to brief periods of ischemia is cardioprotective in an untreated acceptor heart [25].

Irrespective of where the circulating factors originate, our data do suggest that there may be a subgroup of heart failure patients that might respond to RIPC. Although the numbers were small, when we compared those that had significantly improved exercise performance with RIPC, versus those that did not, there was also a

Table 2. Exercise performance of Sham control versus RIPC intervention.

	Sham	RIPC	P value
Peak VO2 (ml/kg/min)	15.6+/−4.2	15.3+/−4.6	0.53
Secondary Endpoints:			
Exercise duration (minutes)	10.3+/−3.0	11.0+/−3.0	0.13
Workload (watts)	108.5+/−29.8	103.0+/−32.6	0.07
AT* (ml/kg/min)	9.6+/−2.6	9.6+/−3.0	0.98
Peak VO2† (L/min)	1.45+/−0.36	1.42+/−0.42	0.39
VE/VECO2‡ slope	28.7+/−4.3	29.9+/−5.4	0.06

(N = 20).
Values expressed as means +/− standard deviation.
*AT: anaerobic threshold.
†VO2: oxygen uptake.
‡VE/VCO2: minute ventilation - carbon dioxide production ratio.

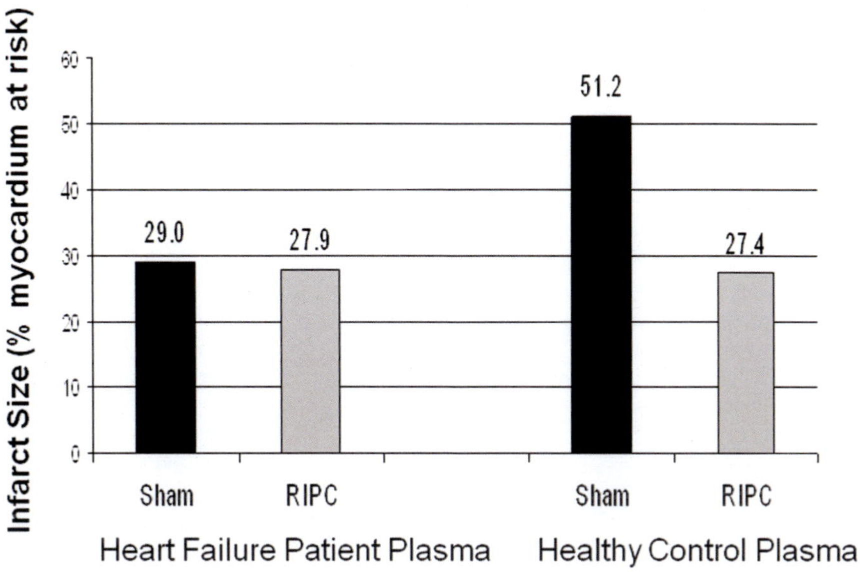

Figure 3. Langendorff mouse heart infarct size after perfusion with dialysate from heart failure patients versus healthy controls. Heart failure patient dialysate, irrespective of RIPC or sham treatment, reduced infarct to the same extent as the dialysate from RIPC-treated healthy controls, as compared to sham treated healthy controls.

significant difference in the level of cardioprotection afforded by their plasma dialysate in the mouse Langendorff studies. Plasma from patients that showed improvement in exercise capacity had lower baseline protection against ischemia, suggesting that their degree of baseline preconditioning was lower, and hence their capacity to respond to RIPC was higher.

It is also important to note, that while we were able to demonstrate the presence of circulating cardioprotective factors in vitro, we cannot confirm that they are the same as those induced by RIPC, nor can we confirm that they have any effect in-vivo in our HF patients. In pre-clinical studies, older age and underlying cardiac dysfunction have been shown to result in abnormal mitochondrial permeability transition pore and kATP channel

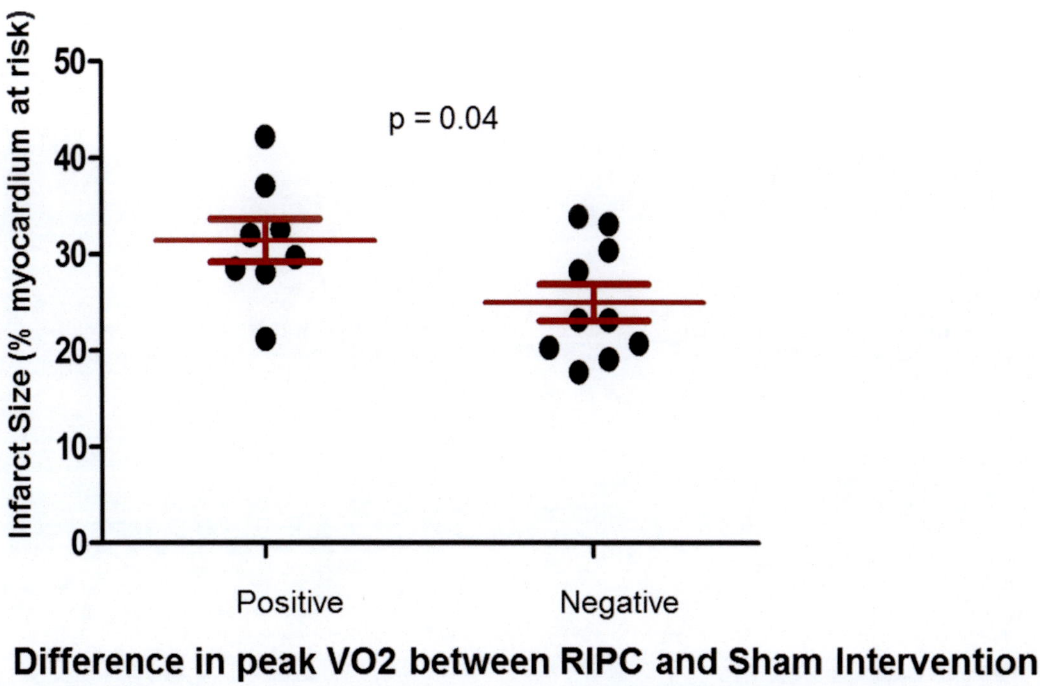

Figure 4. Infarct size stratified by the effect of RIPC on exercise performance. In the Langendorff model, mean infarct size was significantly smaller after perfusion with dialysate from the subgroup of patients who had no improvement in exercise performance following RIPC treatment. Data are presented as mean +/− SD % of infarcted myocardium.

function that may blunt the effects of RIPC [26,27]. There are also well documented ultrastructural changes in peripheral skeletal muscle associated with impairments in oxidative capacity [7–9,28], and the implications for ischemic preconditioning remain unclear. Failing myocardium also undergoes ultrastructural adaptation characterized by fetal gene reprogramming, with a decreased rate of aerobic metabolism and relative resistance to ischemia [29,30]. Coupled with the observation that mitochondrial kATP channels are endogenously activated in heart failure [27], all of this data suggest that in the clinical domain, RIPC may not yield significant additional protection from ischemic stress in a relatively 'preconditioned' HF state. While our pilot data show that there appears to be a subgroup of patients that benefit most from RIPC (those with low baseline preconditioning), in the absence of a clinical test of 'pre-existing preconditioning' the widespread adoption of RIPC as a clinical tool will require demonstration of effect in large, unselected, cohort studies. In this regard, it is likely that our study was underpowered to detect a small, but still meaningful difference in peak VO2 between RIPC intervention and sham control exercise tests. Based on the results from our pilot data, future trials would need an approximately 4–5 fold our sample size to have at least 80% power to detect a clinically important difference of 1–2 mL/kg/min in peak VO2. Smaller degrees of improvement would not likely translate into better transplant free survival [12].

Our study has a number of important limitations that may warrant caution in the interpretation of our results. Our post-hoc subgroup analysis of 'responders' versus 'non-responders' to RIPC, is not only somewhat artificial in terms of examining responses in a binary fashion, but also does not allow meaningful analysis of factors associated with those response, beyond the reported differences in cardioprotective activity of their plasma. A number of comorbidities and medications have been associated with either blunted or enhanced responses to ischemia-reperfusion injury and preconditioning [31,32]. As we did not exclude patients with comorbidities such as hypertension, dyslipidemia or left ventricular hypertrophy, and we did not perform a medication washout prior to testing, it is possible that our results may have been confounded. The impact of residual medications such as ACE inhibitors and statins in the Langendorff perfusate is indeterminate, and it is conceivable that these therapies may have modified the preconditioning response in the mouse heart. Although our model has previously been used to demonstrate the presence of a humoral mediator of RIPC [23], it is also possible that some of the larger sized key mediators of preconditioning were filtered from plasma while preparing the dialysate. For example, Giricz and colleagues recently demonstrated that extracellular vesicles (exosomes and microvesicles) may be necessary to confer protection in a rat heart Langendorff model of ischemic preconditioning [33]. Furthermore, we did not measure lactic acid levels to confirm a state of relative hypoxia with anaerobic metabolism at peak exercise. However, our cardiopulmonary exercise protocol with respiratory gas analysis did allow for an estimation of anaerobic threshold as a surrogate for lactic acidosis. Finally, patients in our trial had considerable variability in their inter-test intervals. Although we attempted to repeat paired exercise tests within 4 weeks from enrollment, we were unable to achieve this for all patients, providing the opportunity for bias due to changes in treatment or clinical status between tests.

In summary, we conducted the first randomized controlled trial of RIPC in ambulatory patients with HF and left ventricular systolic dysfunction. In this study, RIPC was not associated with improvements in objective measures of exercise capacity. The apparent absence of an effect of RIPC may relate to a high degree of baseline preconditioning in our patient population, and those with lesser degrees may be benefit with RIPC. However large, adequately powered clinical trials and further mechanistic translational studies are needed before the effects of RIPC in HF can be established definitively.

Acknowledgments

We wish to thank Michael Walker for his expertise in exercise physiology and cardiopulmonary stress testing

Author Contributions

Conceived and designed the experiments: MM HR AR. Performed the experiments: MM JB JL. Analyzed the data: MM JB JL CM. Contributed reagents/materials/analysis tools: JL HR AR. Wrote the paper: MM CM AR.

References

1. McElroy PA, Janicki JS, Weber KT (1988) Cardiopulmonary exercise testing in congestive heart failure. Am J Cardiol 62: 35A–40A.
2. Mancini DM, Eisen H, Kussmaul W, Mull R, Edmunds LH Jr, et al (1991) Value of peak exercise oxygen consumption for optimal timing of cardiac transplantation in ambulatory patients with heart failure. Circulation 83: 778–86.
3. Pardaens K, Van Cleemput J, Vanhaecke J, Fagard RH (2000) Peak oxygen uptake better predicts outcome than submaximal respiratory data in heart transplant candidates. Circulation 101: 1152–57.
4. O'Neill JO, Young JB, Pothier CE, Lauer MS (2005) Peak oxygen consumption as a predictor of death in patients with heart failure receiving beta-blockers. Circulation 111: 2313–18.
5. Aaronson KD, Schwartz JS, Chen TM, Wong KL, Goin JE, et al (1997) Development and prospective validation of a clinical index to predict survival in ambulatory patients referred for cardiac transplant evaluation. Circulation 95: 2660–67.
6. Wilson JR, Martin JL, Ferraro N (1984) Impaired skeletal muscle nutritive flow during exercise in patients with congestive heart failure: role of cardiac pump dysfunction as determined by the effect of dobutamine. Am J Cardiol 53: 1308–15.
7. Mancini DM, Coyle E, Coggan A, Beltz J, Ferraro N, et al (1989) Contribution of intrinsic skeletal muscle changes to 31P NMR skeletal muscle metabolic abnormalities in patients with chronic heart failure. Circulation 80: 1338–46.
8. Duscha BD, Kraus WE, Keteyian SJ, Sullivan MJ, Green HJ, et al (1999) Capillary density of skeletal muscle: a contributing mechanism for exercise intolerance in class II–III chronic heart failure independent of other peripheral alterations. J Am Coll Cardiol 33: 1956–63.
9. Hambrecht R, Fiehn E, Yu J, Niebauer J, Weigl C, et al (1997) Effects of endurance training on mitochondrial ultrastructure and fibre type distribution in skeletal muscle of patients with stable chronic heart failure. J Am Coll Cardio 29: 1067–73.
10. Haykowsky MJ, Liang Y, Pechter D, Jones LW, McAlister FA, et al (2007) A meta-analysis of the effect of exercise training on left ventricular remodeling in heart failure patients. The benefit depends on the type of training performed. J Am Coll Cardiol 49: 2329–36.
11. O'Connor CM, Whellan DJ, Lee KL, Keteyian SJ, Cooper LS, et al (2009) Efficacy and safety of exercise training in patients with chronic heart failure: HF-ACTION randomized controlled trial. JAMA 301: 1439–50.
12. Stevenson LW, Steimle AE, Fonarow G, Kermani M, Kermani D, et al (1995) Improvement in exercise capacity of candidates awaiting heart transplantation. J Am Coll Cardiol 25: 163–70.
13. Kharbanda RK, Nielsen TT, Redington AN (2009) Translation of remote ischaemic preconditioning into clinical practice. Lancet 374: 1557–65.
14. Shimizu M, Tropak M, Diaz RJ, Suto F, Surendra H, et al (2009) Transient limb ischaemia remotely preconditions through a humoral mechanism acting

directly on the myocardium ; evidence suggesting cross-species protection. Clin Sci (Lond) 117: 191–200.
15. Steensrud T, Li J, Dai X, Manlhiot C, Kharbanda RK, et al (2010) Pretreatment with the nitric oxide donor SNAP or nerve transection blocks humoral preconditioning by remote limb ischemia or intra-arterial adenosine. Am J Physiol 299: H1598–603.
16. Redington KL, Disenhouse T, Strantzas SC Gladstone R, Wei C, et al (2012) Remote cardioprotection by direct peripheral nerve stimulation and topical capsaicin is mediated by circulating humoral factors. Basic Res Cardiol 107: 1–10.
17. Cheung MM, Kharbanda RK, Konstantinov IE, Shimitzu IE, Shimizu M, et al (2006) Randomized controlled trial of the effects of remote ischemic preconditioning on children undergoing cardiac surgery: first clinical application in humans. J Am Coll Cardiol 47: 2277–82.
18. Venugopal V, Hausenloy DJ, Ludman A, Di Salvo C, Kolvekar S, et al (2009) Remote ischaemic preconditioning reduces myocardial injury in patients undergoing cardiac surgery with cold-blood cardioplegia: a randomised controlled trial. Heart 95: 1567–71.
19. Ali ZA, Callaghan CJ, Lim E, Ali AA, Nouraei SA, et al (2007) Remote ischemic preconditioning reduces myocardial and renal injury after elective abdominal aortic aneurysm repair: a randomized controlled trial. Circulation 116(11 Suppl): I98–105.
20. Hoole SP, Heck PM, Sharples L, Khan SN, Duehmke R, et al (2009) Cardiac remote ischemic preconditioning in coronary stenting (CRISP Stent) study: a prospective randomized control trial. Circulation 119: 820–7.
21. Botker HE, Kharbanda R Schmidt MR, Bottcher M, Kaltoft AK, et al (2010) Remote ischaemic conditioning before hospital admission, as a complement to angioplasty, and effect on myocardial salvage in pateints with acute myocardial infarction: a randomized trial. Lancet 375: 727–34.
22. de Groot PC, Thijssen DH, Sanchez M, Ellenkamp R, Hopman MT (2010) Ischemic preconditioning improves maximal performance in humans. Eur J Appl Physio 108: 141–6.
23. Jean-St-Michel E, Manlhiot C, Li J, Tropak M, Michelsen MM, et al (2011) Remote preconditioning improves maximal performance in highly-trained athletes. Med Sci Sports Exerc 43: 1200–6.
24. Michelsen MM, Stottrup NB, Schmidt MR, Lofgren B, Jensen RV, et al (2012) Exercise induced cardioprotection is medicated by a bloodborne, transferable factor. Basic Res Cardiol 107: 1–9.
25. Dickson EW, Lorbar M, Porcaro WA, Lee WJ, Blehar DJ, et al (1999) Rabbit heart can be "preconditioned" via transfer of coronary effluent. Am J Physiol 277:H2451–7.
26. Zhu J, Rebecchi MJ, Tan M, Glass PS, Brink PR, et al (2010) Age-associated differences in activation of Akt/GSK-3beta signaling pathways and inhibition of mitochondrial permeability transition pore opening in the rat heart. J Gerontol A Biol Sci Med Sci 65: 611–9.
27. Maack C, Dabew ER, Hohl M, Schafers HJ, Hohm M (2009) Endogenous activation of mitochondrial katp channels protects human failing myocardium from hydroxyl radical-induced stunning. Circ Res 105: 811–7.
28. Hambrecht R, Niebauer J, Fiehn E, Kalberer B, Offner B, et al (1995) Physical training in patients with stable chronic heart failure: effects on cardiorespiratory fitness and ultrastructural abnormalities of leg muscles. J Am Coll Cardiol 25: 1239–49.
29. Rajabi M, Kassiotis C, Razeghi P, Taegtmeyer H (2007) Return to the fetal gene program protects the stressed heart: a strong hypothesis. Heart Fail Rev 12: 331–43.
30. Ostadal B, Ostadalova I, Kolar F, Charvatova Z, Netuka I (2009) Ontogenetic development of cardiac tolerance to oxygen deprivation – possible mechanisms. Physiol Res 58 Suppl 2: S1–12.
31. Hausenloy DJ, Botker HE, Condorelli G, Ferdinandy P, Garcia-Dorado D, et al (2013) Translating cardioprotection for patient benefit: position paper from the Working Group of Cellular Biology of the Heart of the European Society of Cardiology. Cardiovasc Res 98: 7–27.
32. Ferdinandy P, Schultz R, Baxter GF (2007) Interaction of cardiovascular risk factors with myocardial ischemia/reperfusion injury, preconditioning, and postconditioning. Pharmcol Rev 59: 418–58.
33. Giricz A, Varga ZV, Baranyai T, Sipos P, Paloczi K, et al (2014) Cardioprotection by remote ischemic preconditioning of the rat heart is mediated by extracellular vesicles. J Mol Cell Cardiol 68: 75–78.

25

Resistance Training Improves Hemodynamic Function, Collagen Deposition and Inflammatory Profiles: Experimental Model of Heart Failure

Jadson P. Alves[1], Ramiro B. Nunes[1], Giuseppe P. Stefani[1], Pedro Dal Lago[1,2]*

1 Laboratory of Physiology, Universidade Federal de Ciências da Saúde de Porto Alegre (UFCSPA), Porto Alegre, Rio Grande do Sul, Brazil, **2** Department of Physical Therapy, Universidade Federal de Ciências da Saúde de Porto Alegre (UFCSPA), Porto Alegre, Rio Grande do Sul, Brazil

Abstract

The role of resistance training on collagen deposition, the inflammatory profile and muscle weakness in heart failure remains unclear. Therefore, this study evaluated the influence of a resistance training program on hemodynamic function, maximum strength gain, collagen deposition and inflammatory profile in chronic heart failure rats. Thirty-two male Wistar rats submitted to myocardial infarction by coronary artery ligation or sham surgery were assigned into four groups: sedentary sham (S-Sham, n = 8); trained sham (T-Sham, n = 8); sedentary chronic heart failure (S-CHF, n = 8) and trained chronic heart failure (T-CHF, n = 8). The maximum strength capacity was evaluated by the one maximum repetition test. Trained groups were submitted to an 8-week resistance training program (4 days/week, 4 sets of 10–12 repetitions/session, at 65% to 75% of one maximum repetition). After 8 weeks of the resistance training program, the T-CHF group showed lower left ventricular end diastolic pressure ($P<0.001$), higher left ventricular systolic pressure ($P<0.05$), higher systolic blood pressure ($P<0.05$), an improvement in the maximal positive derivative of ventricular pressure ($P<0.05$) and maximal negative derivative of ventricular pressure ($P<0.05$) when compared to the S-CHF group; no differences were observed when compared to Sham groups. In addition, resistance training was able to reduce myocardial hypertrophy ($P<0.05$), left ventricular total collagen volume fraction ($P<0.01$), IL-6 ($P<0.05$), and TNF-α/IL-10 ratio ($P<0.05$), as well as increasing IL-10 ($P<0.05$) in chronic heart failure rats when compared to the S-CHF group. Eight weeks of resistance training promotes an improvement of cardiac function, strength gain, collagen deposition and inflammatory profile in chronic heart failure rats.

Editor: Xiongwen Chen, Temple University, United States of America

Funding: This work was supported by grants from the following: CAPES and CNPq, Brasília, Brazil, and PROAP/UFCSPA, Porto Alegre, Brazil (http://www.capes.gov.br/; http://www.ufcspa.edu.br/). The funders had no role in study design, data collection and analysis, decision to publish, or preparation of the manuscript.

Competing Interests: The authors have declared that no competing interests exist.

* Email: pdallago@ufcspa.edu.br

Introduction

Chronic heart failure (CHF) is a complex clinical syndrome produced by structural and functional disorders of the heart [1]. Patients with CHF present exercise intolerance; this limitation cannot be solely attributed to cardiac and pulmonary damage [2]. Additionally, abnormalities in skeletal muscle probably contribute to the development of symptoms and exercise intolerance in CHF [3–5].

Damage to the cardiac muscle and to the extracellular matrix leads to changes in the size, shape, and function of the left ventricle, resulting in changes in the entire heart, in a process named cardiac remodeling [6], which affects prognosis and survival in patients with CHF [7]. The increase in fibrous tissue has been observed in animal models of heart failure, and there is also evidence that the same mechanism occurs in human heart failure [8]. Additionally, the extent of damage in collagen is correlated with the degree of expansion of infarction [9]. The accumulation of collagen in places remote to myocardial infarction (MI) is the main negative component of structural remodeling in heart failure of an ischemic origin [10].

The positive effects of exercise on the pathophysiology of CHF have been reported in recent years [11,12], and exercise protocols, such as resistance training (RT), appear to be an auxiliary strategy combined with aerobic training in cardiac rehabilitation programs [13]. The regular practice of physical exercise not only reverses the musculoskeletal changes attributed to physical inactivity, but also inhibits the inflammatory process induced by CHF by increasing anti-inflammatory agents [14].

In response to the effects caused by a physical training program, the heart will develop adaptations of the myocardium, causing a physiological state of cardiac remodeling. These morphological changes may differ depending on the type of training and are clinically characterized by changes in heart size and shape, due to increased load [15]. The RT prescribed with appropriate intensity is associated with a lower hemodynamic load than most of the prescriptions related to submaximal aerobic training, and still may have an additional benefit in reducing the peripheral limitations, which is a common feature found in patients with CHF [16].

Some studies have demonstrated the benefits of RT in patients with CHF [17–20], but the effects of RT on cardiac remodeling and inflammatory profiles are poorly understood. In animal models of CHF, to the best of our knowledge, there are no studies that have evaluated the physiological responses of RT. Therefore, we hypothesized that RT and, consequently, the strength gain could be associated with improvements of cardiac function in rats with CHF. Consequently, the aim of the present study was to evaluate the effects of RT on hemodynamic function, maximal strength gain, collagen deposition and inflammatory profile in rats with CHF.

Methods

Ethical Approval

The investigation followed the ethical rules established by the Guide for the Care and Use of Experimental Animals published by the National Institute of Health (NIH publication no. 85-23, revised in 1996). All of the procedures outlined in this study were approved by the Ethics Committee Research of the UFCSPA (protocol 007-10).Thirty-two male Wistar rats (220 to 270 g; 90 days of age) obtained from the Animal Breeding Unit of the Universidade Federal de Ciências da Saúde de Porto Alegre were housed under standard conditions (food and water *ad libitum*, 12:12-h light-dark cycle; 22°C).

Surgery to induce MI

Rats were anesthetized with xylazine (12 mg/kg i.p.) and ketamine (90 mg/kg i.p.) and artificially ventilated (SamWay VR 15; 60 breaths/min). After thoracotomy, coronary artery ligation (CAL) was performed to induce MI. The sham animals underwent the same procedure without artery ligation, as described previously [21].

Experimental design

After MI, the rats were allowed a minimum of 6 weeks of recovery (the necessary time to achieve the development of the CHF state) [22,23]. The animals were assigned to four experimental groups: sedentary sham (S-Sham, n = 8), trained sham (T-Sham, n = 8), sedentary CHF (S-CHF, n = 8), or trained CHF (T-CHF, n = 8).

Resistance training program

Training groups underwent a 1 week familiarization period (1 set of 10 repetitions, 3 days/week) in the adapted apparatus for RT (Figure 1) [24]. The rats were placed in a neoprene vest leaving it in an upright position on their lower limbs. An electrical stimulus (4–5 mA, 1 second duration, with a 3 second interval between each repetition) was applied to the rat's tail through a surface electrode. As a result, the animals extended their legs repeatedly, which lifted the weight on the exercise apparatus. To determine the training workload, all rats were submitted to a one repetition maximum test (1RM); the 1RM was determined as the maximum weight lifted with the exercise apparatus. The RT program was based on 4 sets of 10–12 repetitions, 65 to 75% of the 1RM, a rest period of 90 s between sets, 4 times per week, for a total of 8 weeks. After the 1RM test, the animals were exercised at 65% of the 1RM in the first week and the workload was increased in the following weeks to 75% of the 1RM. The 1RM test was performed every 2 weeks. The intensities of this protocol are classified as moderate and high intensity for the percentage of 65 to 75% of 1RM according to the guidelines of the American College of Sports Medicine [25].

Surgical preparation for hemodynamic evaluation

Forty-eight hours 48 h after the last exercise session, the animals were anesthetized with xylazine (12 mg/kg i.p.) and ketamine (90 mg/kg i.p.), and a polyethylene catheter (PE-50) was placed into the right carotid artery. The arterial pressure was recorded and the catheter was positioned into the left ventricle to perform

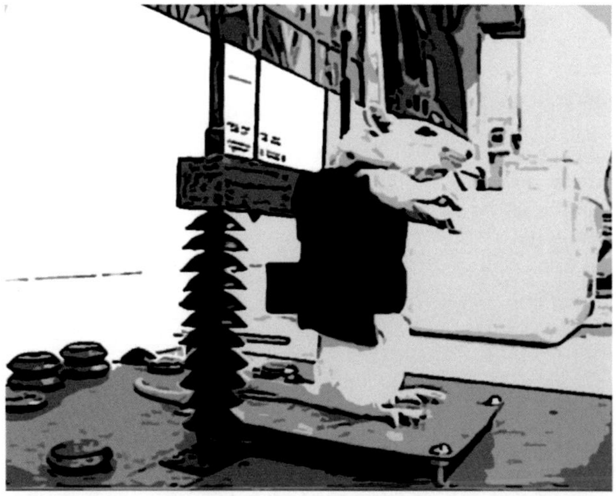

Figure 1. Representative illustration of the apparatus used for resistance training.

the ventricular pressure record. The data were registered by a pressure transducer (strain-gauge, Narco Biosystem Miniature Pulse Transducer RP-155, Houston, Texas, USA), coupled to a pressure amplifier (Stoelting, wood dated, Illinois, USA). Pressure analogical signals were digitalised by a data-acquisition system (CODAS-Data Acquisition System, Akron, OH, USA) with a sampling rate of 2,000 Hz. These data were used to determine diastolic blood pressure (DBP), systolic blood pressure (SBP), mean blood pressure (MBP), heart rate (HR), left ventricular systolic pressure (LVSP), left ventricular end-diastolic pressure (LVEDP), and left ventricular maximum positive and negative dP/dt (+dP/dt_{max}, $-dP/dt_{max}$), as previously described [14].

Blood samples and muscle collection

Blood samples were drawn from the catheter positioned in the right carotid artery, collected into a 1.5 ml tube containing 3.2% sodium citrate (1:9 vol/vol), centrifuged at 500×*g* for 10 min at 4°C and the plasma was stored at −22°C. Animals were killed after blood drawing through an intravenous infusion of an overdose of the anesthetic pentobarbital (80 mg/kg, i.p.) [26].

Infarct size, cardiac hypertrophy and pulmonary and hepatic congestion

Hearts were removed and weighed, without blood within the chamber and without atria. The size of the infarct was determined by the planimetry [27]. To evaluate cardiac hypertrophy, organ weights were expressed as a proportion of body weight (tissue weight/body weight – mg/g). To determine pulmonary and hepatic congestion, the lungs and liver of each animal were removed, weighed, and dehydrated (80°C) for 48 h, and then weighed again to evaluate the water percentage, using the following formula:

$$\text{weight wet-weight dry/weight wet} * 100$$

Analysis of collagen content

The hearts were sectioned in a cryostat (6 μm) and were stained with collagen-specific picrosirius red (PSR) for measurements of the content of interstitial collagen [28]. The images were obtained using a polarized light microscope [29] (Olympus BX51) with a camera attached (Olympus DP72, 40X objective). For image acquisition and quantification, the image pro plus software version 4.5 (Media Cybernetics, Silver Spring, Maryland, USA) was used. For each animal, 40 fields were selected, with the chosen fields being located far from the infarcted area and from the pericardial region, in order to determine the percentage of collagen volume fraction (CVF). The collagen volume fraction was defined as the sum of all stained interstitial collagen tissue areas divided by the entire tissue area [30].

Determination of plasma levels of cytokines

TNF-α, IL-6 and IL-10 plasma levels were determined by a multiplex bead array using Milliplex MAP rat cytokine kits (RCYTO-80K, Millipore - Billerica, MA, USA). Milliplex MAP is based on the Luminex xMAP technology as recommended by the manufacturers. All cytokines are reported as pg/ml.

Statistical analysis

All data are expressed as mean ± SE. The Shapiro–Wilk's normality test was performed. Data were compared among groups by two-way ANOVA followed by the Student-Newman-Keuls post hoc test, and Pearson correlation was also used. A P value of $<$ 0.05 was considered significant. The GraphPad Prism 5.03 program (GraphPad Software, San Diego, CA) and Sigma Plot 12.0 (Systat Software Inc., San Jose, USA) for Windows were used as a computational tool for data analysis.

Results

Total mortality

Mortality in MI-induced CHF rats, during or immediately after surgery, was 35%. There were no deaths or behaviors associated with stress or adverse effects in rats that participated in the RT program in both the sham and CHF groups.

Maximal strength

Figure 2A shows the RM test and a progressive increase in the absolute weight lifted by the trained groups compared to the control groups. All groups had similar values for 1RM at the beginning of the protocol. In the last test of 1RM (the fourth 1RM), the trained groups had an increase in strength when compared to sedentary groups. The S-Sham group had a moderate increase in absolute load when compared to S-CHF, but this difference was not significant when the load was normalized by body weight 1RM/BW (g lifted/g BW; Figure 2B), showing that only the trained groups had a significant increase in the load lifted in the last 1RM test relative to body weight.

Body weight, infarct size, heart hypertrophy, pulmonary and hepatic congestion

All of these data are summarized in Table 1. The initial body weights and final body weights were similar among the four groups in both the pre- and post-training period. There were no differences in the infarcted area between the CHF groups. Pulmonary congestion (PC) was higher in the S-CHF group when compared to Sham groups; however, the T-CHF group showed lower pulmonary congestion when compared to the S-CHF group. Also, there were no differences between the sham groups and the T-CHF group in this variable.

The S-CHF group showed higher cardiac hypertrophy, expressed by the increased weight of the myocardium (MW) normalized by body weight (MW/BW), compared to the sham groups. In addition, the T-CHF group had lower cardiac hypertrophy when compared to S-CHF, which demonstrated that the RT was able to attenuate the pathological hypertrophy. Furthermore, no differences were observed in cardiac hypertrophy between the T-CHF and T-Sham groups. Other comparisons are shown in Table 1.

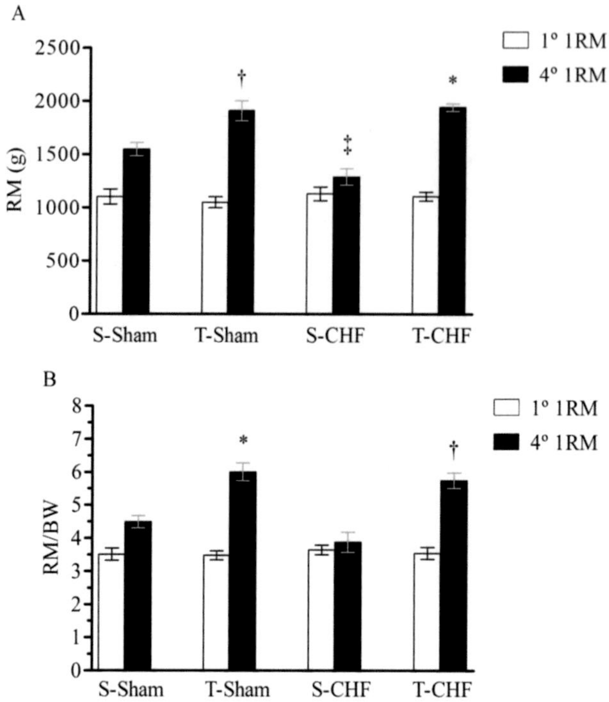

Figure 2. Absolute values for one repetition maximal test (1RM). (**A**). Relative values for one repetition maximal test (1RM) (**B**). Values are means ± SE; n = 8 for all groups. S-Sham, sedentary sham rats; T-Sham, training sham rats; S-CHF, sedentary chronic heart failure rats; T-CHF, training chronic heart failure rats. **P*<0.001 compared to sedentary groups. †*P*<0.01 compared to sedentary groups ‡*P*<0.05 compared to S-Sham group.

The left ventricular hypertrophy, expressed by the increased weight of the left ventricle (LV) normalized by body weight (LVW/BW), was higher in the S-CHF group when compared to the sham groups. However, there were no differences between the T-CHF group and the S-CHF group. No difference was observed in LV hypertrophy between the T-Sham and T-CHF groups. More results are listed in Table 1.

Right ventricle hypertrophy (RVW/BW) was higher in the S-CHF group compared to the sham groups. The T-CHF group showed lower RV hypertrophy when compared to the S-CHF group, suggesting an attenuation of pathological hypertrophy due to training. Moreover, the T-CHF group showed no difference in hypertrophy in RV compared to the sham group.

Hemodynamic parameters

All of these data are summarized in Table 2. The S-CHF group presented values of LVEDP above 20 mmHg, characterizing the presence of significant ventricular dysfunction compared to the sham groups. However, as shown in Table 2, the LVEDP was lower in the T-CHF group when compared to the S-CHF group. No difference was found in the LVEDP in the T-CHF group when compared to the sham groups.

Table 1. Body weight, morphometric cardiac characteristics, infarct area and pulmonary and hepatic congestion of sham-operated rats and rats with left ventricular dysfunction.

Variables	S-Sham	T-Sham	S-CHF	T-CHF
Initial Body Weight, g	253.4±3	250.0±4	253.0±4	258.0±4
Final Body Weight, g	354.0±10	321.0±5	345.0±13	340.0±9
Infarcted Area %	---------	---------	41.5±2	39.3±1
MW/BW mg/g	3.1±0.05†	3.5±0.10	4.2±0.16*	3.8±0.09
LVW/BW mg/g	2.4±0.05†	2.8±0.09	3.2±0.10‡	3.1±0.06
RVW/BW mg/g	0.69±0.03	0.64±0.04	1.02±0.09*	0.74±0.05
Pulmonary Congestion (PC) %	73.2±0.57	70.7±1.2	77.0±1.3*	71.9±1.1
Hepatic Congestion (HC) %	70.8±0.24	70.3±0.19	70.8±0.38	70.2±0.26

Values are means ± SE; n = 8 for all groups. S-Sham, sedentary sham rats; T-Sham, training sham rats; S-CHF, sedentary chronic heart failure rats; T-CHF, training chronic heart failure rats. MW/BW, myocardial weight-to-body weight ratio; LVW/BW, left ventricle-to-body weight ratio and RVW/BW, right ventricle-to-body weight ratio. *$P<0.05$ compared to all groups. †$P<0.05$ compared to trained groups. ‡$P<0.05$ compared to Sham groups.

The LVSP was lower in the S-CHF group when compared to all groups (Table 2). The T-CHF group showed an improvement in $+dP/dt_{max}$ and $-dP/dt_{max}$ when compared to the S-CHF group. The SBP was lower in the S-CHF group when compared to all groups.

Myocardial collagen

Figure 3 shows the sections stained with PSR non-infarcted LV under bright field and polarized light for the S-Sham, T-Sham, S-CHF and T-CHF groups, as well as for the total CVF. Total CVF was higher in the S-CHF group compared to S-Sham, T-Sham and T-CHF groups. Furthermore, the T-CHF group showed no difference in total CVF when compared to the sham groups.

Inflammatory Profile

Figure 4 shows the plasma concentrations of IL-6, IL-10 and TNF-α, as well as the TNF-α to IL-10 and IL-6 to IL-10 ratios. IL-6 was higher in the S-CHF group in comparison with all other groups. In contrast, plasma levels of IL-10 were higher in the T-CHF group when compared to the S-CHF group. We observed a decrease in TNF-α/IL-10 in the T-CHF group when compared with the S-CHF group. In addition, no differences were observed in the TNF-α/IL-10 ratio between the T-CHF group and the Sham groups. The IL-6/IL-10 and plasma levels of TNF-α had no difference among groups. Cytokine analyses were performed only with plasma samples feasible.

Discussion

The main findings of the present study were the improvement of maximal strength gain, hemodynamic function, collagen deposition and the inflammatory profile in rats with CHF subsequent to MI who were submitted to the 8 week RT protocol. We demonstrate that the RT protocol in CHF rats was able to improve cardiac function, as demonstrated by the increased LVSP and SBP, the improved +dP/dtmax and -dP/dtmax, and the decrease in LVEDP. The RT protocol was able to attenuate cardiac hypertrophy, left ventricular collagen volume fraction and reduced IL-6 and the ratio of TNF-α/IL-10; also, there was increased IL-10 in CHF rats. The results presented here are very consistent and only related to the HF animal model; the improvement in cardiac function observed here may not occur in patients with HF. In this context, in the CHF animal model, the injury is mainly central rather than peripheral, which is different in humans with HF syndrome. In fact, this could be, at least in part,

Table 2. Mean blood pressure, diastolic blood pressure, systolic blood pressure, left ventricular end-diastolic pressure, ventricular systolic pressure, left ventricular maximum change in pressure over time and left ventricular minimum change in pressure over time of sham-operated rats and rats with left ventricular dysfunction.

Variables	S-Sham	T-Sham	S-CHF	T-CHF
MBP (mmHg)	99.3±3.9	101.8±4.5	85.7±3.2	99.2±5.8
DBP (mmHg)	85.9±3.8	89.0±4.4	76.4±3.2	88.0±5.5
SBP (mmHg)	112.0±4.3	112.09±4.7	94.19±3.3*	108.08±6.1
LVEDP (mmHg)	5.52±0.65	4.50±0.89	24.20±1.5*	7.62±1.4
LVSP (mmHg)	113.00±6	107.80±4	88.14±3*	102.61±6
+ dP/dtmax (mmHg)	6071±603	5926±750	3548±320*	5290±599
− dP/dtmax (mmHg)	4154±376	4024±358	2495±159*	3519±414

Values are means ± SE; n = 8 for all groups. S-Sham, sedentary sham rats; T-Sham, training sham rats; S-CHF, sedentary chronic heart failure rats; T-CHF, training chronic heart failure rats. Mean blood pressure (MBP), diastolic blood pressure (DBP), systolic blood pressure (SBP), left ventricular end-diastolic pressure (LVEDP) left ventricular systolic pressure (LVSP), maximal positive derivative of ventricular pressure ($+dP/dt_{max}$) and maximal negative derivative of ventricular pressure ($-dP/dt_{max}$). *$P<0.05$ compared to all groups.

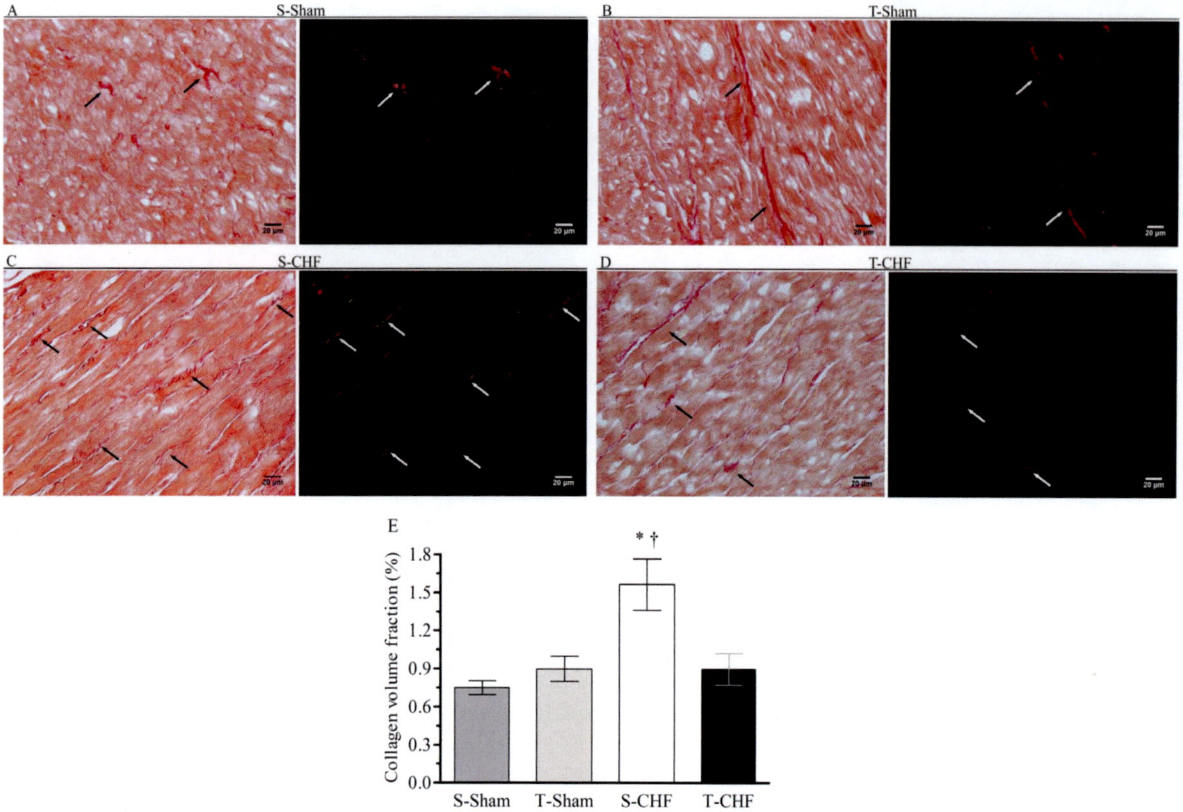

Figure 3. Representative images of ventricular sections stained with Picrosirius (A–D) and statistical analysis (E). Values are means ± SE. The arrows indicate collagen detected in polarized light. **A**. S-Sham, sedentary sham rats (n = 7); **B**. T-Sham, training sham rats (n = 8); **C**. S-CHF, sedentary chronic heart failure rats (n = 8); **D**. T-CHF, training chronic heart failure rats (n = 8). **P*<0.01 compared to trained groups. †*P*<0.001 compared with S-Sham group.

one of the reasons for the results presented here, which demonstrate higher improvements in cardiac function after RT in the animal model [31]. On the other hand, the load during RT in cardiac rehabilitation programs is seated in lower levels (40-60%, 1RM) than that used here (75%, 1RM).

The maximal strength gain in CHF trained rats was an important result found in this study. It is well known that muscle weakness is an independent risk factor for mortality in patients with CHF; therefore, the increased strength becomes a survival predictor in this population suffering from the harmful scenario imposed by CHF [32,33]. In addition, other studies have shown that the increase in muscular strength promotes improvement in clinical status [17], and improvement in functional and physiological capacity to perform activities of daily living [20].

The left coronary artery ligature produces marked left ventricular dysfunction that is directly related to the size of the infarcted area [21,22,34] and simulates the most common cause of CHF, which can negatively alter hemodynamic function. In this model, MI areas greater than 30% represent severe myocardial injury, which results in sustained hemodynamic dysfunction with a higher LVEDP, lower LVSP and heart hypertrophy [14,26]. In the present study, the infarcted area was around 40%, which is associated with severe impairment of the of left ventricular function, producing a severely ill state of the left ventricle, with increases in the end-diastolic pressure higher than 20 mmHg, characterizing the development of severe CHF [35].

In a previous study developed in our laboratory [14], a reduction of 12% in LVEDP was demonstrated in rats with CHF that were submitted to swimming protocol training. More recently, a reduction of 33% in LVEDP and an increase in LVSP of 21% was demonstrated in rats with CHF submitted to respiratory muscle training [26]. These results are similar to the responses found in the present study; therefore, we observed that the RT protocol in rats with CHF was able to reduce 68% in LVEDP and increase 14% in LVSP. Moreover, Pinter *et al.* [36] reported that healthy animals submitted to the RT protocol with intensity of 75% of 1RM test showed an improvement in cardiac performance, probably due to better myocardial perfusion as a result of the increase in systolic pressure of the heart, which increases the dP/dt values during the RT protocol. These results support, in part, the improved cardiac performance found in animals with CHF who underwent the RT protocol in our study. In addition, positive effects of RT on ventricular function, cardiac hypertrophy and maximal strength gain in rats with no left ventricular dysfunction or other cardiovascular disease have been reported [37].

It was also found that RT was able to improve +dP/dtmax and -dP/dtmax (33% and 29%, respectively) in CHF rats. These findings add to those observed in clinical reports, which have clearly demonstrated that RT does not cause a reduction of LV contractility function or enhance myocardial deterioration in the patients with CHF [18,19]. The improvement in cardiac function could be a result of hemodynamic parameters ameliorating the T-CHF group. These results are in agreement with clinical studies which demonstrated that RT can lead to a positive response in

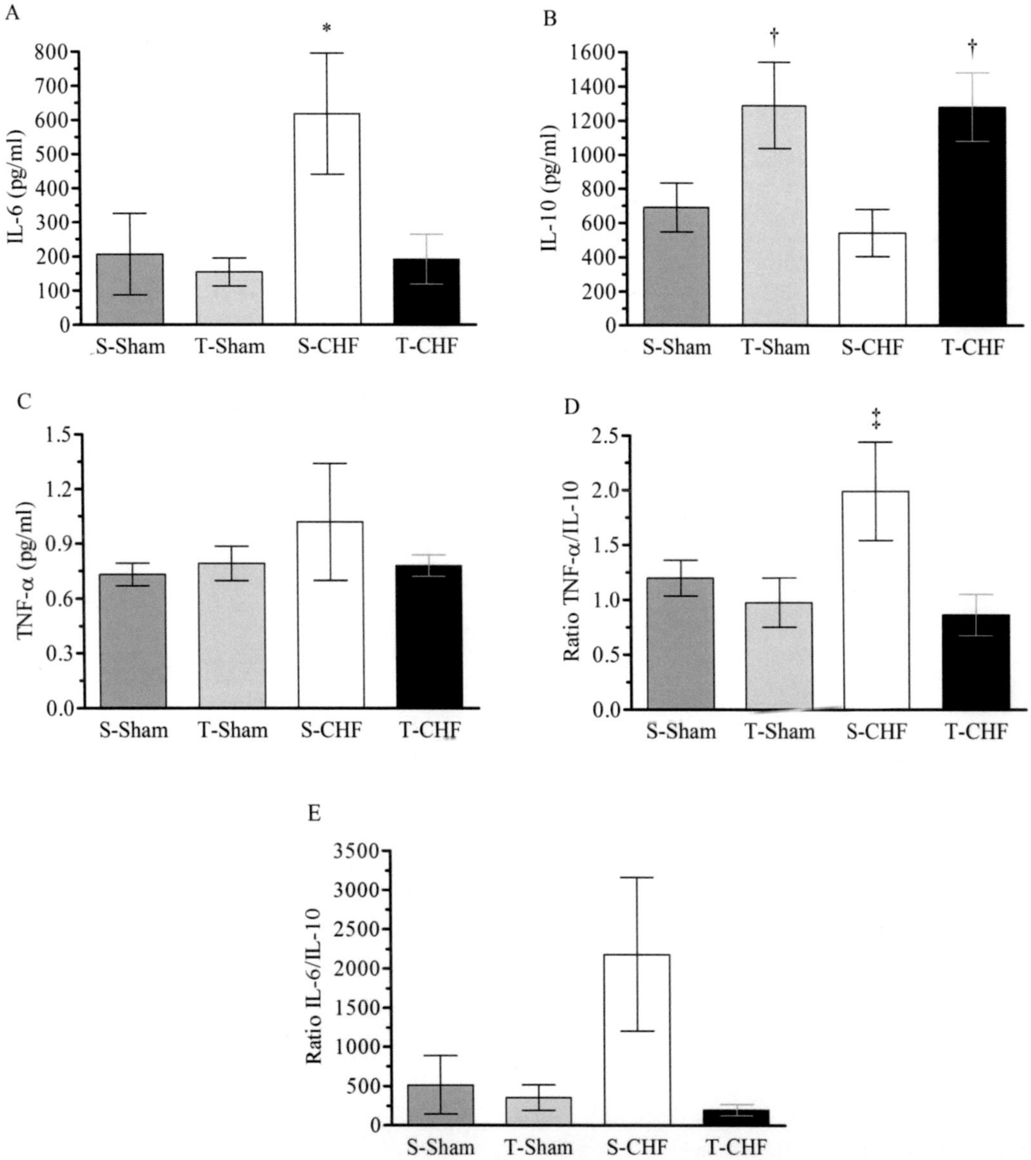

Figure 4. Plasma levels of IL-6, IL-10, TNF-α, TNF- α to IL-10 ratio and IL-6 to IL-10 ratio (A–E). Values are means ± SE. Figure A) S-Sham, sedentary sham rats (n = 5); T-Sham, training sham rats (n = 5); S-CHF, sedentary chronic heart failure rats (n = 5); T-CHF, training chronic heart failure rats (n = 6). Figure B, C and D, n = 6 for all groups. Figure E, n = 5 for all groups. *$P<0.05$ compared to all groups. †$P<0.05$ compared to sedentary groups. ‡$P<0.05$ compared to trained groups.

muscle strength and endurance, without the occurrence of adverse effects on hemodynamics [16,38].

Reduction of the right-ventricle compensatory hypertrophy was found after training (28%) in CHF rats; this is associated with decreased pulmonary congestion ($r = 0.41$; $P = 0.01$). These results demonstrate that pulmonary congestion is negatively associated with the RV hypertrophy. Interestingly, Musch *et al.* [35] reported that rats with severe left ventricular dysfunction, characterized by increasing LVEDP, showed significant pulmonary congestion. In the present study, we observed that the CHF rats undergoing the RT protocol showed reduced pulmonary congestion together with attenuated LVEDP.

The changes in interstitial collagen after MI have gained attention in recent years [8,10,39], but the effects of exercise on changes in interstitial collagen after MI are rarely observed in the literature [28,40], and models of RT for small animals with CHF have not existed until now. Perhaps, higher myocardial collagen content together with the increases in LVEDP are associated with pathologic hypertrophy.

The accumulation of interstitial collagen in rats with CHF after the moderate and high intensity RT protocol (65–75% of 1RM) was able to attenuate the CVF total in comparison to the sedentary group with CHF, suggesting that the reverse of cardiac remodeling occurs. These data corroborate the findings of Xu *et al.* [28], which demonstrated that, after MI, animals submitted to physical exercise had lower CVF totals when compared to sedentary post-MI animals. Our results also corroborate the study of Emter & Baines [40], which demonstrated that physical exercise can prevent pathological remodeling and dysfunctional mitochondria in HF, through attenuation of the accumulation of collagen and the maintenance of a positive inotropic state in pigs with HF.

The increase in ventricular filling pressure has been associated with impaired ventricular systolic function and reduced ventricular compliance by collagen accumulation and fibrosis [41]. In our study, the T-CHF group showed an improvement in ventricular function compared to the S-CHF group, observed by the reduced LVEDP, as previously mentioned, demonstrating that the attenuation of collagen accumulation in animals with CHF that underwent RT may influence the improvement of this parameter. Similar results were observed in the study of Yengo *et al.* [42], who showed that after 10 weeks of training on the treadmill, exercise can minimize the deleterious effects of fibrosis seen post-MI, reducing the stiffness characteristics of the right ventricle that can be associated with abnormalities of diastolic function after heart attack.

The benefits of exercise on inflammatory markers are primarily based on responses to aerobic training, and, to the best of our knowledge, studies demonstrating the inflammatory responses of the isolated practice of RT in CHF have not been performed. Elevated levels of pro-inflammatory cytokines such as TNF-α and IL-6 have been associated with an increased disease severity and poor prognosis in patients with CHF [43]. Interestingly, in our study, we observed that the inflammatory profile in rats with CHF that underwent moderate to high intensity RT protocol (65–75% of 1RM) was able to attenuate the plasma levels of IL-6 when compared with the sedentary CHF group and differences were not observed in the plasma levels of TNF-α between the groups. These results support, in part, the findings of other studies that have shown that aerobic exercise is able to reduce levels of the pro-inflammatory cytokine IL-6 [44,45].

In addition, it was also observed that the RT was able to promote an anti-inflammatory effect in animals with CHF by increasing the plasma levels of IL-10, resembling those observed in aerobic training [14]. Furthermore, in the present study, the TNF-α/IL-10 ratio was lower in the T-CHF group when compared to S-CHF, demonstrating that the RT has a positive effect on the inflammatory process imposed by CHF. Similar responses were found in the study of Batista *et al.* [46], which showed an increase in the IL-10/TNF-α ratio in the skeletal muscle of CHF rats submitted to aerobic training, demonstrating the importance of exercise as an anti-inflammatory strategy. In addition, patients with acute myocardial infarction showed higher TNF-α/IL-10 ratios when compared to the control group, demonstrating an important inflammatory imbalance [47]. Thus, physical exercise can be considered an anti-inflammatory strategy to ameliorate the balance of this immunological complex system.

The limitation of this study was the lack of histological assessment in skeletal muscle. This parameter would help to achieve a better understanding of the effect of RT on skeletal muscle fibers, in both trained and untrained CHF rats. Another limitation was the lack of expression levels of IL-6, IL-10 and TNF-α in the hearts of healthy animals and in those with CHF, which may explain the changes in hemodynamic parameters of the T-CHF group. Also, some animals with a large infarcted area did not present ventricular dysfunction; however, as we can see from the results on LVEDP and LVSP, both were reduced, which probably represents ventricular dysfunction.

In conclusion, a regular program of 8 weeks of RT in Wistar rats with CHF induced by MI was able to improve the hemodynamic function, reduce pulmonary congestion, increase maximum strength gain, attenuate cardiac hypertrophy, and improve collagen deposition in the LV and inflammatory profiles. These results demonstrate an important contribution of the RT in an experimental model of CHF. We suggest that RT may be an effective therapeutic strategy for a cardiac rehabilitation program. Further studies are needed to understand the other possible benefits of RT in CHF through researches that analyze cellular and molecular mechanism-related adaptations of cardiac muscle, skeletal muscle and blood vessels after RT alone or in combination with endurance training.

Acknowledgments

We are very grateful to Terezinha Stein, Rosalva Theresa Meurer, Professor Claudia Ramos Rhoden, PhD, and Graziele Halmenschlager, MSc, for their support during the development of this study.

Author Contributions

Conceived and designed the experiments: JPA RBN GPS PDL. Performed the experiments: JPA RBN GPS PDL. Analyzed the data: JPA RBN GPS PDL. Contributed reagents/materials/analysis tools: JPA RBN GPS PDL. Wrote the paper: JPA RBN GPS PDL.

References

1. Hunt SA, Abraham WT, Chin MH, Feldman AM, Francis GS, et al. (2009) 2009 focused update incorporated into the ACC/AHA 2005 Guidelines for the Diagnosis and Management of Heart Failure in Adults: a report of the American College of Cardiology Foundation/American Heart Association Task Force on Practice Guidelines: developed in collaboration with the International Society for Heart and Lung Transplantation. Circulation 119: e391–479.
2. Piepoli MF, Scott AC, Capucci A, Coats AJ (2001) Skeletal muscle training in chronic heart failure. Acta physiologica Scandinavica 171: 295–303.
3. Georgiadou P, Adamopoulos S (2012) Skeletal muscle abnormalities in chronic heart failure. Curr Heart Fail Rep 9: 128–132.
4. Lunde PK, Sjaastad I, Schiotz Thorud HM, Sejersted OM (2001) Skeletal muscle disorders in heart failure. Acta physiologica Scandinavica 171: 277–294.
5. Jannig PR, Moreira JB, Bechara LR, Bozi LH, Bacurau AV, et al. (2014) Autophagy signaling in skeletal muscle of infarcted rats. PLoS One 9: e85820.
6. McMurray JJ (2010) Clinical practice. Systolic heart failure. The New England journal of medicine 362: 228–238.
7. Pfeffer MA, Braunwald E (1990) Ventricular remodeling after myocardial infarction. Experimental observations and clinical implications. Circulation 81: 1161–1172.
8. Gurtl B, Kratky D, Guelly C, Zhang L, Gorkiewicz G, et al. (2009) Apoptosis and fibrosis are early features of heart failure in an animal model of metabolic cardiomyopathy. International journal of experimental pathology 90: 338–346.
9. Whittaker P, Boughner DR, Kloner RA (1991) Role of collagen in acute myocardial infarct expansion. Circulation 84: 2123–2134.
10. Weber KT, Sun Y, Diez J (2008) Fibrosis: a living tissue and the infarcted heart. Journal of the American College of Cardiology 52: 2029–2031.
11. Smart NA, Dieberg G, Giallauria F (2013) Intermittent versus continuous exercise training in chronic heart failure: a meta-analysis. Int J Cardiol 166: 352–358.
12. Vanzelli AS, Medeiros A, Rolim N, Bartholomeu JB, Cunha TF, et al. (2013) Integrative effect of carvedilol and aerobic exercise training therapies on improving cardiac contractility and remodeling in heart failure mice. PLoS One 8: e62452.
13. Kwan G, Balady GJ (2012) Cardiac rehabilitation 2012: advancing the field through emerging science. Circulation 125: e369–373.
14. Nunes RB, Tonetto M, Machado N, Chazan M, Heck TG, et al. (2008) Physical exercise improves plasmatic levels of IL-10, left ventricular end-diastolic pressure, and muscle lipid peroxidation in chronic heart failure rats. Journal of applied physiology 104: 1641–1647.
15. Mihl C, Dassen WR, Kuipers H (2008) Cardiac remodelling: concentric versus eccentric hypertrophy in strength and endurance athletes. Netherlands heart journal: monthly journal of the Netherlands Society of Cardiology and the Netherlands Heart Foundation 16: 129–133.
16. Cheetham C, Green D, Collis J, Dembo L, O'Driscoll G (2002) Effect of aerobic and resistance exercise on central hemodynamic responses in severe chronic heart failure. Journal of applied physiology 93: 175–180.
17. Jankowska EA, Wegrzynowska K, Superlak M, Nowakowska K, Lazorczyk M, et al. (2008) The 12-week progressive quadriceps resistance training improves

muscle strength, exercise capacity and quality of life in patients with stable chronic heart failure. International journal of cardiology 130: 36–43.
18. Levinger I, Bronks R, Cody DV, Linton I, Davie A (2005) The effect of resistance training on left ventricular function and structure of patients with chronic heart failure. International journal of cardiology 105: 159–163.
19. Palevo G, Keteyian SJ, Kang M, Caputo JL (2009) Resistance exercise training improves heart function and physical fitness in stable patients with heart failure. Journal of cardiopulmonary rehabilitation and prevention 29: 294–298.
20. Savage PA, Shaw AO, Miller MS, VanBuren P, LeWinter MM, et al. (2011) Effect of resistance training on physical disability in chronic heart failure. Medicine and science in sports and exercise 43: 1379–1386.
21. de Leon EB, Bortoluzzi A, Rucatti A, Nunes RB, Saur L, et al. (2011) Neuromuscular electrical stimulation improves GLUT-4 and morphological characteristics of skeletal muscle in rats with heart failure. Acta physiologica 201: 265–273.
22. Pfeffer MA, Pfeffer JM, Fishbein MC, Fletcher PJ, Spadaro J, et al. (1979) Myocardial infarct size and ventricular function in rats. Circulation research 44: 503–512.
23. Francis J, Weiss RM, Wei SG, Johnson AK, Felder RB (2001) Progression of heart failure after myocardial infarction in the rat. Am J Physiol Regul Integr Comp Physiol 281: R1734–1745.
24. Krisan AD, Collins DE, Crain AM, Kwong CC, Singh MK, et al. (2004) Resistance training enhances components of the insulin signaling cascade in normal and high-fat-fed rodent skeletal muscle. Journal of applied physiology 96: 1691–1700.
25. Garber CE, Blissmer B, Deschenes MR, Franklin BA, Lamonte MJ, et al. (2011) American College of Sports Medicine position stand. Quantity and quality of exercise for developing and maintaining cardiorespiratory, musculoskeletal, and neuromotor fitness in apparently healthy adults: guidance for prescribing exercise. Medicine and science in sports and exercise 43: 1334–1359.
26. Jaenisch RB, Hentschke VS, Quagliotto E, Cavinato PR, Schmeing LA, et al. (2011) Respiratory Muscle Training Improves Hemodynamics, Autonomic Function, Baroreceptors Sensitivity and Respiratory Mechanics in Rats with Heart Failure. Journal of applied physiology.
27. Lindpaintner K, Lu W, Neidermajer N, Schieffer B, Just H, et al. (1993) Selective activation of cardiac angiotensinogen gene expression in post-infarction ventricular remodeling in the rat. Journal of molecular and cellular cardiology 25: 133–143.
28. Xu X, Wan W, Powers AS, Li J, Ji LL, et al. (2008) Effects of exercise training on cardiac function and myocardial remodeling in post myocardial infarction rats. Journal of molecular and cellular cardiology 44: 114–122.
29. Whittaker P, Kloner RA, Boughner DR, Pickering JG (1994) Quantitative assessment of myocardial collagen with picrosirius red staining and circularly polarized light. Basic research in cardiology 89: 397–410.
30. Matsubara LS, Matsubara BB, Okoshi MP, Cicogna AC, Janicki JS (2000) Alterations in myocardial collagen content affect rat papillary muscle function. American journal of physiology Heart and circulatory physiology 279: H1534–1539.
31. Houser SR, Margulies KB, Murphy AM, Spinale FG, Francis GS, et al. (2012) Animal models of heart failure: a scientific statement from the American Heart Association. Circ Res 111: 131–150.
32. Anker SD, Ponikowski P, Varney S, Chua TP, Clark AL, et al. (1997) Wasting as independent risk factor for mortality in chronic heart failure. Lancet 349: 1050–1053.
33. Hulsmann M, Quittan M, Berger R, Crevenna R, Springer C, et al. (2004) Muscle strength as a predictor of long-term survival in severe congestive heart failure. Eur J Heart Fail 6: 101–107.
34. Pfeifer PC, Musch TI, McAllister RM (2001) Skeletal muscle oxidative capacity and exercise tolerance in rats with heart failure. Medicine and science in sports and exercise 33: 542–548.
35. Musch TI, Wolfram S, Hageman KS, Pickar JG (2002) Skeletal muscle ouabain binding sites are reduced in rats with chronic heart failure. Journal of applied physiology 92: 2326–2334.
36. de Cassia Cypriano Ervati Pinter R, Padilha AS, de Oliveira EM, Vassallo DV, de Fucio Lizardo JH (2008) Cardiovascular adaptive responses in rats submitted to moderate resistance training. European journal of applied physiology 103: 605–613.
37. Barauna VG, Rosa KT, Irigoyen MC, de Oliveira EM (2007) Effects of resistance training on ventricular function and hypertrophy in a rat model. Clinical medicine & research 5: 114–120.
38. McKelvie RS, McCartney N, Tomlinson C, Bauer R, MacDougall JD (1995) Comparison of hemodynamic responses to cycling and resistance exercise in congestive heart failure secondary to ischemic cardiomyopathy. The American journal of cardiology 76: 977–979.
39. Hutchinson KR, Stewart JA, Jr., Lucchesi PA (2010) Extracellular matrix remodeling during the progression of volume overload-induced heart failure. Journal of molecular and cellular cardiology 48: 564–569.
40. Emter CA, Baines CP (2010) Low-intensity aerobic interval training attenuates pathological left ventricular remodeling and mitochondrial dysfunction in aortic-banded miniature swine. American journal of physiology Heart and circulatory physiology 299: H1348–1356.
41. Yu CM, Sanderson JE, Shum IO, Chan S, Yeung LY, et al. (1996) Diastolic dysfunction and natriuretic peptides in systolic heart failure. Higher ANP and BNP levels are associated with the restrictive filling pattern. European heart journal 17: 1694–1702.
42. Yengo CM, Zimmerman SD, McCormick RJ, Thomas DP (2012) Exercise training post-MI favorably modifies heart extracellular matrix in the rat. Medicine and science in sports and exercise 44: 1005–1012.
43. Anker SD, von Haehling S (2004) Inflammatory mediators in chronic heart failure: an overview. Heart 90: 464–470.
44. Gielen S, Adams V, Mobius-Winkler S, Linke A, Erbs S, et al. (2003) Anti-inflammatory effects of exercise training in the skeletal muscle of patients with chronic heart failure. Journal of the American College of Cardiology 42: 861–868.
45. Adamopoulos S, Parissis J, Karatzas D, Kroupis C, Georgiadis M, et al. (2002) Physical training modulates proinflammatory cytokines and the soluble Fas/soluble Fas ligand system in patients with chronic heart failure. Journal of the American College of Cardiology 39: 653–663.
46. Batista ML, Jr., Rosa JC, Lopes RD, Lira FS, Martins E, Jr., et al. (2010) Exercise training changes IL-10/TNF-alpha ratio in the skeletal muscle of post-MI rats. Cytokine 49: 102–108.
47. Goswami B, Rajappa M, Mallika V, Shukla DK, Kumar S (2009) TNF-alpha/IL-10 ratio and C-reactive protein as markers of the inflammatory response in CAD-prone North Indian patients with acute myocardial infarction. Clin Chim Acta 408: 14–18.

Permissions

All chapters in this book were first published in PLOS ONE, by The Public Library of Science; hereby published with permission under the Creative Commons Attribution License or equivalent. Every chapter published in this book has been scrutinized by our experts. Their significance has been extensively debated. The topics covered herein carry significant findings which will fuel the growth of the discipline. They may even be implemented as practical applications or may be referred to as a beginning point for another development.

The contributors of this book come from diverse backgrounds, making this book a truly international effort. This book will bring forth new frontiers with its revolutionizing research information and detailed analysis of the nascent developments around the world.

We would like to thank all the contributing authors for lending their expertise to make the book truly unique. They have played a crucial role in the development of this book. Without their invaluable contributions this book wouldn't have been possible. They have made vital efforts to compile up to date information on the varied aspects of this subject to make this book a valuable addition to the collection of many professionals and students.

This book was conceptualized with the vision of imparting up-to-date information and advanced data in this field. To ensure the same, a matchless editorial board was set up. Every individual on the board went through rigorous rounds of assessment to prove their worth. After which they invested a large part of their time researching and compiling the most relevant data for our readers.

The editorial board has been involved in producing this book since its inception. They have spent rigorous hours researching and exploring the diverse topics which have resulted in the successful publishing of this book. They have passed on their knowledge of decades through this book. To expedite this challenging task, the publisher supported the team at every step. A small team of assistant editors was also appointed to further simplify the editing procedure and attain best results for the readers.

Apart from the editorial board, the designing team has also invested a significant amount of their time in understanding the subject and creating the most relevant covers. They scrutinized every image to scout for the most suitable representation of the subject and create an appropriate cover for the book.

The publishing team has been an ardent support to the editorial, designing and production team. Their endless efforts to recruit the best for this project, has resulted in the accomplishment of this book. They are a veteran in the field of academics and their pool of knowledge is as vast as their experience in printing. Their expertise and guidance has proved useful at every step. Their uncompromising quality standards have made this book an exceptional effort. Their encouragement from time to time has been an inspiration for everyone.

The publisher and the editorial board hope that this book will prove to be a valuable piece of knowledge for researchers, students, practitioners and scholars across the globe.

List of Contributors

Melissa L. Bates, Emily T. Farrell and Alyssa Drezdon
Department of Pediatrics, Critical Care Division and the John Rankin Laboratory of Pulmonary Medicine, University of Wisconsin School of Medicine and Public Health, Madison, Wisconsin, United States of America

Joseph E. Jacobson
Department of Pediatrics, Critical Care Division and the John Rankin Laboratory of Pulmonary Medicine, University of Wisconsin School of Medicine and Public Health, Madison, Wisconsin, United States of America
Michigan State University College of Human Medicine, East Lansing, Michigan, United States of America

Scott B. Perlman
Department of Radiology, University of Wisconsin School of Medicine and Public Health, Madison, Wisconsin, United States of America

Marlowe W. Eldridge
Department of Pediatrics, Critical Care Division and the John Rankin Laboratory of Pulmonary Medicine, University of Wisconsin School of Medicine and Public Health, Madison, Wisconsin, United States of America
Departments of Biomedical Engineering and Kinesiology, University of Wisconsin School of Medicine and Public Health, Madison, Wisconsin, United States of America

Nikolaos E. Koundourakis
Department of Clinical Chemistry, School of Medicine, University of Crete, Heraklion, Greece

Nikolaos E. Androulakis
Department of Laboratory Haematology, University Hospital, Heraklion, Crete, Greece

Niki Malliaraki and Andrew N. Margioris
Departments of Clinical Chemistry, University of Crete, School of Medicine, and University Hospital, Heraklion, Greece

Jochen Mayer and Ansgar Thiel
Institute of Sports Science, University of Tübingen, Tübingen, Germany

Laura Pérez, Concepción Padilla, Fabrice B. R. Parmentier and Pilar Andrés
Neuropsychology and Cognition Group, Research Institute on Health Sciences and Department of Psychology of the University of the Balearic Islands, Palma, Spain
Neuropsychology and Cognition Group, Instituto de Investigación Sanitaria de Palma, Palma, Spain

Beatriz C. S. Boa, Maria das Graças C. Souza, Richard D. Leite and Eliete Bouskela
Laboratory for Clinical and Experimental Research on Vascular Biology (BioVasc), Biomedical Center, State University of Rio de Janeiro - Rio de Janeiro, RJ - Brazil

Simone V. da Silva and Thereza Christina Barja-Fidalgo
Department of Cell Biology, Institute of Biology Roberto Alcântara Gomes, Biomedical Center, State University of Rio de Janeiro - Rio de Janeiro, RJ - Brazil

Luiz Guilherme Kraemer-Aguiar
Laboratory for Clinical and Experimental Research on Vascular Biology (BioVasc), Biomedical Center, State University of Rio de Janeiro - Rio de Janeiro, RJ - Brazil
Department of Internal Medicine, Faculty of Medical Sciences, Biomedical Center, State University of Rio de Janeiro - Rio de Janeiro, RJ - Brazil

Wilhelm Ammenwerth, Henrik Wurps, Catharina Crolow, Nicolas Schönfeld and Torsten T. Bauer
Department of Pneumology, Lungenklinik Heckeshorn, HELIOS Klinikum Emil von Behring, Berlin, Germany

Mark A. Klemens and Roland C. Bittner
Institute of Radiology and Nuclear Medicine, HELIOS Klinikum Emil von Behring, Berlin, Germany

Jeanette Schulz-Menger
WG Cardiac MRI ECRC a joint institution of the MDC and Charité Medical University Berlin and HELIOS Klinikum Berlin-Buch Department of Cardiology and Nephrology, Berlin, Germany

Christina Backes, Petra Leidinger, Martin Hart and Eckart Meese
Department of Human Genetics, Medical School, Saarland University, Homburg/Saar, Germany

Andreas Keller
Department of Clinical Bioinformatics, Saarland University, Saarbruecken, Germany

Tim Meyer and Anne Hecksteden
Institute of Sports and Preventive Medicine, Saarland University, Saarbruecken, Germany

Tabitha Woolpert, Patrick J. Blair and Dennis Faix
Operational Infectious Diseases, Naval Health Research Center, San Diego, California, United States of America

Christopher J. Phillips, Carter Sevick and Nancy F. Crum-Cianflone
Deployment Health Research, Naval Health Research Center, San Diego, California, United States of America

Heidi J. Syväoja
LIKES - Research Center for Sport and Health Sciences, Jyväskylä, Finland
Department of Psychology, University of Jyväskylä, Jyväskylä, Finland

Tuija H. Tammelin and Anna Kankaanpää
LIKES - Research Center for Sport and Health Sciences, Jyväskylä, Finland

Timo Ahonen
Department of Psychology, University of Jyväskylä, Jyväskylä, Finland

Marko T. Kantomaa
LIKES - Research Center for Sport and Health Sciences, Jyväskylä, Finland
Department of Epidemiology and Biostatistics, MRC–HPA Centre for Environment and Health, Imperial College London, London, United Kingdom

Florence Canou□-Poitrine, Kalaivani Veerabudun and Sylvie Bastuji-Garin
Université Paris Est, Faculté de Médecine, EA 4393, Laboratoire d'Investigation Clinique, Créteil, France
AP-HP, Groupe Henri Mondor-Albert Chenevier, Service de Santé Publique, Créteil, France

Philippe Larmignat
AP-HP, Hôpital Avicenne, Service d'Anesthésie et Réanimation, Bobigny, France

Murielle Letournel
AP-HP, Hôpital Avicenne, Service de Physiologie, Explorations Fonctionnelles et Médecine du Sport, Bobigny, France

Jean-Paul Richalet
Université Paris 13, Sorbonne Paris Cité , EA2363 « Réponses cellulaires et fonctionnelles a` l'hypoxie », U.F.R. SMBH, Bobigny, France
AP-HP, Hôpital Avicenne, Service de Physiologie, Explorations Fonctionnelles et Médecine du Sport, Bobigny, France

Espen Tønnessen, Thomas A. Haugen and Erlend Hem
The Norwegian Olympic Federation, Oslo, Norway

Øystein Sylta and Stephen Seiler
Faculty of Health and Sport Sciences, University of Agder, Kristiansand, Norway

Ida S. Svendsen
School of Sport, Exercise and Health Sciences, Loughborough University, Leicestershire, United Kingdom

Roger Ekeberg Henriksen and Frode Thuen
Centre for Evidence-Based Practice, Bergen University College, Bergen, Norway

Torbjørn Torsheim
Faculty of Psychology, Department of Psychosocial Science, University of Bergen, Bergen, Norway

Vincent Mainguy, Simon Malenfant, Anne-Sophie Neyron, Didier Saey, Franc¸ois Maltais, Sébastien Bonnet and Steeve Provencher
Pulmonary Hypertension Research Group, Centre de recherche de l'Institut universitaire de cardiologie et de pneumologie de Québec, Université Laval, Québec (Québec), Canada

Catherine Sherrington
The George Institute for Global Health, The University of Sydney, Sydney, New South Wales, Australia

Stephen R. Lord, Sandra D. O'Rourke,Elisabeth Ramsay, Elizabeth Barraclough and Robert D. Herbert
Neuroscience Research Australia, University of New South Wales, Randwick, New South Wales, Australia

Constance M. Vogler
Northern Clinical School, The University of Sydney, Sydney, New South Wales, Australia
Department of Aged Care and Rehabilitation, Royal North Shore Hospital, St Leonards, New South Wales, Australia

Jacqueline C. T. Close
Neuroscience Research Australia, University of New South Wales, Randwick, New South Wales, Australia
Prince of Wales Clinical School, University of New South Wales, Randwick, New South Wales, Australia

Kirsten Howard and Robert G. Cumming
School of Public Health, The University of Sydney, Sydney, New South Wales, Australia

Catherine M. Dean
Department of Health Professions, Faculty of Human Sciences, Macquarie University, Macquarie Park, NSW, Australia

Gillian Z. Heller
Department of Statistics, Macquarie University, Macquarie Park, New South Wales, Australia

Lindy Clemson
Discipline of Occupational Therapy, Faculty of Health Sciences, The University of Sydney, Lidcombe, New South Wales, Australia

Norihide Sugisaki
Center for Environment, Health and Field Sciences, Chiba University, Kashiwa, Chiba, Japan
Waseda Institute for Sport Sciences, Waseda University, Tokorozawa, Saitama, Japan

Sadao Kurokawa
Center for Liberal Arts, Meiji Gakuin University, Yokohama, Kanagawa, Japan

Junichi Okada
Faculty of Sport Sciences, Waseda University, Tokorozawa, Saitama, Japan

Hiroaki Kanehisa
National Institute of Fitness and Sports in Kanoya, Kanoya, Kagoshima, Japan

Mads F. Hjorth, Camilla T. Damsgaard, Stine-Mathilde Dalskov, Christian Ritz, Anders Sjödin, Arne Astrup and Kim F. Michaelsen
Department of Nutrition, Exercise and Sports, Faculty of Science, University of Copenhagen, Copenhagen, Denmark

Jean-Philippe Chaput
Healthy Active Living and Obesity Research Group, Children's Hospital of Eastern Ontario Research Institute, Ottawa, Ontario, Canada

Rikke Andersen and Inge Tetens
National Food Institute, Division of Nutrition, Technical University of Denmark, Søborg, Denmark

Francisco García-Rio
Servicio de Neumología, Hospital Universitario La Paz, IdiPAZ, Madrid, Spain, and CIBER de Enfermedades Respiratorias, Madrid, Spain

Joan B. Soriano
Fundación Caubet-CIMERA Illes Balears, Bunyola, Illes Balears, Spain, and CIBER de Enfermedades Respiratorias, Illes Balears, Spain

Marc Miravitlles
Pneumology Department, Hospital Universitario Vall d'Hebron, Barcelona, Spain

Luis Muñoz
Pneumology Department, Hospital Reina Sofía, Córdoba, Spain

Enric Duran-Tauleria
Centro de Investigación en Epidemiología Ambiental - CREAL, Barcelona, Spain

Guadalupe Sánchez
Medical Department, GlaxoSmithkline S.A., Madrid, Spain

Victor Sobradillo
Pneumology Department, Hospital de Cruces, Bilbao, Spain

Julio Ancochea
Servicio de Neumología, Hospital Universitario de La Princesa, Instituto de Investigación Sanitaria Princesa, Madrid, Spain

Shaon Naskar, Kaberi Datta, Arkadeep Mitra, Kanchan Pathak, Ritwik Datta, Trisha Bansal and Sagartirtha Sarkar
Genetics and Molecular Cardiology Laboratory, Department of Zoology, University of Calcutta, Kolkata, West Bengal, India

Azusa Uematsu and Shuji Suzuki
Faculty of Human Sciences, Waseda University, Tokorozawa, Japan

Kazushi Tsuchiya
Graduate School of Human Sciences, Waseda University, Tokorozawa, Japan

Norio Kadono
Advanced Research Center for Human Sciences, Waseda University, Tokorozawa, Japan

Hirofumi Kobayashi
Graduate School of Arts and Sciences, The University of Tokyo, Meguro-ku, Japan

Takamasa Kaetsu
School of Human Sciences, Waseda University, Tokorozawa, Japan

Tibor Hortobágyi
University Medical Center Groningen, University of Groningen, Groningen, The Netherlands
Department of Sport, Exercise and Rehabilitation, Northumbria University, Newcastle-upon-Tyne, United Kingdom

Ramires Alsamir Tibana, Dahan da Cunha Nascimento, Vinicius Carolino de Souza and Jonato Prestes
Catholic University of Brasilia, Graduation Program on Physical Education, Brasilia, Brazil

Nuno Manuel Frade de Sousa
Laboratory of Exercise Physiology, Faculty Estacio of Vitoria, Espirito Santo, Brazil

João Durigan, Amilton Vieira, Martim Bottaro and Otávio de Toledo Nóbrega
University of Brasilia, Brasilia, Brazil

Jeeser Alves de Almeida
Catholic University of Brasilia, Graduation Program on Physical Education, Brasilia, Brazil
University of Brasilia, Brasilia, Brazil

James Wilfred Navalta
Department of Kinesiology and Nutrition Sciences of the University of Nevada, Las Vegas, Nevada, United States of America

Octavio Luiz Franco
Catholic University of Brasilia, Graduation Program on Physical Education, Brasilia, Brazil
Centro de Analises Proteomicas e Bioquimicas. Programa de Pos-Graduaçao em Ciencias Genomicas e Biotecnologia, Universidade Catolica de Brasilia, Brasilia, Brazil

Justin M. Guagliano, Gregory S. Kolt and Emma S. George
School of Science and Health, University of Western Sydney, Sydney, Australia

Chris Lonsdale
Institute for Positive Psychology and Education, Australian Catholic University, Sydney, Australia

Richard R. Rosenkranz
School of Science and Health, University of Western Sydney, Sydney, Australia
Department of Human Nutrition, Kansas State University, Manhattan, Kansas, United States of America

Michael A. McDonald, Juarez R. Braga and Heather J. Ross
Division of Cardiology, Peter Munk Cardiac Centre, University of Toronto, Toronto, Canada

Jing Li, Cedric Manlhiot and Andrew N. Redington
Division of Cardiology, Hospital for Sick Children, University of Toronto, Toronto, Canada

Jadson P. Alves, Ramiro B. Nunes and Giuseppe P. Stefani
Laboratory of Physiology, Universidade Federal de Ciências da Saúde de Porto Alegre (UFCSPA), Porto Alegre, Rio Grande do Sul, Brazil

Pedro Dal Lago
Laboratory of Physiology, Universidade Federal de Ciências da Saúde de Porto Alegre (UFCSPA), Porto Alegre, Rio Grande do Sul, Brazil
Department of Physical Therapy, Universidade Federal de Ciências da Saúde de Porto Alegre (UFCSPA), Porto Alegre, Rio Grande do Sul, Brazil

Index